# Dentistry: Tools, Techniques and Methods

# Dentistry: Tools, Techniques and Methods

Edited by **Kaley Ann**

FOSTER ACADEMICS
New Jersey

Published by Foster Academics,
61 Van Reypen Street,
Jersey City, NJ 07306, USA
www.fosteracademics.com

**Dentistry: Tools, Techniques and Methods**
Edited by Kaley Ann



International Standard Book Number: 978-1-63242-449-5 (Hardback)



Printed in China.

# Contents

# Preface

Dentistry is a field of science which deals with the diagnosis and treatment of disorders, diseases and other problems related to mouth or oral cavity. It consists of treating problems of teeth, gums, etc. This book includes some of the vital pieces of work being conducted across the world, on various topics related to dentistry. Most of the topics covered in it talk about new techniques and their applications in this subject. Scientists and students actively engaged in this field will find this book full of crucial and unexplored concepts. Coherent flow of topics, reader-friendly language and extensive use of examples make it an invaluable source of knowledge.

After months of intensive research and writing, this book is the end result of all who devoted their time and efforts in the initiation and progress of this book. It will surely be a source of reference in enhancing the required knowledge of the new developments in the area. During the course of developing this book, certain measures such as accuracy, authenticity and research focused analytical studies were given preference in order to produce a comprehensive book in the area of study.

This book would not have been possible without the efforts of the authors and the publisher. I extend my sincere thanks to them. Secondly, I express my gratitude to my family and well-wishers. And most importantly, I thank my students for constantly expressing their willingness and curiosity in enhancing their knowledge in the field, which encourages me to take up further research projects for the advancement of the area.

**Editor**

# Evaluation of implant-materials as cell carriers for dental stem cells under *in vitro* conditions

Martin Gosau[1,2], Sandra Viale-Bouroncle[1], Hannah Eickhoff[1], Esthera Prateeptongkum[1], Anja Reck[1], W Götz[3], Christoph Klingelhöffer[1], Steffen Müller[1] and Christian Morsczeck[1*]

## Abstract

**Background:** Dental stem cells in combination with implant materials may become an alternative to autologous bone transplants. For tissue engineering different types of soft and rigid implant materials are available, but little is known about the viability and the osteogenic differentiation of dental stem cells on these different types of materials. According to previous studies we proposed that rigid bone substitute materials are superior to soft materials for dental tissue engineering.

**Methods:** We evaluated the proliferation, the induction of apoptosis and the osteogenic differentiation of dental stem/progenitor cells on a synthetic bone-like material and on an allograft product. The soft materials silicone and polyacrylamide (PA) were used for comparison. Precursor cells from the dental follicle (DFCs) and progenitor cells from the dental apical papilla of retained third molar tooth (dNC-PCs) were applied as dental stem cells in our study.

**Results:** Both dental cell types attached and grew on rigid bone substitute materials, but they did not grow on soft materials. Moreover, rigid bone substitute materials only sustained the osteogenic differentiation of dental stem cells, although the allograft product induced apoptosis in both dental cell types. Remarkably, PA, silicone and the synthetic bone substitute material did not induce the apoptosis in dental cells.

**Conclusions:** Our work supports the hypothesis that bone substitute materials are suitable for dental stem cell tissue engineering. Furthermore, we also suggest that the induction of apoptosis by bone substitute materials may not impair the proliferation and the differentiation of dental stem cells.

**Keywords:** Dental stem cells; Hydroxyapatite; Allograft product; Osteogenic differentiation; Silicone

## Background

While bone substitute materials are routinely used, especially vertical bone, augmentation of the jaws is still a problematic step. Dental stem cells in combination with bone substitute materials may accelerate the augmentation of alveolar bone and perhaps, stem cell-based therapies can become an alternative to autologous, allogenic, or synthetic bone transplants and substitutes [1,2]. However, scaffolds are required for cell delivery, and here, commercially available bone substitute materials could be an excellent source for dental tissue engineering.

For more than 10 years, human dental stem cell research has focused on the identification and characterization of human stem/progenitor cell populations, which can be isolated, for example, from retained third molars of juvenile patients [3]. One example for such type of dental stem cells are undifferentiated cells from the dental follicle (DFCs) [4,5]. These highly proliferative cells can be differentiated *in vitro* into periodontal ligament (PDL) cells, cementoblasts and osteoblasts, and into PDL-like cells *in vivo* [4]. Preliminary results from animal studies suggested that DFCs have also a good osteogenic differentiation potential and could be an excellent source for the regeneration of craniofacial bone [6]. Another excellent source for cellular therapies of mineralized tissues is progenitor cells from the dental apical papilla of retained third molar tooth (dNC-PCs) [7]. These dental

* Correspondence: christian.morsczeck@ukr.de
[1]Department of Cranio- and Maxillofacial Surgery, Hospital of the University of Regensburg, Franz-Josef-Strauss-Allee 11, 93053 Regensburg, Germany
Full list of author information is available at the end of the article

cells differentiate into osteoblast-like cells after the induction with osteogenic differentiation medium under *in vitro* conditions and under *in vivo* conditions in immunocompromised mice [8].

For the osteogenic differentiation under *in vivo* conditions, stem cells are combined actually with hydroxylapatite (HAP) or β tricalcium phosphate (TCP) scaffolds [4,9]. Although this is routinely applied, we know only little about the adherence and the viability of dental progenitor cells on these implant materials. Conversely, an optimal bone substitute material has not been identified so far for different dental stem cell types. In a recent study, we investigated, therefore, cell survival/proliferation and cell differentiation of DFCs in combination with a commercially available TCP [10]. Here, DFCs attached on TCP and cell numbers increased after 6 days of cultivation. We showed that DFCs had a typical flattened-shaped morphology with close contacts to the bone substitute material [10]. Interestingly, the gene expression of osteogenic markers such as osteopontin or RUNX2 was increased, and the alkaline phosphatase (ALP) activity was induced on TCP in differentiated DFCs [10]. All these data support the assumption that TCP could be the optimal scaffold for a successful differentiation protocol of DFC.

Unfortunately, an additional study showed that TCP induced apoptosis in DFCs [11]. However, the induction of apoptosis exposed a risk for cellular therapies. We decided therefore to evaluate additional implant materials for the identification of a suitable scaffold for dental stem cells. Soft materials such as silicone are successfully used in regenerative medicine, and they are suitable for tissue engineering, but, however, we propose that rigid and bone-like materials are superior for dental tissue engineering than soft implant materials. Therefore, this study evaluated and compared solid bone substitute materials with elastic materials such as silicone or polyacrylamide (PA). This study investigated the proliferation, the induction of apoptosis, and the osteogenic differentiation of DFCs and dNC-PCs after the attachment on implant-materials.

## Methods

### Cell culture

The isolation and characterization of DFCs and dNC-PCs were described in previous studies [4,7,12]. DFCs were routinely cultivated in DMEM (Sigma-Aldrich, St. Louis, MO, USA) supplemented with 10% fetal bovine serum (Sigma-Aldrich, St. Louis, MO, USA) and 100 μg/ml penicillin/streptomycin (standard cell culture medium). dNC-PCs were cultivated in DMEM (Sigma-Aldrich) supplemented with 15% fetal bovine serum (Sigma-Aldrich) and 100 μg/ml penicillin/streptomycin (standard cell culture medium). For experiments, both cell types were used after passage 6. DFCs and dNC-PCs expressed typical markers for dental stem cells such as CD105, Nestin, and STRO-1 (Additional file 1: Figure S1).

### Preparation of polyacrylamide materials

Five milliliter of PA gel solution with the concentration of 8% acrylamide and 0.06% bis-acrylamide (Bio-Rad, Hercules, CA, USA) were mixed and degas under vacuum for at least 20 min to remove oxygen. Then, 30 μl of 0.1 mg/mL ammonium persulfate (Sigma-Aldrich, St. Louis, MO, USA) and 20 μl TEMED (Applichem, Omaha, NE, USA) were added and placed into the mini protean casting strand and frame (Bio-Rad) to form 1-mm thickness of substrate. After letting the gel to polymerize for 30 to 45 min, gently remove and rinse gel with 50-mM HEPES, pH 8.5 (Applichem, Omaha, NE, USA). PA gel was then cut into circular shape with 14 mm diameters and placed in 24 well plates for the experiment. Sulfo-SANPAH (Pierce Biotechnologies, Rockford, IL USA) 0.5 mg/mL in 50-mM HEPES, pH 8.5 was pipetted onto the surface and exposed to the UV light for photoactivation procedure. After photoactivation, the substrate was washed several times in 50-mM HEPES. A 0.2 mg/mL of type I collagen (Sigma-Aldrich, St. Louis, MO, USA) was then layered onto the surface of gel and incubated 4 h at room temperature or overnight at 4°C on a shaker. After washing with PBS, the gels were stored in PBS at 4°C. Before platting the cells, the gel was exposed to UV for 15 min for the sterilization and replace PBS with complete culture medium for 1 h at 37°C.

### Implant materials

The bone substitutes Maxgraft® (AP) and Maxresorb® (SB) were obtained from the company Botiss (botiss dental GmbH, Berlin, Germany). Maxgraft® is a sterile, high-safety allograft product (AP), derived from human donor bone. It is processed by an audited and certified bone bank (Cells$^+$ Tissue Bank Austria, Berlin, Germany). In contrast, Maxresorb® is a fully synthetic bone graft substitute (SB) with controlled resorption properties. It is a homogenous composition of 60% hydroxyapatite and 40% beta-tri-calcium phosphate. SB maintains the volume and mechanical stability over a long time period. The osteoconductivity of SB is achieved by a matrix of interconnecting pores and a very high porosity of approximately 80%, as well as pore sizes from 200 to 800 μm (www.botiss.com). Experiments with AP and SB were done with solid blocks (10 × 10 × 20 mm cancellous block). PA was produced in our lab (see above), and silicone-based implant materials were obtained from Vivomed (Downpatrick, UK) as tubes. Silicone tubes were cut in pieces with a size which is similar to that of AP and SB.

Implant materials were washed with PBS or cell culture medium before use. DFCs and dNC-PCs were seeded onto materials for indicated periods of time. For the isolation of total RNA and the estimation of vital cell numbers, implant materials with cells were transferred to a fresh well with cell culture medium.

For the evaluation of apoptosis induction, cell culture eluates were produced by incubating 0.1 mL of bone substitutes or soft materials in 1-mL standard medium at 37°C for 24 h. This incubation step with the implant material was repeated twice with fresh cell culture media. Three eluates were pooled for cell culture experiments. DFCs were seeded onto cell culture plates and cultivated in standard cell culture media. After cell seeding (12 to 24 h), cell culture media were changed, and cells were cultivated in cell culture media with material eluates. After 24 h of cultivation, cells were harvested for flow cytometry analyses or protein isolation for Western blots (see below).

### Cell counting kit 8 assay

Numbers of vital cells were evaluated after days 1, 2, 3, and 6. For cell counting, cell cultures were incubated with the cell counting kit 8 (CCK8) ready to use solution according to manufactures instructions (Dojindo, Rockville, MD, USA). The optical density (O.D.) was measured at a wavelength of 450 nm. For the evaluation of the cell adherence (normalized to standard cell culture dishes), cell proliferation (normalized to cell number at day 1 of cell culture) relative cell numbers were calculated.

### Flow cytometry analysis

The induction of apoptosis in DFCs and dNC-PCs was evaluated by measuring the Cell Event® Caspase3/7 Green Flow cytometry assay (Life Technologies, Carlsbad, CA, USA). For the Caspase3/7assay, cells were cultivated in eluates as described above. After 24 h, cells were harvested by trypsin-EDTA treatment, washed with PBS, and stained first with Caspase3/7 Green Detection Reagent (25 min, 37°C). After this step 1-mM SYTOX® AADvanced dead cell stain solution was added to the sample (5 min, 37°C). Cell fluorescence was analyzed at 488-nm excitation and applied to standard fluorescence compensation. Emission of fluorescence was measured with 530/30 BP (Caspase3/7 Green Detection Reagent) and with 690/50 BP (SYTOX® AADvanced dead cell stain) filters. Cells positive for Caspase3/7 Green Detection Reagent were identified as apoptotic cells, while dead cells were positive for SYTOX® AADvanced dead cell stain. However, vital cells were negatively stained for both staining solutions.

### Western blotting

For protein isolation, cells were treated with lysis buffer (250 µl phosphatase, 100 mM Na3VO4, 137 mM NaCl, 200 mM Tris, 480 mM NaF, 1% NP-40, 10% Glycerol) on ice for 2 min. A protease-inhibitor (1 Protease Inhibitor Cocktail tablet from Roche) was included to minimize protein degradation. Cell lysates were placed on ice for 10 min. Protein samples were separated by SDS-polyacrylamide gel electrophoresis in pre-casted 12% Tris-glycine gels (Invitrogen, Waltham, MA, USA) and blotted to nitrocellulose membranes. Membranes were blocked with skimmed milk for 1 h and incubated with primary antibodies that were specific for proteins BAX (pro apoptotic protein), BCL2 (anti apoptotic protein), and β-Actin (housekeeper protein). Washed membranes were then incubated with a horseradish peroxidase-labeled secondary antibody. The detection of the secondary antibody was performed via chemiluminescence and X-ray films (GE Healthcare, Pewaukee, WI, USA).

### Osteogenic differentiation

DFCs were cultivated until sub-confluence (>80%) in standard cell culture medium before the differentiation starts with the osteogenic differentiation medium (ODM) comprised DMEM (PAA) supplemented with 10% fetal bovine serum (Sigma-Aldrich), 100 µmol/L ascorbic acid 2-phosphate, 10 mmol/L $KH_2PO_4$, $1 \times 10^{-8}$ mol/L dexamethasone sodium phosphate (Sigma-Aldrich, St. Louis, MO, USA), HEPES (20 mmol/L) and 100 µg/ml penicillin/streptomycin. The differentiation was evaluated by qRT-PCR and ALP activity detection.

### ALP activity detection

Cells were washed with PBS buffer and lysed by shock freezing (−80°C). Diluted 1:1 in 1 × PBS, 100 mM p-nitrophenyl phosphate (Sigma) was added to each sample. After incubation at 37°C for 60 min, the reaction was stopped by adding 300 µL of 0.3 M NaOH and the liberated p-nitrophenol was measured at 405 nm. ALP activity values were normalized to total DNA concentration, which were determined by the Quant-iT PicoGreen dsDNA Assay (Invitrogen).

### Prime PCR arrays

For the evaluation of osteogenic marker expression, the Biorad PrimePCR array (Development - Hedgehog and PTH signaling pathways in bone and cartilage development) was used, which consists of the most important markers for the osteogenic differentiation. Total RNAs, which were isolated from differentiated dental cells at day 7, were reverse-transcripted with the iScript™ Advanced cDNA Synthesis Kit for RT-qPCR (Biorad) according to the manufacturers protocol. PCRs were made with SsoAdvanced™ Universal SYBR® Green Supermix (Biorad) on the StepOne real-time PCR machine (Life Technologies, Carlsbad, CA, USA). Results were analyzed with the PrimePCR™ Analysis Software (Biorad), and the output is presented as Clustergrams. While red tiles signify a high gene expression, black/gray and green

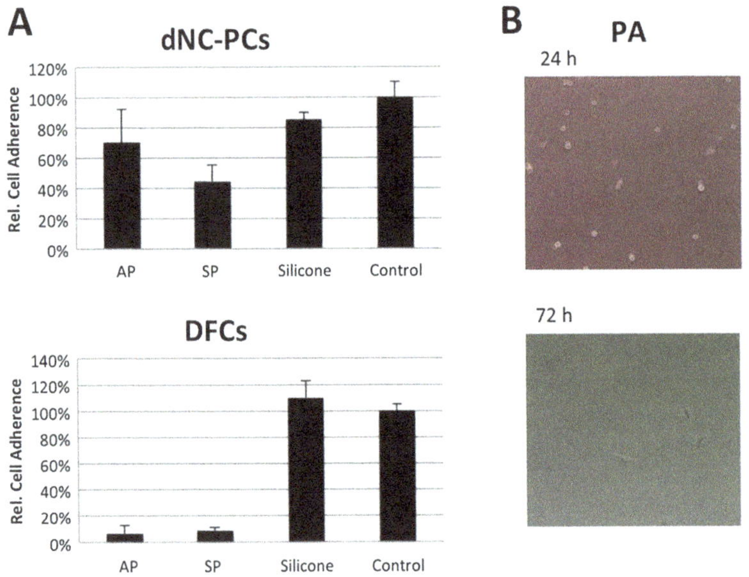


**Figure 1 Cell attachment on tested materials.** **(A)** Relative cell adherence of DFCs and dNC-PCs; **(B)** dental cells did little adhere on PA; representative pictures of DFCs.

tiles show a middle gene expression and a low gene expression, respectively. Black tiles with a cross designate no gene expression.

### Histology

Combinations of SB with dNC-PCs and AP with dental cells yielded from cell cultures after 7 days of osteogenic differentiation were fixed in 4% formaldehyde/0.1 M PBS at 4°C for at least 24 h. Tissues were decalcified with EDTA and subsequently dehydrated in an ascending series of ethanol and embedded in paraffin. Serial sections of 5 μm were cut in different planes for orientation and stained with hematoxylin-eosin (HE).

## Results

### Cell viability

Dental cells were cultivated in standard cell culture media until passage 6. Cell adherence and cell proliferation/growth were measured for the estimation of cell viability on tested rigid and soft materials. In Figure 1, the cell adherence of dNC-PCs on bone substitute materials was better than that of DFCs. However, both dental cells types

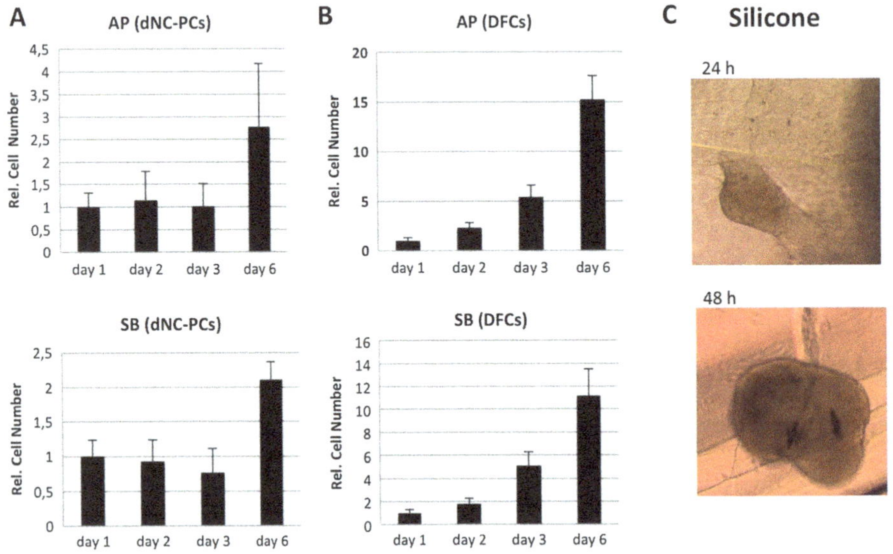


**Figure 2 Cell proliferation of dNC-PCs and DFCs on tested materials.** **(A)** and **(B)** Relative cell numbers; **(C)** spheroid cell clusters on silicone (representative pictures for DFCs); Silicone (24 and 48 h).

adhered very well on silicone. Unluckily, dental cells did not adhere on PA; only single cells survived for longer than 48 h (Figure 1B). For the evaluation of cell proliferation, relative cell numbers on implant materials were measured (Figure 2). While cell proliferation of dNC-PCs was moderate (Figure 2A), relative cell numbers of DFCs increased dramatically on bone substitute materials (Figure 2B). However, these results proved the viability of dNC-PCs and DFCs on SB and AP. Interestingly, dental cells formed large spheroid cell clusters on silicone, but cells lost their adherence to this material (Figure 2C), so numbers of silicone adherent cells decreased until day 6 of cell culture (data not shown).

The induction of apoptosis and/or cell death was estimated by flow cytometry and western-blot analyses (Figure 3). While eluates of SB, PA, and silicone did neither induce cell death nor apoptosis, AP induced both cell death and apoptosis in DFCs and dNC-PCs. Both dental cell types expressed the pro-apoptotic marker BAX and the anti-apoptosis marker BCL2 under standard cell culture conditions (Figure 3B). However, BCL2 was not expressed on AP. Interestingly, BCL2 was also not expressed in DFCs after cultivation on SB. The low expression of BCL2 in DFCs may explain the low cell adherence on SB and AP (Figure 1).

## Osteogenic differentiation

We measured the normalized ALP activity in dNC-PCs and DFCs after cultivation on tested materials (Figure 4). While ALP activities in dental cells on bone substitutes were increased or comparable to that of differentiated

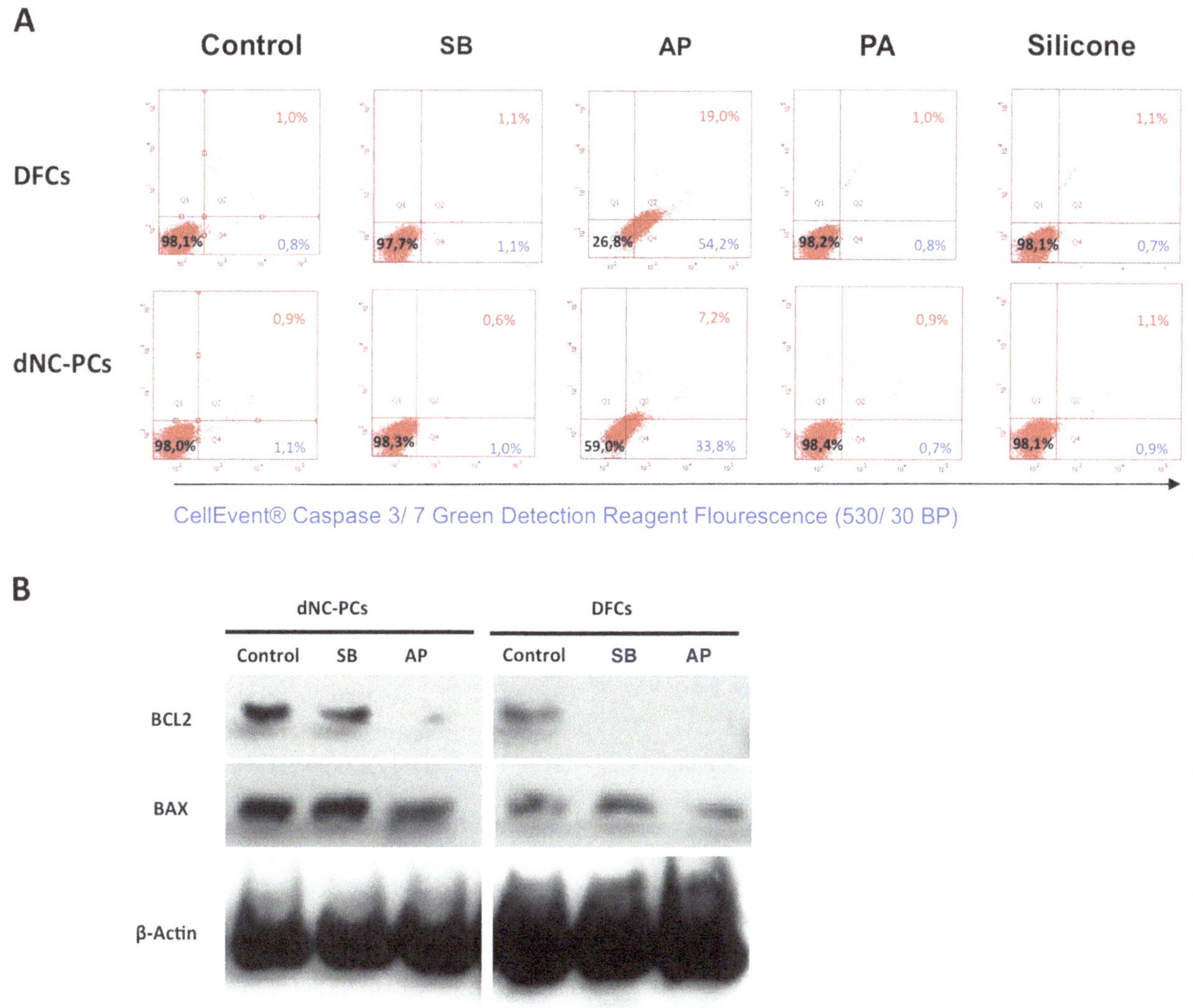


**Figure 3 Evaluation of programmed cell death (apoptosis) in dental stem cells. (A)** Flow cytometry analyses (for details materials and methods) show percentage of vital cells (black number), apoptotic cells (blue number), and dead cells (red number). **(B)** Western blot analyses show the expression of the pro-apoptotic marker BAX and the anti-apoptotic marker BCL2.

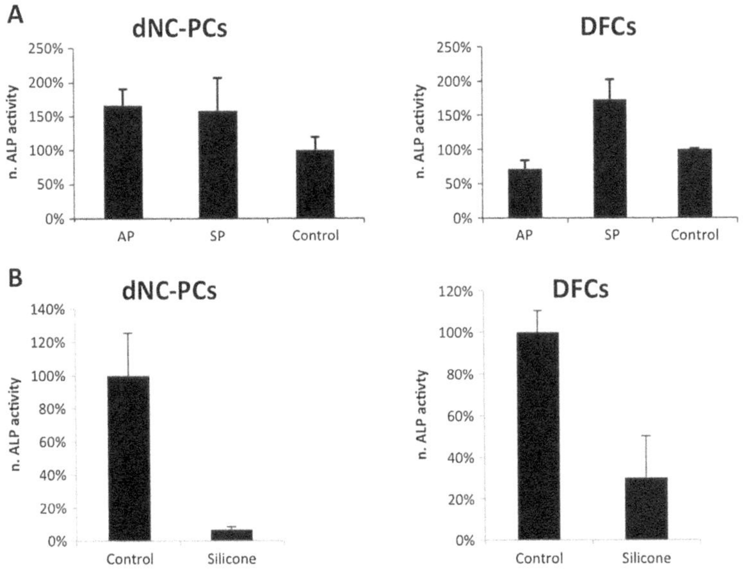


**Figure 4 Osteogenic differentiation of dental stem cells.** Normalized ALP activity of dNC-PCs and DFCs on AP and SB **(A)** and on silicone **(B)**. Cells were differentiated on standard cell culture dishes for control.

cells in standard cell culture dishes (control), the specific ALP activity was decreased on silicone (Figure 4B). A PCR array analysis showed that AP induced the expression of osteogenic differentiation markers (Figure 5A). Moreover, differentiated cells formed thick connective tissue like matrices on bone substitute materials (Figure 5B). These results reminded on the differentiation of osteogenic progenitor cells.

### PA after collagen I modification

The soft material PA was also treated with the extracellular matrix protein collagen to improve cell adherence. We tested representatively DFCs with collagen I modified PA. DFCs adhered and proliferated on modified PA, but, however, the specific ALP activity was reduced in comparison to that of DFCs on standard cell culture dishes (Figure 6). This reduction of the specific ALP activity was similar to that of silicone.

## Discussion

Scaffolds play an important role in tissue engineering. However, little is known about the proliferation and differentiation of DFCs and dNC-PCs on different types of materials. As we have learned from previous studies mechanical properties such as surface stiffness are decisive for a successful osteogenic differentiation of dental stem cells [13,14]. Moreover, we showed that bone substitute materials such as β-tricalcium phosphate (TCP) supports the osteogenic differentiation [10]. Our study proposed therefore that bone-like materials such as commercially available bone substitutes are superior for dental tissue engineering. Therefore, bone substitute materials SB and AP were compared with soft or connective tissue like materials. SB is synthetic and consists of 60% HAP and 40% TCP. In contrast, AP is an allograft product, which was derived from human donor bone. For comparison, two different soft materials silicone or PA were used in our study. Whereas silicone is routinely applied in regenerative medicine, the self-made PA scaffold has been very often used in cell biology studies [15].

dNC-PCs and DFCs attached on SB, AP, and silicone, but not on PA unless it was untreated. A modification with the extracellular matrix protein collagen permitted the attachment of dental cells. Interestingly, cell proliferation on silicone was hampered, because dental cells grew in non-attached spheroid cell clusters. This formation of spheroid cell clusters reminds on the neurogenic differentiation of DFCs [16-18]. The proliferation of DFCs on SB and AP was better than that of dNC-PCs, because the attachment of DFCs on these materials was lower than that of dNC-PCs. However, we conclude that bone substitute materials are suitable for dental cell attachment and proliferation. Our results for bone substitute materials are comparable to that of previous studies with different dental cell types. Kasaj and co-workers showed that cell adherence and cell proliferation of PDL cells on nanostructured HAP bone replacement grafts *in vitro* [19]. In another study, PDL cells adhere and proliferate on chitosan or on a combination of chitosan and nanostructured HAP [20]. In this setting, the combination of chitosan and nanostructured HAP was even favored by PDL cells. The adhesion and proliferation of dental pulp derived cells on HAP was demonstrated by Abe et al. [21].

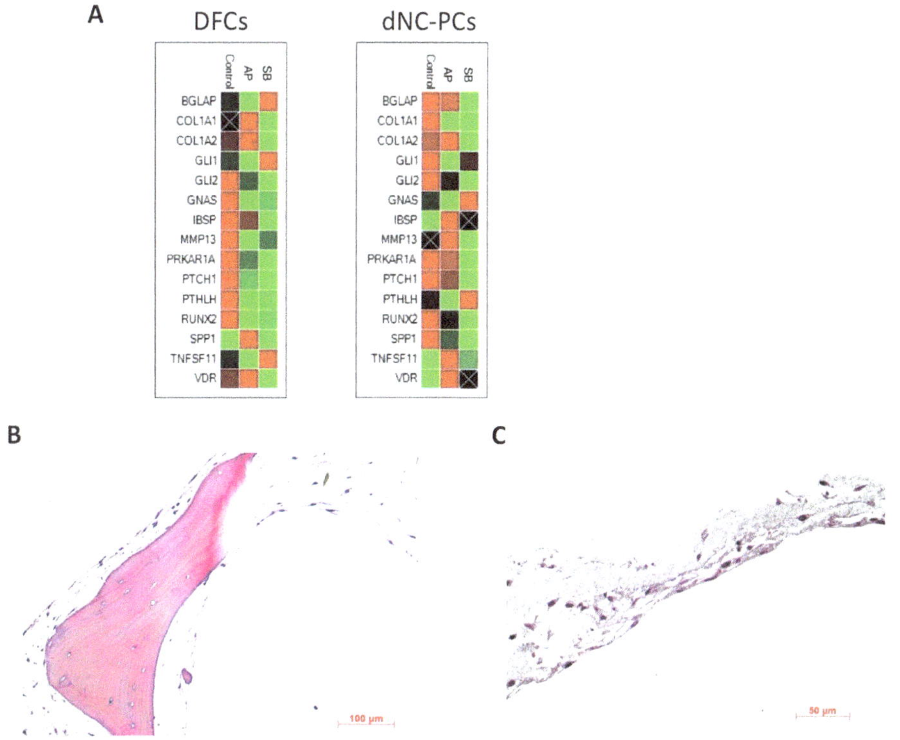


**Figure 5 Evaluation of osteogenic differentiation.** **(A)** Clustergram of PCR-array results; **(B-C)** histology of differentiated dental cells on AP **(B)** and SB **(C)**. Representative results are shown for dNC-PCs.

In a previous study, we showed that TCP induced the programmed cell death (apoptosis) in DFCs [11]. Our new study investigated therefore the induction of apoptosis in dental cells. While SB and soft materials did not induce apoptosis or cell death, AP induced obviously cell death and apoptosis in dental cells. Here, the results for dNC-PCs and DFCs were almost the same. Interestingly, neither silicone nor PA induced the apoptosis in dental cells but did not also sustain the osteogenic differentiation of dental cells. Here, the ALP activity was strongly inhibited. Although no explanation for the induction of apoptosis by AP is available, the induction of apoptosis by AP does not correlate with the induction of the osteogenic differentiation. Both bone substitute materials sustained the differentiation, but only AP induced the expression of typical osteogenic differentiation markers. The induction of both osteogenic markers and apoptosis is very similar to that of our previous studies with TCP [10,11]. Interestingly, a study with pre-differentiated human cord blood stem cells showed also very similar effects on TCP [22]. They discovered a reduced number of pre-differentiated stem cells after long term cultures on TCP [22]. But although cell numbers decreased between days 1 and 7, the gene expression of osteogenic cell differentiation markers was increased [22]. In contrast, Marino et al. demonstrated that TCP scaffolds promoted

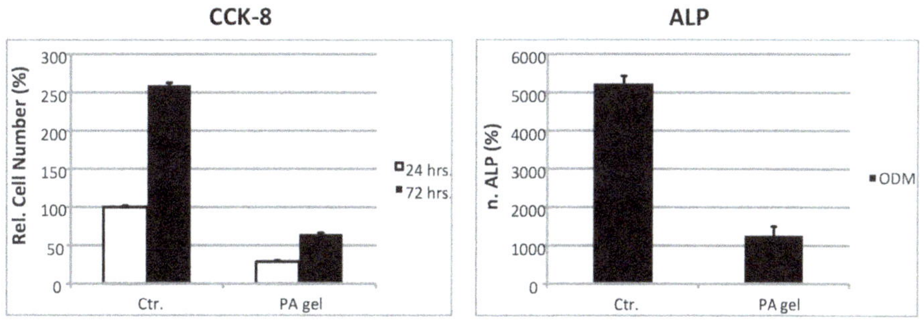


**Figure 6 Cultivation and osteogenic differentiation of DFCs on PA after modification with collagen I.** (Left) Relative cell number and (Right) normalized ALP activity.

both cell proliferation and osteogenic differentiation of human adipose stem cells [23]. However, additional studies are required to disclose the molecular relationship between apoptosis and the osteogenic differentiation.

Finally, we could show that surface modifications are important for the attachment and cell proliferation of dental cells (Figure 6). Our results are in accordance to the results obtained in previous studies. For example, modifications such as fibronectin coating of TCP or composites with a combination of polymer of poly glycolic-lactic acid (PGLA) with TCP may also influence cell attachment and proliferation of seeded cells [24,25]. Moreover, Seebach et al. showed that TCP products from different suppliers differ substantially in their morphology and that surface or porous structure seems to be of importance for the cell seeding and proliferation [25]. Unfortunately, a modification of PA with collagen did not improve the osteogenic differentiation of dental stem cells.

## Conclusions

In conclusion, our work supports our hypothesis that soft implant materials are not suitable for dental tissue engineering. Moreover, our study also supports the results of our previous studies with DFCs and TCP that induction of apoptosis did not impair the proliferation and the differentiation in dental stem cells.

#### Competing interests

Martin Gosau, Sandra Viale-Bouroncle, Hannah Eickhoff, Esthera Prateeptongkum, Anja Reck, W Götz, Christoph Klingelhöffer, Steffen Müller and Christian Morsczeck declare that they have no competing interests.

#### Authors' contributions

SVB, HE, and EP carried out all cell biology experiments, performed real-time PCRs, Western blots, and the statistical analysis and made figures for the manuscript. AR carried out and analyzed the flow cytometry experiments and made figures. SM participated in study design and supervised the research team. MG, CK, and CM designed experiments, supervised the research team, and prepared the manuscript. WG evaluated the histology of dental stem cells on biomaterials. All authors read and approved final version of the manuscript.

#### Acknowledgement

This study was supported by a grant from the Deutschen Gesellschaft für Implantologie (DGI) e.V.

#### Author details

[1]Department of Cranio- and Maxillofacial Surgery, Hospital of the University of Regensburg, Franz-Josef-Strauss-Allee 11, 93053 Regensburg, Germany. [2]Department of Oral and Maxillofacial Surgery, Paracelsus Medical University Nuernberg, Breslauer Str., 201, 90471 Nürnberg, Germany. [3]Department of Orthodontics, Oral Biology Laboratory, Dental Clinic, University of Bonn, Regina-Pacis-Weg 3, 53113 Bonn, Germany.

#### References

1. Kagami H, Agata H, Tojo A. **Bone marrow stromal cells (bone marrow-derived multipotent mesenchymal stromal cells) for bone tissue engineering: basic science to clinical translation.** *Int J Biochem Cell Biol.* 2011; **43**:286–89.
2. Robey PG. **Cell sources for bone regeneration: the good, the bad, and the ugly (but promising).** *Tissue Eng Part B Rev.* 2011; **17**:423–30.
3. Morsczeck C, Shi S, Huang G. **Stem/progentinor cells of dental and gingival tissue origin.** In: Huang; Thesleff, editor. *Stem Cells in Craniofacial Development, Regeneration and Repair.* New York: Wiley-Blackwell John Wiley & Sons; 2013.
4. Morsczeck C, Gotz W, Schierholz J, Zeilhofer F, Kuhn U, Mohl C, Sippel C, Hoffmann KH. **Isolation of precursor cells (PCs) from human dental follicle of wisdom teeth.** *Matrix Biol.* 2005; **24**:155–65.
5. Morsczeck C, Schmalz G, Reichert TE, Völlner F, Saugspier M, Viale-Bouroncle S, Driemel O. **Gene expression profiles of dental follicle cells before and after osteogenic differentiation in vitro.** *Clin Oral Invest.* 2009; **13**:383–91.
6. Honda MJ, Imaizumi M, Tsuchiya S, Morsczeck C. **Dental follicle stem cells and tissue engineering.** *J Oral Sci.* 2010; **52**:541–52.
7. Degistirici O, Jaquiery C, Schönebeck B, Siemonsmeier J, Götz W, Martin I, Thie M. **Defining properties of neural crest-derived progenitor cells from the apex of human developing tooth.** *Tissue Eng Part A.* 2008; **14**:317–30.
8. Degistirici O, Grabellus F, Irsen S, Schmid KW, Thie M. **Using human neural crest-derived progenitor cells to investigate osteogenesis: an in vitro study.** *Matrix Biol J Int Soc Matrix Biol.* 2010; **29**:219–27.
9. Gronthos S, Mankani M, Brahim J, Robey PG, Shi S. **Postnatal human dental pulp stem cells (DPSCs) in vitro and in vivo.** *Proc Natl Acad Sci USA.* 2000; **97**:13625–30.
10. Viale-Bouroncle S, Bey B, Reichert TE, Schmalz G, Morsczeck C. **β-tricalcium-phosphate stimulates the differentiation of dental follicle cells.** *J Mater Sci Mater Med.* 2011; **22**:1719–24.
11. Viale-Bouroncle S, Buergers R, Morsczeck C, Gosau M. **β-tricalcium phosphate induces apoptosis on dental follicle cells.** *Calcif Tissue Int.* 2013; **92**:412–17.
12. Felthaus O, Gosau M, Morsczeck C. **ZBTB16 induces osteogenic differentiation marker genes in dental follicle cells independent from RUNX2.** *J Periodontol.* 2014; **85**:e144–51.
13. Viale-Bouroncle S, Gosau M, Küpper K, Möhl C, Brockhoff G, Reichert TE, Schmalz G, Ettl T, Morsczeck C. **Rigid matrix supports osteogenic differentiation of stem cells from human exfoliated deciduous teeth (SHED).** *Differ Res Biol Divers.* 2012; **84**:366–70.
14. Viale-Bouroncle S, Völlner F, Möhl C, Küpper K, Brockhoff G, Reichert TE, Schmalz G, Morsczeck C. **Soft matrix supports osteogenic differentiation of human dental follicle cells.** *Biochem Biophys Res Commun.* 2011; **410**:587–92.
15. Engler AJ, Sen S, Sweeney HL, Discher DE. **Matrix elasticity directs stem cell lineage specification.** *Cell.* 2006; **126**:677–89.
16. Völlner F, Ernst W, Driemel O, Morsczeck C. **A two-step strategy for neuronal differentiation in vitro of human dental follicle cells.** *Differ Res Biol Divers.* 2009; **77**:433–41.
17. Beck HC, Petersen J, Felthaus O, Schmalz G, Morsczeck C. **Comparison of neurosphere-like cell clusters derived from dental follicle precursor cells and retinal Müller cells.** *Neurochem Res.* 2011; **36**:2002–07.
18. Beck HC, Gosau M, Kristensen LP, Morsczeck C. **A site-specific phosphorylation of the focal adhesion kinase controls the formation of spheroid cell clusters.** *Neurochem Res.* 2014; **39**:1199–205.
19. Kasaj A, Willershausen B, Reichert C, Gortan-Kasaj A, Zafiropoulos G-G, Schmidt M. **Human periodontal fibroblast response to a nanostructured hydroxyapatite bone replacement graft in vitro.** *Arch Oral Biol.* 2008; **53**:683–89.
20. Zhang Y-F, Cheng X-R, Chen Y, Shi B, Chen X-H, Xu D-X, Ke J. **Three-dimensional nanohydroxyapatite/chitosan scaffolds as potential tissue engineered periodontal tissue.** *J Biomater Appl.* 2007; **21**:333–49.
21. Abe S, Yamaguchi S, Watanabe A, Hamada K, Amagasa T. **Hard tissue regeneration capacity of apical pulp derived cells (APDCs) from human tooth with immature apex.** *Biochem Biophys Res Commun.* 2008; **371**:90–3.
22. Naujoks C, Langenbach F, Berr K, Depprich R, Kübler N, Meyer U, Handschel J., Kögler G. **Biocompatibility of osteogenic predifferentiated human cord blood stem cells with biomaterials and the influence of the biomaterial on the process of differentiation.** *J Biomater Appl.* 2011; **25**:497–512.
23. Marino G, Rosso F, Cafiero G, Tortora C, Moraci M, Barbarisi M, Barbarisi A. **Beta-tricalcium phosphate 3D scaffold promote alone osteogenic**

differentiation of human adipose stem cells: in vitro study. *J Mater Sci Mater Med.* 2010; **21**:353–63.
24. Arnold U, Lindenhayn K, Perka C. In vitro-cultivation of human periosteum derived cells in bioresorbable polymer-TCP-composites. *Biomaterials.* 2002; **23**:2303–10.
25. Seebach C, Schultheiss J, Wilhelm K, Frank J, Henrich D. Comparison of six bone-graft substitutes regarding to cell seeding efficiency, metabolism and growth behaviour of human mesenchymal stem cells (MSC) in vitro. *Injury.* 2010; **41**:731–38.

# Current status of implant prosthetics in Japan: a survey among certified dental lab technicians

Yoshiyuki Hagiwara[1*], Tatsuya Narita[1], Yohei Shioda[1], Keisuke Iwasaki[1], Takayuki Ikeda[1], Shunsuke Namaki[1] and Thomas J Salinas[2]

## Abstract

**Background:** There are many implant cases in which dental technicians take initiative with regard to the design of implant prostheses, and to a certain extent, this area of care is one in which dentists do not necessarily play the leading role. Moreover, inadequate communication between dental technicians and dentists and insufficient instructions for technicians has been highlighted as issues in the past. The purpose of this questionnaire is to improve the quality of implant prostheses and thereby contribute to patient service by clarifying, among other aspects of treatment, problem areas and considerations in the fabrication of implant prostheses, conceptual-level knowledge, and awareness of prosthodontics on the part of the dentists in charge of treatment and methods for preventing prosthetic complications.

**Methods:** A cross-sectional survey was given to 120 certified dental technicians. To facilitate coverage of a broad range of topics, we classified the survey content into the following four categories and included detailed questions for (1) the conditions under which implant technicians work, (2) implant fixed prostheses, (3) implant overdentures, and (4) prosthetic complications.

**Results:** Out of 120 surveys sent, 74 technicians responded resulting in a response rate of 61.6%.

**Conclusions:** This survey served to clarify the current state of implant prosthodontics, issues, and considerations in the fabrication of implant prostheses, and the state of prosthetic complications and preventive initiatives, all from a laboratory perspective. The results of this survey suggested that, to fabricate prostheses with a high level of predictability, functional utility, and aesthetic satisfaction, it is necessary to reaffirm the importance for dentists to increase their prosthetic knowledge and work together with dental technicians to develop comprehensive treatment plans, implement an organized approach to prosthesis design, and accomplish occlusal reconstruction.

**Keywords:** Questionnaire; Survey; Implant prosthesis; Certified dental technicians; Prosthetic complications

## Background

Currently, dental implant treatment is evaluated on the basis not only of restoring masticatory function, but also a variety of other factors, including the implant and superstructure survival rate and psychological impacts [1-3]. Numerous factors must be taken into account, to offer highly predictable implant treatment, and there is no doubt that prosthetic-related factors such as the type and compatibility of the prosthesis, as well as occlusion, make a major contribution to that goal [4-9].

Recently, a restoration-driven approach to implant treatment has gained recognition and is being put into practice on a broad basis [10,11]. However, an increasingly diverse range of patient cases has led to a situation in which it is impossible to ascertain such aspects of actual practice as prosthesis type and design, making it necessary to reaffirm the importance of treatment carried out from a prosthetic perspective [12]. Many surveys querying dentists or patients with regard to implant treatment have been reported in the literature, addressing such topics as the state of implant treatment in particular countries and regions [13,14], quality of life and patient satisfaction [15-17], peri-implantitis and mucositis [18], and implant education [19,20]. However, very few surveys have queried

* Correspondence: hagiwara.yoshiyuki@nihon-u.ac.jp
[1]Implant Dentistry, Nihon University School of Dentistry, Dental Hospital, 1-8-13 Kandasurugadai, Chiyoda-ku, Tokyo 101-8310, Japan
Full list of author information is available at the end of the article

dental technicians, whose job it is to fabricate implant prostheses [21,22].

Dental technicians play a major role in current implant treatment because of increases in both the importance of their participation as part of the treatment team from the treatment planning stage [21] and the frequency of prosthesis repairs, refabrication, and related procedures in the event of prosthetic complications. In particular, the types of prosthetic complications being experienced and associated trends are becoming clear thanks to numerous systematic reviews undertaken recently to investigate the implant complications. Fixed prostheses are prone to issues such as screw loosening, crown detachment, and fracturing of the veneering material on a frequent basis [23-27]. Similarly, implant overdentures are frequently affected by progressive loosening of attachments, denture base fractures, and a sequential need for relining [28,29]. However, because understanding the status of these complications is based on the results of surveys targeting dentists, information is needed on the situation as seen from the standpoint of implant technicians, to clarify the causes of these complications and the techniques for dealing with them. Issues including inadequate communication between dental technicians and dentists and insufficient instructions for technicians have been pointed out in the past [21,30,31]. These reports derive from surveys targeting older fixed or removable prosthesis designs, leaving it unclear not only whether those issues have been rectified in the face of expanding use of implant prostheses in recent years, but also to what degree the opinions and wishes of dental technicians are being reflected in implant treatment.

This survey consists of a questionnaire targeting the certified dental technicians of the Japanese Society of Oral Implantology (JSOI) [32] who are primarily involved in fabricating dental implant restorations. It was formulated to clarify the current status of implant prostheses from a prosthetic and technician-oriented standpoint through questions addressing current trends among dental implant technicians, fixed prostheses, implant overdentures, and prosthetic complications and measures. The certified dental technicians of JSOI queried by the survey are involved in implant-related laboratory work on a comparatively frequent basis, and the responses they provided can be expected to accurately reflect the current state of implant laboratory practice in Japan. Our goal through this questionnaire is ultimately to improve the quality of implant prostheses and thereby contribute to patient service. We aim to do this by clarifying, among other aspects of treatment, problem areas, and considerations in the fabrication of implant prostheses, the conceptual-level knowledge base and awareness of prosthodontics on the part of the dentists in charge of treatment and methods for preventing prosthetic complications.

## Methods

This cross-sectional questionnaire survey was performed among the certified dental technicians of JSOI from September to December in 2011. Selected were 120 out of 285 certified dental technicians of JSOI using a random number table and mailing each questionnaire directly to the participant. To facilitate coverage of a broad range of topics, the survey classified content into the following four categories and included detailed questions for each: (1) the conditions under which implant technicians work (questions 1 and 2); (2) implant fixed prostheses (methods of retention, abutment, and prosthesis types; questions 3–6); (3) implant overdentures (questions 7 and 8); and (4) prosthetic complications (complication types, methods of treatment and prevention; questions 9–14). Details of the questions and results are provided in Tables 1, 2, 3, and 4. Given that no previous survey regarding implant dental technician data had been developed, an original form for this purpose was constructed following suggested guidelines [33,34]. Important to the construction validity, both the questionnaire authors and their audience were clinical specialists and were aware of the topic content. The content sought in the questionnaire was a measure of responder demographics, clinical experiences, and subjective perceptions. Additionally, interpretation errors were minimized because of content familiarity and standardization, which improved reliability, and no pretest measures were obtained given the mail-based assessment method.

## Results and discussion

Out of 120 surveys sent, 74 technicians responded, resulting in a response rate of 61.6%. A summary of the responses is provided in Tables 1, 2, 3, and 4 and Figures 1, 2, 3, 4, 5, 6, 7, 8, and 9.

**Table 1 Conditions characterizing implant laboratories**

| Question | | Values |
|---|---|---|
| Q1. The years of experience working as a dental technician, and the number of dentists from whom job orders are received. | | Mean (SD)<br>17.0 (6.8) years<br>36.5(12.4)/Lab. |
| Q2. Who takes the leading role in treatment planning and prosthetic design (initiative with regard to prostheses)? | Dentists mainly exercise initiative | 39.3% |
| | Technicians mainly exercise initiative | 15.0% |
| | Technicians are often consulted when it comes to specific cases and parts | 16.8% |
| | Decisions are made in collaboration with each other | 28.9% |

**Table 2 Implant fixed prostheses**

| Question | | Values |
|---|---|---|
| Q3. The percentages of implant fixed prostheses: | Cement-retained | 61.4% |
| | Screw-retained | 38.6% |
| Q4. What are the proportions of abutments used with cement-retained prostheses? | CAD/CAM (titanium) | 19.7% |
| | CAD/CAM (zirconia) | 12.1% |
| | Custom abutments (UCLA-type abutment + gold alloy) | 33.2% |
| | Two-piece-type titanium (prepable type) | 28.3% |
| | Other | 6.5% |
| Q5. What types of materials (i.e. veneer, coping) are used to make implant prostheses in the anterior region? | Porcelain fused to metal crown | 43.4% |
| | All ceramic crown (zirconia) | 27.1% |
| | All ceramic crown (other materials) | 6.6% |
| | Indirect composites (facing crown) | 21.3% |
| | Indirect composites (jacket crown) | 2.4% |
| Q6. What types of implant fixed prostheses are used in the posterior region? | Porcelain fused to metal crown (full bake) | 31.4% |
| | Porcelain fused to metal crown (metal occlusal) | 9.1% |
| | All ceramic crown (zirconia) | 14.3% |
| | Indirect composite veneer crown (full bake) | 22.3% |
| | Indirect composite veneer crown (metal occlusal) | 12.6% |
| | Metal crown | 10.3% |

Because implant treatment (implant prostheses) requires a significant amount of specialized, high-precision laboratory procedures, this area of dental care exhibits slightly different trends than prosthetic treatment as it was practiced in the past, and this work is concentrated at specialized fabrication labs. Moreover, there are many

**Table 3 Implant overdentures (IODs)**

| Question | | Values |
|---|---|---|
| Q7. The design of the implant overdenture: | Decision made according to instructions of dentist | 43.2% |
| | Work is left to technicians | 19.3% |
| | Decided upon through consultation with each other | 37.5% |
| Q8. What are the proportions of attachment types used with IODs? | Bar and clip | 35.6% |
| | Magnet | 30.2% |
| | Ball and socket | 19.0% |
| | Locator | 5.2% |
| | ERA | 2.3% |
| | Other | 7.7% |

**Table 4 Prosthetic complications**

| Question | | Values |
|---|---|---|
| Q9. What are the main issues generally encountered? | Compatibility precision issues | 29.6% |
| | Aesthetic issues | 33.2% |
| | Occlusal issues | 37.2% |
| Q10. What are the main fabrication challenges faced? | Poor implant location and orientation | 42.4% |
| | Inadequate consideration of occlusion | 17.0% |
| | Defects and inaccuracies in impression and bite registration | 29.0% |
| | Defective or unreasonable prosthesis design | 10.6% |
| | Other | 1.0% |
| Q11. What are the frequently received repair requests involving implant fixed prostheses? | Facing damage and chipping | 54.5% |
| | Facing discoloration and wear (indirect composite veneer crowns) | 17.0% |
| | Bridge connector fracture | 10.0% |
| | Design changes and modification associated with additional implants | 13.9% |
| | Other | 4.6% |
| Q12. What kind of creative steps do you take in order to prevent veneer fracture and chipping in the molar region? | Use of metal occlusal designs | 15.1% |
| | Use of indirect composite resin material | 15.7% |
| | Devise metal coping designs | 36.3% |
| | Cover the distal-most part with metal | 24.0% |
| | Nothing in particular | 8.9% |
| Q13. What are the frequently received repair requests for IODs? | Fracturing of the denture base or denture tooth detachment/fracture | 53.8% |
| | Mesostructure (attachment) damage | 8.4% |
| | Occlusal reconstruction due to denture wear or attrition | 24.1% |
| | Replacement of the attachment system (transition to another system) | 8.1% |
| | Other | 5.6% |
| Q14. Do you have any requests for dentists who practice implant treatment? | To consult technicians or allow technicians to participate from the treatment planning stage | 28.3% |
| | To use suitable implant location and orientation | 31.8% |
| | To improve treatment and condition of soft tissue | 21.8% |
| | To study more about prostheses and occlusion | 14.5% |
| | Other | 3.6% |

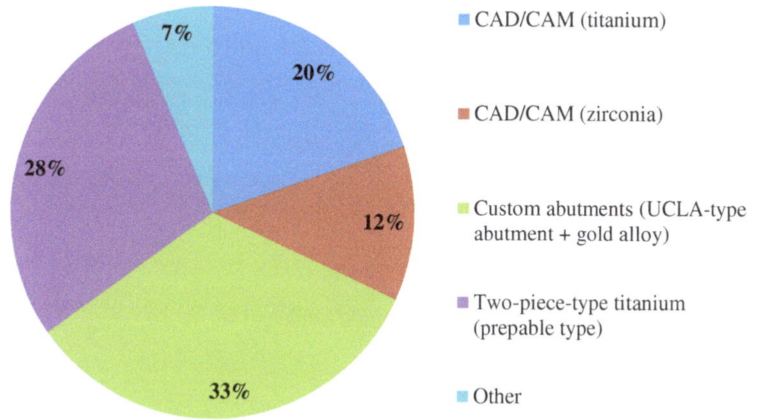


**Figure 1 Q4. What are the proportions of abutments used with cement-retained prostheses?**

cases in which dental technicians take initiative with regard to the design of implant prostheses, and to a certain extent, this area of care is one in which dentists do not necessarily play the leading role. In light of these circumstances, it was intended for this questionnaire to verify trends in implant treatment from a different perspective than has been used in the past, by investigating the current state of practice in the field from the dental technician perspective. By evaluating implant treatment from the standpoint of dental technology/prosthodontics and identifying current trends and problem areas, it was expected to gain information that enables highly predictable implant treatment.

1. Conditions characterizing implant laboratories (Table 1)
   The dental technicians who responded to this questionnaire have an average of about 17 years of experience in the field, indicating that they possess an adequate level of fabrication experience. In light of the reality that dental implant treatment is a comparatively new field, these personnel can be proficient with digital techniques as they differ from past generations of technicians who practiced the craft. On average, each dental technician serves about 36.5 customers, although that number varies depending on the scale of the fabrication lab at which they work. While implant laboratory work consists of complex processes, the fees are high, and labs generate a stable flow of revenue given a constant stream of work requests (Q1).
   Dentists play a leading role in 39.3% of the time in implant treatment planning and prosthetic design, and dental technicians are consulted concerning cases and part usage 34.7% of the time, suggesting the approach to implants is driven by prosthetic considerations (by dentists) to some degree. However, because dental technicians indicated that they take the initiative 15% of the time, it is impossible to ignore issues involving the care, skill, and judgment of dentists offering implant treatment. This is distinct from the question of whether communication or

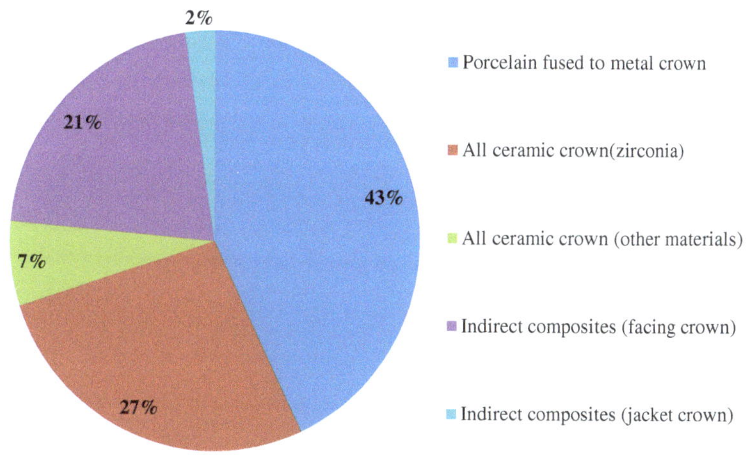


**Figure 2 Q5. What types of materials (i.e. veneer, coping) are used to make implant prostheses in the anterior region?**

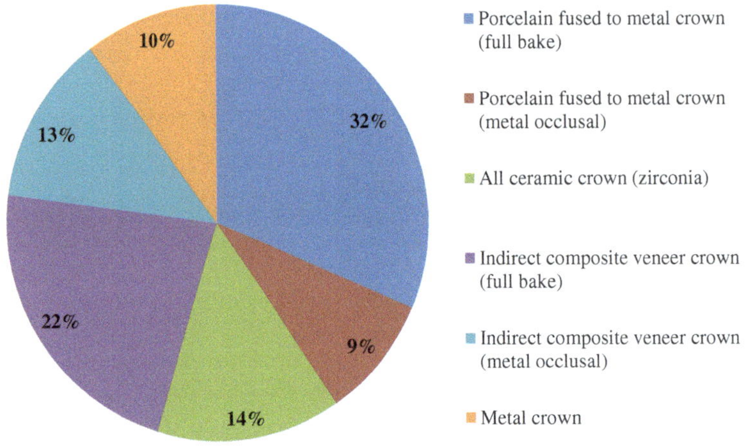


**Figure 3** Q6. What types of implant fixed prostheses are used in the posterior region?

information transmission between dentists and dental technicians is adequate, but rather relates to implant treatment knowledge, especially decisions about which prostheses and other treatment tools to use. The repercussions of this problem extend to the rate of incidence of prosthetic complications occurring after the start of functional use, their prevention, and the measures that are undertaken to address them (Q2).

Education of dental technicians varies by country, and there are a variety of means by which personnel master fabrication knowledge and skills. For example, a survey of dental technicians in the UK conducted by Bower et al. [35] reveals that while subjects read commercial magazines published for dental technicians, they rarely subscribed to academic journals in the field of prosthodontics, and two thirds of the survey's respondents had never attended a training course on fabrication practices. By contrast, certified dental technicians of JSOI are required to belong to an academic society and to participate in society meetings and certification courses to maintain their credentials. Subscription to JSOI's journal is an example of the advantages of membership for continuing education.

2. Implant fixed prostheses (Table 2)

Implant fixed prostheses employ either cement or screw retention. While there are a variety of reports comparing the two methods in terms of such metrics as their respective prognoses, success rates, and advantages and disadvantages [7,36-38], no reports have been published concerning their relative frequency of use. Our questionnaire indicated a distribution of 61.4% cement-retained versus 38.6% screw-retained prostheses (Q3), suggesting that cement retention is used more frequently in Japan. Unfortunately, the fabrication-oriented focus of this survey prevented clarification of the types of cement used for cement retention and the breakdown between provisional and definitive cement.

Next, concerning the types of abutments used with cement-retained prostheses (Q4) (Figure 1), CAD/CAM abutments accounted for about one third of the total (titanium, 19.7%; zirconia, 12.1%), and custom

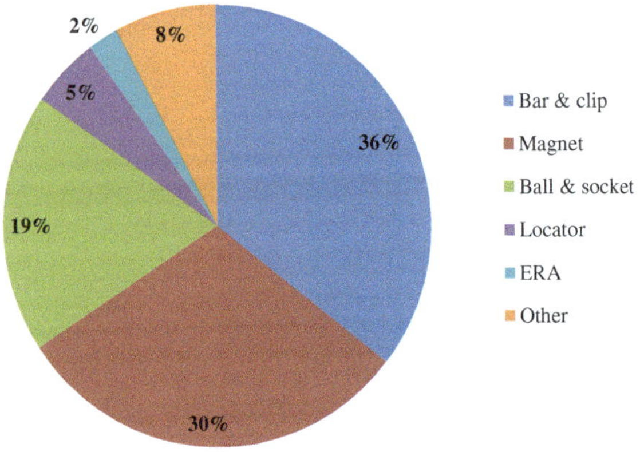


**Figure 4** Q8. What are the proportions of attachment types used with IODs?

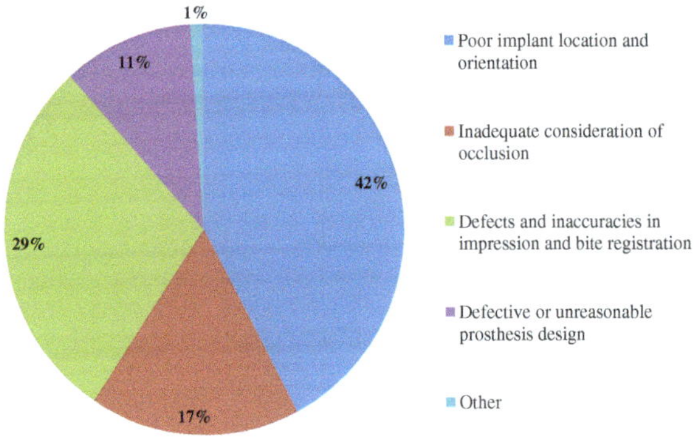


**Figure 5** Q10. What are the main fabrication challenges faced?

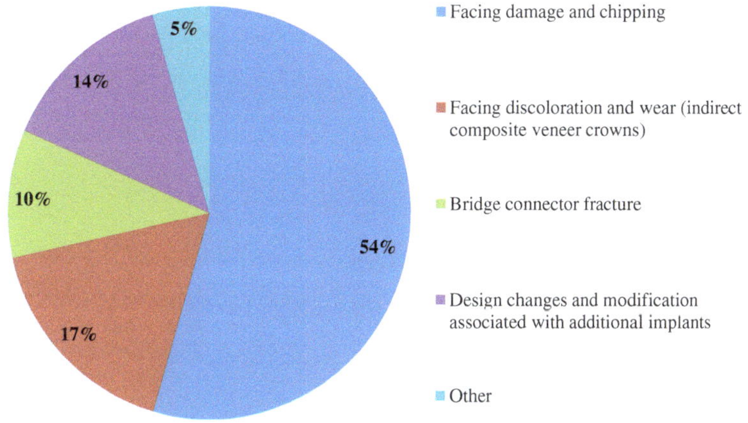


**Figure 6** **Q11. What are the frequently received repair requests involving implant fixed prostheses?**

UCLA-type abutments made from cast gold alloy accounted for about the same proportion. It is likely that this breakdown is because, in many cases, implant systems using fabricated crowns are not supported by CAD/CAM abutments. CAD/CAM system use is also subject to numerous limitations because of the licensing process imposed by the Ministry of Health, Labour and Welfare (MHLW) in Japan, which is strict when compared with its constituents in other countries. The questionnaire also indicated that titanium two-piece abutments (preparable type) are used in about the same proportion; 28% of the time. This reflects such factors as efforts to keep laboratory costs down and to shorten delivery time frames, in addition to the above reasons.

Concerning the types of prostheses used in the anterior region (i.e., veneering materials), the questionnaire indicated a trend toward selection of roughly the same materials for both single crowns and bridges (Q5) (Figure 2). As a rule, porcelain fused to metal (PFM) crowns accounted for 43.7% of the total, but selection of metal-free restorations using zirconia has been increasing in recent years, reaching approximately 27.1%. Incidentally, veneering porcelain was also used as the veneer material for zirconia copings. The questionnaire also indicated that while highly filled indirect composites such as Estenia (Kuraray, Osaka, Japan) were used 21.3% of the time, primarily for facing crowns, these materials were used infrequently for jacket crowns (2.4%). There is a low risk of facing damage and chipping for prostheses in the anterior region. Nonetheless, the questionnaire revealed the unexpected result that indirect composite facing crowns accounted for 21.3% of the total. This may be because there are many indirect composite resins (Estenia, Ceramage, etc.) available in Japan, and crowns and bridges in the anterior region (natural abutment teeth) are covered by certain types of insurance in the country (National Health Insurance and Social Insurance), with the result that Japanese

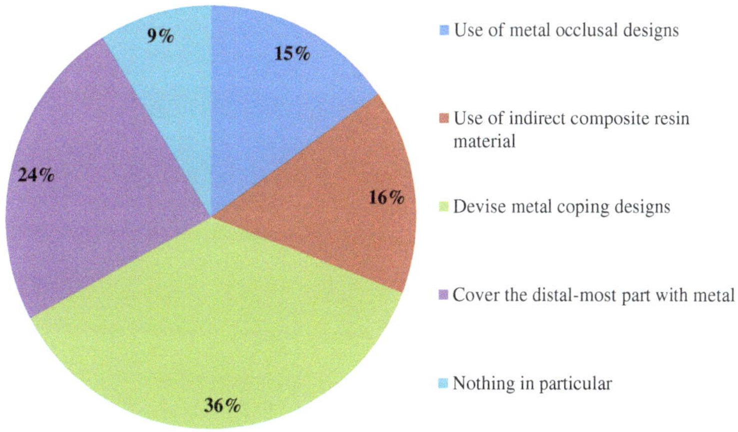


**Figure 7** **Q12. What kind of creative steps do you take in order to prevent veneer fracture and chipping in the molar region?**

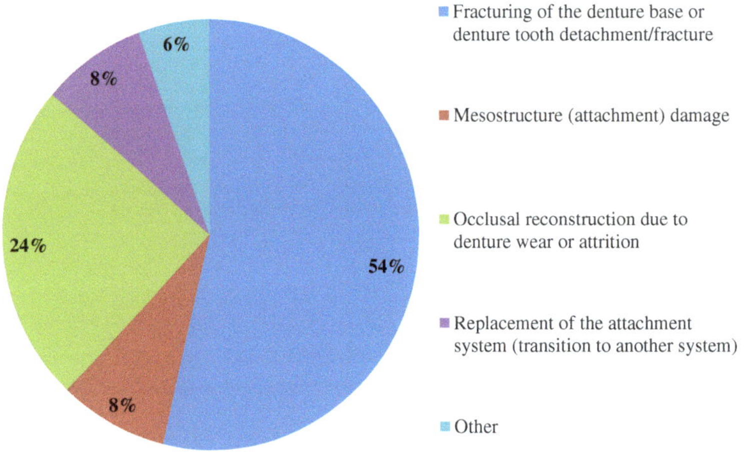


**Figure 8** Q13. What are the frequently received repair requests for IODs?

dentists are familiar with these materials and use them frequently. Consequently, it can be surmised that using these materials in implant prostheses is more common than in Europe and the USA. However, no survey of prosthesis selection has yet been carried out, and future research on that subject is expected. Concerning the types of prostheses used in the posterior region (Q6) (Figure 3), PFM design accounts for about 40% of the total, although the questionnaire also revealed a trend (in 9.1% of all cases) toward metal occlusal designs to avoid fracture and chipping of the veneer material. The same trend is evident in indirect composite facing crowns, where metal occlusal designs are used in about 35% of all cases that this type of prosthesis represents. In the past, the PFM crown was frequently used in implant crowns and bridges. However, a trend is seen toward increasing indirect composite resin use as a veneer material for implant superstructures. In addition to improvements in the physical properties (strength, wear resistance, and discoloration resistance) of indirect composites in recent years, their selection as veneer materials that chemically bond to titanium against the backdrop of increasing CAD/CAM-designed titanium frameworks, because of the low reliability of veneering porcelain, in terms of bonding strength, when used with titanium frames. There is also a greater possibility of direct (in-mouth) repair of failed veneering materials and greater shock-absorbing potential relative to occlusal force in comparison with porcelain [39]. The trend to adhere resin materials instead of porcelain, from Brånemark and colleagues' recommendations for acrylic resin as an occlusal surface material in the

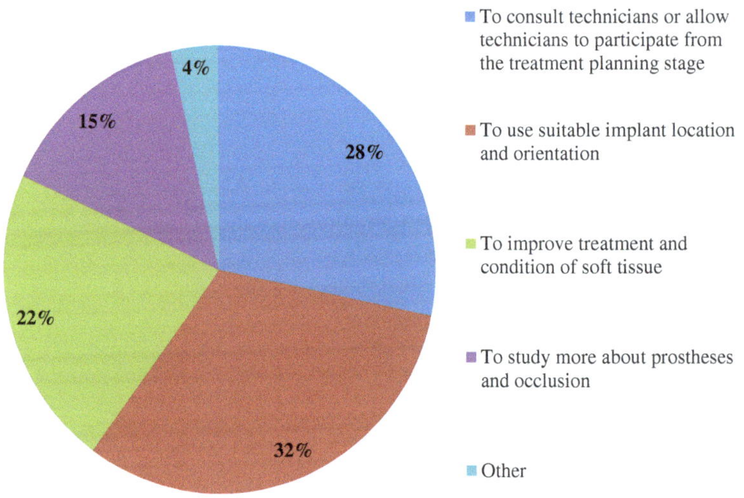


**Figure 9** Q14. Do you have any requests for dentists who practice implant treatment?

early 1980s, also cannot be ignored [40]. All metal crowns were used about 10.3% of the time in molar regions because of a lack of strong aesthetic requirements. Zirconia, however, accounted for 14.3%; only about half of its use in the anterior region. Possible reasons include this region not being an aesthetic area and veneer material fracture and chipping problems that have yet to be completely resolved [23,41,42].

3. Implant overdentures (IODs) (Table 3)
Some 19% of IOD design work is left to technicians, while 80% is performed according to the instructions of, or in consultation with, dentists (Q7). As was the case with the question concerning overall prosthesis design described above, these results indicate that a team approach is being put into practice.
Bar and clip attachments were most commonly used for IODs, followed by magnet, ball, and socket, and Locator attachments (Q8) (Figure 4). It is noteworthy among the questionnaire results that magnetic attachment use is highest in Asian countries, including Japan [43]. Additionally, it is thought that the low use of Locators (5.2%) is strongly influenced by Japan's strict pharmaceutical regulations and because the MHLW in Japan had not yet licensed the device at the time the questionnaire was administered. Conversely, ball and socket attachments have been standardized by major implant manufacturers, and the freedom with which prefabricated parts can be used has led to their comparatively broad use. IOD use in Japan is by no means widespread; a survey of IOD use in ten countries by Carlsson et al. [44] revealed that the adoption rate of these devices in Japan was just 7% for individuals with mandibular edentulism. This number was lower than in any of the other nine countries, and future changes in IOD use in Japan are a topic that remains interesting.

4. Prosthetic complications (Table 4)
According to Papaspyridakos et al. [2], indicators such as implant level (the relationship between the implant and bone) and the state of soft tissue around the implant are the most frequently used indices of implant success, followed by the presence and status of any implant prosthetic complication. Implant prosthetic complications include materials science-related factors, biomechanical and occlusion-related factors, and aesthetic factors. A systematic review of numerous complications that have been reported recently reveals the prostheses, restoration methods, materials, and areas most susceptible to complications [2,23-29]. Additionally, the frequency of prosthesis repairs, and repair costs cannot be ignored from a medical economic standpoint [2].
Of the problems and issues generally encountered on the laboratory side, compatibility precision, aesthetic issues, and occlusal issues each accounted for about one third of the total (Q9). When these results are examined in connection with laboratory challenges (Q10) (Figure 5), it becomes clear that technicians regard poor implant location and orientation (42.4%) as obstacles to success. Many other issues derived from factors such as dentists' skill level and treatment planning knowledge are directly related to quality implant treatment, such as defects and inaccuracies in impression-taking and bite registration (29%), inadequate establishment of appropriate occlusal schemes (17%), and deficient or unreasonable prosthesis design (10.6%). These issues can easily give rise to a variety of prosthetic complications after initiating functional use (and may also lead to biological complications), and dentists who offer dental implant treatment should reflect on improving their techniques. In particular, unsuitable implant locations, positions, and orientations can be prevented through appropriate preoperative examination and planning based on diagnostic wax-ups and surgical templates.
Looking at repair requests (i.e., complications) involving the superstructures of fixed implant prostheses (Q11) (Figure 6), facing damage and chipping accounted for more than half of all requests (54.5%). Generally speaking, there are many reports that indicate a high incidence of complications related to fixed prostheses involving abutment screw loosening, detachment of cement-retained crowns, and veneer (porcelain/composite resin) fracturing and damage. Because this question addressed repair of implant prostheses, we did not obtain information about complications that can be resolved in a chair-side setting. However, the high rate of requests for facing repairs makes it clear that veneer material chipping and similar issues are occurring at a high frequency [25-27].
Although the literature includes reports indicating a greater incidence of chipping and fractures for veneering porcelain than hardened resin [45,46] and for bridges than single crowns [26,27], this questionnaire does not shed light on the relative repair rates for porcelain and composite resin, nor the types of prostheses most likely to experience these issues. In the future, it would be worthwhile to conduct follow-up surveys on the differences among veneering materials and prostheses as well as veneer material failure trends.
Other cases requiring repair seen by technicians include facing discoloration (veneering composite resin) (17%) (Figure 7) and design changes and modification requests associated with additional implants (13.9%). Studies have pointed to issues

related to degradation of materials science characteristics for veneering composites that are distinct from those associated with porcelain, including loss of glossiness because of the deterioration of the surface and discoloration, wear, and attrition due to long-term use [47]. It is interesting to note how relatively frequently repairs are performed to address these issues. It has become clear that no small number of laboratory work requests deal with these issues experienced by patients undergoing implant treatment because of changes over time in the area surrounding existing implant treatments that occasionally necessitate additional implants and superstructure design changes or modifications.

The questionnaire revealed several creative steps, based on laboratory considerations, being taken to prevent veneer chipping and fractures, a frequent and problematic prosthetic complication (Q12) (Figure 7). Technicians were taking into account metal (including zirconia) coping designs (36.3%), covering only the distal-most part of the molar region with metal (24%), using veneering composite resin (15.7%), and using metal occlusal designs (15.1%). The type of coping is important in preventing veneer fractures, and it is necessary to secure adequate veneering material thickness and to consider the dispersion of stress [48]. Particularly as zirconia becomes more common, there has been a move to improve coping designs using CAD/CAM and to exercise care concerning the prevention of veneering porcelain fracture [49,50]. Responses to this survey support the idea that this concept has been gaining popularity among technicians in recent years. Conversely, it was not expected that 15.7% of respondents would indicate that they use composite resin to prevent veneering material fractures. Moreover, there is no evidence that veneering composites are more resistant to fracture than porcelain (as they are more prone to chipping) [45,46]. As noted above, veneering composites are often used in Japan, and one theory is that this trend is driven by a conceptual assumption that veneering composites are softer than porcelain and less likely to fracture from a materials science standpoint. It can be concluded that the ability to repair prostheses directly in the mouth is also a deciding factor.

More than half of all repair requests for IODs (i.e., complications) (Q13) (Figure 8) involve fracturing of the denture base or denture tooth detachment (53.8% of all repair requests). The questionnaire also revealed that reconstruction of occlusion because of wear or attrition of denture teeth (24.1%) is a frequent issue leading to laboratory orders. While the literature includes reports of frequent IOD-related prosthetic complications such as attachment-related compromised retention, detachment or fracturing of denture teeth, relining, and attachment damage [25,28,29], this survey showed a somewhat different trend. It can be inferred that these results differ from actual complication trends because they constitute responses to cases sent to labs as repair requests, and because the survey targeted dental technicians. The causes of this phenomenon can be found in responses to other questions as described above. In short, the questionnaire suggested the possibility that inadequate awareness of prosthetics is making IOD complications in Japan more complex, with issues including the comparatively frequent use of resin bases, problems with implant location and orientation, and inadequate consideration of occlusion by dentists.

Finally, technicians gave voice to the several requests for dentists, who are their customers, as a result of their daily experiences accomplishing implant laboratory procedures (Q14) (Figure 9). These included asking dentists to use suitable implant location and orientation (31.8%), to allow technicians to participate and consult with technicians from the treatment planning stage (28.3%), to improve consideration of soft tissue as well as its condition (21.8%), and to add more in-depth knowledge of prosthesis and occlusal design (14.5%). As observed, implant location and orientation issues in particular not only complicate technical work, but may also cause a variety of complications after the initiation of loading. For cases involving a broad range of implant prostheses and occlusal reconstruction, if not all cases, the dental technicians should be a part of the team from the treatment planning stage to enable restoration-driven implant treatment in the true sense of the term. At the same time, a dentist with an extensive understanding of prosthodontics should play the leading role in treatment of such cases. This survey succeeded in identifying prosthetic problems by examining implant prosthetic complications from the dental technician's perspective. As stated in the description of the survey's purpose, it is hoped that dentists make use of this report to reaffirm prosthetic concepts and awareness so that there is achievement of predictable implant prosthetic treatment.

## Conclusions

This survey served to clarify the current status of implant prosthodontics, issues, and considerations in their fabrication, and the status of prosthetic complications and preventive initiatives, all from a laboratory perspective.

1. Concerning implant treatment, it was concluded that dentists either play the leading role or work in collaboration with technicians, including in the formulation of treatment direction and that a team approach has been achieved to a certain extent.
2. This survey identified the problems that technicians address on a frequent basis in the fabrication of prostheses (these should be noted by dentists), including implant location and angulation, impression and bite registration precision, and occlusal considerations.
3. Concerning prevention of veneer fractures, it was also concluded that the best approach consists of metal occlusal (including a metal backing for the distal-most area) and coping designs.
4. The results of this survey suggest that, to fabricate prostheses with a high level of predictability, functional utility, and aesthetic satisfaction, it is necessary to reaffirm the importance of dentists increasing their prosthetic knowledge and working together with dental technicians to develop comprehensive treatment plans, design prostheses, and accomplish occlusal reconstruction.

### Competing interests

The authors have declare that they have no competing interests.

### Authors' contributions

TN, YS, KI, TI and SN were compiled and aggregate of the questionnaire. YH and TS conceived of the study and participated in its design and coordination and helped to draft the manuscript. All authors read and approved the final manuscript.

### Acknowledgements

This paper was partially supported by a Grant-in-Aid for Scientific Research (C) (No. 24592935) from the Japan Society for the Promotion of Science.

### Author details

[1]Implant Dentistry, Nihon University School of Dentistry, Dental Hospital, 1-8-13 Kandasurugadai, Chiyoda-ku, Tokyo 101-8310, Japan. [2]Department of Dental Specialties, Mayo Clinic, Mayo Clinic, 200 First Street SW, Rochester, MINN 55905, USA.

### References

1. Att W, Stappert C. Implant therapy to improve quality of life. Quintessence Int. 2003;34:573–81.
2. Papaspyridakos P, Chen CJ, Singh M, Weber HP, Gallucci GO. Success criteria in implant dentistry: a systematic review. J Dent Res. 2012;91:242–8.
3. Shumaker ND, Metcalf BT, Toscano NT, Holtzclaw DJ. Periodontal and periimplant maintenance: a critical factor in long-term treatment success. Compend Contin Educ Dent. 2009;30:388–90.
4. Abduo J, Bennani V, Waddell N, Lyons K, Swain M. Assessing the fit of implant fixed prostheses: a critical review. Int J Oral Maxillofac Implants. 2010;25:506–15.
5. Weber HP, Sukotjo C. Does the type of implant prosthesis affect outcomes in the partially edentulous patient? Int J Oral Maxillofac Implants. 2007;22:140–72.
6. Monteiro DR, Goiato MC, Gennari Filho H, Pesqueira AA. Passivity in implant-supported prosthesis. J Craniofac Surg. 2010;21:2026–9.
7. Chaar MS, Att W, Strub JR. Prosthetic outcome of cement-retained implant-supported fixed dental restorations: a systematic review. J Oral Rehabil. 2011;38:697–711.
8. Klineberg IJ, Trulsson M, Murray GM. Occlusion on implants - is there a problem? J Oral Rehabil. 2012. doi:10.1111/j.1365-2842.2012.02305.x
9. Taylor TD, Wiens J, Carr AB. Evidence-based considerations for removable prosthodontic and dental implant occlusion: a literature review. J Prosthet Dent. 2005;94:555–60.
10. Levine RA, Nack G. Team treatment planning for the replacement of esthetic zone teeth with dental implants. Compend Contin Educ Dent. 2011;32:44–50.
11. Elian N, Ehrlich B, Jalbout Z, Cho SC, Froum S, Tarnow D. A restoratively driven ridge categorization, as determined by incorporating ideal restorative positions on radiographic templates utilizing computed tomography scan analysis. Clin Implant Dent Relat Res. 2009;11:272–8.
12. Bartlett D. Implants for life? A critical review of implant-supported restorations. J Dent. 2007;35:768–72.
13. Patel PM, Lynch CD, Sloan AJ, Gilmour AS. Treatment planning for replacing missing teeth in UK general dental practice: current trends. J Oral Rehabil. 2010;37:509–17.
14. Lang-Hua BH, Lang NP, Lo EC, McGrath CP. Attitudes of general dental practitioners towards implant dentistry in an environment with widespread provision of implant therapy. Clin Oral Implants Res. 2012. doi:10.1111/j.1600-0501.2012.02537.x. [Epub ahead of print].
15. Gatten DL, Riedy CA, Hong SK, Johnson JD, Cohenca N. Quality of life of endodontically treated versus implant treated patients: a University-based qualitative research study. J Endocrinol. 2011;37:903–9.
16. Johannsen A, Wikesjö U, Tellefsen G, Johannsen G. Patient attitudes and expectations of dental implant treatment—a questionnaire study. Swed Dent J. 2012;36:7–14.
17. Pavel K, Seydlova M, Dostalova T, Zdenek V, Chleborad K, Jana Z, et al. Dental implants and improvement of oral health-related quality of life. Community Dent Oral Epidemiol. 2012;40 Suppl 1:65–70. doi:10.1111/j.1600-0528.2011.00668.x.
18. Mattheos N, Collier S, Walmsley AD. Specialists' management decisions and attitudes towards mucositis and peri-implantitis. Br Dent J. 2012;212(1):E1. doi:10.1038/sj.bdj.2012.1.
19. Vasak C, Fiederer R, Watzek G. Current state of training for implant dentistry in Europe: a questionnaire-based survey. Clin Oral Implants Res. 2007;18:668.
20. De Bruyn H, Koole S, Mattheos N, Lang NP. A survey on undergraduate implant dentistry education in Europe. Eur J Dent Educ. 2009;13:3–9.
21. Afsharzand Z, Rashedi B, Petropoulos VC. Dentist communication with the dental laboratory for prosthodontic treatment using implants. J Prosthodont. 2006;15:202–7.
22. Lang M. Professional cooperation between dentist and laboratory technician. Implant Dent. 1999;8:25–8.
23. Raigrodski AJ, Hillstead M, Meng GK, Chung KH. Survival and complications of zirconia-based fixed dental prostheses: a systematic review. J Prosthet Dent. 2012;107:170–7.
24. Papaspyridakos P, Chen CJ, Chuang SK, Weber HP, Gallucci GO. A systematic review of biologic and technical complications with fixed implant rehabilitations for edentulous patients. Int J Oral Maxillofac Implants. 2012;27:102–10.
25. Goodacre CJ, Bernal G, Rungcharassaeng K, Kan JY. Clinical complications with implants and implant prostheses. J Prosthet Dent. 2003;90:121–32.
26. Jung RE, Pjetursson BE, Glause R, Zembic A, Zwahlen M, Lang NP. A systematic review of the 5-year survival and complication rates of implant-supported single crowns. Clin Oral Implants Res. 2008;19:119–30.
27. Vere J, Bhakta S, Patel R. Prosthodontic complications associated with implant retained crowns and bridgework: a review of the literature. Br Dent J. 2012;212:267–72.
28. Andreiotelli M, Att W, Strub JR. Prosthodontic complications with implant overdentures: a systematic literature review. Int J Prosthodont. 2010;3:195–203.
29. Cehreli MC, Karasoy D, Kokat AM, Akca K, Eckert SE. Systematic review of prosthetic maintenance requirements for implant-supported overdentures. Int J Oral Maxillofac Implants. 2010;25:163–80.
30. Hatzikyriakos A, Petridis HP, Tsiggos N, Sakelariou S. Considerations for services from dental technicians in fabrication of fixed prostheses: a survey of commercial dental laboratories in Thessaloniki, Greece. J Prosthet Dent. 2006;96:362–6.
31. Afsharzand Z, Rashedi B, Petropoulos VC. Communication between the dental laboratory technician and dentist: Work authorization for fixed partial dentures. J Prosthodont. 2006;15:123–8.
32. Kawazoe T. Introduction of Japanese Society of Oral Implantology. Int J Oral Sci. 2009;1:13–5.

33. Boynton PM, Greenhalgh T. Selecting designing, and developing your questionnaire. Br Med J. 2004;328:1312–5.
34. Boynton PM. Administering, analyzing, and reporting your questionnaire. Br Med J. 2004;328:1372–5.
35. Bower EJ, Newton PD, Gibbons DE, Newton JT. A national survey of dental technicians: Career development, professional status and job satisfaction. Br Dent J. 2004;197:144–8.
36. Nissan J, Narobai D, Gross O, Ghelfan O, Chaushu G. Long-term outcome of cemented versus screw-retained implant-supported partial restorations. Int J Oral Maxillofac Implants. 2011;26:1102–7.
37. Salvi GE, Brägger U. Mechanical and technical risks in implant therapy. Int J Oral Maxillofac Implants. 2009;24(Suppl):69–85.
38. Michalakis KX, Hirayama H, Garefis PD. Cement-retained versus screw-retained implant restorations: a critical review. Int J Oral Maxillofac Implants. 2003;18:719–28.
39. Conserva E, Menini M, Tealdo T, Bevilacqua M, Ravera G, Pera F, et al. The use of a masticatory robot to analyze the shock absorption capacity of different restorative materials for prosthetic implants: a preliminary report. Int J Prosthodont. 2009;22:53–5.
40. Sahin S, Cehreli MC, Yalçin E. The influence of functional forces on the biomechanics of implant-supported prostheses—a review. J Dent. 2002;30:271–82.
41. Augstin-Panadero R, Fons-Font A, Roman-Rodriguez JL, Granell-Ruiz M, Del Rio-Highsmith J, Sola-Ruiz MF. Zirconia versus metal: a preliminary comparative analysis of ceramic veneer behavior. Int J Prosthodont. 2012;25:294–300.
42. Larsson C. Vult von Steyern P. Five-year follow-up of implant-supported Y-TZP and ZTA fixed dental prostheses. A randomized, prospective clinical trial comparing two different material systems. Int J Prosthodont. 2010;23:555–61.
43. Gonda T, Maeda Y. Why are magnetic attachments popular in japan and other asian countries? Jpn Dental Sci Rev. 2011;47:124–30.
44. Carlsson GE, Kronström M, de Baat C, Cune M, Davis D, Garefis P, et al. A survey of the use of mandibular implant overdentures in 10 countries. Int J Prosthodont. 2004;17:211–7.
45. Pjetursson BE, Lang NP. Prosthetic treatment planning on the basis of scientific evidence. J Oral Rehabil. 2008;35:72–9.
46. Kreissl ME, Gerds T, Muche R, Heydecke G, Strub JR. Technical complications of implant-supported fixed partial dentures in partially edentulous cases after an average observation period of 5 years. Clin Oral Implants Res. 2007;18:720–6.
47. Drummond JL. Degradation, fatigue, and failure of resin dental composite materials. J Dent Res. 2008;87:710–9.
48. Geminiani A, Lee H, Feng C, Ercoli C. The influence of incisal veneering porcelain thickness of two metal ceramic crown systems on failure resistance after cyclic loading. J Prosthet Dent. 2010;103:275–382.
49. Schmitter M, Mueller D, Rues S. Chipping behaviour of all-ceramic crowns with zirconia framework and CAD/CAM manufactured veneer. J Dent. 2012;40:154–62.
50. Lorenzoni FC, Martins LM, Silva NR, Coelho PG, Guess PC, Bonfante EA, et al. Fatigue life and failure modes of crowns systems with a modified framework design. J Dent. 2010;38:626–34.

# 3

# Inter- and intraobserver reproducibility of buccal bone measurements at dental implants with cone beam computed tomography in the esthetic region

Kirsten W Slagter[1], Gerry M Raghoebar[1], Arjan Vissink[1] and Henny J A Meijer[1,2*]

**Abstract**

**Background:** Sufficient buccal bone is important for optimal esthetic results of implant treatment in the anterior region. It can be measured with cone beam computed tomography (CBCT), but background scattering and problems with standardization of the measurements are encountered. The aim was to develop a method for reliable, reproducible measurements on CBCTs.

**Methods:** Using a new method, buccal bone thickness was measured on ten CBCTs at six positions along the implant axis. Inter- and intraobserver reproducibility was assessed by repeated measurements by two examiners.

**Results:** Mean buccal bone thickness measured by observers 1 and 2 was 2.42 mm (sd: 0.50) and 2.41 mm (sd: 0.47), respectively. Interobserver intraclass correlation coefficient was 0.96 (95% CI 0.93 to 0.98). The mean buccal bone thickness of the first measurement and the second measurement of observer 1 was 2.42 mm (sd: 0.50) and 2.53 mm (sd: 0.49), respectively, with an intraobserver intraclass correlation coefficient of 0.93 (95% CI 0.88 to 0.96). The mean buccal bone thickness of the first measurement and the second measurement of observer 2 was 2.41 mm (sd: 0.47) and 2.52 mm (sd: 0.47), respectively, with an intraobserver intraclass correlation coefficient of 0.96 (95% CI 0.93 to 0.97).

**Conclusions:** Applying the methods used in this study, CBCTs are suitable for reliable and reproducible measurements of buccal bone thickness at implants.

**Keywords:** Dental implants; Esthetic region; CBCT; Bone thickness

## Background

Single-tooth implant placement in the esthetic zone is a highly reliable treatment option for replacing a failing tooth [1-4]. Yet, research interest has shifted from implant survival towards optimal preservation of soft and hard tissues [5-7]. Especially in the esthetic region, buccal bone and its preservation is one of the key factors in esthetic outcome [8].

Computerized tomography (CT) scans and cone beam CTs (CBCTs) are commonly used for presurgical planning and to predict bone density and potential stability of dental implants [9]. Next to this, CTs and CBCTs also allow for measuring bone at dental implants during follow-up [10,11]. The quality and accuracy of a three-dimensional (3D) model derived from a (CB)CT is dependent on scanner-related factors such as type of scanner, field of view (FoV), artifacts, and voxel size [12]. In addition, patient-related factors such as patient position and metal artifacts [13] and operator-related factors such as the segmentation process or interpretation of the (CB) CT are of influence [14]. It has been reported that buccal bone thickness at implant sites can be measured with

* Correspondence: h.j.a.meijer@umcg.nl
[1]Department of Oral and Maxillofacial Surgery, University of Groningen, University Medical Center Groningen, PO Box 30.001, 9700RB Groningen, The Netherlands
[2]Department of Fixed and Removable Prosthodontics, University of Groningen, University Medical Center Groningen, PO Box 30.001, 9700RB Groningen, The Netherlands

CBCT, but background scattering and problems with standardization of the measurements are frequently encountered [15]. In view of the aforementioned factors, there is need for a reliable, reproducible method to facilitate measurements. The use of 3D image diagnostic and treatment planning software programs in combination with software programs for tracking and registration of the exact position of existing dental implants in radiographs can be of help [16].

The aim of the current study was to develop a reproducible method based on 3D image diagnostic and treatment planning software programs for buccal bone measurements at implants on CBCTs.

## Methods

Ten patients with a dental implant in the esthetic zone (regions 13 to 23) were included (Figures 1 and 2). Research was carried out in compliance with the Helsinki Declaration. Patients were part of a randomized controlled trial on esthetics; the study was approved by the Medical Ethic Board of the University Medical Center Groningen, University of Groningen (METC 2010.246) as well as that written informed consent was obtained from all patients. The CBCT scans were made with an iCAT 3D exam scanner (KaVo Dental GmbH, Biberach, Germany), which scanner was validated for measuring bone thickness by Fourie et al. [17]. The method error of this scanner is very small, i.e., 0.05 mm (95% CI 0.03 to 0.07). The standard used voxel size was 0.30 and FoV was 100 × 100 mm on the CBCT scans. Bone measurements at implants on the CBCT scans was done using 3D image diagnostic and treatment planning software (NobelClinician, version 2.1 (Nobel Biocare - Guided Surgery Center, Mechelen, Belgium). A novelty is that this program, regularly used preoperatively, was employed to measure the buccal bone thickness (in mm), after implant surgery. To allow for reproducible measurements, a CBCT imaging and software protocol was developed.

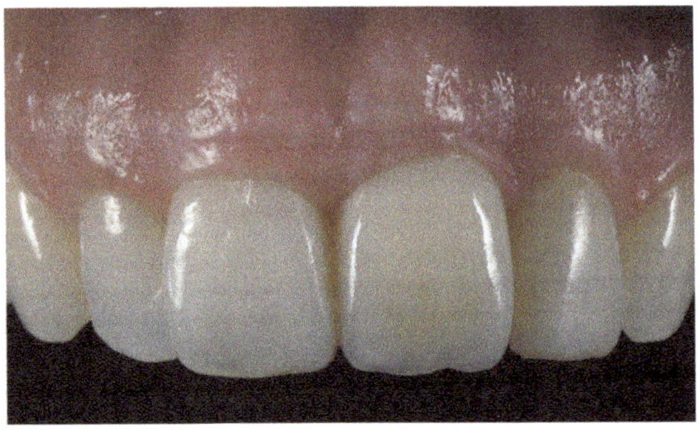

**Figure 1** Clinical photograph of implant-supported restoration at position 21.

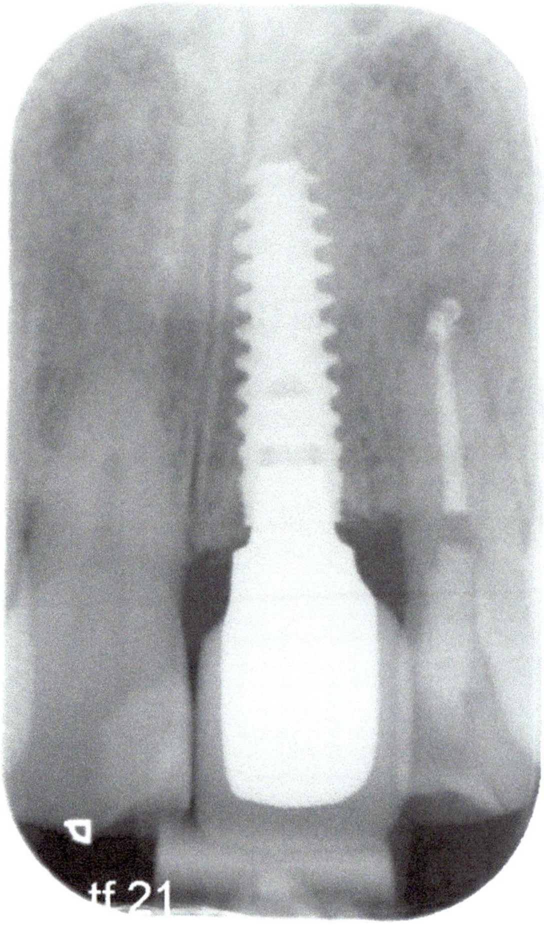

**Figure 2** Conventional intra-oral radiograph of same patient with implant-supported restoration at position 21.

### CBCT imaging and software protocol

Acquired CBCT Digital Imaging and Communications in Medicine (DICOM) datasets were transferred to a computer. The CBCT images were exported in DICOM multi-file format and imported into Maxilim, version 2.3 (Medicim, Sint-Niklass, Belgium). Maxilim is a medical image computing program assessing the patients head anatomy and is used for diagnostics and preoperative planning of maxillofacial surgery. The input information for Maxilim is a 3D dataset, often (CB)CT data. The DICOM files of all patients were set continuously on Hounsfield unit (HU) isovalue 280. The implant used was set on HU isovalue 130. With Multimodality Image Registration using Information Theory (MIRIT), which has an accuracy of a subvoxel, the exact position of the implant could be recognized, determined and implemented in the patients DICOM files [16]. The MIRIT procedure is based on recognizing image similarities. The degree of similarity between intensity patterns in two images is determined, and consequently, the recognized image is registered automatically into one coordinate system. Image similarities are broadly used in medical imaging to enhance diagnostics. In the software program NobelClinician, the patients DICOM files were opened with the same HU isovalue of 280. An extra research tool was added to this software program by the program makers, so that the DICOM file from Maxilim was recognized by this program and the exact position of the implant, as determined in Maxilim, could be aligned with a planning implant in NobelClinician. Due to the alignment of a planning implant (with a known configuration) and an actual inserted implant into one image, measurements could take place at the exact buccal midline of the implant (Figure 3). The display of the implant and surrounding structures was set on bone value, so that the outline of the bony structures could be seen and measured. The buccal bone measurements at midline of the implant were performed with the standard provided measurement tools in the software program of NobelClinician.

### Measuring procedure

The implant and patient dataset were exactly aligned by the MIRIT method, so that the distance from the central axis of the implant to the outer contour of the buccal bone could be measured. Area of interest was the upper 5 mm section of the implant, beginning at the neck of the implant towards the apical direction. Exact dimensions along the implant axis of each implant configuration used in the study were provided by the manufacturer. Buccal bone measurements (in mm) were performed calculating the distance to the buccal bone outline minus the radius of the interior contour of the implant. These buccal bone measurements were done for 5 mm at each millimeter along the axis, beginning at the neck of the implant (Figure 4). Measurements were repeated twice (with time interval to prevent recollection) by two independent operators (HJAM and KWS, both dentists) in a random order. Flow diagram of the consecutive steps has been depicted in Figure 5.

### Statistical analysis

Continuous variables were expressed as a mean with standard deviation. Interobserver and intraobserver variability was assessed using two-way mixed intraclass correlation coefficient single measures analysis [18]. All analyses were performed using SPSS software (version 20.0).

## Results

The mean buccal bone thickness measured by observers 1 and 2 was 2.42 mm (sd: 0.50) and 2.41 mm (sd: 0.47), respectively. Interobserver intraclass correlation coefficient was 0.96 (95% CI 0.93 to 0.98). The mean buccal bone thickness of the first measurement and the second measurement of observer 1 was 2.42 mm (sd: 0.50) and 2.53 mm (sd: 0.49), respectively, with an intraobserver intraclass correlation coefficient of 0.93 (95% CI 0.88 to 0.96). The mean buccal bone thickness of the first measurement and the second measurement of observer two was 2.41 mm (sd: 0.47) and 2.52 mm (sd: 0.47), respectively, with an intraobserver intraclass correlation coefficient of 0.96 (95% CI 0.93 to 0.97).

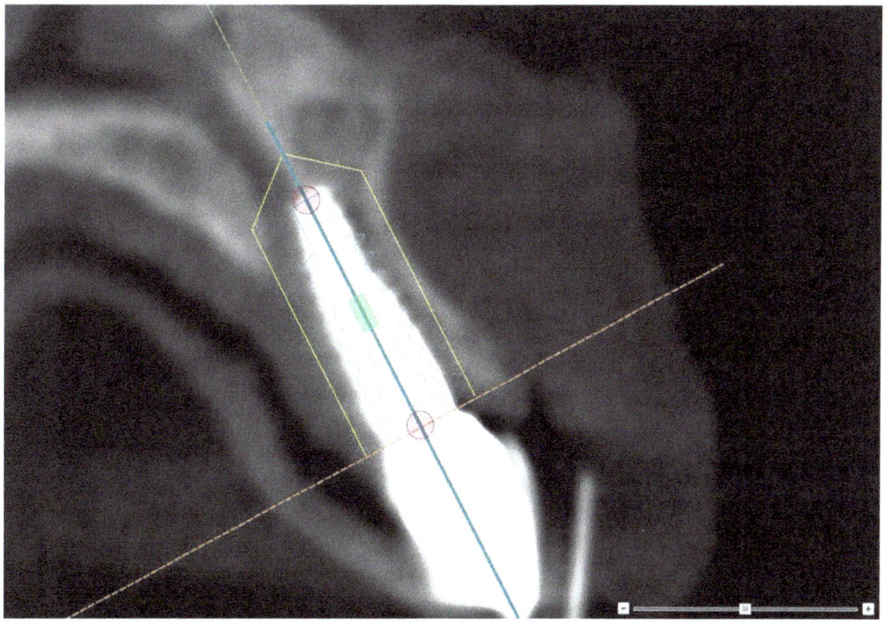

**Figure 3 Implant position.** Due to the alienation of the patients' DICOM files by MIRIT, the exact position of the implant was defined. As such, the measurements could take place in the exact correct buccal direction.

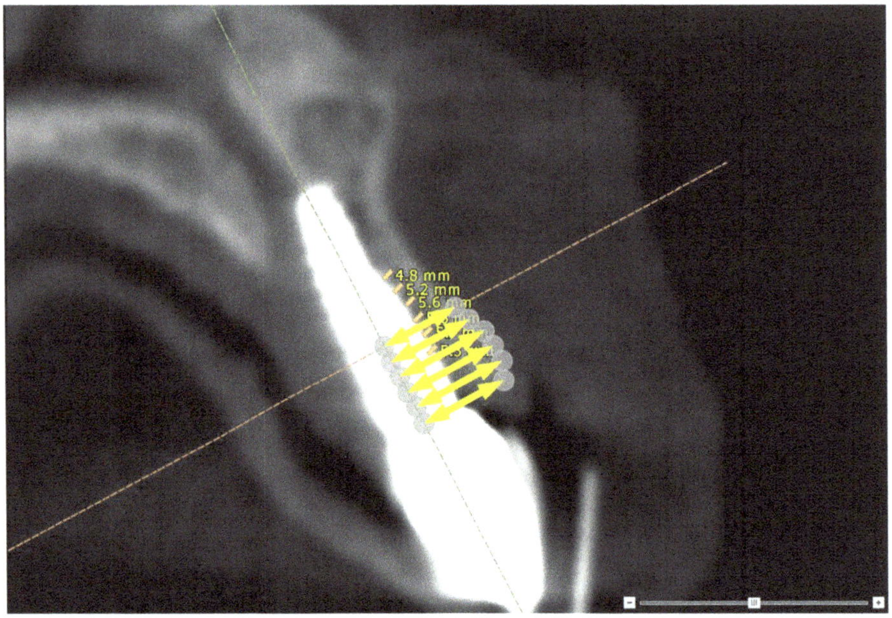


**Figure 4 Implant measurements.** Measurements were performed at each millimeter along the axis of the implant for 5 mm, beginning at the neck of the implant.

## Discussion

Intraobserver and interobserver agreement was very high with measurements on CBCTs of bone buccally of dental implants. Apparently, the method is clear and measurements can be performed reproducibly. Moreover, measurements are not observer dependent, meaning that results of different observers in different studies can be compared with each other.

In previous studies, buccal bone thickness was also measured, but the exact position of these measurements at the

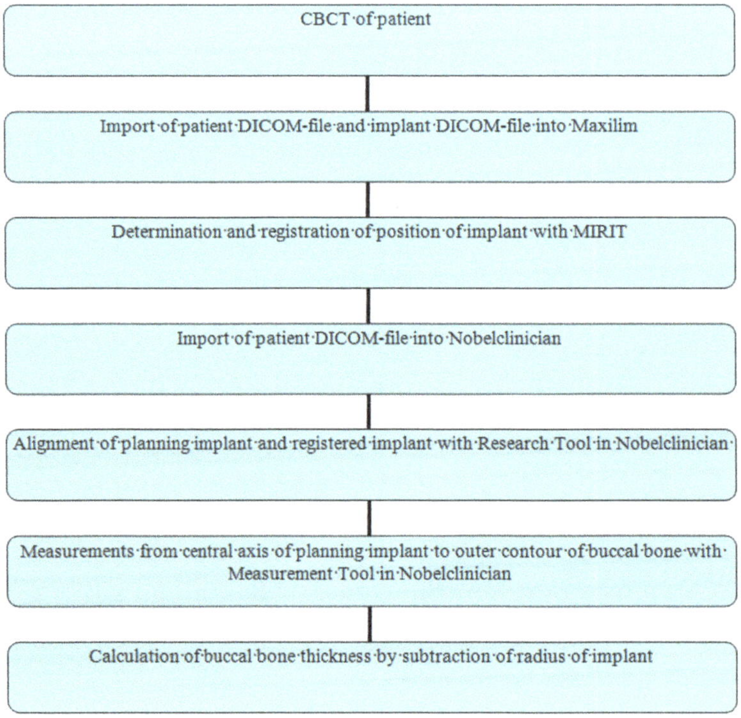


**Figure 5 Flow diagram of CBCT imaging and measurements to calculate bone thickness buccally of implants.**

surface of the implant was not determined by 3D image-based diagnostic and treatment planning software programs [10,11,15]. It is important to perform measurements of bone thickness at the same position at implants to make comparison in time possible. Because of the cylindrical contour of the implant, thickness of bone can vary considerably in the mesio-distal direction. The combination of the software programs MIRIT (for determination and registration of the implant position in Maxilim) and Research Tool in NobelClinician (for alignment of planning implant and registered implant) makes the method reproducible.

Scattering of the titanium dental implant makes it difficult to perform measurements from the bone-to-implant boundary to the buccal outer contour of the bone [19]. The combination of Research Tool in NobelClinician (exact positioning of the planning implant) and Measurement Tool in NobelClinician (for measurements from central axis of the implant) makes it possible to bypass the scattering area. Measurements are corrected by subtraction of the known radius of implant, resulting in the actual thickness of bone.

Measurements are not directly possible in NobelClinician, because the image-recognizing program MIRIT can only be executed in the configuration of Maxilim. It would be desirable if the total procedure could be carried in one program, being NobelClinician.

## Conclusions

When applying 3D image-based software programs according to the set-up used in this study, CBCTs are suitable for reliable and reproducible measurements of buccal bone thickness at implants.

#### Abbreviations

3D: three-dimensional; CBCT: cone beam computed tomography; CT: computerized tomography; DICOM: Digital Imaging and Communications in Medicine; FoV: field of view; HU: Hounsfield unit; MIRIT: Multimodality Image Registration using Information Theory.

#### Competing interests

Kirsten W. Slagter, Gerry M. Raghoebar, Arjan Vissink, Henny JA. Meijer declare that they have no competing interests.

#### Authors' contributions

KWS, GMR, AV, and HJAM provided substantial contributions to the conception or design of the work, or the acquisition, analysis, or interpretation of data for the work; drafted the paper or revised it critically; gave final approval of the version to be published; and agreed to be accountable for all aspects of the work in ensuring that questions related to accuracy or integrity of any parts of the work are appropriately investigated and resolved. All authors read and approved the final manuscript.

#### References


1. Den Hartog L, Slater JJ, Vissink A, Meijer HJ, Raghoebar GM. Treatment outcome of immediate, early and conventional single-tooth implants in the aesthetic zone: a systematic review to survival, bone level, soft-tissue, aesthetics and patient satisfaction. J Clin Periodontol. 2008;35:1073–86.
2. De Rouck T, Collys K, Cosyn J. Single-tooth replacement in the anterior maxilla by means of immediate implantation and provisionalization: a review. Int J Oral Maxillofac Implants. 2008;23:897–904.
3. Esposito M, Grusovin MG, Polyzos IP, Felice P, Worthington HV. Timing of implant placement after tooth extraction: immediate, immediate-delayed or delayed implants? A Cochrane systematic review. Eur J Oral Implantol. 2010;3:189–205.
4. Jung RE, Zembic A, Pjetursson BE, Zwahlen M, Thoma DS. Systematic review of the survival rate and the incidence of biological, technical, and aesthetic complications of single crowns on implants reported in longitudinal studies with a mean follow-up of 5 years. Clin Oral Implants Res. 2012;23 Suppl 6:2–21.
5. Hammerle CH, Araujo MG, Simion M, Osteology Consensus Group 2011. Evidence-based knowledge on the biology and treatment of extraction sockets. Clin Oral Implants Res. 2012;23 Suppl 5:80–2.
6. Botticelli D, Berglundh T, Lindhe J. Hard-tissue alterations following immediate implant placement in extraction sites. J Clin Periodontol. 2004;31:820–8.
7. Jemt T. Regeneration of gingival papillae after single-implant treatment. Int J Periodontics Restorative Dent. 1997;17:326–33.
8. Meijer HJ, Stellingsma K, Meijndert L, Raghoebar GM. A new index for rating aesthetics of implant-supported single crowns and adjacent soft tissues–the implant crown aesthetic index. Clin Oral Implants Res. 2005;16:645–9.
9. Sennerby L, Andersson P, Pagliani L, Giani C, Moretti G, Molinari M, et al. Evaluation of a novel cone beam computed tomography scanner for bone density examinations in preoperative 3D reconstructions and correlation with primary implant stability. Clin Implant Dent Relat Res. 2013. doi:10.1111/cid.12193.
10. Kan JY, Roe P, Rungcharassaeng K, Patel RD, Waki T, Lozada JL, et al. Classification of sagittal root position in relation to the anterior maxillary osseous housing for immediate implant placement: a cone beam computed tomography study. Int J Oral Maxillofac Implants. 2011;26:873–6.
11. Miyamoto Y, Obama T. Dental cone beam computed tomography analyses of postoperative labial bone thickness in maxillary anterior implants: comparing immediate and delayed implant placement. Int J Periodontics Restorative Dent. 2011;31:215–25.
12. Kamburoglu K, Murat S, Kilic C, Yuksel S, Avsever H, Farman A, et al. Accuracy of CBCT images in the assessment of buccal marginal alveolar peri-implant defects: effect of field of view. Dentomaxillofac Radiol. 2014;43:20130332.
13. Ritter L, Mischkowski RA, Neugebauer J, Dreiseidler T, Scheer M, Keeve E, et al. The influence of body mass index, age, implants, and dental restorations on image quality of cone beam computed tomography. Oral Surg Oral Med Oral Pathol Oral Radiol Endod. 2009;108:e108–16.
14. Besimo CE, Lambrecht JT, Guindy JS. Accuracy of implant treatment planning utilizing template-guided reformatted computed tomography. Dentomaxillofac Radiol. 2000;29:46–51.
15. Roe P, Kan JY, Rungcharassaeng K, Caruso JM, Zimmerman G, Mesquida J. Horizontal and vertical dimensional changes of peri-implant facial bone following immediate placement and provisionalization of maxillary anterior single implants: a 1-year cone beam computed tomography study. Int J Oral Maxillofac Implants. 2012;27:393–400.
16. Maes F, Collignon A, Vandermeulen D, Marchal G, Suetens P. Multimodality image registration by maximization of mutual information. IEEE Trans Med Imaging. 1997;16:187–98.
17. Fourie Z, Damstra J, Schepers RH, Gerrits PO, Ren Y. Segmentation process significantly influences the accuracy of 3D surface models derived from cone beam computed tomography. Eur J Radiol. 2012;81:e524–30.
18. Shrout PE, Fleiss JL. Intraclass correlations: uses in assessing rater reliability. Psychol Bull. 1979;86:420–8.
19. Parsa A, Ibrahim N, Hassan B, Syriopoulos K, van der Stelt P. Assessment of metal artefact reduction around dental titanium implants in cone beam CT. Dentomaxillofac Radiol. 2014;43:20140019.

# 4

# Efficacy of intravenous sedation and oral nifedipine in dental implant patients with preoperative hypertension - a retrospective study of 516 cases

Motoshi Kimura[1*], Yoshihiro Takasugi[2], Shigeyoshi Hanano[1], Katsuyuki Terabe[3] and Yuko Kimura[4]

**Abstract**

**Background:** To examine the effects of intravenous sedation and oral nifedipine on blood pressure and pulse rate in patients with perioperative high blood pressure undergoing implant surgery, the clinical records of dental implant patients managed by intravenous sedation at our outpatient dental offices were retrospectively evaluated.

**Methods:** A total of 516 clinical charts were evaluated. The subjects were divided into two groups: a normotensive group with no history of hypertension and a hypertensive group with a history of hypertension. The patients in the hypertensive group were further divided into two subgroups: with or without nifedipine administration before operation. Systolic blood pressure (SBP), diastolic blood pressure (DBP), pulse rate (PR), and rate pressure product (RPP) were assessed.

**Results:** In 30 patients (33%) of the hypertensive group, the high blood pressure on arrival obviously declined to around or less than 160 mmHg; in the remaining patients in the group who showed a mean SBP of 182.1 ± 13.8 mmHg on arrival, the blood pressure did not decrease after a 30-min rest. Oral nifedipine administered to the patients with sustained high blood pressure decreased SBP to 144.7 ± 23.1 mmHg in 28.1 ± 9.3 min after administration, comparable to that in hypertensive patients without nifedipine.

**Conclusions:** For patients with stage 2 hypertension before operation, it may be difficult to maintain the recommended blood pressure during surgery by only intravenous sedation; reduction of blood pressure by antihypertensive drugs may be necessary.

**Keywords:** Oral surgery; Dental implant; Hemodynamics; Intravenous sedation; Nifedipine administration

## Background

Osseointegrated dental implants were introduced in Japan in 1983, and the procedures are now performed very frequently. Dental implants are placed in a wide age range of patients, including elderly patients with hypertension. Patients with very high blood pressure are at great risk for acute medical problems when undergoing stressful dental procedures, such as oral surgery, periodontal surgery, and placement of dental implants [1].

Patients with normal blood pressure (<120/80 mmHg), prehypertension (120 to 139/80 to 89 mmHg), or stage I hypertension (140 to 159/90 to 99 mmHg) may receive regular dental care, but those with stage 2 hypertension (≥160/≥100 mmHg) should receive noninvasive treatment only and be referred to the physician for immediate follow-up [2]. Normotensive individuals may develop signs of hypertensive encephalopathy at blood pressures as low as 160/100 mmHg, whereas chronically hypertensive patients can tolerate higher blood pressure and may not do so until the blood pressure rises to 220/110 mmHg or above [3]. Although no recommendation has been presented on the optimal level of blood pressure to avoid hypertensive complications during invasive dental treatments, blood pressure in hypertensive patients should be maintained below 160/100 mmHg.

Pain, stress, or anxiety-related dental procedures can raise blood pressure in both hypertensive and normotensive

* Correspondence: kimkimkim0719@yahoo.co.jp
[1]Hanano Dental Clinic, 4-2-3 Yamanoue, Hirakata, Osaka 573-0047, Japan
Full list of author information is available at the end of the article

patients [4]. We have employed intravenous sedation to manage patients with hypertension as well as dental anxiety and phobia. The oral antihypertensive agent nifedipine is mainly administered to patients with high systolic blood pressure (SBP) ≥160 mmHg prior to implant placement. To examine the effects of intravenous sedation and oral nifedipine on blood pressure and pulse rate in patients with perioperative high blood pressure, the clinical records of dental implant patients managed by intravenous sedation at our outpatient dental offices were retrospectively evaluated. The purpose of this clinical study is to examine whether intravenous sedation and oral administration of nifedipine is efficient for the hemodynamic for the patient with hypertension. The authors expect that it is possible not only to obtain a hemodynamic blood stable but also to prevent the medical sequelae by performing intravenous sedation and oral nifedipine for patients with hypertension.

## Methods

A retrospective review of the clinical records was conducted for 336 patients who received dental implant-related surgeries combined with intravenous sedation between January 2008 and February 2012 at our outpatient dental offices. Among the patients, 125 patients received multiple surgeries during the observation period: 4 patients underwent surgery five times, 7 patients four times, 29 patients three times, 85 patients twice, and others once. The following surgical procedures were performed in a total of 516 patients: dental implant placement (466 patients), sinus lift surgery and dental implant (28 patients), socket lift and dental implant (10 patients), and guided bone regeneration and dental implant (12 patients).

We performed surgeries after medical consultation when patients had a history of hypertension or cardiovascular or cerebrovascular diseases. History of ischemic heart disease, renal dysfunction, diabetes mellitus, cerebral infarction, or articular rheumatism was documented in 17 patients in the hypertensive group and 16 patients in the normotensive group. They were confirmed stable and well controlled for implant surgery. For patients who received therapeutic drugs, surgery was performed following daily medication.

The patients were allowed to have water or snacks until 2 h before the visit. On arrival at the office, systolic blood pressure (SBP), diastolic blood pressure (DBP), and pulse rate (PR) were measured using an automatic blood pressure monitor with an oscillometric method (HEM-1010, Omron Healthcare, Kyoto, Japan). The cephalic vein was cannulated with a 22-G disposable intravenous catheter. Nifedipine capsule (10 mg) was orally administered to patients with sustained increases in SBP ≥160 mmHg for 30 min from baseline measurement. A noninvasive blood pressure monitoring system with electrocardiogram (ECG) monitor and pulse oximeter (Moneo BP-88, Omron Healthcare, Kyoto, Japan) was mounted, and blood pressure was measured at 2- to 5-min intervals. In patients with a history of cardiovascular disease, ECG was continuously monitored. Following confirmation of a definite decline of blood pressure or SBP <160 mmHg, infiltration anesthesia and/or conduction anesthesia was administered using 1 to 3 cartridges (1.8 to 5.4 ml) of 2% lidocaine containing 1/80,000 epinephrine.

Following confirmation of a sufficient anesthetic effect, intravenous sedation with continuous infusion of propofol 1 to 2 mg/kg/h and midazolam 20 to 40 μg/kg bolus together with inhalation of oxygen 3 L/min via nasal cannula was initiated. After confirming Verrill sign, implant surgery was initiated. During operation, the propofol dose was adjusted to maintain the optimum conscious sedative condition (level 2 on the Ramsay sedation scale) [5], and local anesthesia was added when the patient complained of pain. On completion of surgery, administration of oxygen and propofol were terminated and the patient was observed for about 1 h, until normal cognitive and motor functions were restored.

The subjects were divided into two groups: a normotensive group with no history of hypertension and a hypertensive group with a history of hypertension. Thirteen patients who had no history of hypertension were included in the hypertensive group, since they indicated SBP ≥160 mmHg on arrival at the office and were later diagnosed with essential hypertension by cardiologists. Furthermore, the patients in the hypertensive group were divided into two subgroups: with or without nifedipine administration.

From the clinical chart, data of SBP, DBP, PR, and percutaneous oxygen saturation ($SpO_2$) were sampled at the point of arrival to the office, prior to the initiation of sedation, 30 min after the initiation of operation, and on completion of operation. Furthermore, rate pressure product (RPP: SBP × PR) was calculated.

There were two primary outcome measures: (1) incidence of improved hypertension following oral nifedipine and (2) incidence of normal ranges of hemodynamic parameters during surgery. The secondary outcome variable was incidence of hypertension related to perioperative complications.

### Statistical analysis

In this study, we used data from all cases (516 cases) for statistical analysis.

Data were described as mean ± standard deviation. The unpaired *t* test was used to compare demographic variables between groups. Fisher's exact test was used to compare ratios of patients in hypertensive group between subgroups. One-way analysis of variance (ANOVA) followed by Tukey's multiple comparison test was performed to examine the change in the values of parameters. Repeated measures

ANOVA followed by Dunnett's multiple comparison test was used to compare the values of parameters in groups at each time point. Statistical analysis was performed using Prism 5 for Windows Ver. 5.01 (GraphPad Software Inc., San Diego, CA, USA). The significance level was set at $p < 0.05$.

### Ethical approval

This study protocol was approved by the ethics committee of Japanese Dental Society of Anesthesiology (No. 2015–4).

## Results

Patient demographics and clinical characteristics are summarized in Table 1. There were significant differences in age ($p < 0.0001$) and duration of surgery ($p = 0.025$) between normotensive and hypertensive groups. On arrival at the office, values of all hemodynamic parameters, including SBP, DBP, PR, and RPP, were higher in the hypertensive group than in the normotensive group ($p < 0.0001$).

Tables 2 and 3 indicate incidences of patients with SBP ≥160 mmHg and RPP ≥12,000 bpm × mmHg, and perioperative hemodynamic changes, respectively. On arrival at the office, 66 patients (62%) in the hypertensive group and 41 patients (10%) in the normotensive group revealed high SBP ≥160 mmHg. Thirty minutes later, SBP declined to less than 160 mmHg in most of the patients in the normotensive group. On the other hand, in 30 patients (33%) in the hypertensive group, high blood pressure on arrival obviously declined to around or less than 160 mmHg, while in the remaining patients in the group who showed a mean SBP of 182.1 ± 13.8 mmHg on arrival, the blood pressure did not clearly decrease after 30 min of rest. Oral nifedipine administered to patients with sustained high blood pressure decreased SBP to 144.7 ± 23.1 mmHg by 28.1 ± 9.3 min after administration, which was similar to that in hypertensive patients without nifedipine.

Although the mean SBP in the hypertensive group was significantly higher than that in the normotensive group during operation, SBP <160 mmHg was maintained in all patients except three in the hypertensive group (2.8%) and one in the normotensive group (0.2%). The values of DBP in patients in the hypertensive group were higher than those in the normotensive group throughout the observation course, and changes in DBP in each group were similar to those in SBP.

On arrival at the office, RPP ≥12,000 bpm × mmHg was found in 74 patients (70%) in the hypertensive group and 111 patients (27%) in the normotensive group. More than 90% of the patients with preoperative nifedipine showed high RPP on arrival at the office. Among patients with high RPP, all patients in the normotensive group, 10% of the patients without nifedipine in the hypertensive group and 35% of patients with nifedipine in the hypertensive group had RPP <12,000 bpm × mmHg until initiation of intravenous sedation. The values of RPP during operation under intravenous sedation were maintained at a normal range except in nine patients (8.5%) in the hypertensive group and one patient (0.2%) in the normotensive group.

In patients with oral nifedipine in the hypertensive group, the PR value slightly increased prior to initiation of intravenous sedation ($p = 0.224$) and then significantly decreased until completion of the operation ($p < 0.001$).

All patients stated a pleasant feeling and amnesia during surgery. No complication occurred during surgery, and no cognitive and motor dysfunctions were observed 1 h after surgery. The patients revealed SBP of >160 mmHg during and at completion of operation showed maximum SBP of 180 mmHg in the normotensive group, 190 mmHg on the hypertensive group without preoperative oral nifedipine, and 180 mmHg in the hypertensive group with preoperative oral nifedipine. They did not complaint any symptom such as headache, confusion, and chest pain. Upon leaving

**Table 1 Demographic and clinical characteristics**

| | Normotensive group | Hypertensive group | *p* value |
|---|---|---|---|
| Number (male: female) | 410 (127: 283) | 106 (37: 69) | 0.170 |
| Age (year mean ± SD) | 59 ± 11 | 65 ± 10 | <0.0001 |
| Weight (kg) | 54.5 ± 9.2 | 57.1 ± 10.9 | 0.204 |
| Values of circulation parameters on arrival at office | | | |
| SBP (mmHg) | 133 ± 19 | 165 ± 22 | <0.0001 |
| DBP (mmHg) | 76 ± 13 | 99 ± 20 | <0.0001 |
| PR (bpm) | 79 ± 13 | 90 ± 19 | <0.0001 |
| RPP (bpm × mmHg) | 10,574 ± 2,614 | 12,367 ± 5,771 | <0.0001 |
| Preoperative oral nifedipine | 0 | 44 (42%) | <0.0001 |
| Duration of surgery (min) | 40 ± 20 | 35 ± 17 | 0.025 |
| Duration of sedation (min) | 69 ± 25 | 65 ± 22 | 0.114 |

SBP, systolic blood pressure; DBP, diastolic blood pressure; PR, pulse rate; RPP. rate pressure product.

**Table 2 Incidence of high blood pressure and high rate pressure product**

| | SBP (>160 mmHg) | RPP (>12,000 bpm × mmHg) |
|---|---|---|
| Normotensive group (*N* = 410) | | |
| On arrival at the office | 41 (10.0%) | 111 (27.1%) |
| Prior to sedation | 31 (7.6%) | 72 (17.6%) |
| During operation | 1 (0.2%) | 1 (0.2%) |
| Completion of operation | 3 (0.7%) | 9 (2.2%) |
| Hypertensive group without preoperative oral nifedipine (*N* = 62) | | |
| On arrival at the office | 22 (35.5%)** | 34 (54.8%)** |
| Prior to sedation | 13 (21.0%)** | 27 (43.5%)** |
| During operation | 2 (3.2%)* | 5 (8.1%)** |
| Completion of operation | 5 (8.1%)** | 6 (9.7%)** |
| Hypertensive group with preoperative oral nifedipine (*N* = 44) | | |
| On arrival at the office | 44 (100%)** | 40 (90.9%)** |
| Prior to sedation | 8 (18.2%)* | 24 (54.5%)** |
| During operation | 1 (2.2%) | 4 (9.1%)** |
| Completion of operation | 3 (6.8%)* | 8 (18.2%)** |

*$p$ <0.05, **$p$ <0.01 vs normotensive group (Fisher's exact test). SBP, systolic blood pressure; RPP, rate pressure product.

the office, high SBP of the patients decreased to the level on arrival without any antihypertensive treatment.

## Discussion

In 44 (8.5%) of the 516 implant surgery cases, oral nifedipine had to be administered, since preoperative SBP was higher than 160 mmHg in these patients. Within 30 min of administration of nifedipine, SBP of hypertensive patients decreased to a similar range as that of hypertensive patients who did not need administration of oral nifedipine. Intravenous sedation after nifedipine administration to hypertensive patients resulted in stable hemodynamics during implant surgery.

The Seventh Report of the Joint National Committee on Prevention, Detection, Evaluation, and Treatment of High Blood Pressure [6] classified hypertensive patients into five categories based on systolic or diastolic blood pressure. Patients with normal blood pressure (<120/80 mmHg), prehypertension (120 to 139/80 to 89 mmHg), or stage I hypertension (140 to 159/90 to 99 mmHg) can receive

**Table 3 Changes in values of hemodynamic parameters**

| | SBP (mmHg) | DBP (mmHg) | PR (bpm) | RPP (bpm × mmHg) |
|---|---|---|---|---|
| Normotensive patients (*N* = 410) | | | | |
| On arrival at the office | 133.0 ± 18.4 | 76.4 ± 12.5 | 79.2 ± 13.4 | 10,603 ± 2,623 |
| Prior to sedation | 128.5 ± 18.3* | 70.5 ± 11.9* | 76.8 ± 13.0* | 9,927 ± 2,485* |
| During operation | 109.7 ± 11.9* | 62.7 ± 10.0* | 70.6 ± 10.2* | 7,768 ± 1,555* |
| Completion of operation | 115.9 ± 14.2* | 66.1 ± 11.3* | 70.4 ± 10.7* | 8,196 ± 1,796* |
| Hypertensive patients without preoperative oral nifedipine (*N* = 62) | | | | |
| On arrival at the office | 152.5 ± 17.6 | 88.3 ± 11.8 | 84.6 ± 14.3 | 12,972 ± 3,055 |
| Prior to sedation | 143.2 ± 18.1* | 77.4 ± 9.6* | 82.7 ± 13.4 | 11,874 ± 2,540* |
| During operation | 118.9 ± 15.5* | 67.2 ± 10.0* | 75.2 ± 12.8* | 8,977 ± 2,164* |
| Completion of operation | 125.4 ± 19.1* | 68.8 ± 12.6* | 74.7 ± 10.9* | 9,360 ± 1,977* |
| Hypertensive patients with preoperative oral nifedipine (*N* = 44) | | | | |
| On arrival at the office | 182.1 ± 13.8 | 102.8 ± 12.5 | 87.2 ± 17.1 | 15,901 ± 3,623 |
| Prior to sedation | 144.7 ± 23.1* | 77.3 ± 15.9* | 89.3 ± 16.1 | 12,986 ± 3,437* |
| During operation | 119.8 ± 16.5* | 65.8 ± 10.0* | 78.0 ± 12.3* | 9,413 ± 2,265* |
| Completion of operation | 130.1 ± 18.8* | 71.4 ± 13.2* | 78.4 ± 13.6* | 10,294 ± 2,728* |

*$p$ <0.01 vs value on arrival at the office (Dunnett's multiple comparison test). SBP, systolic blood pressure; DBP, diastolic blood pressure; PR, pulse rate; RPP, rate pressure product.

regular dental care, though a stress reduction protocol is necessary for stage I hypertension [2,7]. In accordance with the guidelines during oral surgery, the blood pressure of hypertensive patients should be maintained at a normal or prehypertension level. RPP is a reliable predictor of myocardial oxygen consumption [8], and RPP >12,000 bpm × mmHg is associated with myocardial ischemia [9,10]. In this study, although blood pressure was managed by a physician, hypertensive patients showed SBP >160 mmHg when they visited the dental office for dental implant surgery, and 50% of hypertensive patients showed high RPP after 30 min of rest. In patients presenting with high blood pressure and high RPP, anxiety and fear must be reduced by conscious sedation and antihypertensives to prevent cardiovascular complications during dental implant surgery.

Increases in SBP due to psychological stress are proportional to age and baseline blood pressure [4]. Intravenous sedation stabilizes measurable changes in blood pressure and pulse rate due to fear and anxiety about dental treatment and has been used to manage patients with ischemic heart disease and hypertension [11]. In this study, the effect of intravenous sedation was as follows: SBP and RPP, compared with those prior to intravenous sedation, were decreased by 15% and 20% in patients with normal blood pressure, 15% and 25% in hypertensive patients without oral nifedipine, and 15% to 20% and 20% to 30% in hypertensive patients with administered nifedipine, respectively. That is, SBP and myocardial oxygen consumption of prehypertension and stage I hypertension can be reduced to the levels recommended for dental treatment before surgery by intravenous sedation.

For patients with stage 2 hypertension before operation, it is difficult to maintain the recommended blood pressure during surgery using only intravenous sedation, and it is necessary to decrease blood pressure by antihypertensive drugs. In this study, the blood pressure of patients with sustained hypertension was reduced to stage I hypertension about 30 min after administration of oral nifedipine. On the other hand, the decrease in RPP after oral nifedipine administration was not less than 12,000 bpm × mmHg, which could be due to the fact that an increase in pulse rate with nifedipine by reflex tachycardia. Thereafter, blood pressure and RPP during surgery under intravenous sedation has remained at levels similar to those of hypertensive patients with well-controlled blood pressure. Maximum effect (21.4% decreases in SBP) appears in 30 to 60 min and lasts about 3 h on oral administration of nifedipine [12]. The half-lives of oral nifedipine, diltiazem and verapamil, and calcium antagonists are 0.2 to 1 h, 6 to 8 h, and 6 to 8 h, respectively [13]. Since oral nifedipine has the properties of fast onset (30 to 45 min) [14] and relatively short duration, it is suitable for outpatient dental implant surgery and is useful in perioperative management of patients with hypertension.

The overdose of vasoconstrictor that is added to the local anesthetic in order to prolong the anesthetic effect and hemostatic action may cause increased blood pressure and arrhythmias. Elevation of blood pressure in hypertensive patients is greater than that in normotensive patients during dental surgery [15]. Although there is an increase in blood pressure and tachycardia when using three cartridges of local anesthetic containing epinephrine 1:10,000 (5.4 ml), there are no adverse symptoms in patients with normal blood pressure [16]. Little recommended that the amount of local anesthetic solution administered should be less than two cartridges (3.6 ml) for patients with hypertension [1]. Nakamura et al. reported that patients with essential hypertension who have been administered nifedipine can receive less than 3.6 cartridges of local anesthetic containing epinephrine 1:80,000 (6.4 ml) [17]. The administration of exogenous epinephrine with local anesthesia produces the highest plasma concentration in 3 to 6 min and lasts for 20 min [18]. It has been reported that the anesthetic rate of 2% lidocaine containing 1:10,000 epinephrine is 47% 45 min after administration and 27% 60 min after administration [19]. During dental implant surgery which requires a relatively long duration and a wide field in patients with hypertension, administration of conduction anesthesia including inferior alveolar block and posterior superior alveolar nerve block is desirable. When the patient complains of pain, it is important to add local anesthesia while monitoring blood pressure to prevent increased blood pressure caused by pain.

Implant surgery is performed in patients with a wide age range, including elderly patients with hypertension. Dentists or oral surgeons often encounter hypertensive patients who are undiagnosed or noncompliant. Among Japanese over the age of 30, 60% of men and 44.6% of women suffer from high blood pressure, and 33.8% of men and 25.6% of women with a history of hypertension have not been managed medically [20]. In this study, though 13 of the patients did not have a history of hypertension, they were diagnosed with essential hypertension by a physician because they had high blood pressure before surgery. Among patients with a history of high blood pressure, 31 patients (29%) showed high blood pressure before surgery. Because there are many of dental patients with undiagnosed or noncompliant hypertension, blood pressure measurement before treatment, particularly invasive surgery, is indispensable.

For dental implant surgery in hypertensive patients who are not adequately controlled, the application of intravenous sedation and preoperative antihypertensive medication would be useful in order to prevent perioperative hypertension crisis including hypertension emergency with end-organ damage or hypertension urgency without end-organ damage. Since sublingual administration of immediate-release (IR) nifedipine may cause side effects such as significant decrease in blood pressure, reflex tachycardia, and acute myocardial infarction [21], the sublingual administration of IR nifedipine to hypertension crisis has not been approved by the Food and Drug Administration (1985) and Japanese Society of Hypertension Guidelines for the Management of Hypertension (2000). Since we could manage patients with high blood pressure without any cerebrovascular complications by oral administration of nifedipine under closely monitoring, it may be concluded that preoperative administration of oral nifedipine to patients with high blood pressure may be effective to prevent hypertensive crisis due to sudden rise in blood pressure during surgery. Further studies are necessary to evaluate the usefulness of captopril, clonidine, and labetalol, which have been reported as alternatives to nifedipine in emergency hypertension [22-24] in patients with high blood pressure.

## Conclusions

In this study, we showed that the stable hemodynamic was obtained by performing intravenous sedation and oral administration of nifedipine for patients with hypertension. It is important not only to understand the systemic management of the patient but also to obtain stabled hemodynamic by performing intravenous sedation and oral administration of nifedipine for patients with hypertension in order to perform the implant surgery safely, and it could be possible to prevent the medical sequelae.

### Abbreviations

SBP: Systolic blood pressure; DBP: Diastolic blood pressure; PR: Pulse rate; RPP: Rate pressure product; ECG: Electrocardiogram; $SpO_2$: Percutaneous oxygen saturation; ANOVA: Analysis of variance; IR: Immediate-release.

### Competing interests

Motoshi Kimura, Yoshihiro Takasugi, Shigeyoshi Hanano, Katsuyuki Terabe and Yuko Kimura declare that they have no competing interests.

### Authors' contributions

YT and MK designed the study; MK, SH, and KT performed the surgeries; YT performed the intravenous sedation. YT, MK, and YK collected and analyzed the data; MK wrote the manuscript. YT revised the manuscript. All authors read and approved the final manuscript.

### Author details

[1]Hanano Dental Clinic, 4-2-3 Yamanoue, Hirakata, Osaka 573-0047, Japan. [2]Department of Anesthesiology, Kinki University Faculty of Medicine, 377-2 Ohno-Higashi, Osaka-Sayama, Osaka 589-8511, Japan. [3]Terabe Dental Clinic, 4-249 Sakae-cho, Tsu, Mie 514-0004, Japan. [4]First Department of Internal Medicine, Osaka Medical College, 2-7 Daigaku-machi, Takatsuki, Osaka 569-8686, Japan.

### References

1. Little JW. The impact on dentistry of recent advances in the management of hypertension. Oral Surg Oral Med Oral Pathol Oral Radiol Endod. 2000;90:591–9.
2. Aubertin MA. The hypertensive patient in dental practice: updated recommendations for classification, prevention, monitoring, and dental management. Gen Dent. 2004;52:544–52.
3. Vaughan CJ, Delanty N. Hypertensive emergencies. Lancet. 2000;356:411–7.
4. Tsuchihashi T, Takata Y, Kurokawa H, Miura K, Maruoka Y, Kajiyama M, et al. Blood pressure response during dental surgery. Hypertens Res. 1996;19:189–94.
5. Ramsay MA, Savege TM, Simpson BR, Goodwin R. Controlled sedation with alphaxalone-alphadolone. Br Med J. 1974;2:656–9.
6. Chobanian AV, Bakris GL, Black HR, Cushman WC, Green LA, Izzo Jr JL, et al. The seventh report of the Joint National Committee on Prevention, Detection, Evaluation, and Treatment of High Blood Pressure: the JNC 7 report. JAMA. 2003;289:2560–72.
7. Holm SW, Cunningham Jr LL, Bensadoun E, Madsen MJ. Hypertension: classification, pathophysiology, and management during outpatient sedation and local anesthesia. J Oral Maxillofac Surg. 2006;64:111–21.
8. Gobel FL, Norstrom LA, Nelson RR, Jorgensen CR, Wang Y. The rate-pressure product as an index of myocardial oxygen consumption during exercise in patients with angina pectoris. Circulation. 1978;57:549–56.
9. White WB. Heart rate and the rate-pressure product as determinants of cardiovascular risk in patients with hypertension. Am J Hypertens. 1999;12:50S–5.
10. Urban MK, Gordon MA, Harris SN, O'Connor T, Barash PG. Intraoperative hemodynamic changes are not good indicators of myocardial ischemia. Anesth Analg. 1993;76:942–9.
11. Ichinohe T, Kaneko Y, Nakakuki T, Aida H, Abe H. Systemic management of dental patients with cardiovascular disease. Anesth Prog. 1989;36:219–21.
12. Kuwajima I, Ueda K, Kamata C, Matsushita S, Kuramoto K, Murakami M, et al. A study on the effects of nifedipine in hypertensive crises and severe hypertension. Jpn Heart J. 1978;19:455–67.
13. Elliott WJ, Ram CV. Calcium channel blockers. J Clin Hypertens (Greenwich). 2011;13:687–9.
14. Cohan JA, Checcio LM. Nifedipine in the management of hypertensive emergencies: report of two cases and review of the literature. Am J Emerg Med. 1985;3:524–30.
15. Abraham-Inpijn L, Borgmeijer-Hoelen A, Gortzak RAT. Changes in blood pressure, heart rate, and electrocardiogram during dental treatment with use of local anesthesia. J Am Dent Assoc. 1988;116:531–6.
16. Brand HS, Gortzak RA, Palmer-Bouva CC, Abraham RE, Abraham-Inpijn L. Cardiovascular and neuroendocrine responses during acute stress induced by different types of dental treatment. Int Dent J. 1995;45:45–8.
17. Nakamura K, Shionoya Y, Furuya H. The effect of a sublingually administered calcium antagonist, nifedipine, on the action of epinephrine in patients with essential hypertension. J Jpn Dent Soc Anesthesiol. 1987;15:244–53 (In Japanese with English abstract).
18. Knoll-Köhler E, Knöller M, Brandt K, Becker J. Cardiohemodynamic and serum catecholamine response to surgical removal of impacted mandibular third molars under local anesthesia: a randomized double-blind parallel group and crossover study. J Oral Maxillofac Surg. 1991;49:957–62.
19. Katz S, Drum M, Reader A, Nusstein J, Beck M. A prospective, randomized, double-blind comparison of 2% lidocaine with 1:100,000 epinephrine, 4% prilocaine with 1:200,000 epinephrine, and 4% prilocaine for maxillary infiltrations. Anesth Prog. 2010;57:45–51.
20. Ministry of Health, Labour and Welfare, Japan. National health and nutrition survey Japan, 2012. (in Japanese)
21. Grossman E, Messerli FH, Grodzicki T, Kowey P. Should a moratorium be placed on sublingual nifedipine capsules given for hypertensive emergencies and pseudoemergencies? JAMA. 1996;276:1328–31.
22. Thach AM, Schultz PJ. Nonemergent hypertension, new perspectives. Adv Updat Cardiovasc Emerg. 1995;13:1009–23.
23. Murphy C. Hypertensive emergencies. Adv Updat Cardiovasc Emerg. 1995;13:973–1007.
24. Hirschl M. Guidelines for the drug treatment of hypertensive crises. Drugs. 1995;50:991–1000.

# Three-dimensional analysis of incisive canals in human dentulous and edentulous maxillary bones

Masayuki Fukuda*, Satoru Matsunaga, Kento Odaka, Yuuya Oomine, Masaaki Kasahara, Masahito Yamamoto and Shinichi Abe

**Abstract**

**Background:** The purpose of this study was to reveal the structural properties that need to be considered in dental implant treatment by investigating differences between dentulous and edentulous maxillae in the three-dimensional (3D) microstructure of the incisive canals (ICs) and their surrounding bone.

**Methods:** A total of 40 maxillary bones comprising 20 dentulous maxillae and 20 edentulous maxillae were imaged by micro-CT for 3D observation and measurement of the IC and alveolar bone in the anterior region of the IC.

**Results:** The Y-morphology canal was most frequently observed at 60% in dentulous maxilla and 55% in edentulous maxilla. There was a significant difference between dentulous and edentulous maxillae in IC diameter and volume, but no significant difference between the two in the major axis of the ICs.

**Conclusions:** The anatomic structure surrounding the IC has limited area for implant placement. Therefore, where esthetic and long-term maintenance requirements are taken into account, careful attention is needed when setting the placement position. Also, due to the resorption of bone, edentulous maxillae have a different IC morphology from dentulous maxillae, and therefore, a cautious approach is required.

**Keywords:** Anatomy; Dental implant; Incisive canal; Maxilla; Micro-computed tomography; Three-dimensional structure

## Background

In recent years, with the rapid spread of dental implant treatment and a dramatic increase in accidents, the importance of precise 3D data on the human jaw is ever-increasing [1-3]. Bone resorption after tooth extraction is an unavoidable event, and the morphological features of the jawbone change greatly after tooth loss [4-7]. Moreover, the maxilla has a thinner cortical bone than the mandible and presents with a structure where cancellous bone predominates [8]. Therefore, implants have a lower survival rate than the mandible, and the search for sites suitable for implant placement has become an urgent need [9]. The position of the incisive canal (IC) is one of the most important factors for implant placement in the premaxillary region, not only in terms of survival rate but also from an esthetic point of view [10-17]. The incisive canals tend to increase in size with aging and after tooth extraction [18]. If there is a possibility of perforating the incisive canals during implant placement, then a cortical bone/cancellous bone block graft can be adapted to the incisive fossa without removing the contents of the fossa. The contents are pushed posteriorly, thus allowing proper implant placement [19].

The ICs are located in the maxillary midline posterior to the maxillary central incisors, and through them descend the nasopalatine nerve and nasopalatine artery, so they are anatomically important structures [20,21]. Mardinger et al. classified IC morphology as observed from sagittal sections into four types: cylinder-shaped, funnel-shaped, hourglass-shaped, and banana-shaped [18]. Song et al. confirmed one to four branches at the midpoint of the length of the IC and made classifications depending on the number of branches. They reported that the major type of canal shape for the IC is Y-morphology, with four other types - spindle-shaped, very large, cystic, and narrowed - existing as minor types [22]. Tolga et al. ran 2D bone measurements on the IC and

* Correspondence: fukudam@tdc.ac.jp
Department of Anatomy, Tokyo Dental College, 2-9-18, Misaki-cho, Chiyoda-ku, Tokyo 101-0061, Japan

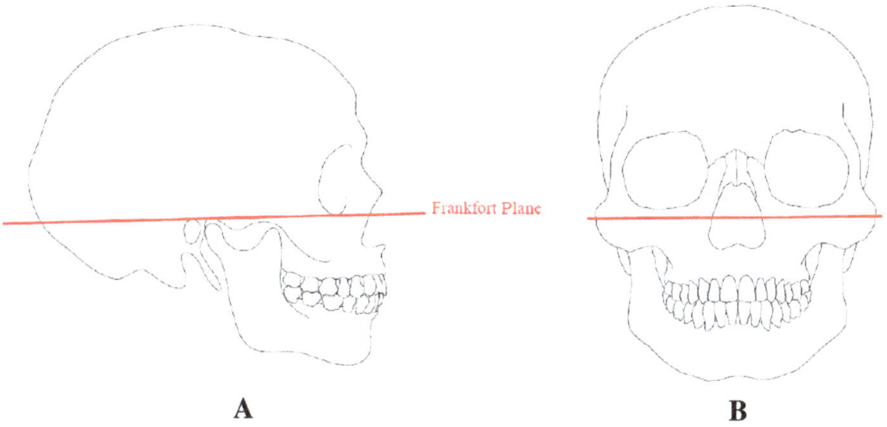


**Figure 1** Method of collecting samples. **(A)** The skull was secured to a device and the Frankfort plane served as a reference. **(B)** A cut was made at the location of the zygomatic bone center, parallel to the Frankfort plane, and the maxillary bone was detached.

surrounding bone of the IC and observed the differences between dentulous and edentulous maxillary bone [23]. Accumulating more finely detailed data directly connected to clinical practice necessitates 3D structure analysis of the bone surrounding the IC.

Kim et al. reported on the usefulness of micro-CT in analyzing the internal microstructure of bones [24]. 3D analysis using micro-CT, which has an imaging resolution of 5 μm at the maximum, makes it possible to reveal very complex structural properties, including even the trabecular bone.

The purpose of the present study is therefore to reveal the structural properties that need to be considered in dental implant treatment by investigating the differences in the IC and their surrounding bone structures between dentulous and edentulous maxillary bones.

## Methods

### Specimens

A total of 20 dentulous human maxillae and 20 edentulous maxillae samples were resected from dried adult skull bones obtained from the Department of Anatomy, Tokyo Dental College. Dentulous jaw samples with maxillary central incisors present on both sides and no midline diastema were selected to ensure they had no tooth loss.

The skull was secured to a device, and the Frankfort plane was marked with India ink; this served as the reference for cutting in parallel from the position of the zygomatic bone center to collect the sample (Figure 1).

### Micro-CT imaging

The samples were imaged with a micro-CT system (HMX-225 Actis4; TESCO, Tokyo, Japan). Imaging

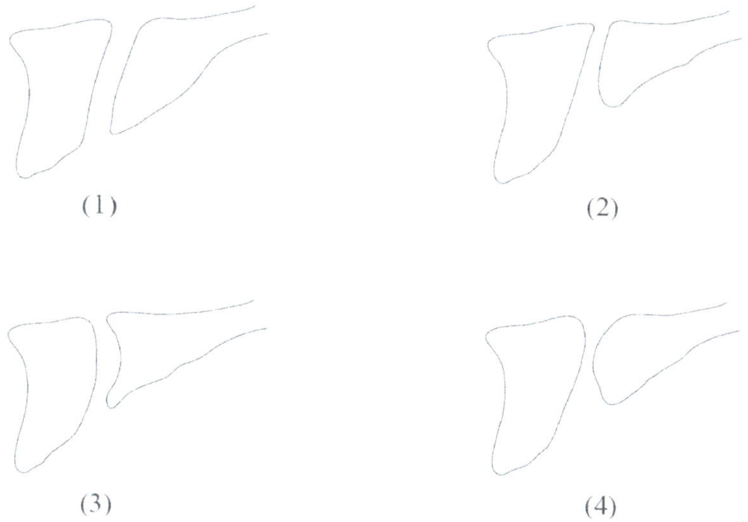


**Figure 2** Morphological variations of IC as observed from the side [18]. **(1)** Cylinder-shaped. **(2)** Funnel-shaped. **(3)** Banana-shaped. **(4)** Hourglass-shaped.

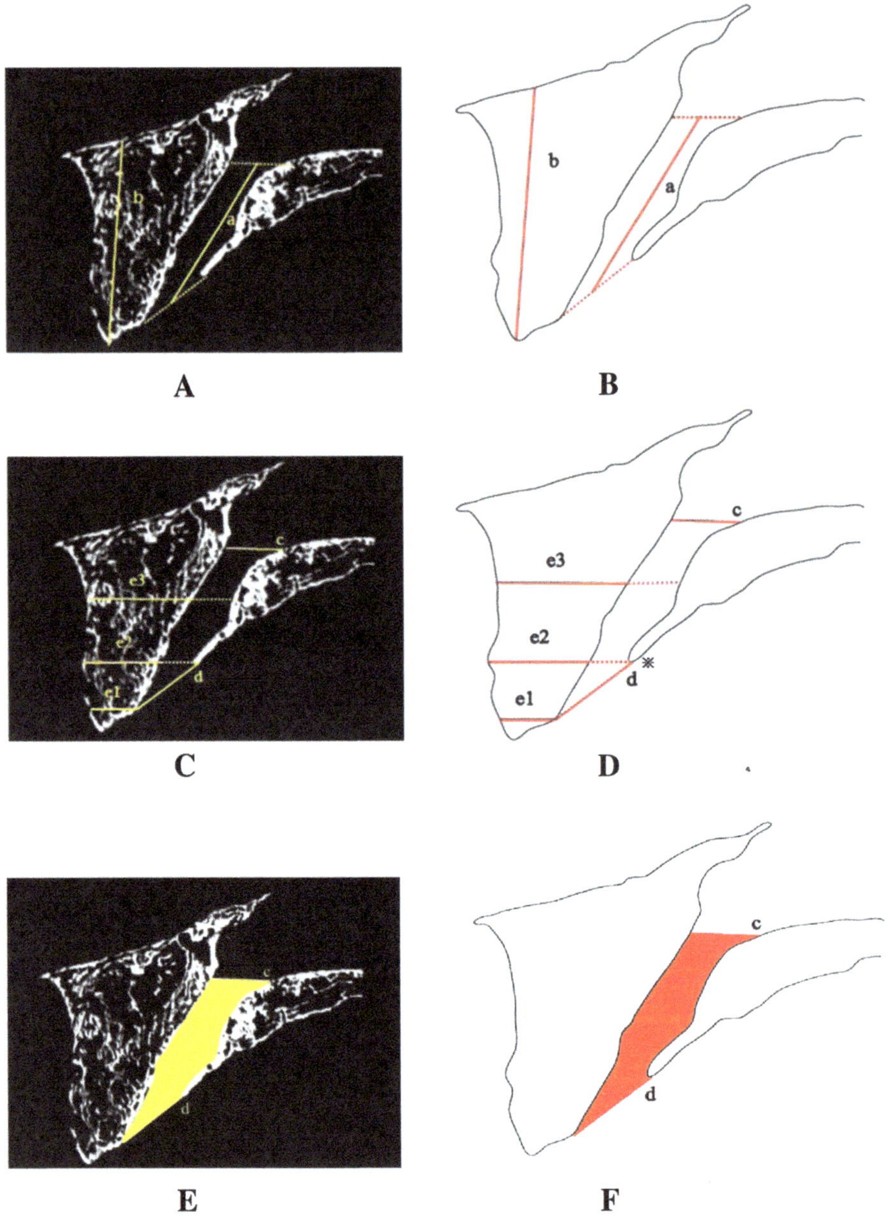


**Figure 3** IC measurement items. **(A, C, E)** CT slice images observed from the side, with sagittal sections of the IC at the middle. **(B, D, F)** Schematic diagrams of A, C, and E. a: IC length, distance between the midpoint of c and midpoint of d. b: Height of the anterior alveolar bone of the IC, distance to the alveolar crest from a line passing through the anterior nasal spine, in parallel with the virtual plane. c: Diameter of the nasopalatine foramina, IC diameter passing over a line connecting the anterior nasal spine and the floor of the nasal cavity, in parallel with the virtual plane. d: Diameter of the incisive foramen, maximum distance from the point (asterisk) where the superoposterior angle changes significantly. e: Width of the IC anterior alveolar bone, distance of the anterior alveolar bone parallel to the virtual plane. (e1: position of the anteroinferior point matching the diameter of the incisive foramen; e2: position of the intermediate part (asterisk); e3: position of 50% of the major axis of the upper IC). f: Total volume from c to d.

conditions were as follows: matrix size 512 × 512, tube voltage 120 kV, and tube current 80 μA. The micro-CT imaging intensifier (I.I.) had a 1-in. CCD camera with a 4-in., 16-bit 1,024 × 1,024 scanning line. A total of 1,200 images of raw data were output with this camera. On the basis of this raw data, a back projection method was used to produce 2D slice data.

**Region of interest**

Measurement was performed by preparing three-dimensional constructed models and thereafter taking a sagittal section at the region with maximum IC diameter. The region of interest was the distance from the anterior nasal spine to the maxillary first premolar. Taken as a reference plane at the time of measurement, the virtual plane was set so as to be a plane connecting

**Table 1 Number of individuals and proportions based on classification of the principal item**

| | | Classification of the IC from the overall appearance | |
|---|---|---|---|
| | | Y-morphology | Cylindrical |
| Dentulous | *n* | 12 | 7 |
| | % | 60 | 35 |
| Edentulous | *n* | 11 | 5 |
| | % | 55 | 25 |
| Dentulous + edentulous | *n* | 23 | 12 |
| | % | 58 | 30 |

the points of the largest bulge of the left/right maxillary tuberosities and the point of the incisive foramen, parallel to the Frankfort plane.

### Image processing

3D construction software (VG Studio; Volume Graphics, Heidelberg, Germany) was used to observe the internal structure of the bone by 3D construction with volume rendering from the slice data. At the same time, image processing software (Mimics; Materialise, Leuven, Belgium) was used to separate the IC and other structures, followed by reconstruction with the IC shown in red.

### Classification of IC morphologies and calculation of their incidences

As the principal item, those that divided completely in two by a bony wall following the nasal septum at a point approximately one fifth to the nasal side of the nasopalatine foramina were set as Y-morphology type, and those that did not were set as cylindrical type. As a secondary item, local IC morphologies in the sagittal cross section were taken as cylinder-shaped, funnel-shaped, banana-shaped, or hourglass-shaped, in accordance with Mardinger and Mraiwa classifications [18,25]. The incidence was calculated for both the principal item and the secondary item (Figure 2).

### Measurements of surrounding bone

Measurement software (TRI-3D/BON; Ratoc System Engineering, Tokyo, Japan) was used for the following bone measurements: IC length (a), IC anterior alveolar bone height (b), IC diameter (c, d), bone width of the IC anterior alveolar bone (e1, e2, e3), and IC volume (f) (Figure 3).

### Statistical analysis

PASW Statistics 18 for Windows (SPSS Inc., Tokyo, Japan) was used for statistical processing. Student's *t*-test was used to test for comparison between dentulous and edentulous maxillary bones. The $p$ value was set to <0.05.

## Results

Overall, 58% of all samples presented with the Y-morphology, divided completely in two by a bony wall following the nasal septum at a point approximately one fifth to the nasal side of the IC length, with two nasopalatine foramina opening on the floor of the nasal cavity. The incidence of each classification in the dentulous maxilla was as follows: 60% Y-morphology and 35% cylindrical. The corre sponding values in the edentulous maxilla were 55% and 25%. Next, the shape of the IC from the sagittal cross section was most often funnel-shaped for both dentulous and edentulous maxilla, at 50% and 45%, respectively. The cylinder-shaped was observed most frequently after the funnel-shaped morphology. Otherwise, 7.5% overall had two to four branches observed at the middle point of the length of the IC (Tables 1 and 2) (Figures 4 and 5).

### Observation of bone structure

Alveolar bone in the anterior region of the IC tended to be extremely thin on the cortical bone. In association with this, the trabecular bone structure of the alveolar process was such that in dentulous maxilla, the trabecular bone runs

**Table 2 Number of individuals and proportions based on classification of the secondary item**

| | | Classification of the IC from the sagittal cross section | | | |
|---|---|---|---|---|---|
| | | Cylinder-shaped | Funnel-shaped | Banana-shaped | Hourglass-shaped |
| Dentulous | *n* | 9 | 10 | 0 | 1 |
| | % | 45 | 50 | 0 | 5 |
| Edentulous | *n* | 9 | 9 | 1 | 1 |
| | % | 45 | 45 | 5 | 5 |

Morphologies of the classification match those in Figure 2.

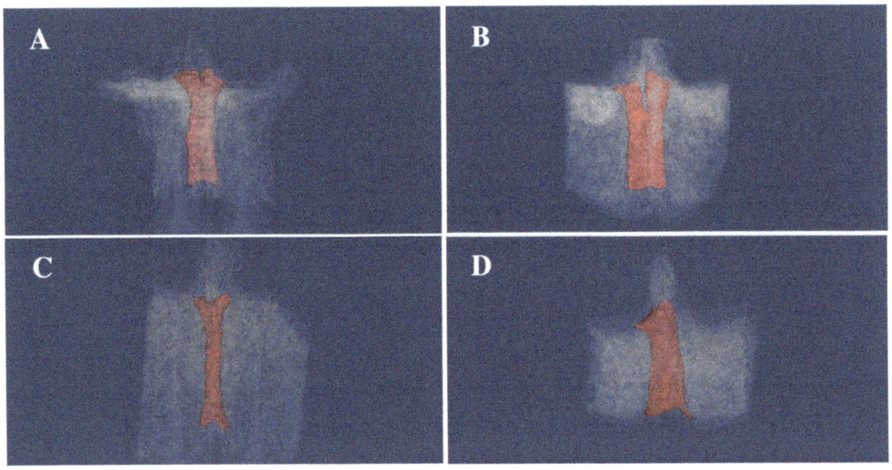


**Figure 4** 3D image constructions of the IC in dentulous maxilla and edentulous maxilla. After imaging by micro-CT, the slice data was used for 3D construction, with the IC shown in red. IC morphology as observed from the front view was classified into Y-morphology and cylindrical [22]. **(A)** Y-morphology of dentulous maxilla. **(B)** Y-morphology of edentulous maxilla. **(C)** Cylindrical of dentulous maxilla. **(D)** Cylindrical of edentulous maxilla.

parallel to the longitudinal axis of the tooth and was distributed sparsely. In the edentulous maxilla, however, the arrangement of trabecular bone structure was irregular and very dense, representing a difference in bone structure characteristics (Figure 6).

### Descriptive analysis of the IC and alveolar bone

The mean IC length (a) was 11.75 mm for dentulous maxilla and 10.84 mm for edentulous maxilla. The mean alveolar bone height (b) anterior to the IC was 17.97 mm for dentulous maxilla and 14.01 mm for edentulous maxilla. The mean IC diameter in (c) showed results of 2.84 mm for dentulous maxilla and 3.56 mm for edentulous maxilla; in (d), it was 4.28 mm for dentulous maxilla and 5.40 mm for edentulous maxilla. The mean bone width for IC anterior alveolar bone was 5.80 mm for dentulous maxilla and 4.06 mm for edentulous maxilla at (e1), 5.61 mm for dentulous maxilla and 5.08 mm for edentulous maxilla at (e2), and 8.45 mm for dentulous maxilla and 8.42 mm for edentulous maxilla at (e3). The mean IC volume (f) was 60.67 $mm^3$ for dentulous maxilla and 87.05 $mm^3$ for edentulous maxilla (Table 3).

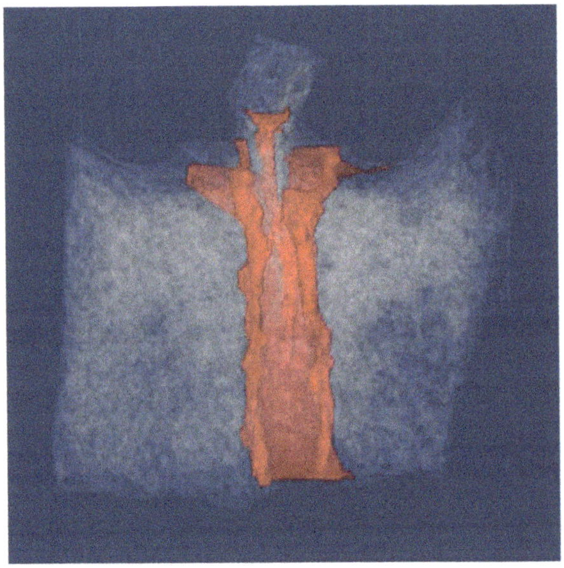

**Figure 5** 3D image constructions of IC showing a unique morphology. IC morphology with three or four branches was observed in one sample.

## Discussion

Dental implant surgery in the premaxillary region often has limited bone for implant placement, and as a result, there is the risk of a poor prognosis in some instances [26]. In particular, the ICs are located in the anterior part of the hard palate, and the probability of adverse effects during implant placement in the premaxillary region is about 4% [27]. Therefore, practitioners must be aware of the risks of accidents and avoid them by using precise, detailed research data on the IC.

Close to 60% of all ICs exhibit Y-morphology. However, according to the report by Michael et al., the frequency of a cylindrical morphology of IC was 50% or more [28]. Otherwise, in terms of rare cases, Frederico et al. studied prospective implant patients using CBCT and reported that two ICs that are completely independent exist [29]. In the present study, instances where two or more IC branches existed accounted for 7.5% of the whole sample, and this suggests the possibility that they vary depending on various factors such as ethnicity or environment.

Regarding IC morphology as observed from the sagittal plane, on the other hand, funnel-shaped predominated, at

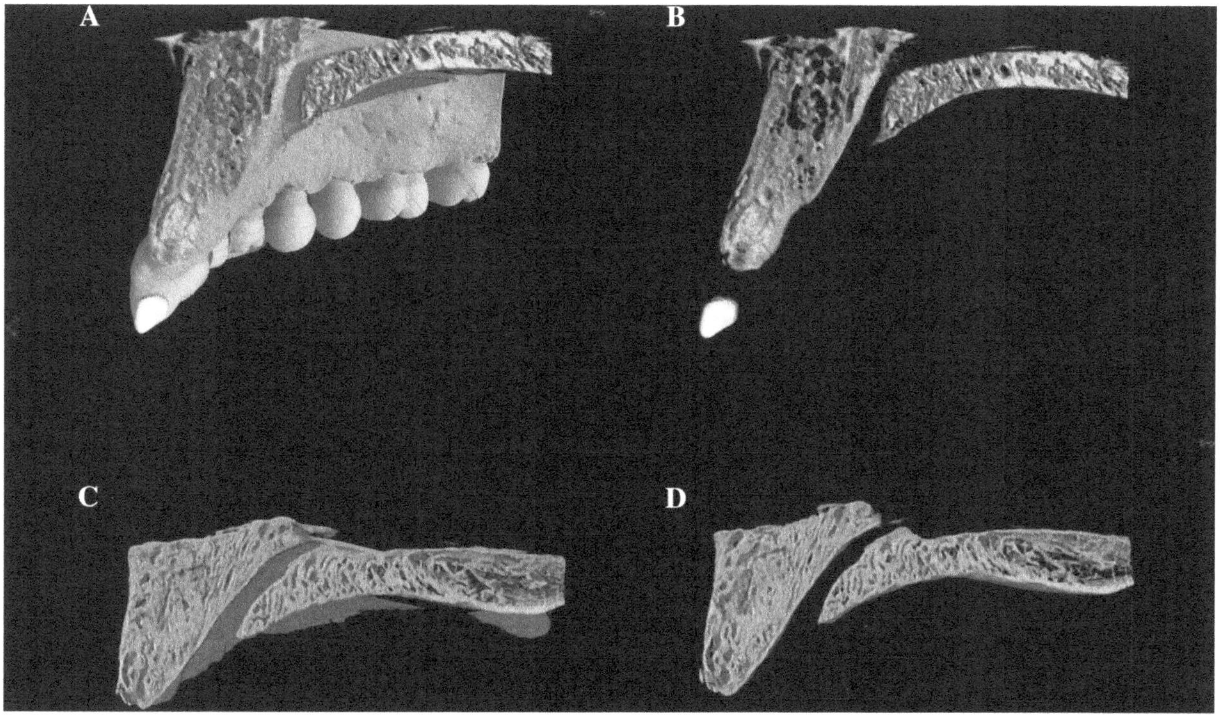


**Figure 6** Representative images of bone internal structure of the bone surrounding the IC. In **(A-D)**, the 3D image constructions of dentulous maxilla and edentulous maxilla were cut in the labiopalatal direction and differences in properties pertaining to the structure of bone were observed. In (B) and (D), the samples were further sliced and observed in detail. (A, B) Relatively thick cortical bone; the cancellous bone travels in a direction parallel to the longitudinal axis of the tooth, and the density is low. (C, D) Cortical bone is especially thin in edentulous maxilla, and the cancellous bone travels with irregular arraying of fine trabecular bone. The density is very high.

55% in dentulous maxilla and 50% in edentulous maxilla, followed by cylinder-shaped at 45% in dentulous maxilla and 45% in edentulous maxilla. This result is largely consistent with Mardinger et al.'s findings, namely, the principal shapes of the IC were shown to be funnel-shaped and cylinder-shaped, whether it be for dentulous or for edentulous maxilla. With funnel-shaped, expansion of the incisive foramen is observed, so depending on the angle of implant placement, there is a risk of perforating the IC and damaging the nasopalatine nerves and arteries. Next, the IC diameter (c, d) and volume (f) showed significant differences between dentulous and edentulous maxilla. This suggests that bone resorption due to the loss of teeth also has an impact on the IC. Bhola et al. reported that in order to obtain initial stability of the implant, there are two requisites: an implant fixture measuring 10 mm or longer must be used, and at the time of placement, there needs to be at least 3 mm or more alveolar bone from the implant body tip [30]. In the present study, where attention is limited to the alveolar bone height (b) in the anterior region of the IC, adequate bone for implant placement was present in 60% of edentulous maxilla. It is, however, desirable for there to be a thickness of 2 mm or more of hard tissue on the labial side (buccal side) of the implant, when the long-term prognosis is taken into account [31]. The mean bone width of the IC anterior alveolar bone was 4.05 mm in edentulous maxilla at e1. Considering the placement of an implant with a diameter of 4 mm, which is now commonly used, there are still comparatively many cases with high risk.

**Table 3 Comparative analysis of measurements items in dentulous maxilla and edentulous maxilla**

| Measurements | Dentulous ($n$ = 20) Mean ± SD | Edentulous ($n$ = 20) Mean ± SD | $p$ |
|---|---|---|---|
| a | 11.75 ± 1.70 (mm) | 10.84 ± 2.42 | 0.241 |
| b | 17.97 ± 3.16 (mm) | 14.01 ± 3.50 | 0.001* |
| c | 2.84 ± 0.79 (mm) | 3.56 ± 0.91 | 0.022* |
| d | 4.28 ± 1.49 (mm) | 5.40 ± 1.44 | 0.020* |
| e1 | 5.80 ± 1.21 (mm) | 4.06 ± 1.77 | 0.002* |
| e2 | 5.61 ± 1.13 (mm) | 5.08 ± 1.87 | 0.358 |
| e3 | 8.45 ± 1.84 (mm) | 8.42 ± 1.59 | 0.972 |
| f | 60.67 ± 36.25 ($mm^3$) | 87.05 ± 32.34 | 0.036* |

*$p < 0.05$. Measurements a to f match those in Figure 3.

Typically, in implant surgery, a platform is prepared at the top of the alveolar bone [32]. However, there are reported cases where a slight gap created at the platform after placement became a space for bacteria to grow, resulting in about 1 to 2 mm of bone resorption due to inflammation of the peri-implant gingiva [33-35]. As gingival recession affects the esthetics, it seems possible that long-term prognosis could be affected by the fine cancellous bone and thin cortical bone observed in the present study.

## Conclusions

The structure surrounding the IC, anatomically, has limited area for implant placement, and when esthetic and long-term maintenance requirements are taken into account, careful attention is needed in setting the placement position. Also, due to the resorption of bone, edentulous maxillae have a different IC morphology from dentulous maxillae, and therefore, a cautious approach is required.

This study demonstrated that the IC displays many morphological as well as dimensional variations. These findings may assist clinicians in understanding the morphology and planning treatment.

### Competing interests

Masayuki Fukuda, Satoru Matsunaga, Kento Odaka, Yuuya Oomine, Masaaki Kasahara, Masahito Yamamoto, and Shinichi Abe declare that they have no competing interests.

### Authors' contributions

MF had the discussion and analysis of incisive canals. SM participated in the design of the study and helped to draft the manuscript. KO carried out image processing. YO carried out micro-CT imaging. MK helped conduct the statistical analysis. MY participated in the bone structure analysis of the incisive canals. SA conceived the idea for the study, participated in its design and coordination, and helped draft the manuscript. All authors have read and approved the final manuscript.

### Acknowledgements

This study was supported by an Oral Health Science Center Grant (#5A10: Satoru Matsunaga) from Tokyo Dental College and by a Grant-in Aid for Scientific Research (no. 22791905: Satoru Matsunaga) from the Ministry of Education, Culture, Sports, Science and Technology, Japan. We thank all staff of the Department of Anatomy, Tokyo Dental College for their whole-hearted cooperation.

### References

1. Feldkamp LA, Goldstein SA, Parfitt AM, Jesion G, Kleerekoper M. The direct examination of three-dimensional bone architecture in vitro by computed tomography. J Bone Miner Res. 1989;4(1):3–11.
2. Ruegsegger P, Koller B, Muller R. A microtomographic system for the nondestructive evaluation of bone architecture. Calcif Tissue Int. 1996;58(1):24–9.
3. Sawada K, Nakahara K, Matsunaga S, Abe S, Ide Y. Evaluation of cortical bone thickness and root proximity at maxillary interradicular sites for mini-implant placement. Clin Oral Implants Res. 2013;24(A100):1–7. doi:10.1111/j.1600-0501.2011.02354.x.
4. Atwood DA. Some clinical factors related to rate of resorption of residual ridges. 1962. J Prosthet Dent. 2001;86(2):119–25.
5. Atwood DA, Coy WA. Clinical, cephalometric, and densitometric study of reduction of residual ridges. J Prosthet Dent. 1971;26(3):280–95.
6. Atwood DA. Bone loss of edentulous alveolar ridges. J Periodontol. 1979;50:11–21.
7. Araújo MG, Lindhe J. Dimensional ridge alterations following tooth extraction. An experimental study in the dog. J Clin Periodontol. 2005;32(2):212–8.
8. Huang H, Richards M, Bedair T, Fields HW, Palomo JM, Johnston WM, et al. Effects of orthodontic treatment on human alveolar bone density distribution. Clin Oral Investig. 2013;17(9):2033–40. doi:10.1007/s00784-012-0906-y.
9. van Steenberghe D. A retrospective multicenter evaluation of the survival rate of osseointegrated fixtures supporting fixed partial prostheses in the treatment of partial edentulism. J Prosthet Dent. 1989;61(2):217–23.
10. Saadoun AP, Sullivan DY, Krischek M, Le Gall M. Single tooth implant–management for success. Pract Periodontics Aesthet Dent. 1994;6(3):73–80.
11. Mecall RA, Rosenfeld AL. Influence of residual ridge resorption patterns on implant fixture placement and tooth position. 1. Int J Periodontics Restorative Dent. 1991;11(1):8–23.
12. Lazzara RJ. Criteria for implant selection: surgical and prosthetic considerations. Pract Periodontics Aesthet Dent. 1994;6(9):55–62.
13. Daftary F, Bahat O. Prosthetically formulated natural aesthetics in implant prostheses. Pract Periodontics Aesthet Dent. 1994;6(9):75–83.
14. Parel SM, Sullivan DY. Esthetics and osseointegration. Dallas: Taylor Publishing Co.; 1989. p. 19–122.
15. Rosenquist JB, Nystrom E. Occlusion of the incisal canal with bone chips. A procedure to facilitate insertion of implants in the anterior maxilla. Int J Oral Maxillofac Surg. 1992;21(4):210–1.
16. Scher EL. Use of the incisive canal as a recipient site for root form implants: preliminary clinical reports. Implant Dent. 1994;3(1):38–41.
17. Jacobs R, Lambrichts I, Liang X, Martens W, Mraiwa N, Adriaensens P, et al. Neurovascularization of the anterior jaw bones revisited using high-resolution magnetic resonance imaging. Oral Surg Oral Med Oral Pathol Oral Radiol Endod. 2007;103(5):683–93.
18. Mardinger O, Namani-Sadan N, Chaushu G, Schwartz-Arad D. Morphologic changes of the nasopalatine canal related to dental implantation: a radiologic study in different degrees of absorbed maxillae. J Periodontol. 2008;79(9):1659–62. doi:10.1902/jop.2008.080043.
19. Artzi Z, Nemcovsky CE, Bitlitum I, Segal P. Displacement of the incisive foramen in conjunction with implant placement in the anterior maxilla without jeopardizing vitality of nasopalatine nerve and vessels: a novel surgical approach. Clin Oral Implants Res. 2000;11(5):505–10.
20. Standring S. Gray's anatomy. 39th ed. Edinburgh: Churchill Livingstone; 2005. p. 583–4.
21. Rodella LF, Buffoli B, Labanca M, Rezzani R. A review of the mandibular and maxillary nerve supplies and their clinical relevance. Arch Oral Biol. 2012;57(4):323–34. doi:10.1016/j.archoralbio.2011.09.007.
22. Song WC, Jo DI, Lee JY, Kim JN, Hur MS, Hu KS, et al. Microanatomy of the incisive canal using three-dimensional reconstruction of microCT images: an ex vivo study. Oral Surg Oral Med Oral Pathol Oral Radiol Endod. 2009;108(4):583–90. doi:10.1016/j.tripleo.2009.06.036.
23. Tözüm TF, Güncü GN, Yildirim YD, Yilmaz HG, Galindo-Moreno P, Velasco-Torres M, et al. Evaluation of maxillary incisive canal characteristics related to dental implant treatment with computerized tomography: a clinical multicenter study. J Periodontol. 2012;83(3):337–43. doi:10.1902/jop.2011.110326.
24. Kim YJ, Henkin J. Micro-computed tomography assessment of human alveolar bone: bone density and three-dimensional micro-architecture. Clin Implant Dent Relat Res. 2013. doi:10.1111/cid.12109.
25. Mraiwa N, Jacobs R, Van Cleynenbreugel J, Sanderink G, Schutyser F, Suetens P, et al. The nasopalatine canal revisited using 2D and 3D CT imaging. Dentomaxillofac Radiol. 2004;33(6):396–402.
26. Liang X, Jacobs R, Lambrichts I. An assessment on spiral CT scan of the superior and inferior genial spinal foramina and canals. Surg Radiol Anat. 2006;28(1):98–104.
27. Kraut RA, Boyden DK. Location of incisive canal in relation to central incisor implants. Implant Dent. 1998;7(3):221–5.
28. Bornstein MM, Balsiger R, Sendi P, Von Arx T. Morphology of the nasopalatine canal and dental implant surgery: a radiographic analysis of 100 consecutive patients using limited cone-beam computed tomography. Clin Oral Implants Res. 2011;22(3):295–301. doi:10.1111/j.1600-0501.2010.02010.x.
29. Neves FS, Oliveira LK, Ramos Mariz AC, Crusoé-Rebello I, De Oliveira-Santos C. Rare anatomical variation related to the nasopalatine canal. Surg Radiol Anat. 2013;35(9):853–5. doi:10.1007/s00276-013-1089-1.
30. Bhola M, Neely AL, Kolhatkar S. Immediate implant placement: clinical decisions, advantages, and disadvantages. J Prostho. 2008;17(7):576–81. doi:10.1111/j.1532-849X.2008.00359.x.
31. Grunder U, Gracis S, Capelli M. Influence of the 3-D bone-to-implant relationship on esthetics. Int J Periodontics Restorative Dent. 2005;25(2):113–9.
32. Alonso-González R, Aloy-Prósper A, Peñarrocha-Oltra D, Peñarrocha-Diago MA, Peñarrocha-Diago M. Marginal bone loss in relation to platform switching implant insertion depth: an update. J Clin Exp Dent. 2012;4(3):e173–9. doi:10.4317/jced.50743.

33. Esposito M, Ekestubbe A, Gröndahl K. Radiological evaluation of marginal bone loss at tooth surfaces facing single Brånemark implants. Clin Oral Implants Res. 1993;4(3):151–7.
34. Paul SJ, Jovanovic SA. Anterior implant-supported reconstructions: a prosthetic challenge. Pract Proced Aesthet Dent. 1999;11(5):585–90.
35. Saadoun AP, LeGall M, Touati B. Selection and ideal tridimensional implant position for soft tissue aesthetics. Pract Proced Aesthet Dent. 1999;11(9):1063–72.

# Real-time PCR analysis of fungal organisms and bacterial species at peri-implantitis sites

Frank Schwarz[1], Kathrin Becker[2*], Sebastian Rahn[3], Andrea Hegewald[1], Klaus Pfeffer[3] and Birgit Henrich[3]

**Abstract**

**Background:** The potential role of fungal organisms and their co-aggregation with either periodontopathogens or opportunistic pathogens at peri-implantitis sites is unknown. The aim of the present study was to qualitatively/quantitatively analyze and correlate fungal organisms and bacterial species at peri-implantitis sites.

**Methods:** In a total of 29 patients, submucosal/subgingival plaque samples were collected at peri-implantitis and healthy implant sites as well as teeth with a history of periodontitis (controls). A real-time PCR assay was established for the qualification of fungal organisms and a TaqMan assay for the quantification of *Porphyromonas gingivalis*, *Parvimonas micra*, *Tannerella forsythia*, *Mycoplasma salivarium*, *Veillonella parvula*, and *Staphylococcus aureus*.

**Results:** Fungal organisms were more frequently identified at peri-implantitis (31.6%) (i.e., *Candida albicans*, *Candida boidinii*, *Penicillium* spp., *Rhodotorula laryngis*, *Paelicomyces* spp., *Saccharomycetes*, *Cladosporium cladosporioides*) and healthy implant sites (40% - *Candida dubliniensis*, *C. cladosporioides*) than at selected teeth (20% - *C. albicans*, *Fusarium solani*). At implant sites, fungal organisms were significantly correlated with *P. micra* and *T. forsythia*.

**Conclusions:** *Candida* spp. and other fungal organisms were frequently identified at peri-implantitis as well as healthy implant sites and co-colonized with *P. micra* and *T. forsythia*.

**Keywords:** Peri-implantitis; Diagnosis; Microbiology; Fungal organisms

## Background

There is considerable evidence supporting the view that peri-implant diseases are infectious in nature and mainly linked to an uncontrolled accumulation of bacterial plaque biofilms [1]. Basically, diseased implant sites are dominated by gram-negative anaerobic bacteria and therefore feature microbiological characteristics similar to those noted for chronic periodontal infections [2]. Even though the history of periodontitis is a documented risk indicator for peri-implant diseases [3,4], the diversity of microbiota at diseased tooth sites was reported to be higher than that noted at diseased implant sites [5]. Common periodontopathogenic bacteria could be isolated at both healthy and diseased implant sites [6], and the microbiological analysis of 40 species did not markedly differ by the clinical implant status (i.e., healthy, mucositis, peri-implantitis) [7]. However, a most recent analysis of 78 species has pointed to higher counts of 19 bacterial species at peri-implantitis - when compared with healthy implant sites, mainly including *Porphyromonas gingivalis* (*P. gingivalis*) and *Tannerella forsythia* (*T. forsythia*) [4].

In addition, peri-implantitis was linked with opportunistic pathogens such as *Pseudomonas aeruginosa* and *Staphylococcus aureus* (*S. aureus*), thus pointing to a rather complex and heterogenous 'polymicrobal infection'. Yeasts are frequently isolated from the oral cavity [8] and were also identified in the submucosal plaque of patients with peri-implantitis [9,10]. These studies, however, mainly focused on the assessment of *Candida albicans*, and at the time being, a qualitative evaluation of other fungal organisms is lacking. Moreover, the potential role of yeasts and their co-aggregation with either periodontopathogens or other opportunistic bacteria at peri-implantitis sites is unknown.

Therefore, the aim of the present study was to analyze and correlate fungal organisms and bacterial species at peri-implantitis and healthy implant sites as well as teeth

* Correspondence: kathrin.becker@med.uni-dueseldorf.de
[2]Department of Orthodontics, Westdeutsche Kieferklinik, Heinrich Heine University, Moorenstraße 5, D-40225 Düsseldorf, Germany
Full list of author information is available at the end of the article

with a history of periodontitis using real-time polymerase chain reaction (PCR).

## Methods

### Study population

A total of 29 partially or fully edentulous patients were consecutively recruited from the Department of Oral Surgery, Heinrich Heine University, Düsseldorf, Germany, between April 2013 and July 2014. Nineteen patients (7 men and 13 women; mean age 58.8 ± 12.6 years) suffered from initial to moderate or advanced peri-implantitis, while ten patients (6 men and 4 women; mean age 55.2 ± 11.3 years) revealed clinically healthy implant sites. Prior to participation, each patient was given a detailed description of the procedure and was required to sign informed consent forms. The study was in accordance with the Helsinki Declaration of 2008 and the study protocol was approved by the ethics committee of the Heinrich Heine University.

### Patient selection

For patient selection, the following inclusion criteria were defined: 1) partially or fully edentulous, 2) presence of one screw-type titanium implant either exhibiting healthy (absence of bleeding on probing (BOP), probing depth (PD) <4 mm) or established peri-implantitis (i.e., bleeding on probing with or without suppuration/pus, pocketing, and radiographic bone loss - initial to moderate: <50%/advanced: >50% of the implant length relative to baseline) [11], 3) presence of a sufficiently dimensioned (>2 mm) keratinized mucosa, 4) no implant mobility, 5) no systemic antibiotic medication within the last 3 months, 6) no history of malignancy, radiotherapy, chemotherapy, or immunodeficiency within the last 4 years, 7) proper recall/periodontal maintenance care, 8) non-smoker or light smoking status in smokers (<10 cigarettes per day).

### Plaque samples

After a gentle supramucosal cleaning, submucosal plaque samples and peri-implant sulcus fluid were collected at the deepest aspect of each implant site by means of sterile paper points (i.e., each was left in place for 30 s). The paper point was transferred into 200 µl G2 buffer of the EZ1 DNA Tissue Kit (Qiagen, Hilden, Germany) and stored at −20°C until transportation to the Institute of Medical Microbiology and Hospital Hygiene at the Heinrich Heine University for analysis.

In the peri-implantitis group, one additional subgingival plaque sample was obtained from partially edentulous patients with a history of periodontitis ($n = 10$) and obtained at a tooth exhibiting the highest PD but no signs of acute periodontal disease (i.e., BOP/no suppuration). None of these teeth were located adjacent to the sampled implant sites. The control samples were also prepared for PCR analysis.

### Genomic DNA preparation

At the Institute of Medical Microbiology and Hospital Hygiene, the specimens were re-suspended in the buffer by vortexing. After the addition of 10 µl Proteinase K solution (100 µg/ml Proteinase K), the samples were incubated for 30 min at 56°C. Total genomic DNA was isolated from 200 µl of the Proteinase K-digested samples by semiautomatic DNA preparation on an EZ1 biorobot machine (Qiagen) and the eluted 100 µl DNA samples stored at −20°C until use.

### TaqMan PCR

*In house* TaqMan PCRs for the quantification of *Mycoplasma salivarium* (*M. salivarium*) [12], *Veillonella parvula* (*V. parvula*) [13], *S. aureus* [14], *P. gingivalis* [15], *Parvimonas micra* (*P. micra*) [16], and *T. forsythia* [15] (Table 1) were carried out in a total volume of 25 µl consisting of 1× Eurogentec qPCR MasterMix (Eurogentec, Seraing, Belgium) without ROX (containing buffer, dNTPs (including dUTP), HotGoldStar DNA polymerase, 5 mM $MgCl_2$, uracil-N-glycosylase and stabilizers (RT-QP2X-03NR, Eurogentec)), 300 nM each forward and reverse primer, 200 nM labeled probe, and 2.5 µl of template DNA (primer and probes are listed in Tables 1 and 2). Amplicon carrying plasmids were used in concentrations of $10^5$ and $10^2$ copies/µl as quantification standards. Thermal cycling conditions were as follows: 1 cycle at 50°C for 10 min, 1 cycle at 95°C for 10 min followed by 45 cycles at 95°C for 15 s, and 60°C for 1 min. Cycling and fluorescent data collection and analysis were carried out with an iCycler from BioRad (BioRad Laboratories, Munich, Germany) according to the manufacturer's instructions.

### Real-time PCR

Real-time PCR assays for the detection of fungal DNA (Table 2) were carried out in a total volume of 25 µl consisting of 1× MesaGreen qPCR MasterMix Plus for SYBR Assay (containing Buffer, dNTPs (including dUTP), Meteor Taq DNA polymerase, 4 mM MgCl2, uracil-N-glycosylase, SYBR Green I, stabilizers and passive reference (RT-SY2X-06 + WOU); Eurogentec, Seraing, Belgium), 300 nM each forward and reverse primer and 2.5 µl of template DNA. In multiplex assays with three forward primers, each primer was adjusted to 100 mM. Positive detection was verified by sequencing [17] and BLAST analysis [18]. Thermal cycling conditions were as follows: 10 min at 50°C, 10 min at 95°C followed by 40 cycles of 15 s at 95°C, and 1 min at 60°C. Subsequent melting point analysis followed after 15 s at 95°C and

**Table 1 Overview of bacterial species, corresponding genes, primers/probes, and DNA sequences**

| Species | Gene | Primer/probe | Sequences (5′-3′) |
|---|---|---|---|
| *Mycoplasma salivarium* | *rpoB* | msali-F | CCG TCA AAT GAT TTC GAT TGC |
| | | msali-R | GAA CTG CTT GAC GTT GCA TGT T |
| | | msali-S | Hex-ATG ATG CTA ACC GTG CGC TTA TGG GTG-BHQ1 |
| *Veillonella parvula* | 16S rDNA | vpar-F | TGC TAA TAC CGC ATA CGA TCT AAC C |
| | | vpar-R | GCT TAT AAA TAG AGG CCA CCT TTC A |
| | | vpar-S | HEX-CTA TCC TCG ATG CCG A-BHQ1 |
| *Staphylococcus aureus* | *nuc* | saur-F | CAA AGC ATC CTA AAA AAG GTG TAG AGA |
| | | saur-R | TTC AAT TTT CTT TGC ATT TTC TAC CA |
| | | saur-S | FAM-TTT TCG TAA ATG CAC TTG CTT CAG GAC CA-BHQ1 |
| *Porphyromonas gingivalis* | Arg-gingipain | pgin-F | CCT ACG TGT ACG GAC AGA GCT ATA |
| | | pgin-R | AGG ATC GCT CAG CGT AGC ATT |
| | | pgin-S | TexRed-TCG CCC GGG AAG AAC TTG TCT TCA-BHQ2 |
| *Parvimonas micra* | 16S rDNA | pmic-F | TCG AAC GTG ATT TTT GTG GAA A |
| | | pmic-R | GGT AGG TTG CTC ACG TGT TAC TCA |
| | | pmic-S | FAM-CCC GTT CGC CAC TT-BHQ1 |
| *Tannerella forsythia* | bspA | tfor-F | TCC CAA AGA CGC GGA TAT CA |
| | | tfor-R | ACG GTC GCG ATG TCA TTG T |
| | | tfor-S | FAM-CCG CGA CGT GAA ATG GTA TTC CTC-BHQ1 |
| | | tfor-S II | HEX-TCG CGA CGT GAA ATG GTA TTC CTC-BHQ1 |

1 min at 60°C from 65°C to 95°C with an increment of 0.5°C for 15 s and plate read.

### Statistical analysis

The statistical analysis was performed using a commercially available software program (SPSS Statistics 22.0, IBM Corp., Ehningen, Germany). Kendall-Tau-b correlation coefficients were calculated to evaluate the dependence between fungal organisms, bacterial species as well as disease severity (i.e., initial to moderate and advanced sites). Results were considered statistically significant at $P < 0.05$.

## Results

According to the given definition, the present analysis was based on a total of $n = 13$ initial to moderate and $n = 6$ advanced peri-implantitis lesions ($n = 19$ patients), 10 healthy implant sites ($n = 10$ patients), as well as 10 teeth

**Table 2 Overview of fungal organisms, corresponding genes, primers/probes, and DNA sequences**

| Species | Gene | Primer/probe | Sequences (5′-3′) |
|---|---|---|---|
| *Aspergillus* spp. plus | ITS2 | aspe-F | CTG TCC GAG CGT CAT TG |
| *Penicillium* spp. | | pen1-F | GTC CGA GCG TCA TTT CTG |
| | | pen2-F | TCC GAG CGT CAT TGC TG |
| | | its2-R | TCC TCC GCT TAT TGA TAT GC |
| *Rhizomucor* spp. plus | ITS2 | muco-F | GAA CGC AWC TTG CGC TCA |
| *Mucor* spp. plus | | rhi1-F | TCA TCC ATT GGG TAC GTC TAG |
| *Rhizopus* spp. | | its2-R | TCC TCC GCT TAT TGA TAT GC |
| *Absidia* spp. plus | ITS2 | absi-F | ATY TTT GAA CGC ATC TTG CA |
| *Cunninghamella* spp. plus | | lic1-F | ATT YAG TTG CTG TCA TGG CC |
| *Lichtheimia* spp. | | lic2-F | CAT TCA GTT GCT CTC ATG GTC |
| | | its2-R | TCC TCC GCT TAT TGA TAT GC |
| *Candida* spp. | ITS2 | cand-F | CCT GTT TGA GCG TCR TTT |
| | | its2-R | TCC TCC GCT TAT TGA TAT GC |

with a history of periodontitis ($n = 10$ out of 19 patients suffering from peri-implantitis).

### Fungal and bacterial analysis

The analysis of fungal organisms as well as of *M. salivarium, V. parvula, S. aureus, P. gingivalis, P. micra,* and *T. forsythia* at peri-implantitis as well as healthy implant and selected tooth sites is presented in Tables 3, 4, and 5.

#### *Peri-implantitis sites*

Fungal organisms were identified in 31.6% (six sites) of the patients and equally distributed between initial to moderate (three sites) and advanced (two sites) peri-implantitis sites. The respective plaque samples were dominated ($n = 3$) by *Candida* spp. (i.e., *C. albicans* and *Candida boidinii*) and at two sites co-colonized with *Penicillium* spp. and *Rhodotorula laryngis. Paelicomyces* spp. (67% homologous), *Saccharomycetes* (76% homologous), and *Cladosporium cladosporioides* were identified at three sites (Table 3). The Kendall-Tau-b coefficients failed to reveal any significant correlations between the presence of fungal organisms and the proportions of *M. salivarium* (−0.26), *V. parvula* (0.26), *S. aureus* (0.34), and *P. gingivalis* (0.09) as well as disease severity (0.26) ($P > 0.05$, respectively). However, a significant correlation was noted with respect to the proportions of *P. micra* (−0.42) and *T. forsythia* (−0.44) ($P < 0.05$, respectively).

#### *Healthy implant sites*

In the selected partially edentulous patients, fungal organisms were identified at four implant sites (*Candida dubliniensis* and *C. cladosporioides*), corresponding to a frequency of 40.0% (Table 4). The Kendall-Tau-b coefficients failed to reveal any significant correlations between the presence of fungal organisms and the proportions of *M. salivarium* (0.38), *V. parvula* (−0.24), *S. aureus* (−0.33), and *P. gingivalis* (−0.51) ($P > 0.05$, respectively). However, a significant correlation was noted with respect to the proportions of *P. micra* (0.65) and *T. forsythia* (0.65) ($P < 0.05$, respectively).

#### *Selected tooth sites*

In the selected partially edentulous patients, fungal organisms were identified at two tooth sites (*C. albicans* and *Fusarium solani*), corresponding to a frequency of 20.0% (Table 5).

The Kendall-Tau-b coefficients failed to reveal any significant correlations between the presence of fungal organisms and the proportions of *M. salivarium* (0.25), *V. parvula* (0.34), *P. gingivalis* (0.60), *P. micra* (0.32), *T. forsythia* (0.12), and *S. aureus* (0.66) ($P > 0.05$, respectively).

## Discussion

The present study aimed at analyzing and correlating fungal organisms with several periodontopathogenic and opportunistic bacterial species at peri-implantitis

**Table 3 Bacterial and fungal analysis: peri-implantitis sites ($n = 19$ patients)**

| Patient | Severity | *M. salivarium* | *V. parvula* | *S. aureus* | *P. gingivalis* | *P. micra* | *T. forsythia* | Fungal organisms |
|---|---|---|---|---|---|---|---|---|
| 1 | i-m | - | 7.96E + 04 | - | - | 6.29E + 01 | 2.14E + 01 | *Paelicomyces* spp. |
| 2 | i-m | 3.31E + 02 | 4.59E + 03 | - | - | 1.94E + 04 | 6.60E + 01 | - |
| 3 | i-m | 1.80E + 01 | 5.25E + 02 | - | 3.07E + 05 | 7.67E + 04 | 9.28E + 04 | - |
| 4 | i-m | 1.02E + 01 | 3.23E + 03 | - | 1.16E + 02 | 1.98E + 02 | 3.33E + 01 | *Candida boidinii, Penicillium* spp. |
| 5 | i-m | - | 2.08E + 03 | - | - | 1.11E + 01 | 1.51E + 01 | - |
| 6 | i-m | 1.23E + 02 | 2.29E + 03 | - | 4.40E + 04 | 1.45E + 03 | 1.33E + 04 | - |
| 7 | i-m | 1.17E + 03 | 9.02E + 02 | - | 6.37E + 03 | 3.71E + 03 | 4.28E + 01 | - |
| 8 | i-m | - | 3.13E + 03 | - | - | - | 3.87E + 00 | *Candida albicans* |
| 9 | i-m | - | 1.13E + 02 | - | 7.67E + 01 | 4.26E + 03 | 5.20E + 03 | - |
| 10 | i-m | 1.46E + 04 | 5.58E + 04 | - | 1.24E + 01 | 1.29E + 03 | 5.33E + 04 | - |
| 11 | i-m | - | 8.22E + 03 | - | - | - | 1.06E + 02 | - |
| 12 | i-m | 1.48E-01 | 4.98E + 03 | 37.43 | 2.31E + 02 | 3.10E + 01 | 5.33E + 01 | *Cladosporium cladosporioides* |
| 13 | i-m | 8.46E + 02 | 1.76E + 02 | - | - | 1.33E + 04 | 2.99E + 03 | - |
| 14 | a | 1.66E + 03 | 3.90E + 04 | - | 1.28E + 05 | 6.75E + 03 | 1.02E + 04 | *Rhodotorula laryngis, Candida alb.* |
| 15 | a | 1.91E + 02 | 1.13E + 03 | - | 1.51E + 01 | 6.33E + 03 | 1.56E + 01 | |
| 16 | a | 1.29E + 05 | 1.27E + 04 | - | - | 3.85E + 05 | 1.29E + 05 | - |
| 17 | a | 6.82E + 01 | 5.43E + 01 | - | - | 3.00E + 04 | 1.17E + 04 | - |
| 18 | a | 1.95E + 04 | 1.35E + 05 | - | 1.46E + 04 | 2.25E + 03 | 4.44E + 03 | - |
| 19 | a | - | 7.43E + 03 | - | 3.08E + 01 | 1.26E + 02 | 1.33E + 02 | - |

i-m, initial to moderate; a, advanced.

**Table 4 Bacterial and fungal analysis: healthy implant sites (*n* = 10 patients)**

| Patient | *M. salivarium* | *V. parvula* | *S. aureus* | *P. gingivalis* | *P. micra* | *T. forsythia* | Fungal organisms |
|---|---|---|---|---|---|---|---|
| 1 | - | 2.26E + 03 | - | 1.64E + 01 | 8.02E + 00 | 7.58E + 01 | - |
| 2 | 1.46E + 04 | 3.94E + 04 | 36.45 | - | 4.00E + 04 | 1.14E + 04 | *Candida dubliniensis* |
| 3 | - | 3.16E + 04 | 37.49 | 1.62E + 01 | 8.88E + 01 | 4.90E + 01 | - |
| 4 | - | 3.42E + 04 | - | - | 1.62E + 04 | 7.78E + 01 | - |
| 5 | - | 1.78E + 04 | - | - | 1.81E + 02 | 3.66E + 03 | - |
| 6 | - | 2.74E + 03 | - | - | 1.38E + 01 | 1.40E + 02 | *Cladosporium cladosporioides* |
| 7 | - | 2.50E + 02 | 36.90 | - | 1.03E + 03 | 6.19E + 01 | - |
| 8 | 9.34E + 01 | 1.37E + 03 | 36.61 | 8.52E + 02 | 1.15E + 03 | 2.84E + 01 | - |
| 9 | 2.04E + 01 | 1.29E + 03 | - | - | 8.06E + 01 | 8.79E + 02 | *Cladosporium cladosporioides* |
| 10 | - | - | - | - | 4.48E + 02 | 8.69E + 02 | *Cladosporium cladosporioides* |

sites using real-time PCR. These outcomes were compared with those noted at healthy implant sites as well as teeth with a history of periodontitis.

Basically, the present analysis has pointed to a high prevalence of fungal organisms in submucosal plaque samples obtained at both peri-implantitis (31.6%) and healthy (40%) implant sites. Peri-implantitis sites were dominated by *Candida* spp. (i.e., *C. albicans* and *C. boidinii*) and occasionally co-colonized with *Penicillium* spp. and *R. laryngis*, while at three additional sites, *Paelicomyces* spp., *Saccharomycetes*, and *C. cladosporioides* were identified. Healthy implant sites were mainly associated with *C. dubliniensis* and *C. cladosporioides*.

In this context, it must be emphasized that this is the first report on *Penicillium spp.*, *R. laryngis*, *Paelicomyces* spp., *Saccharomycetes*, and *C. cladosporioides* at implant sites, and therefore, any comparison with previous findings is not feasible. However, the high proportions of *Candida* spp. noted in the present analysis corroborate previous data also pointing to a frequency of 55% at peri-implantitis sites [9], while a most recent study merely identified *C. albicans* in 3% of the patients investigated [10].

In contrast to the present data, Leonhardt et al. failed to identify *Candida* spp. in a total of 51 patients with clinically healthy mucosal conditions [9]. In this context, however, it is also important to emphasize that the presence of *C. albicans* per se does not necessarily cause symptomatic oral mucosal lesions (i.e., stomatitis) [19]. Host susceptibility to these infections is commonly triggered either by local or systemic (e.g., HIV infection, antibiotic medication) factors [20,21]. Furthermore, *Candida* spp. possess a high potential to colonize and invade gingival tissues [22] and co-aggregate with other oral microorganisms such as *Pg* [23,24]. The present microbiological analysis also has identified high proportions of periodontopathogenic bacteria associated with peri-implant diseases, thus corroborating previous analyses [4,7,9,25,26]. However, at both peri-implantitis and healthy implant sites, fungal organisms were only correlated with *P. micra* and *T. forsythia*. Unfortunately, the PCR analysis employed did not allow for a quantification of yeasts, and therefore, further studies are needed to determine relative differences in the composition of these specific organisms at healthy and diseased implant sites.

Furthermore, the present analysis failed to identify any significant correlation of either fungal organisms or disease severity with opportunistic bacteria, such as *M. salivarium*, *V. parvula*, and *S. aureus*. At tooth sites, *M.*

**Table 5 Bacterial and fungal analysis: tooth sites (*n* = 10 patients)**

| Patient | *M. salivarium* | *V. parvula* | *S. aureus* | *P. gingivalis* | *P. micra* | *T. forsythia* | Fungal organisms |
|---|---|---|---|---|---|---|---|
| 1 | 7.05E + 01 | 7.00E + 01 | - | - | - | 4.67E + 01 | - |
| 5 | - | 1.18E + 04 | - | 6.30E + 00 | 5.02E + 02 | 1.51E + 01 | - |
| 6 | 4.08E + 03 | 6.71E + 02 | - | - | 5.23E + 03 | 4.89E + 04 | *Fusarium solani* |
| 7 | 4.55E + 02 | 7.06E + 03 | - | 1.43E + 05 | 1.47E + 04 | 6.36E + 04 | - |
| 10 | - | 1.79E + 02 | - | 1.76E + 01 | 5.49E + 00 | 2.40E + 00 | - |
| 12 | 1.79E + 03 | 1.92E + 03 | - | - | 1.43E + 04 | 3.59E + 03 | *Candida albicans* |
| 13 | - | 1.26E + 02 | - | - | - | 1.21E + 02 | - |
| 16 | - | 3.19E + 03 | - | 1.07E + 04 | 3.44E + 03 | 3.01E + 04 | - |
| 17 | 2.69E + 01 | 2.68E + 03 | 28.25 | 6.82E + 01 | 2.08E + 02 | 4.83E + 01 | - |
| 19 | 1.03E + 01 | 1.33E + 02 | - | - | 9.81E + 01 | 4.08E + 01 | - |

*salivarium* was mainly isolated from the sulcus area and associated with gingivitis lesions [27]. Interestingly, *S. aureus* has only been identified at one single peri-implantitis - but several healthy implant sites, which is contradictory to the higher prevalence at peri-implantitis sites noted in larger cohorts [4,7,9]. When further analyzing the present data, it was also noted that at several sites, the frequency of selected periodontopathogenic bacteria was below the detection thresholds, irrespective of disease severity. These findings clearly corroborate previous data indicating that these periodontopathogenic bacteria may not necessarily be related to peri-implantitis [6].

Fungal organisms have also been isolated from periodontal pockets in chronic periodontitis patients. The reported prevalence of yeast-positive samples varied between 15.6% and 17.5% [28,29]. These untreated periodontal pockets were also dominated by *C. albicans*. Other species, such as *Candida parapsilosis*, *C. dubliniensis*, *Candida tropicalis*, and *Rhodotorula* spp., were rarely observed [30]. Even though the prevalence of *C. albicans* tended to be higher in chronic periodontitis (30%) when compared with healthy patients (15%), this difference did not reach statistical significance [30]. The present frequency of fungal organisms in subgingival plaque samples obtained from teeth with a history of periodontitis basically corroborates the above reported data but was markedly lower when compared with all implant sites investigated. However, the frequency distribution of periodontopathogenic and opportunistic bacteria did not seem to differ between tooth and implant sites, which is basically in line with a recent analysis assessing *Aggregatibacter actinomycetemcomitans*, *Pg*, *Prevotella intermedia*, *Tf*, *Treponema denticola*, *S. aureus*, enteric bacteria, and *P. aeruginosa* [10]. In this context, it must be emphasized that the present analysis just focused on the most relevant periodontopathogens associated with peri-implantitis [4] as well as a few opportunistic bacteria [4,7,9,27] that were linked to the oral cavity. Therefore, future analyses should consider a broader spectrum of potential pathogens.

## Conclusions

Within the limitations of the present analysis, it was concluded that *Candida* spp. and other fungal organisms were frequently identified at peri-implantitis as well as healthy implant sites and co-colonized with *P. micra* and *T. forsythia*.

### Abbreviations

BOP: Bleeding on probing; *M. salivarium*: *Mycoplasma salivarium*; *P. gingivalis*: *Porphyromonas gingivalis*; *P. micra*: *Parvimonas micra*; PD: Probing pocket depth; *S. aureus*: *Staphylococcus aureus*; *T. forsythia*: *Tannerella forsythia*; *V. parvula*: *Veillonella parvula*.

### Competing interests

Frank Schwarz, Kathrin Becker, Sebastian Rahn, Andrea Hegewald, Klaus Pfeffer, and Birgit Henrich declare that they have no competing interests.

### Authors' contributions

FS, BH, and KP have made substantial contributions to study conception and design, analysis, and interpretation of data as well as manuscript preparation. KB performed the statistical analysis. AH and SR were involved in data acquisition. All authors read and approved the final manuscript.

### Acknowledgements

We kindly appreciate the skills and commitment of Ms. Dana Belick (Institute of Medical Microbiology and Hospital Hygiene, Heinrich Heine University, Düsseldorf) in the DNA preparation and bacterial analysis and the Jürgen Manchot Foundation for financial support.

### Author details

[1]Department of Oral Surgery, Westdeutsche Kieferklinik, Heinrich Heine University, Moorenstraße 5, D-40225 Düsseldorf, Germany. [2]Department of Orthodontics, Westdeutsche Kieferklinik, Heinrich Heine University, Moorenstraße 5, D-40225 Düsseldorf, Germany. [3]Institute of Medical Microbiology and Hospital Hygiene, Heinrich Heine University, Universitätsstraße 1, D-40225 Düsseldorf, Germany.

### References

1. Lindhe J, Meyle J, Group DoEWoP. Peri-implant diseases: consensus report of the sixth European workshop on periodontology. J Clin Periodontol. 2008;35:282–5.
2. Mombelli A, Decaillet F. The characteristics of biofilms in peri-implant disease. J Clin Periodontol. 2011;38 Suppl 11:203–13.
3. Heitz-Mayfield LJ. Peri-implant diseases: diagnosis and risk indicators. J Clin Periodontol. 2008;35:292–304.
4. Persson GR, Renvert S. Cluster of bacteria associated with peri-implantitis. Clin Implant Dent Relat Res. 2014;16:783–93.
5. Heuer W, Kettenring A, Stumpp SN, Eberhard J, Gellermann E, Winkel A, et al. Metagenomic analysis of the peri-implant and periodontal microflora in patients with clinical signs of gingivitis or mucositis. Clin Oral Investig. 2012;16:843–50.
6. Casado PL, Otazu IB, Balduino A, de Mello W, Barboza EP, Duarte ME. Identification of periodontal pathogens in healthy periimplant sites. Implant Dent. 2011;20:226–35.
7. Renvert S, Roos-Jansaker AM, Lindahl C, Renvert H, Rutger PG. Infection at titanium implants with or without a clinical diagnosis of inflammation. Clin Oral Implants Res. 2007;18:509–16.
8. Oliveira MA, Carvalho LP, Gomes Mde S, Bacellar O, Barros TF, Carvalho EM. Microbiological and immunological features of oral candidiasis. Microbiol Immunol. 2007;51:713–9.
9. Leonhardt A, Renvert S, Dahlen G. Microbial findings at failing implants. Clin Oral Implants Res. 1999;10:339–45.
10. Albertini M, Lopez-Cerero L, O'Sullivan MG, Chereguini CF, Ballesta S, Rios V, et al. Assessment of periodontal and opportunistic flora in patients with peri-implantitis. Clin Oral Implants Res. 2014; Apr 10. doi: 10.1111/clr.12387. [Epub ahead of print]
11. Lang NP, Berglundh T, Working Group 4 of Seventh European Workshop on P. Periimplant diseases: where are we now?–Consensus of the Seventh European Workshop on Periodontology. J Clin Periodontol. 2011;38 Suppl 11:178–81.
12. Henrich B, Schmitt M, Bergmann N, Zanger K, Kubitz R, Haussinger D, et al. Mycoplasma salivarium detected in a microbial community with Candida glabrata in the biofilm of an occluded biliary stent. J Med Microbiol. 2010;59:239–41.
13. Bizhang M, Ellerbrock B, Preza D, Raab W, Singh P, Beikler T, et al. Detection of nine microorganisms from the initial carious root lesions using a TaqMan-based real-time PCR. Oral Dis. 2011;17:642–52.
14. McDonald RR, Antonishyn NA, Hansen T, Snook LA, Nagle E, Mulvey MR, et al. Development of a triplex real-time PCR assay for detection of Panton-Valentine leukocidin toxin genes in clinical isolates of methicillin-resistant Staphylococcus aureus. J Clin Microbiol. 2005;43:6147–9.

15. Morillo JM, Lau L, Sanz M, Herrera D, Martin C, Silva A. Quantitative real-time polymerase chain reaction based on single copy gene sequence for detection of periodontal pathogens. J Clin Periodontol. 2004;31:1054–60.
16. Price RR, Viscount HB, Stanley MC, Leung KP. Targeted profiling of oral bacteria in human saliva and in vitro biofilms with quantitative real-time PCR. Biofouling. 2007;23:203–13.
17. Sanger F, Nicklen S, Coulson AR. DNA sequencing with chain-terminating inhibitors. Proc Natl Acad Sci U S A. 1977;74:5463–7.
18. Morgulis A, Coulouris G, Raytselis Y, Madden TL, Agarwala R, Schaffer AA. Database indexing for production MegaBLAST searches. Bioinformatics. 2008;24:1757–64.
19. Arendorf TM, Walker DM. The prevalence and intra-oral distribution of Candida albicans in man. Arch Oral Biol. 1980;25:1–10.
20. Helovuo H, Hakkarainen K, Paunio K. Changes in the prevalence of subgingival enteric rods, staphylococci and yeasts after treatment with penicillin and erythromycin. Oral Microbiol Immunol. 1993;8:75–9.
21. Odden K, Schenck K, Koppang H, Hurlen B. Candidal infection of the gingiva in HIV-infected persons. J Oral Pathol Med. 1994;23:178–83.
22. Nikawa H, Egusa H, Makihira S, Okamoto T, Kurihara H, Shiba H, et al. An in vitro evaluation of the adhesion of Candida species to oral and lung tissue cells. Mycoses. 2006;49:14–7.
23. Jabra-Rizk MA, Falkler Jr WA, Merz WG, Kelley JI, Baqui AA, Meiller TF. Coaggregation of Candida dubliniensis with Fusobacterium nucleatum. J Clin Microbiol. 1999;37:1464–8.
24. Thein ZM, Samaranayake YH, Samaranayake LP. Effect of oral bacteria on growth and survival of Candida albicans biofilms. Arch Oral Biol. 2006;51:672–80.
25. Shibli JA, Melo L, Ferrari DS, Figueiredo LC, Faveri M, Feres M. Composition of supra- and subgingival biofilm of subjects with healthy and diseased implants. Clin Oral Implants Res. 2008;19:975–82.
26. Hultin M, Gustafsson A, Hallstrom H, Johansson LA, Ekfeldt A, Klinge B. Microbiological findings and host response in patients with peri-implantitis. Clin Oral Implants Res. 2002;13:349–58.
27. Engel LD, Kenny GE. Mycoplasma salivarium in human gingival sulci. J Periodontal Res. 1970;5:163–71.
28. Jarvensivu A, Hietanen J, Rautemaa R, Sorsa T, Richardson M. Candida yeasts in chronic periodontitis tissues and subgingival microbial biofilms in vivo. Oral Dis. 2004;10:106–12.
29. Reynaud AH, Nygaard-Ostby B, Boygard GK, Eribe ER, Olsen I, Gjermo P. Yeasts in periodontal pockets. J Clin Periodontol. 2001;28:860–4.
30. Canabarro A, Valle C, Farias MR, Santos FB, Lazera M, Wanke B. Association of subgingival colonization of Candida albicans and other yeasts with severity of chronic periodontitis. J Periodontal Res. 2013;48:428–32.

# 7

# Is the presence of keratinized mucosa associated with periimplant tissue health? A clinical cross-sectional analysis

Catharina Ladwein, Rainer Schmelzeisen, Katja Nelson, Tabea Viktoria Fluegge and Tobias Fretwurst*

**Abstract**

**Background:** Long-term data concerning the impact of missing keratinized mucosa (KM) on periimplant tissue health are rare. The importance of KM for implant success remains unclear.

**Methods:** Two hundred eleven patients with 967 dental implants were analyzed up to 15 years after implant placement. Implants were divided into two groups: no keratinized mucosa (NKM) and KM. Evaluated parameters were plaque index (mAPI), bleeding index (mSBI), bleeding on probing (BOP), probing depth (PD), width of KM, and radiographic vertical bone level.

**Results:** mAPI, mSBI, and BOP were significantly higher for the NKM group. Implants of both groups showed no significant difference in PD and vertical bone level. Of the implants in the posterior regions ($n = 261$), 40.3% (regions 37 to 34, 44 to 47, 27 to 24, 17 to 14) showed NKM, whereas 30.4% of the implants in the anterior regions (regions 13 to 23; regions 33 to 43) presented NKM ($n = 97$).

**Conclusions:** Results indicate that the presence of KM has a positive effect on periimplant tissue health, but does not seem to have an influence on the periimplant bone level.

**Keywords:** Periimplantitis; Keratinized mucosa; Attached gingiva; Dental implants; Implantology

## Background

Various factors influence the long-term success of dental implants are bone quality and quantity, oral hygiene, medical conditions, mechanical factors such as the surgical procedure, and the subsequent prosthetic treatment [1-6]. The importance of keratinized mucosa (KM) surrounding the implant as a barrier against microorganisms and subgingival plaque as a factor for long-term success is discussed [7,8]. KM includes the gingival margin and the mucogingival junction [9]. A width of ≥2 mm of masticatory mucosa with ≥1 mm of attached gingiva has been proposed as adequate for gingival health [10]. Periimplant soft tissue differs from periodontal tissue [11-14]. The mucosa adjacent to the implant has been described to consist a marginal layer of junctional epithelium with a height (length) of 2 mm and a more apical zone of connective tissue with a height (length) of about 1.5 mm [11,15]. Periimplant mucosa is akin to scar tissue, and its fibers are orientated parallel to the implant surface [12,16]. Animal and human studies showed that the early soft tissue response to plaque is similar around teeth and implants, although periimplant tissue is supposed to be less resistant [17-22].

Hitherto the influence of KM on periimplant health remains to be discussed controversial [8,23,24]. One clinical study investigating implants failed to show the influence of the existence of KM on periimplant soft tissue health [23]. Current studies with moderate examination periods up to 5 years reported that higher plaque accumulation and gingival inflammation were associated with the absence of KM [25,26]. This statement is supported by several systematic reviews [27-29]. Dental implants with less than 2 mm of KM seem to be more prone to recession and alveolar bone loss, measured

* Correspondence: tobias.fretwurst@uniklinik-freiburg.de
Department of Oral and Craniomaxillofacial Surgery, Center for Dental Medicine, University Medical Center Freiburg, Hugstetter Straße 55, D-79106 Freiburg, Germany

between the crestal bone level and a reference point on the implant surface [26,30]. To determine the clinical periimplant status, defined parameters are available: implant mobility, radiographic bone level, probing depth (PD), plaque and gingival indices, bleeding on probing (BOP), and width of the KM [7,30].

The aim of the present study was to evaluate the relationship between the existence of KM and periimplant health regarding a larger collective in the long-term.

## Methods

This clinical cross-sectional study was conceived in accordance with the Helsinki Declaration of 1964, as revised in 2013. The study has been approved by the local ethical committee (University Medical Center Freiburg, no. 326_09).

### Population

Between February 1995 and December 2005, patients of the Clinic of Oral and Maxillofacial Surgery (Freiburg, Germany) who received endosseous dental implants (Tissue Level Standard Plus/Standard) of the Straumann-Dental Implant System (Straumann AG, Basel, Switzerland) were included in this monocentric clinical study. With the database PROMetheus Version III (KRZ, University medical center Freiburg), 620 patients with 2,667 dental implants were identified. Only those patients were evaluated who were available for follow-up investigation in 2009 to 2010. An evaluation of the incidence and reason for 'lost of follow-up' were not performed.

### Exclusion criteria

Exclusion criteria were diabetes, diseases of bone metabolism like osteoporosis, plasmozytoma, and osseous metastases, further malignant diseases in the head and neck region, bisphosphonat-, chemo-, or radiotherapy in the anamnesis, immunosuppressive diseases/therapies, pregnancy, and patient's age <18 years.

### Clinical parameters and measurements

Patients and implant-related parameters including gender, age at implant insertion, time of implant insertion, region of insertion, implant length, and implant diameter were assessed. The clinical examination was performed three times, with independent time points by a single examiner. Please refer to Tables 1, 2, and 3 for the description of the evaluated parameters.

Measurements were performed manually using a plastic periodontal probe (Plast-o-Probe®, Dentsply, York, PA, USA). All clinically measured distances were rounded to the nearest millimeter. Panoramic radiographs were used to assess the radiographic vertical bone level [31,32]. To account for dimensional distortions, the length of each implant was measured and correlated to the actual implant length. The vertical distance of the rough/smooth border of the implant to the first implant-bone contact was measured at the mesial and distal of each implant to define vertical bone level. The smooth-rough border is located either 2.8 mm (Tissue Level Standard) or 1.8 mm (Tissue Level Standard Plus) from the implant shoulder; this was regarded when radiologic measurements were performed. All examinations were performed on digital radiographs with a virtual measurement tool (SIDEXIS neXt Generation 2.4©, Sirona Dental Systems GmbH, Bensheim, Germany). Standardized radiographic examinations (orthopantomograms) were performed immediately after implant placement, before implant uncovery, in the first year every 6 months, and thereafter annually. The radiological analysis was performed by a single examiner (CL).

Case definition (Healthy, Mucositis, Periimplantitis) was performed according to the criteria of the seventh and eighth Workshop of the European Federation of Periodontology: 'In absence of previous radiographic records, a threshold vertical distance of 2 mm from the expected marginal bone level following remodeling post-implant placement is recommended, provided peri-implant inflammation is evident' [33]. If several implants were placed in a single patient, these were considered as individual implants, independent of each other.

### Statistical analysis

Implants were divided into two groups: no keratinized mucosa (NKM) = 0 mm of keratinized mucosa and

**Table 1 Evaluated implant parameters**

| Clinical | Radiological |
|---|---|
| mAPI [41] (see Table 2) | Radiographic bone level (vertical bone defect) |
| mSBI [41] (see Table 3) | |
| PD in millimeters at four sites of the implant [42] | |
| Presence or absence of BOP | |
| Width of the KM in millimeters at the mid-facial aspects of the implants marked with iodide solution [10,42] | |
| Implant mobility for single-tooth restorations [43] | |

**Table 2 Assessment of plaque accumulation by the mAPI**

| | Assessment of plaque accumulation |
|---|---|
| Score 0 | No detection of plaque |
| Score 1 | Plaque recognized by running a probe across the smooth marginal surface of the implant |
| Score 2 | Plaque can be seen by the naked eye |
| Score 3 | Abundance of soft matter |

**Table 3 Assessment of bleeding tendency by the mSBI**

| | Assessment of bleeding tendency |
|---|---|
| Score 0 | No bleeding when a periodontal probe is passed along the gingival margin adjacent to the implant |
| Score 1 | Isolated bleeding spots visible |
| Score 2 | Blood forms a confluent red line on margin |
| Score 3 | Heavy or profuse bleeding |

KM > 0 mm of keratinized mucosa. All quantitative parameters are shown as mean ± standard deviation. Statistical analyses were performed with Mann-Whitney *U* test and the chi-squared test using the software program SPSS 18.0 (PASW® Statistics, SPSS Inc., IBM Company, Chicago, IL, USA). A $p$ value < 0.05 was considered significant.

## Results

Two hundred eleven patients (97 = male, 114 = female) with 967 dental implants were available for follow-up examination. The mean observation period was 7.78 years ± 1.92 (4 to 15 years); the mean age at implant insertion was 54.63 years ± 13.58 (maximum 78 years).

Two hundred seventy-five implants were placed in the posterior regions of the lower jaw (34 to 37, 44 to 47), and 143 implants were placed in the anterior region of the lower jaw (33 to 43). In the maxilla, 373 implants were placed in the posterior regions (14 to 17, 24 to 27) and 176 implants were inserted in regions 13 to 23. Three hundred fifty-eight implants (37.02 %) did show NKM and 609 implants (62.98 %) showed KM. Of the implants in the posterior regions, 40.3% ($n$ = 261) did not present KM, whereas 59.7% ($n$ = 387) of posterior implants had KM (see Table 4). In the anterior regions, 30.4% ($n$ = 97) of the implants were classified NKM and 59.7% ($n$ = 222) were classified KM.

The mean width of KM was 1.87 ± 1.82 mm. Considering plaque index (mAPI), bleeding index (mSBI), and BOP implants with NKM showed significantly more plaque accumulation and bleeding than implants with KM (see Table 5). PD and vertical bone defect were not significantly different between both groups (PD mesial 3.78 ± 1.57 mm (NKM) vs. 3.61 ± 1.48 mm (KM), $p$ = 0.28) (see Table 6).

**Table 4 Distribution of presence of keratinized/non-keratinized gingiva with regard to the region**

| Region | Number of implants | NKM<br>*n* (%) | KM<br>*n* (%) |
|---|---|---|---|
| Posterior region maxilla | 373 | 134 (13.9) | 239 (24.7) |
| Anterior region maxilla | 176 | 54 (5.6) | 122 (12.6) |
| Posterior region mandible | 275 | 127 (13.1) | 148 (15) |
| Anterior region mandible | 143 | 43 (4.5) | 100 (10.3) |

**Table 5 Results for mAPI, mSBI, and BOP for implants with either keratinized mucosa or no keratinized mucosa**

| | | NKM (%) | KM (%) | *p* value |
|---|---|---|---|---|
| mAPI | Score 0 | 24.3 | 32.8 | <0.05 |
| | Score 1 | 19.0 | 36.1 | |
| | Score 2 | 23.9 | 18.1 | |
| | Score 3 | 32.7 | 12.9 | |
| mSBI | Score 0 | 32.9 | 46.3 | <0.05 |
| | Score 1 | 20.8 | 28.4 | |
| | Score 2 | 31.1 | 18.5 | |
| | Score 3 | 15.2 | 6.8 | |
| BOP | Distal | 46.1 | 35.9 | <0.05 |
| | Buccal | 43.7 | 32.1 | <0.05 |
| | Mesial | 57.7 | 50.6 | 0.55 |

## Discussion

Multiple investigators discussed the necessity of KM around dental implants [28]. But still, there is a lack of evidence whether KM has an impact on periimplant tissue health and periimplant bone level, respectively [27,29]. The main reason for this limitation is the heterogeneity in study designs and data extraction; consecutively, there is a lack of a synoptic statistical analysis [34]. The present study examined the aforementioned issue in a large collective in the long-term. According to a recent review comparing 19 relevant publications out of 217 articles, only 1 study has a comparable, slightly larger, collective with a similar observation period (>10 years) [34,35]. Roos-Jansaker et al. demonstrated with a univariate and multivariate analyses that the presence of KM is associated with a mucositis [35].

The influence of KM on oral plaque accumulation and hygiene measures is discussed controversially in literature. In the present study, patients with NKM show significantly more plaque accumulation than patients with

**Table 6 PD and bone level for implants regarding the soft tissue condition**

| | NKM<br>Mean SD<br>(mm) | KM<br>Mean SD<br>(mm) | *p* value |
|---|---|---|---|
| PD distal | 3.3 ± 1.4 | 3.5 ± 1.5 | 0.21 |
| PD buccal | 2.9 ± 1.3 | 2.9 ± 1.3 | 0.81 |
| PD mesial | 3.8 ± 1.6 | 3.6 ± 1.5 | 0.28 |
| Vertical bone defect distal | 0.8 ± 1.4 | 0.7 ± 1.2 | 0.70 |
| Vertical bone defect mesial | 0.9 ± 1.2 | 0.8 ± 1.3 | 0.31 |

KM. Human studies with substantially smaller cohorts confirm these results and reported even higher plaque scores at implant sites in the absence of KM [7,25,26,30,36,37] On the other hand, several longitudinal studies revealed no significant association between higher plaque scores and KM level [11,23,38,39].

A similar ambivalence exists for the bleeding after probing parameter in literature [34]. The present study shows significantly higher values of BOP and mSBI in the absence of KM. KM is supposed to be a physical barrier, and the absence of it seems to provide easier apical migration of inflammation [28,30]. KM has been assumed to prevent mechanical damage evoked by toothbrushing and/or masticatory forces [20,39].

In this study, only one implant type (Straumann, Tissue Level) with a polished neck was examined. Therefore, the acquired data may not represent different implant designs and emergence profiles. Some authors established studies with a range of different implant surfaces like sandblasted with large grit and acid-etched surfaces or anodized surfaces. Other authors give no description of the implant surface conditions [7,39]. The implant type and material may influence the periimplant parameters especially the bone level. It is discussed whether machined surfaces are more favorable for periimplant soft tissue parameters [40]. But different implant surface conditions may alter the effect on KM [28,40]. To identify influencing factors like implant surface or occlusal overload, longitudinal prospective studies with a standardized protocol are needed.

In the present study, the mean width of KM was $1.87 \pm 1.82$ mm. Thus, our results suggest that even smaller amounts of KM may be sufficient for periimplant health, in contrast to the values claimed by other authors [7,10]. According to our state of knowledge, no data exist on the amount of KM remaining after the removal of a tooth with consideration of the anatomical region. Our data reveal no difference in the amount of KM in certain anatomical regions of the maxilla and mandible.

There was no significant difference in PD and vertical bone defect between both groups. A 4-year prospective longitudinal study confirms these results and showed no significant difference in the proximal periimplant bone level between implants with KM or NKM, respectively [36]. Cross-sectional studies reported an impact of missing KM on the mean loss of alveolar bone around implants [30,39]. Large, randomized, and long-term multicenter studies with regard to the different implant surfaces and materials are necessary to investigate further association between the existence of KM and periimplant bone level.

## Conclusions

The present findings indicate a correlation between periimplant soft tissue health and the presence of KM. Dental implants lacking KM showed significantly more plaque accumulation and BOP than implants with a zone of KM. The presence of KM did not have a significant influence on the vertical periimplant bone level.

**Competing interests**

The study was supported by a research grant of the ITI foundation (ITI Research Grant No. 704_2010). Catharina Ladwein, Rainer Schmelzeisen, Katja Nelson, Tabea Viktoria Fluegge, and Tobias Fretwurst declare that they have no competing interests.

**Authors' contributions**

CL, KN, and TF conceived the study. CL, TVF, and TF participated in the design of the study and performed the statistical analysis. CL, RS, KN, TVF, and TF drafted the manuscript. All authors read and approved the final manuscript.

**Acknowledgements**

The authors gratefully acknowledge Lioudmila Bogatyreva of the Institute for Medical Biometry and Medical Informatics of Albert-Ludwigs-University of Freiburg for her assistance with statistics.

**References**

1. Belibasakis GN. Microbiological and immuno-pathological aspects of peri-implant diseases. Arch Oral Biol. 2014;59(1):66–72.
2. Cappiello M, Luongo R, Di Iorio D, Bugea C, Cocchetto R, Celletti R. Evaluation of peri-implant bone loss around platform-switched implants. Int J Periodontics Restorative Dent. 2008;28(4):347–55.
3. Cehreli M, Sahin S, Akça K. Role of mechanical environment and implant design on bone tissue differentiation: current knowledge and future contexts. J Dent. 2004;32(2):123–32.
4. Karthik K, Sivakumar S, Thangaswamy V. Evaluation of implant success: a review of past and present concepts. J Pharm Bioallied Sci. 2013;5 Suppl 1:117–9.
5. Peñarrocha-Diago MA, Flichy-Fernández AJ, Alonso-González R, Peñarrocha-Oltra D, Balaguer-Martínez J, Peñarrocha-Diago M. Influence of implant neck design and implant-abutment connection type on peri-implant health. Radiological study. Clin Oral Implants Res. 2013;24(11):1192–200.
6. Steigenga JT, Al-Shammari KF, Nociti FH, Misch CE, Wang HL. Dental implant design and its relationship to long-term implant success. Implant Dent. 2003;12(4):306–17.
7. Adibrad M, Shahabuei M, Sahabi M. Significance of the width of keratinized mucosa on the health status of the supporting tissue around implants supporting overdentures. J Oral Implantol. 2009;35(5):232–7.
8. Wennström JL, Bengazi F, Lekholm U. The influence of the masticatory mucosa on the peri-implant soft tissue condition. Clin Oral Implants Res. 1994;5(1):1–8.
9. Orban B. Clinical and histologic study of the surface characteristics of the gingiva. Oral Surg Oral Med Oral Pathol. 1948;1(9):827–41.
10. Lang NP, Löe H. The relationship between the width of keratinized gingiva and gingival health. J Periodontol. 1972;43(10):623–7.
11. Abrahamsson I, Berglundh T, Wennström J, Lindhe J. The peri-implant hard and soft tissues at different implant systems. A comparative study in the dog. Clin Oral Implants Res. 1996;7(3):212–9.
12. Berglundh T, Lindhe J, Ericsson I, Marinello CP, Liljenberg B, Thomsen P. The soft tissue barrier at implants and teeth. Clin Oral Implants Res. 1991;2(2):81–90.
13. Berglundh T, Lindhe J, Jonsson K, Ericsson I. The topography of the vascular systems in the periodontal and peri-implant tissues in the dog. J Clin Periodontol. 1994;21(3):189–93.
14. Ericsson I, Lindhe J. Probing depth at implants and teeth. An experimental study in the dog. J Clin Periodontol. 1993;20(9):623–7.
15. Berglundh T, Lindhe J. Dimension of the periimplant mucosa. Biological width revisited. J Clin Periodontol. 1996;23(10):971–3.
16. Buser D, Weber HP, Donath K, Fiorellini JP, Paquette DW, Williams RC. Soft tissue reactions to non-submerged unloaded titanium implants in beagle dogs. J Periodontol. 1992;63(3):225–35.

17. Ericsson I, Berglundh T, Marinello C, Liljenberg B, Lindhe J. Long-standing plaque and gingivitis at implants and teeth in the dog. Clin Oral Implants Res. 1992;3(3):99–103.
18. Leonhardt A, Berglundh T, Ericsson I, Dahlén G. Putative periodontal pathogens on titanium implants and teeth in experimental gingivitis and periodontitis in beagle dogs. Clin Oral Implants Res. 1992;3(3):112–9.
19. Schou S, Holmstrup P, Stoltze K, Hjørting-Hansen E, Fiehn NE, Skovgaard LT. Probing around implants and teeth with healthy or inflamed peri-implant mucosa/gingiva. A histologic comparison in cynomolgus monkeys (Macaca fascicularis). Clin Oral Implants Res. 2002;13(2):113–26.
20. Schou S, Holmstrup P, Hjørting-Hansen E, Lang NP. Plaque-induced marginal tissue reactions of osseointegrated oral implants: a review of the literature. Clin Oral Implants Res. 1992;3(4).149–61.
21. Zitzmann NU, Berglundh T, Marinello CP, Lindhe J. Experimental peri-implant mucositis in man. J Clin Periodontol. 2001;28(6):517–23.
22. Pontoriero R, Tonelli MP, Carnevale G, Mombelli A, Nyman SR, Lang NP. Experimentally induced peri-implant mucositis. A clinical study in humans. Clin Oral Implants Res. 1994;5(4):254–9.
23. Adell R, Lekholm U, Rockler B, Brånemark PI, Lindhe J, Eriksson B, et al. Marginal tissue reactions at osseointegrated titanium fixtures (I). A 3-year longitudinal prospective study. Int J Oral Maxillofac Surg. 1986;15(1):39–52.
24. Mericske-Stern R, Steinlin Schaffner T, Marti P, Geering AH. Peri-implant mucosal aspects of ITI implants supporting overdentures. A five-year longitudinal study. Clin Oral Implants Res. 1994;5(1):9–18.
25. Chung DM, Oh TJ, Shotwell JL, Misch CE, Wang HL. Significance of keratinized mucosa in maintenance of dental implants with different surfaces. J Periodontol. 2006;77(8):1410–20.
26. Schrott AR, Jimenez M, Hwang JW, Fiorellini J, Weber HP. Five-year evaluation of the influence of keratinized mucosa on peri-implant soft-tissue health and stability around implants supporting full-arch mandibular fixed prostheses. Clin Oral Implants Res. 2009;20(10):1170–7.
27. Gobbato L, Avila-Ortiz G, Sohrabi K, Wang CW, Karimbux N. The effect of keratinized mucosa width on peri-implant health: a systematic review. Int J Oral Maxillofac Implants. 2013;28(6):1536–45.
28. Brito C, Tenenbaum HC, Wong BK, Schmitt C, Nogueira-Filho G. Is keratinized mucosa indispensable to maintain peri-implant health? A systematic review of the literature. J Biomed Mater Res B Appl Biomater. 2014;102(3):643–50.
29. Lin GH, Chan HL, Wang HL. The significance of keratinized mucosa on implant health: a systematic review. J Periodontol. 2013;84(12):1755–67.
30. Bouri Jr A, Bissada N, Al-Zahrani MS, Faddoul F, Nouneh I. Width of keratinized gingiva and the health status of the supporting tissues around dental implants. Int J Oral Maxillofac Implants. 2008;23(2):323–6.
31. Kullman L, Al-Asfour A, Zetterqvist L, Andersson L. Comparison of radiographic bone height assessments in panoramic and intraoral radiographs of implant patients. Int J Oral Maxillofac Implants. 2007;22(1):96–100.
32. Zechner W, Watzak G, Gahleitner A, Busenlechner D, Tepper G, Watzek G. Rotational panoramic versus intraoral rectangular radiographs for evaluation of peri-implant bone loss in the anterior atrophic mandible. Int J Oral Maxillofac Implants. 2003;18(6):873–8.
33. Sanz M, Chapple IL, Working Group 4 of the VIII European Workshop on Periodontology. Clinical research on peri-implant diseases: consensus report of Working Group 4. J Clin Periodontol. 2012;39 Suppl 12:202–6.
34. Wennström JL, Derks J. Is there a need for keratinized mucosa around implants to maintain health and tissue stability? Clin Oral Implants Res. 2012;23 Suppl 6:136–46.
35. Roos-Jansåker AM, Renvert H, Lindahl C, Renvert S. Nine- to fourteen-year follow-up of implant treatment. Part III: factors associated with peri-implant lesions. J Clin Periodontol. 2006;33(4):296–301.
36. Crespi R, Capparè P, Gherlone E. A 4-year evaluation of the peri-implant parameters of immediately loaded implants placed in fresh extraction sockets. J Periodontol. 2010;81(11):1629–34.
37. Boynueğri D, Nemli SK, Kasko YA. Significance of keratinized mucosa around dental implants: a prospective comparative study. Clin Oral Implants Res. 2013;24(8):928–33.
38. Heckmann SM, Schrott A, Graef F, Wichmann MG, Weber HP. Mandibular two-implant telescopic overdentures. Clin Oral Implants Res. 2004;15(5):560–9.
39. Kim BS, Kim YK, Yun PY, Yi YJ, Lee HJ, Kim SG, et al. Evaluation of peri-implant tissue response according to the presence of keratinized mucosa. Oral Surg Oral Med Oral Pathol Oral Radiol Endod. 2009;107(3):e24–8.
40. Lee S, Goh BT, Wolke J, Tideman H, Stoelinga P, Jansen J. Soft tissue adaptation to modified titanium surfaces. J Biomed Mater Res A. 2010;95(2):543–9.
41. Mombelli A, van Oosten MA, Schurch Jr E, Land NP. The microbiota associated with successful or failing osseointegrated titanium implants. Oral Microbiol Immunol. 1987;2(4):145–51.
42. Buser D, Weber HP, Brägger U. The treatment of partially edentulous patients with ITI hollow-screw implants: presurgical evaluation and surgical procedures. Int J Oral Maxillofac Implants. 1990;5(2):165–75.
43. Lindhe J, Nyman S. The role of occlusion in periodontal disease and the biological rationale for splinting in treatment of periodontitis. Oral Sci Rev. 1977;10:11–43.

# Temperature rise during removal of fractured components out of the implant body: an *in vitro* study comparing two ultrasonic devices and five implant types

Eric W Meisberger[1*], Sjoerd J G Bakker[1] and Marco S Cune[1,2]

**Abstract**

**Background:** Ultrasonic instrumentation under magnification may facilitate mobilization of screw remnants but may induce heat trauma to surrounding bone. An increase of 5°C is considered detrimental to osseointegration. The objective of this investigation was to examine the rise in temperature of the outer implant body after 30 s of ultrasonic instrumentation to the inner part, in relation to implant type, type of ultrasonic equipment, and the use of coolants *in vitro*.

**Methods:** Two ultrasonic devices (Satelec Suprasson T Max and Electro Medical Systems (EMS) miniMaster) were used on five different implant types that were provided with a thermo couple (Astra 3.5 mm, bone level Regular CrossFit (RC) 4.1 mm, bone level Narrow CrossFit (NC) 3.3 mm, Straumann tissue level regular body regular neck 3.3 mm, and Straumann tissue level wide body regular neck 4.8 mm), either with or without cooling during 30 s. Temperature rise at this point in time is the primary outcome measure. In addition, the mean maximum rise in temperature (all implants combined) was assessed and statistically compared among devices, implant systems, and cooling mode (independent *t*-tests, ANOVA, and post hoc analysis).

**Results:** The Satelec device without cooling induces the highest temperature change of up to 13°C, particularly in both bone level implants ($p < 0.05$) but appears safe for approximately 10 s of continuous instrumentation, after which a cooling down period is rational. Cooling is effective for both devices. However, when the Satelec device is used with coolant for a longer period of time, a rise in temperature must be anticipated after cessation of instrumentation, and post-operational cooling is advised.

**Conclusions:** The in vitro setup used in this experiment implies that care should be taken when translating the observations to clinical recommendations, but it is carefully suggested that the EMS device causes limited rise in temperature, even without coolant.

**Keywords:** Implant; Abutment; Complication; Fracture

* Correspondence: e.w.meisberger@umcg.nl
[1]University Medical Center Groningen, Center for Dentistry and Oral Hygiene, Department of Fixed and Removable Prosthodontics and Biomaterials, The University of Groningen, Gebouw 3216, kamer 206, A. Deusinglaan 1, 9713 AV Groningen, The Netherlands
Full list of author information is available at the end of the article

## Background

Complications in implant dentistry are generally divided into biological and mechanical complications. Mechanical complications include fracture of the implant body or prosthetic components such as chipping of ceramic material as well as loosening or fracture of implant abutments or fixation screws. This has a documented prevalence of 6 to 13% and 0.4 to 2% respectively after 5 years [1-7].

With respect to the etiology of screw loosening, several causes are to be considered [8]. Screw-nut systems generally become unstable when the load that is applied to the system exceeds that of the preload of the screw that causes a clamping force preventing separation of the joint [9]. Preload is proportional to the tightening torque at placement. Hence, tightening torque on the one hand has a significant effect on screw loosening [10]. Embedment relaxation or settling can be overcome by retorquing abutment screws after a certain period of time, increasing joint stability [9,11]. On the other hand, the magnitude of forces applied to the system is of major influence. The transfer of high forces can be generated by bruxers, through non-occlusal loading or because of a non-passive fit of suprastructures [8,12-15]. Other factors that are of influence of a systems' resistance to screw loosening include lubrication, screw design, screw material, and surface characteristics [16-20]. Especially implant designs with an external hex configuration are prone to abutment screw loosening [21].

Fracture of abutments or abutment screws can be contributed to acute trauma, chronic overload, production flaws, or errors in screw-nut design. If fractured screw components cannot be removed, it may render the implant unrestorable or forces the dentist to creative solutions, such as cementable components. Fortunately, fractured screw components will generally be loose because the preload has not been retained. In that case, they may be removed by manipulating them counter clockwise with a straight probing instrument. On occasion, screw remnants cannot be mobilized, and removal remains a clinical challenge. Careful instrumentation when attempting to remove them should prevent damage to the internal thread of the implant and its surrounding tissues. The use of a fine-tipped hand instrument, a round burr turning counter clockwise, or drilling a slot in the screw in order to get more grip can be attempted to loosen the fragment. Specific instrumentation to remove broken screws from implants is available from most implant suppliers.

The use of ultrasonic equipment under adequate magnification may facilitate removal. It generates heat. Instrumentation without a coolant likely increases the temperature of the implant body and could cause tissue damage, in particular be harmful to osseointegration. The use of a coolant could be effective, but compromises visibility considerably, hence increases the risk of damaging the internal configuration of the implant.

Results from an experimental heat conduction model investigating the ranges of temperature gradients occurring in implants demonstrate that a 60°C heat source causes a heat front exceeding 47°C and advances more than 3 mm down an implant within 1 s [22]. Temperatures over 47°C for more than a minute cause necrosis of cortical bone [23-25]. Some studies investigating the potential harmfulness of intraoral abutment preparation or plaster on implants to osseointegration mention this threshold as harmful [26-28]. It has been postulated that a rise in temperature to 42°C causes denaturation of osteoblasts and should be considered the temperature threshold of transient changes in bone [25]. This threshold was used by others when investigating the potentially damaging effect to the implant-bone interface as a result of drinking hot beverages [29-31]. Also from endodontic literature regarding the removal of metal endodontic posts, concerns have been raised based on observations from *in vitro* experiments with respect to potentially detrimental heat transformation through dentine while ultrasonically manipulating the post [32-37].

The objective of this investigation is to examine the rise in temperature of the outer surface of an implant body after 30 s of ultrasonic instrumentation of its inner part in relation to type of ultrasonic equipment, implant type, and the use of coolants *in vitro*.

## Methods

Two different types of commercially available ultrasonic devices, set at their lowest intensity for endodontic purpose, were used to instrument the internal portion of five different implant types, either with or without cooling. Intermittent anti-clockwise strokes were made, assuring that the tip was constantly in contact with the inner implant wall, as much as possible mimicking the motion that would have been used in clinical practice.

The ultrasonic devices used were the Satelec Suprasson T Max (Acteon Group, Merignac, France) and the EMS miniMaster (EMS, Electro Medical Systems SA, Nyon, Switzerland) with non-diamant, non-cutting tips ET 20, Satelec, and Instrument A (EMS). The device allowed for internal cooling of the tip with the cooling liquid at 31°C during instrumentation.

The implants used were from different brands; all 8-mm long but with various diameters and designs: Astra 3.5 mm (Dentsply Implants, Mölndal, Sweden), bone level Regular CrossFit (RC) 4.1 mm, bone level Narrow CrossFit (NC) 3.3 mm, Straumann tissue level regular body regular neck 3.3 mm (Straumann, Basel, Switzerland), and Straumann tissue level wide body regular neck 4.8 mm (Straumann AG, Basel, Switzerland). A single implant per group was used. They were embedded in epoxy resin, with a thermocouple (TC-08, Pico Technology, St. Neots, Great Britain) glued to the outer implant surface, at a level corresponding with the anticipated marginal bone level in uncompromised conditions. The change in temperature was registered for 30 s, followed by a 30-s cooling down period, at 5-s intervals (Figure 1).

### Statistical analysis

The primary outcome variable was defined as the difference in temperature between the start of instrumentation and after 30 s when comparing the different implants and the maximum rise in temperature (deltaTmax) where results were averaged per experimental condition (type of device, with or without coolant). All tests were performed three times, and the results were averaged per condition. Differences between several experimental conditions were analyzed by means of independent *t*-tests and univariate analysis of variance, after verification of normal distribution by human eyeballing and the Kolmogorov-Smirnov test. Where appropriate, post hoc analysis was performed using the Student-Newman-Keuls multiple comparison test. The value for $\alpha$ was set at 0.05 to distinguish statistical significancy.

## Results

The results for all implants instrumented with the two tested ultrasonic devices, either with or without cooling, are presented in Figure 2a,b,c,d.

For the Satelec device, applied *without* coolant, only the temperature of the Straumann wide body regular neck implant never exceeded the 50 threshold. The data proved normally distributed (Kolmogorov-Smirnov test, $p > 0.05$). Analysis of variance indicated statistically significant differences among the implant types ($F = 33.3$, *df* 4, $p < 0.001$). The highest mean temperature increase at 30 s was seen around the 3.3-mm bone level implant (13.0°C), followed by the 4.1-mm bone level implant (9.5°C), and subsequently by the other three implant types (Student-Newman-Keuls (SNK) test, Figure 2a). When coolant was used during instrumentation, an increase of temperature exceeding 5°C was not seen. There were some differences between the implant types (ANOVA, $F = 6.4$, *df* 4, $p < 0.01$), primarily between the bone level 3.3 mm and Astra 3.5-mm implant on the one hand and both Straumann tissue level implants on the other hand (SNK test). Interestingly, when instrumentation and cooling had stopped, the outer temperature of all implants raised markedly above the 5°C critical threshold during the following 10 s, for both bone level implant types up to approximately 10°C (Figure 2b).

For the EMS device when applied *without* cooling, an increase at 30 s above the threshold was only seen for the 3.3- and 4.1-mm bone level implant types (approximately 6°C), which was statistically significantly higher than the rise in temperature seen in the other three implant types (ANOVA, $F = 3.4$, $df = 4$, $p = 0.04$, and SNK test, Figure 2c). Cooling the EMS device proved pretty efficient at 30 s, without differences between the groups. Only a mild increase of the outer temperature was observed to a maximum of 2°C. It takes some time for cooling to take effect. When instrumentation and cooling is stopped, no increase of outer implant temperature occurs, which contrasts the findings with the Satelec device (Figure 2d).

The mean maximum rise in temperature (deltaTmax, all implants averaged per experimental condition) was reached at 30 to 40 s for all conditions. There was a significant difference for the Satelec device without cooling (mean 9.6, SD 1.6°C) and the EMS device without cooling (mean 4.3, SD 2.0°C) (*t*-test, $t(28) = 4.7$, $p < 0.001$). When using coolant, the deltaTmax for the Satelec device (mean 8.3, SD 1.3°C) was significantly higher than for the EMS device (mean 1.6, SD 0.6°C) (*t*-test, $t(28) = 17.9$, $p < 0.001$).

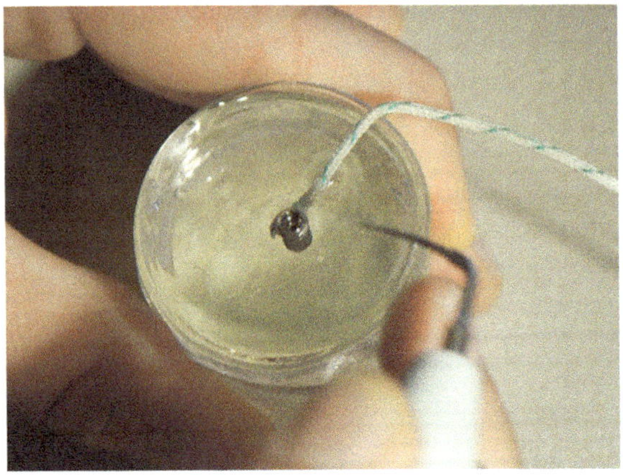

**Figure 1** Implant embedded in epoxy resin with thermocouple at the outer surface.

## Discussion

Several techniques have been described to deal with biomechanical complications. Acquiring adequate visibility and access is essential to success which will require the use of a dental microscope.

Several mechanical approaches to remove screw remnants can be employed. Generally, after identifying the position and condition of the screw remnant, it can be carefully removed using manual instrumentation. A fine-tipped hand instrument may be wedged between screw and implant. If this fails to do the trick, the use of a round burr applying occlusal pressure and turning counter clockwise may loosen the fragment. When a flared burr is wedged between implant and screw remnant, the drill should make a clockwise action, to direct the screw

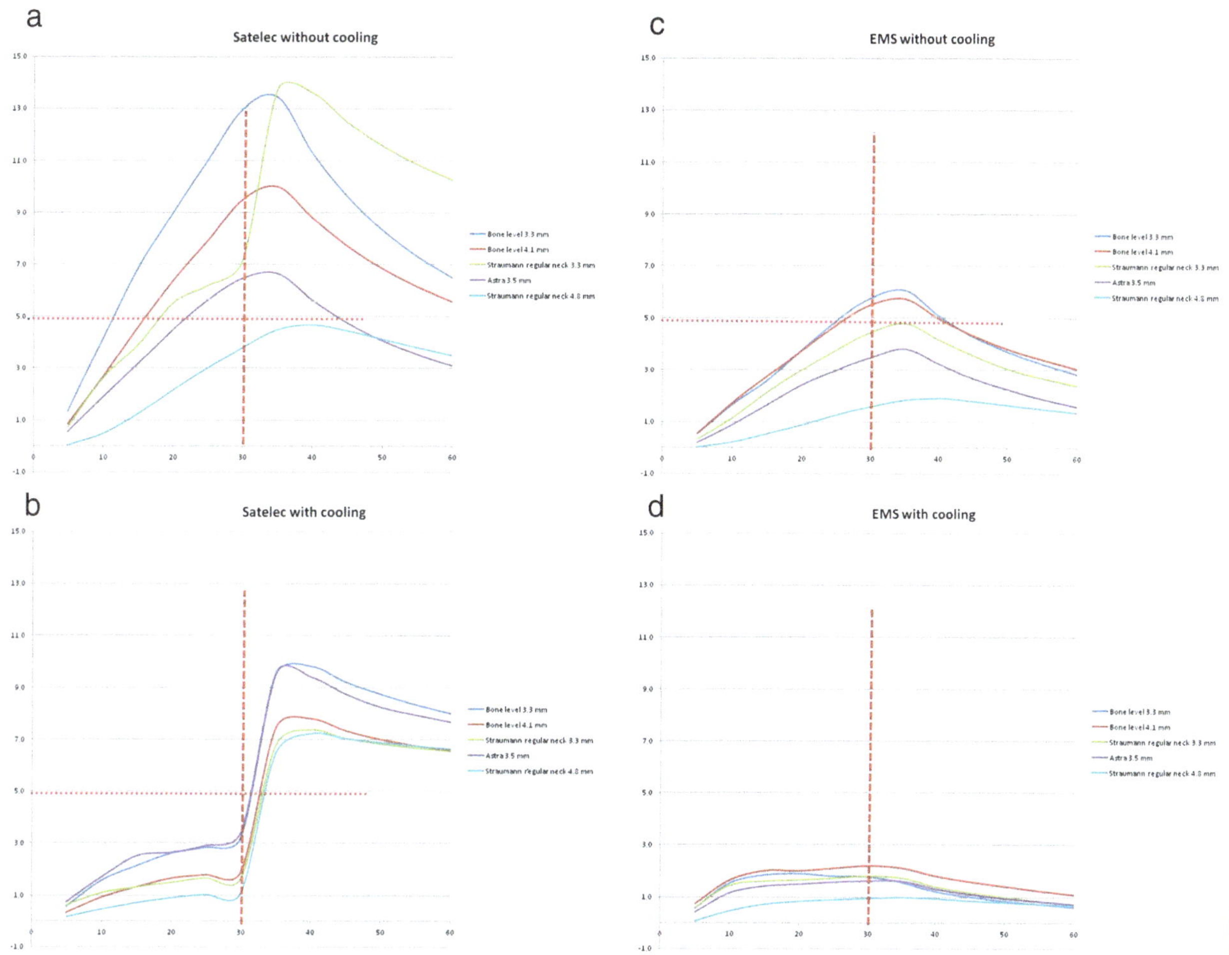


**Figure 2 Results for all implants instrumented with two tested ultrasonic devices, either with or without cooling. (a)** Temperature rise when instrumenting with the Satelec ultrasonic device without cooling. The horizontal dotted line denotes the assumed critical rise in temperature. Temperature rise at 30 s: bone level 3.3 mm > bone level 4.1 mm > Straumann regular neck 3.3 mm = Astra 3.5 mm = Straumann regular neck 4.8 mm. **(b)** Temperature rise when instrumenting with the Satelec ultrasonic device with cooling. The horizontal dotted line denotes the assumed critical rise in temperature. Temperature rise at 30 s: bone level 3.3 mm = Astra 3.5 implant > Straumann regular neck 3.3 mm = Straumann regular neck 4.8 mm. Temperature rise at the bone level 4.1 implant lies in between the bone level 3.3 mm and Astra 3.5 mm implant and both Straumann implants, but not significantly different from either of these implants. **(c)** EMS without cooling. Temperature rise at 30 s: bone level 3.3 mm = bone level 4.1 mm > Straumann regular neck 3.3 mm = Astra 3.5 mm = Straumann regular neck 4.8 mm. **(d)** EMS with cooling. No statistically significant differences between the implant types at 30 s.

in the counterclockwise direction. Cutting a deep slot in the screw and subsequently removing it with a bladed screw driver has also been advised. The use of rotary instrumentation may cause damage to the cranial inner portion of the implant body. If that occurs, even when the fragment (finally) loosens, it will not screw out, and this complicates matters considerably.

Most implant suppliers, and also some third parties, provide specific instrumentation to remove broken screws from implants (i.e., Certain screw removal kit, Biomet 3I, Palm Beach Gardens, United States; screw removal kit NobelReplace, Nobel Biocare, Göteborg, Sweden; Neo screw remover kit, Neobiotech Co, South Korea). In general, they screw into the center of the screw remnant, which facilitates another burr to grip it and remove it counter clockwise or fragmentate the screw remnant.

The use of ultrasonic equipment has also proven to be effective in dislodging fixed screw remnants at the risk of damaging the inner portion or overheating the implant. Hence, the use of magnification is a must and cooling may be advisable, but compromises the vision of the operator. The present study evaluated heat accumulation *in vitro* and the efficiency of cooling when using two types of ultrasonic equipment to the inner portion of several implants.

The degree to which a material is able to transfer heat is called thermal conductivity. It can be defined as the time rate of transfer by conduction, through unit thickness, across unit area for unit temperature gradient. Differences in design and wall thickness of the implants used in the present study account for the variation in outcome (i.e., Straumann tissue level 4.8 implant less effected), considering the fact that all implant types used are made from the same material: grade 4 commercially pure (CP) titanium. The thermal conductivity of CP titanium is relatively low compared to, for instance, that of steel (1/4) and aluminum (1/13). On the other hand, it is approximately 60% higher than that of grade 5 titanium alloy (16.3 $W \cdot m^{-1} \cdot K^{-1}$ for grade 4 CP titanium compared to 7.2 $W \cdot m^{-1} \cdot K^{-1}$ for grade 5 Ti-6Al-4 V). The former material is used in several other implant brands than the ones used here [38], and as a consequence, the results cannot be extrapolated to those systems. The data from this *in vitro* experiment can only be generalized to the clinical situation bearing in mind some inherent limitations and assumptions. The epoxy resin used does not resemble alveolar bone, its structure, water content, and potential to cope with thermal challenges. It is unlikely that wall thickness, design, and material between different implants from the same implant type will vary because of the high degree of current precision and standardization achieved during the fabrication of implants. Consequently, only one specimen per brand was used. To correct for variation during the instrumentation of the ultrasonic device, the experiment was performed three times.

The results show that both 1. the type of implant and 2. the type of ultrasonic device (and in especially the use of coolant) affect the amount of temperature rise to the outer implant surface. Both bone level implants in particular appear to heat up the most. Without the use of coolant, the heat accumulation was much higher with the Satelec compared to the EMS device and exceeded the theoretical threshold for permanent biological damage after 10 to 15 s of continuous instrumentation (Figure 2a, c) and differed statistically significant at deltaTmax. There may be several explanations for this, but most likely, the produced energy at the point of the tip for the Satelec device was higher. Both devices were set at their lowest possible level. The present authors have not been able to verify what energy levels are actually produced. The former is presumed linear to the frequency and the deflection/amplitude of the tip. The frequency is mentioned in the product documentation (Satelec: 27 to 33 kHz and the EMS: 24 to 32 kHz) but the amplitudes differ per tip and are not disclosed. The effect of the difference in coolant spray between the two instruments is also a factor that needs considering when interpreting the data.

Cooling proves effective for both systems, increasing the outer implant temperature by an acceptable 1°C to 3°C during continued instrumentation; however, as already stated, the spray will blur the vision of the operator.

One would expect the temperature to drop immediately after cessation of instrumentation and cooling, but the peak temperature is reached some seconds later for all experimental conditions, so regardless of device, use of coolant, or implant type (Figure 2a,b,c,d). Others, instrumenting endodontic posts in natural teeth [32,33], also saw a 'lag' period with a rise in temperature after cessation that lasted up to 9 s post-instrumentation. They left it unexplained. We offer two possible explanations. Firstly, ultrasonic instrumentation causes the implant wall and its surrounding tissues (in this case, resin and thermocouple, but *in vivo*, this would be surrounding alveolar bone) to vibrate and generate heat. Vibration continues some time after cessation of instrumentation, explaining the continued rise in temperature. Secondly, after cooling has stopped, generated and stored heat in the surrounding 'tissues' may flow back to the outer wall of the implant that is no longer cooled from the inside and raises the temperature. The potentially damaging rise in temperature ('explosion') seen for the Satelec device, but not for the EMS device when instrumentation and cooling was stopped, could be explained by these phenomena on the one hand and by the fact that energy produced by the Satelec device was presumably higher on the other hand (Figure 2b).

## Conclusions

It is concluded from this *in vitro* study that heat accumulation and transfer is dependent on the type of ultrasonic device, the use of coolant, and the implant type. The highest rise in temperature is seen when using the Satelec device without coolant on the smaller diameter implants. The EMS device causes limited rise in temperature when used without coolant for less than 10 s, but presumably delivers less energy to the tip, and consequently may be not as effective. A cooling down period is sensible. When used with coolant for a longer period of time, the clinician should anticipate a considerable rise in temperature after cessation of instrumentation, and post-operational cooling is advised.

### Competing interests

This research was made possible by the support of the authors' institutions. Eric W Meisberger, Sjoerd JG Bakker and Marco S Cune declare that they have no competing interests.

### Authors' contributions

EM and SB carried out the experiment. MC participated in the design of the study and performed the statistical analysis and helped to draft the manuscript. All authors read and approved the final manuscript.

### Acknowledgements

The input of Prashant K. Sharma PhD, material scientist of the Department of Biomedical Engineering (Kolff Institute) of the UMC Groningen is greatly appreciated for his help interpreting the data. Michael Kars, DDS assisted during the collection of the data.

**Author details**
[1]University Medical Center Groningen, Center for Dentistry and Oral Hygiene, Department of Fixed and Removable Prosthodontics and Biomaterials, The University of Groningen, Gebouw 3216, kamer 206, A. Deusinglaan 1, 9713 AV Groningen, The Netherlands. [2]Department of Oral-Maxillofacial Surgery, Prosthodontics and Special Dental Care, St. Antonius Hospital Nieuwegein, Koekoekslaan 1, 3435 CM Nieuwegein, The Netherlands.

## References

1. Sailer I, Philipp A, Zembic A, Pjetursson BE, Hammerle CH, Zwahlen M. A systematic review of the performance of ceramic and metal implant abutments supporting fixed implant reconstructions. Clin Oral Implants Res. 2009;20 Suppl 4:4–31.
2. Romeo E, Storelli S. Systematic review of the survival rate and the biological, technical, and aesthetic complications of fixed dental prostheses with cantilevers on implants reported in longitudinal studies with a mean of 5 years follow-up. Clin Oral Implants Res. 2012;23 Suppl 6:39–49.
3. Jung RE, Pjetursson BE, Glauser R, Zembic A, Zwahlen M, Lang NP. A systematic review of the 5-year survival and complication rates of implant-supported single crowns. Clin Oral Implants Res. 2008;19:119–30.
4. Hsu YT, Fu JH, Al-Hezaimi K, Wang HL. Biomechanical implant treatment complications: a systematic review of clinical studies of implants with at least 1 year of functional loading. Int J Oral Maxillofac Implants. 2012;27:894–904.
5. Goodacre CJ, Bernal G, Rungcharassaeng K, Kan JY. Clinical complications with implants and implant prostheses. J Prosthet Dent. 2003;90:121–32.
6. Pjetursson BE, Bragger U, Lang NP, Zwahlen M. Comparison of survival and complication rates of tooth-supported fixed dental prostheses (FDPs) and implant-supported FDPs and single crowns (SCs). Clin Oral Implants Res. 2007;18 Suppl 3:97–113.
7. Kreissl ME, Gerds T, Muche R, Heydecke G, Strub JR. Technical complications of implant-supported fixed partial dentures in partially edentulous cases after an average observation period of 5 years. Clin Oral Implants Res. 2007;18:720–6.
8. Cranin AN, Dibling JB, Simons A, Klein M, Sirakian A. Report of the incidence of implant insert fracture and repair of Core-Vent dental implants. J Oral Implantol. 1990;16:184–8.
9. Siamos G, Winkler S, Boberick KG. Relationship between implant preload and screw loosening on implant-supported prostheses. J Oral Implantol. 2002;28:67–73.
10. Lee J, Kim YS, Kim CW, Han JS. Wave analysis of implant screw loosening using an air cylindrical cyclic loading device. J Prosthet Dent. 2002;88:402–8.
11. Bakaeen LG, Winkler S, Neff PA. The effect of implant diameter, restoration design, and occlusal table variations on screw loosening of posterior single-tooth implant restorations. J Oral Implantol. 2001;27:63–72.
12. Assenza B, Tripodi D, Scarano A, Perrotti V, Piattelli A, Iezzi G, et al. Bacterial leakage in implants with different implant-abutment connections: an *in vitro* study. J Periodontol. 2011;83:491–7.
13. Ha CY, Lim YJ, Kim MJ, Choi JH. The influence of abutment angulation on screw loosening of implants in the anterior maxilla. Int J Oral Maxillofac Implants. 2011;26:45–55.
14. Spazzin AO, Henrique GE, Nobilo MA, Consani RL, Correr-Sobrinho L, Mesquita MF. Effect of retorque on loosening torque of prosthetic screws under two levels of fit of implant-supported dentures. Braz Dent J. 2010;21:12–7.
15. Khraisat A. bu-Hammad O, Dar-Odeh N, Al-Kayed AM. Abutment screw loosening and bending resistance of external hexagon implant system after lateral cyclic loading. Clin Implant Dent Relat Res. 2004;6:157–64.
16. Farina AP, Spazzin AO, Pantoja JM, Consani RL, Mesquita MF. An *in vitro* comparison of joint stability of implant-supported fixed prosthetic suprastructures retained with different prosthetic screws and levels of fit under masticatory simulation conditions. Int J Oral Maxillofac Implants. 2012;27:833–8.
17. Diez JS, Brigagao VC, Cunha LG, Neves AC, da Silva-Concilio LR. Influence of diamondlike carbon-coated screws on the implant-abutment interface. Int J Oral Maxillofac Implants. 2012;27:1055–60.
18. Kim SK, Koak JY, Heo SJ, Taylor TD, Ryoo S, Lee SY. Screw loosening with interchangeable abutments in internally connected implants after cyclic loading. Int J Oral Maxillofac Implants. 2012;27:42–7.
19. Tsuge T, Hagiwara Y. Influence of lateral-oblique cyclic loading on abutment screw loosening of internal and external hexagon implants. Dent Mater J. 2009;28:373–81.
20. Tzenakis GK, Nagy WW, Fournelle RA, Dhuru VB. The effect of repeated torque and salivary contamination on the preload of slotted gold implant prosthetic screws. J Prosthet Dent. 2002;88:183–91.
21. Bidra AS, Rungruanganunt P. Clinical outcomes of implant abutments in the anterior region: a systematic review. J Esthet Restor Dent. 2013;25:159–76.
22. Wong K, Boyde A, Howell PG. A model of temperature transients in dental implants. Biomaterials. 2001;22:2795–7.
23. Eriksson AR, Albrektsson T. Temperature threshold levels for heat-induced bone tissue injury: a vital-microscopic study in the rabbit. J Prosthet Dent. 1983;50:101–7.
24. Benington IC, Biagioni PA, Briggs J, Sheridan S, Lamey PJ. Thermal changes observed at implant sites during internal and external irrigation. Clin Oral Implants Res. 2002;13:293–7.
25. Li S, Chien S, Branemark PI. Heat shock-induced necrosis and apoptosis in osteoblasts. J Orthop Res. 1999;17:891–9.
26. Huh JB, Eckert SE, Ko SM, Choi YG. Heat transfer to the implant-bone interface during preparation of a zirconia/alumina abutment. Int J Oral Maxillofac Implants. 2009;24:679–83.
27. Nissan J, Gross M, Ormianer Z, Barnea E, Assif D. Heat transfer of impression plasters to an implant-bone interface. Implant Dent. 2006;15:83–8.
28. Gross M, Laufer BZ, Ormianer Z. An investigation on heat transfer to the implant-bone interface due to abutment preparation with high-speed cutting instruments. Int J Oral Maxillofac Implants. 1995;10:207–12.
29. Feuerstein O, Zeichner K, Imbari C, Ormianer Z, Samet N, Weiss EI. Temperature changes in dental implants following exposure to hot substances in an *ex vivo* model. Clin Oral Implants Res. 2008;19:629–33.
30. Ormianer Z, Laufer BZ, Nissan J, Gross M. An investigation of heat transfer to the implant-bone interface related to exothermic heat generation during setting of autopolymerizing acrylic resins applied directly to an implant abutment. Int J Oral Maxillofac Implants. 2000;15:837–42.
31. Ormianer Z, Feuerstein O, Assad R, Samet N, Weiss EI. *In vivo* changes in dental implant temperatures during hot beverage intake: a pilot study. Implant Dent. 2009;18:38–45.
32. Huttula AS, Tordik PA, Imamura G, Eichmiller FC, McClanahan SB. The effect of ultrasonic post instrumentation on root surface temperature. J Endod. 2006;32:1085–7.
33. Davis S, Gluskin AH, Livingood PM, Chambers DW. Analysis of temperature rise and the use of coolants in the dissipation of ultrasonic heat buildup during post removal. J Endod. 2010;36:1892–6.
34. Ettrich CA, Labossiere PE, Pitts DL, Johnson JD. An investigation of the heat induced during ultrasonic post removal. J Endod. 2007;33:1222–6.
35. Satterthwaite JD, Stokes AN, Frankel NT. Potential for temperature change during application of ultrasonic vibration to intra-radicular posts. Eur J Prosthodont Restor Dent. 2003;11:51–6.
36. Horan BB, Tordik PA, Imamura G, Goodell GG. Effect of dentin thickness on root surface temperature of teeth undergoing ultrasonic removal of posts. J Endod. 2008;34:453–5.
37. Dominici JT, Clark S, Scheetz J, Eleazer PD. Analysis of heat generation using ultrasonic vibration for post removal. J Endod. 2005;31:301–3.
38. Jokstad A, Braegger U, Brunski JB, Carr AB, Naert I, Wennerberg A. Quality of dental implants. Int Dent J. 2003;53:409–43.

# 9

# Immediate placement and provisionalization of an implant after removal of an impacted maxillary canine: two case reports

Elise G Zuiderveld[1*], Henny J A Meijer[1,2], Arjan Vissink[1] and Gerry M Raghoebar[1]

**Abstract**

Single immediate implant replacement is accompanied by excellent survival rates and a favorable esthetic outcome. The objective of this report was to describe a surgical approach for removal of a buccal or palatally located impacted secondary canine, combined with extraction of the failing primary canine, and immediate placement and provisionalization of an implant. A window technique was applied for surgical removal of the impacted canine. The alveolar crest was preserved. After extraction of the primary canine, the implant was inserted with primary stability. Finally, the exposed surfaces of the implant were covered with a 1:1 mixture of autologous bone and Bio-Oss®. At the 1-year evaluation, both implants were successfully osseointegrated and in function. Esthetics were excellent. It is concluded that under premise of preservation of sufficient bone to achieve primary stability of the implant, removal of the canines can be combined with immediate placement and provisionalization of the implant.

**Keywords:** Dental implants; Maxillary impacted canine; Immediate implant; Immediate placement; Immediate provisionalization

## Background

Maxillary canines are the second most impacted teeth (20 % of all impacted teeth); the prevalence in general population is approximately 2 %. Most impacted cuspids are located palatally, with a palatal/buccal ratio of 8:1 [1–4].

There are several known treatment options for impacted canines to align them into the dental arch. The most widely used option is orthodontic traction after surgical exposure. An alternative is autotransplantation of the impacted canine optionally combined with orthodontic treatment, e.g., when only orthodontic repositioning is not possible or unsuccessful [4–6]. In general, these treatment options use the patient's own teeth to encounter the clinical problem. The advantages of this aspect are functioning as normal teeth, normal dentofacial development, and maintenance of the alveolar bone. Prognosis of autotransplantation is significantly dependent on the stage of root development, with lower risk of failure in teeth with open apex [7]. Success rates for autotransplantation, mentioned in the literature, lie between 82 and 99 % [8]. Disadvantages of both treatment options for alignment of impacted canines into the dental arch are a long treatment time and high costs, not to mention the unpredictable final outcome [2, 9, 10]. Surgical exposure followed by orthodontic traction is associated with damage to supporting structures such as bone loss, root resorption, and gingival recession [2, 10]. The most frequently reported complications in autotransplantation are root resorption or ankylosis, pulp necrosis, and reduction of final root length [5, 7]. Replacement of a failing single tooth, such as a failing primary canine with an impacted secondary canine, through a single implant is another reasonable treatment option [3, 4, 6]. Single implant treatment in this respect is not widely applied yet, but should be considered, if orthodontic treatment and autotransplantation are not feasible because of factors such as canine location, severity of impaction and age of the patient, or when the patient is not willing to encounter conventional treatment options because of treatment duration, morbidity, and costs [4, 6, 9]. With regard to

* Correspondence: e.zuiderveld@umcg.nl
[1]Department of Oral and Maxillofacial Surgery, University of Groningen, University Medical Center Groningen, P.O. Box 30.001, NL-9700 RB Groningen, the Netherlands
Full list of author information is available at the end of the article

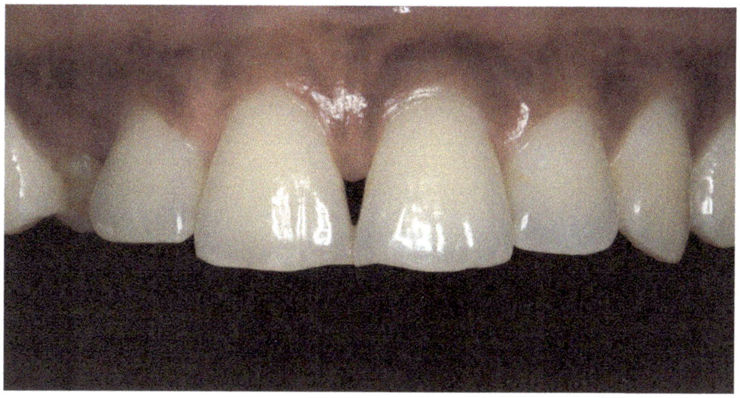

**Fig. 1** Clinical view showing the failing right primary canine

prosthodontic rehabilitation of a single implant, the concept of immediate single implant placement and provisionalization is not yet a standard treatment [11], but there is a growing interest in immediate tooth replacement, particularly in the esthetic region.

Applying an immediate protocol means shortening of the treatment duration as only one surgical intervention is needed and no need for a temporary prosthesis. Thus morbidity and costs of the treatment are reduced [12–14].

According to the literature, immediate implant placement is accompanied by survival rates comparable to conventionally placed implants [12, 15]. With regard to immediate provisionalization, it is not yet set that the esthetic outcome is more favorable [12]. However, immediate provisionalization of the immediately placed implant is presumed to give better support to the surrounding peri-implant tissue for preservation of the original architecture, conditions which are in favor for an optimal esthetic result [3, 11, 15, 16].

The objective of the present report was to describe a surgical approach for removal of an impacted secondary canine, either located buccally or palatally, combined with extraction of the primary canine and immediate placement and provisionalization of an implant.

## Case presentation

### Case 1

A 36-year-old woman consulted the Department of Oral and Maxillofacial Surgery of the University Medical Center Groningen, Groningen, the Netherlands, with a persisting upper right primary canine and impacted secondary canine (Fig. 1). The primary canine had to be removed because of fracture of the crown. The patient did not want to undergo orthodontic treatment, and autotransplantation was no treatment option. She asked for a fixed restoration without involvement of the adjacent teeth and chose for a single implant treatment. She was healthy and non-smoker.

Intra-oral examination revealed a healthy, well maintained dentition. Clinically, adequate bone volume was thought to be present at the future implant site as well as favorable conditions for an implant crown with an anatomical design.

Radiographic examination, consisting of a standardized digital intra-oral radiograph and a cone beam computer tomography (CBCT) image (i-CAT® 17–19; Imaging Sciences International, LLC, Hatfield, USA), was done prior to localize the impacted canine. The CBCT image revealed an impacted right maxillary canine, situated on the buccal side (Fig. 2) with sufficient bone volume on the apical part of the future implant site. Removal of the impacted canine seemed to be possible with maintenance of sufficient bone at the future implant site for

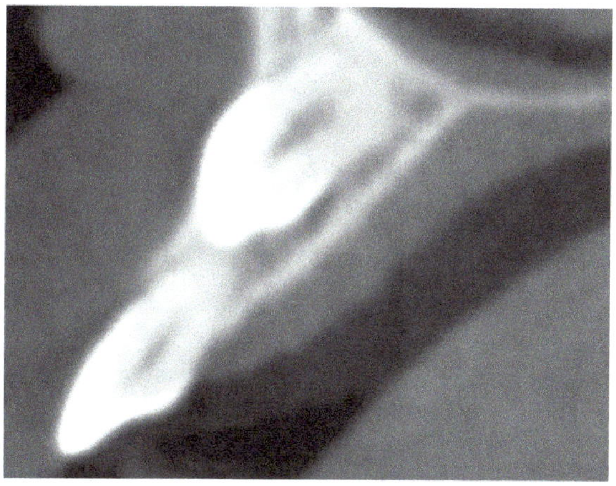

**Fig. 2** CBCT image showing the buccal location of the impacted secondary canine

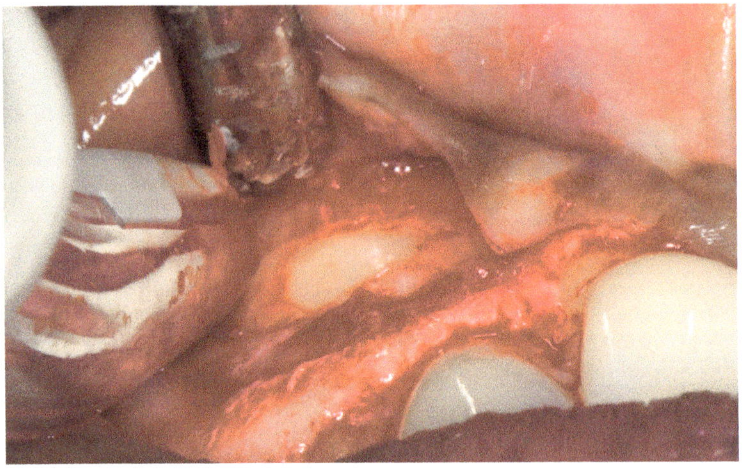

**Fig. 3** The impacted canine has become visible after elevation of a full-thickness buccal mucoperiosteal flap and removing overlying bone

immediate implant placement. Furthermore, no pathology of the dentition was pre-existent. Because of this favorable starting point, it was decided to extract the primary canine and to surgically remove the secondary canine, immediately followed by insertion of an implant according to an immediate loading protocol.

Preoperatively, a cast was made for planning the preferred position of the implant from a prosthodontic perspective. Next, a transparent acrylic resin template (Vertex Castapress; Vertex-Dental BV, Zeist, the Netherlands) was made of this cast with the future implant crown in the preferred position. This template was transferred to a surgical guide. Care was taken to design the surgical guide as such that the guide channel allowed for screw retaining of the provisional restoration.

One day before surgery, the patient started taking antibiotics (amoxicillin 500 mg, three times daily for 7 days) and using a 0.2 % chlorhexidine mouthwash (Corsodyl; GlaxoSmithKline, Utrecht, the Netherlands) for oral disinfection. Following the administering of local anesthesia (Ultracaine D-S Forte; Aventis Pharma Deutschland GmbH, Frankfurt am Main, Germany), an incision was made on the palatal side of the crest with extensions in the buccal and palatal sulcus of the adjacent teeth. For good access to the impacted maxillary canine, a full-thickness buccal mucoperiosteal flap was elevated. After

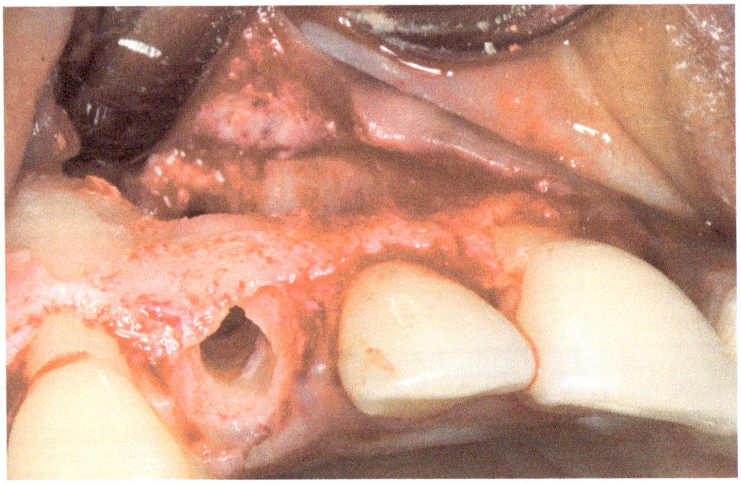

**Fig. 4** The prepared implant socket and osseous defect resulting from removal of the buccally impacted secondary canine and the primary canine. Note that the upper part of the alveolar crest is intact

removal of bone overlying the impacted canine with a round drill and a disposable bone scraper (Safescraper® TWIST Cortical Bone Collector, Biomet 3i, Palm Beach Gardens, USA), the impacted tooth (Fig. 3) was extracted with preservation of the alveolar crest. The roots of the adjacent teeth were not exposed. Finally, the primary canine was extracted with a forceps in order to preserve the alveolar crest as long as possible.

Sufficient bone was left on the buccal and palatal side of the alveolus to allow for immediate implant placement (Fig. 4). After drilling the implant site according to the implant system applied, the final twist drill was placed in the prepared socket. Next, the space between the twist drill and the palatal bone wall was augmented with a 1:1 mixture of autologous bone, harvested from the retro molar area, and Bio-Oss® (Geistlich Pharma AG, Wolhusen, Switzerland). Next, the twist drill was carefully removed and an implant (NobelActive RP, 18 mm; Nobel Biocare AB, Göteborg, Sweden) was placed into the prepared implant socket according to the procedure prescribed by the manufacturer, guided by the surgical template (Fig. 5). An 18-mm implant was chosen for good primary stability because of the bone defect. The shoulder of the implant was placed at a depth of 3 mm apical to the buccal and cervical aspect of the prospective clinical crown to provide soft tissue to develop an adequate emergence profile. Good primary implant stability of >45 Ncm was obtained, determined with the measuring device for implant site preparation (Osseocare; Nobel Biocare AB).

Next, an open tray impression was made at implant level using a custom acrylic resin impression tray (Lightplast base plates; Dreve Dentamid GmbH, Unna, Germany) and a polyether impression material (Impregum Penta; 3 M ESPE, St. Paul, USA). Finally, a healing abutment (NobelReplace; Nobel Biocare AB) was placed, and any remaining residual space between the implant and the buccal bone wall was filled with a 1:1 mixture of autologous bone and Bio-Oss® (Geistlich Pharma AG) (Fig. 6). A Geistlich Bio-Gide (Geistlich Pharma AG) was used to cover the reconstructed alveolar process. The wound was closed with Ethilon 5–0 nylon sutures (Johnson & Johnson Gateway, Piscatatway, USA).

Six hours following implant placement, the healing abutment was removed, and a provisional crown was placed and torqued to 32 Ncm (Fig. 7). Special care was taken to prevent any contact with the antagonist teeth as well as that the provisional restoration was contoured for optimal support of the peri-implant soft tissue. In particular, the interproximal papillae were given sufficient space to regenerate.

The patient was instructed to follow a soft diet, to avoid exerting force on the provisional restoration, and to continue the chlorhexidine rinse (Corsodyl; GlaxoSmithKline) for 7 days. For pain control, 600 mg ibuprofen (Brufen Bruis 600; Abott BV, Hoofddorp, the Netherlands) was prescribed, to be taken three times daily for the time period needed. Two weeks following surgery, the sutures were removed.

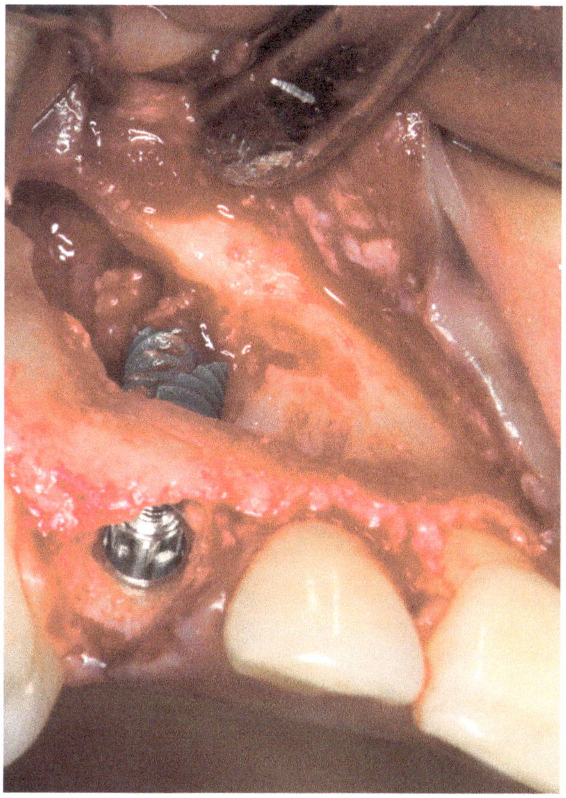

**Fig. 5** The implant is placed in the prepared socket

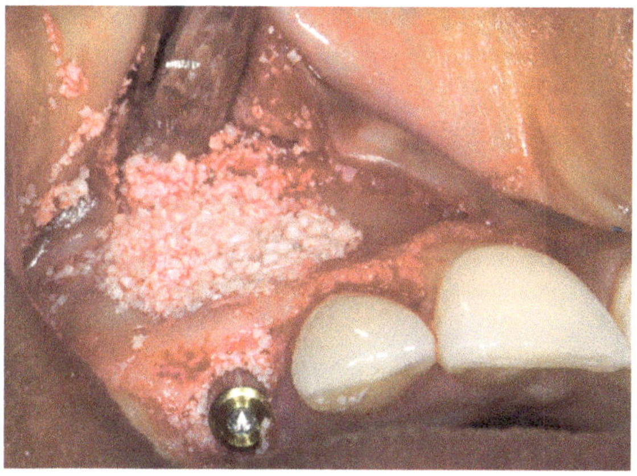

**Fig 6** Situation after implant placement and restoration of the bony defect with a 1:1 mixture of Bio-Oss® and autologous bone

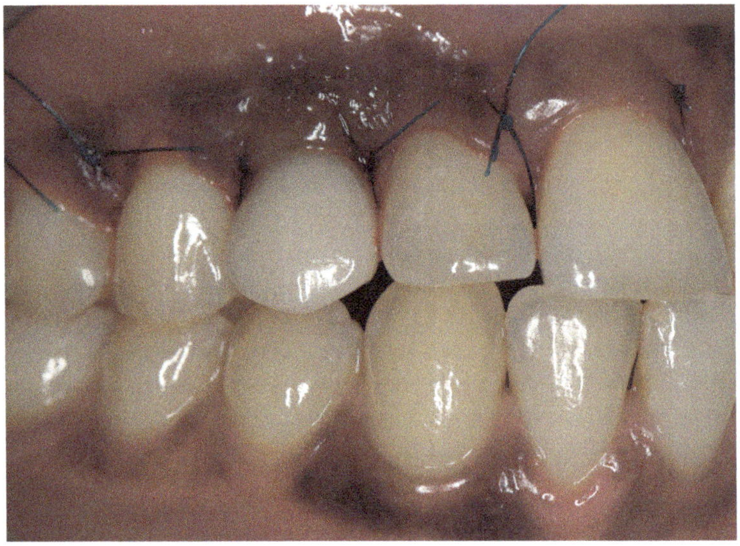

**Fig. 7** Clinical view immediately after placement of the provisional implant crown

Three months later, a screw-retained definitive all-ceramic crown was placed. Follow-up appointments were scheduled 1 and 12 months after installation of the definitive implant crown (Fig. 8) and consisted of intra-oral examination and radiographic assessment of the peri-implant bone level. At both follow-up visits, intra-oral examination revealed healthy peri-implant tissues. Radiographic examination showed minimal bone resorption mesial and distal of the implant (Fig. 9).

### Case 2

A 45-year-old man consulted our department with an impacted right maxillary canine and a persistent primary canine with evident mobility and in need of removal (Fig. 10). The patient chose for a single implant treatment because he wanted to have a long lasting and fixed solution for the failing tooth. All general health prerequisites were met and intra-oral examination revealed a healthy, well-maintained dentition. Clinically, adequate bone volume was present at the future implant site. In all dimensions, sufficient space was available for an implant crown with an anatomical design. The CBCT image (i-CAT® 17–19) revealed an impacted canine situated on the palatal side (Fig. 11) without any other pathology of the dentition as well as sufficient bone volume on the apical part of the future implant site.

Preoperative preparations were the same as for the first case. Next, after administration of local anesthesia (Ultracaine D-S Forte), a full-thickness palatal flap, by an intrasulcular incision on the palatal gingiva from the distal margin of the first premolar to the mesial margin of

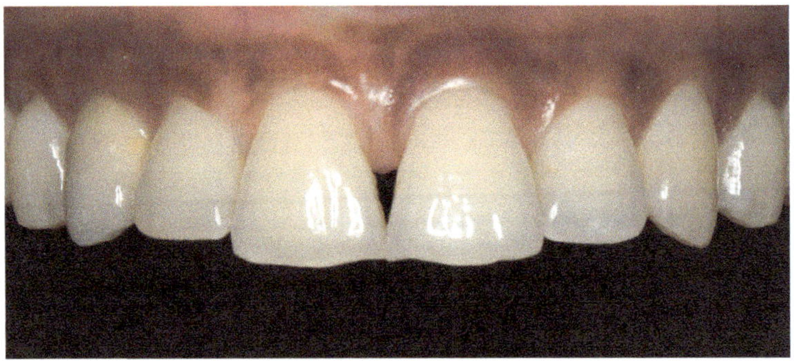

**Fig. 8** Clinical view showing optimal esthetics around the screw-retained definitive all-ceramic crown

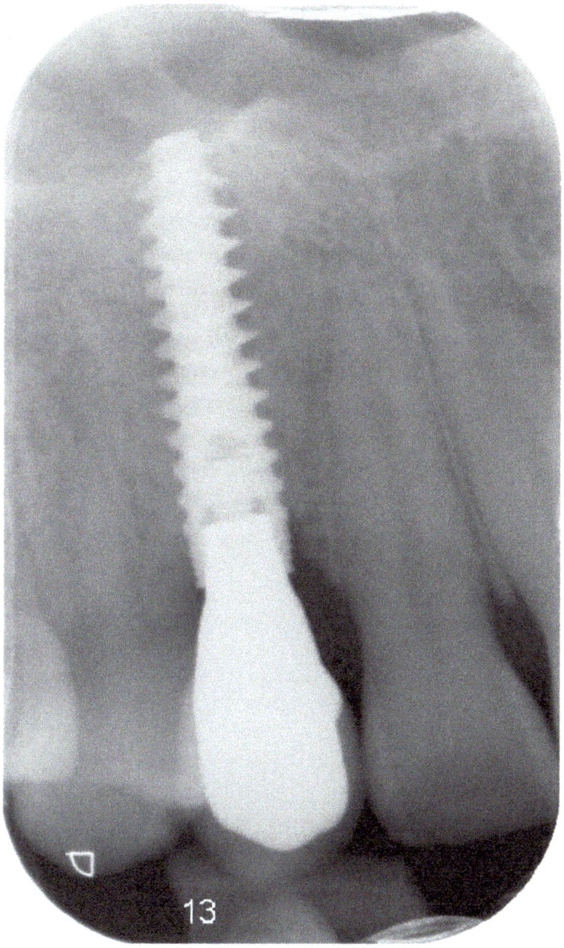


**Fig. 9** Intra-oral radiograph showing the implant 12 months after placement

the central incisor, was elevated for good access to the impacted canine (Fig. 12). Extraction was done carefully, again using a round drill and a bone scraper (Safescraper®), with preservation of the alveolar crest and buccal bone wall. The roots of the neighboring teeth were not exposed. Afterwards, the primary canine was extracted using a forceps.

Because of sufficient bone remaining, an implant (NobelActive NP, 18 mm) was placed immediately into the extraction socket according to the prescribed manufacturer's procedure and guided by the surgical template, with good primary stability of >45 Ncm. An 18-mm implant was chosen for good primary stability because of the bone defect. Bone augmentation was done as described in the first case (Fig. 13). Installation of the provisional implant crown, about six hours following implant placement, was also done according to the procedure described for the first case and with special attention to avoid any contact to the antagonist and contour of the crown. Post-operative care instruction was identical to the first case too. Sutures were removed two weeks after implant placement. Three months after implant installation, the definitive implant crown was placed.

During both follow-up appointments, scheduled 1 and 12 months after installation of the final implant crown (Fig. 14), intra-oral examination revealed healthy peri-implant tissues. Radiographic examination showed minimal bone resorption mesial and distal of the implant (Fig. 15).

## Discussion

This case report describes two approaches for immediate replacement of a failing primary canine and an impacted secondary canine, viz. one for impacted cuspids located at the buccal side of the maxilla and one for impacted cuspids located at the palatal side of the maxilla, by an

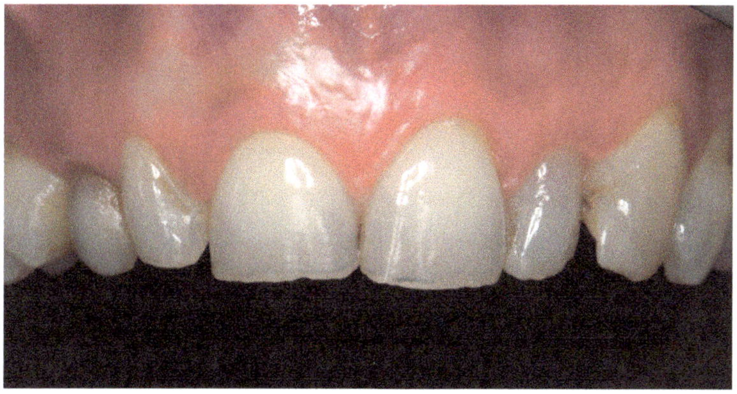

**Fig. 10** Clinical view showing the failing right primary canine

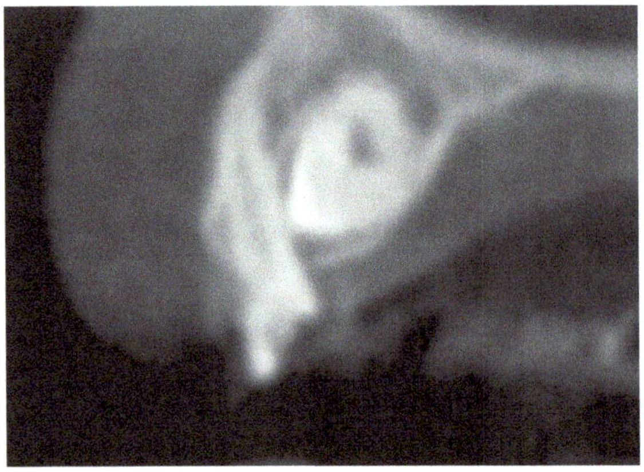

Fig. 11 CBCT image showing the palatal location of the impacted secondary canine

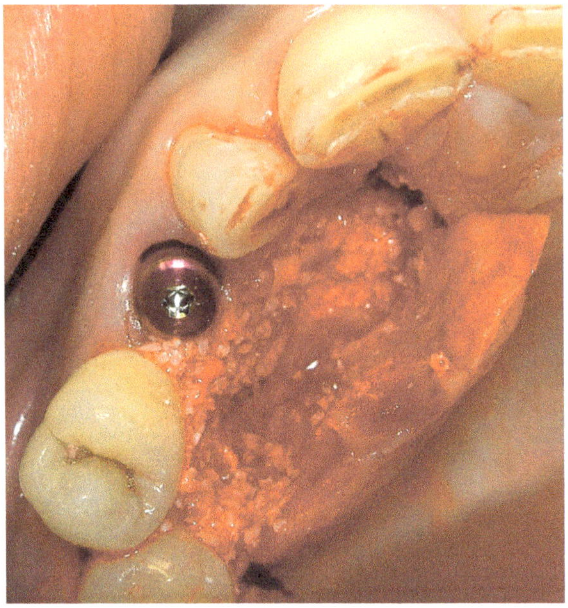

Fig. 13 Situation after implant placement and repair of the bony defect with a 1:1 mixture of Bio-Oss® and autologous bone

immediately placed and provisionalized single implant. With both approaches, esthetically satisfying results were achieved, comparable with other case reports [3, 6, 10]. Removal of an impacted canine causes an evident bone defect, which can be a possible limitation of the proposed technique, because it may be difficult or even not possible to place the implant with enough primary stability [6].

In order to preserve as much bone as possible during the surgical removal of the impacted tooth, it is important to localize the impacted tooth and to judge whether a buccal or palatal approach will preserve most of the native bone by three-dimensional radiographical imaging. Such an approach is supported by recent literature claiming that evaluation of a CBCT image favors treatment planning [5, 9]. Even though in both cases, a significant amount of bone had to be removed to expose the impacted cuspid, proper pre-operative planning still allowed for immediate implant placement and immediate provisionalization because of enough primary stability of the implant.

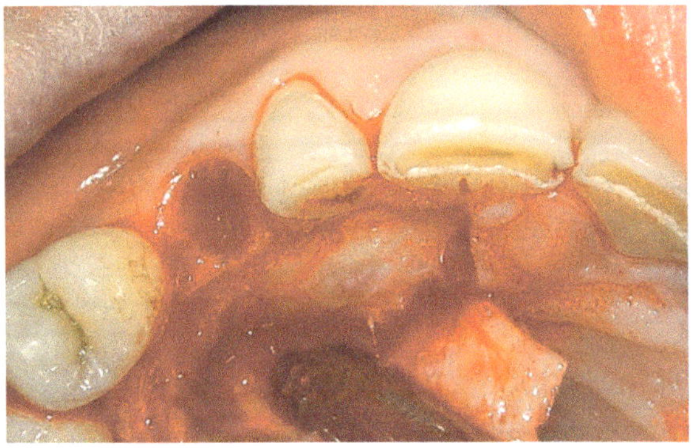

Fig. 12 The impacted canine has become visible after elevation of a full-thickness palatal flap and removing overlying bon

Characteristic for the bone defect in both cases was preservation of the coronal part of the alveolar crest, especially the labial bone plate. According to Kan et al. the presence of ideal pre-existent soft and hard conditions are a prerequisite for immediate implant placement and provisionalization. Particularly, an intact labial bone plate is important to minimize facial gingival recession [17, 18].

Furthermore, an implant system was used, which claims to achieve good primary stability in a small amount of bone, which allowed for immediate provisionalization [19, 20]. This is consistent with recent literature that claims when good primary implant stability is achieved, in the presence of sufficient bone volume, single implants should be provisionalized immediately for preservation of the pre-operatively existing tissue conditions in order to achieve a favorable esthetic outcome [12, 21–24].

But, in order to avoid significant facial hard and soft tissue loss due to the remodeling process after tooth extraction, jeopardizing the final esthetic result, a bone grafting procedure is necessary [17].

Although immediate implant placement and provisionalization is a desired treatment option, it is not possible to apply to young still growing patients. In this case, orthodontic treatment or autotransplantion are indicated [8].

In addition, a primary canine is smaller in all dimensions, but especially in its mesio-distal dimension,

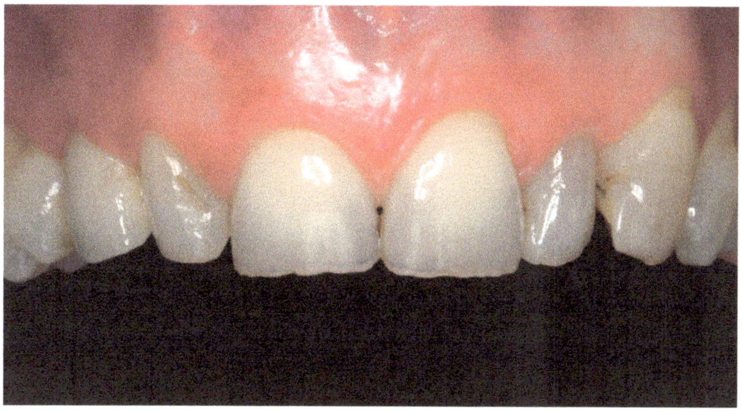

**Fig. 14** Clinical view showing optimal esthetics around the screw-retained definitive all-ceramic crown

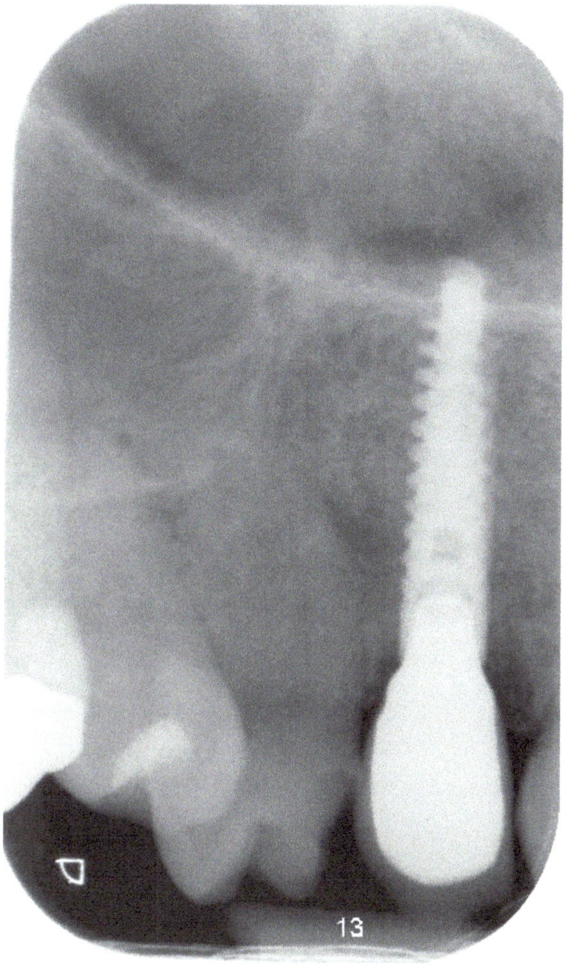


**Fig. 15** Intra-oral radiograph showing the implant 12 months after placement

compared to a secondary canine. In order to place an implant crown with comparable dimensions as the contralateral secondary canine to achieve symmetry, sufficient mesio-distal space is needed. This can be a limitation of the proposed technique because when insufficient space is available, orthodontic treatment is still needed to create enough space for an implant crown with an anatomical design.

## Conclusions

It is concluded that under premise of preservation of sufficient bone to achieve primary stability of the implant, removal of the canines can be combined with immediate placement and provisionalization of the implant.

## Consent

Written informed consent was obtained from the patient for publication of this case report and any accompanying images. A copy of the written consent is available for review by the Editor-in-Chief of this journal.

### Abbreviations

CBCT: cone beam computed tomography; RP: regular platform; NP: narrow platform.

### Competing interests

Elise G. Zuiderveld, Henny J.A. Meijer, Arjan Vissink, and Gerry M. Raghoebar declare that they have no competing interests.

### Authors' contributions

EGZ, HJAM, AV, GMR have substantial contributions to the conception or design of the work and the acquisition, analysis, or interpretation of data for the work. EGZ, HJAM, AV, GMR were involved in rafting the paper and revising it critically. EGZ, HJAM, AV, and GMR gave final approval of the version to be published. EGZ, HJAM, AV, and GMR agreed to be accountable for all aspects of the work in ensuring that questions related to accuracy or integrity of any parts of the work are appropriately investigated and resolved.

**Author details**
[1]Department of Oral and Maxillofacial Surgery, University of Groningen, University Medical Center Groningen, P.O. Box 30.001, NL-9700 RB Groningen, the Netherlands. [2]Department of Fixed and Removable Prosthodontics, University of Groningen, University Medical Center Groningen, P.O. Box 30.001, 9700RB, Groningen, the Netherlands.

**References**

1. Alqerban A. Root resorption of the maxillary lateral incisor caused by impacted canine: a literature review. Clin Oral Investig. 2009;13:247–55.
2. Litsas G, Acar A. A review of early displaced maxillary canines: etiology, diagnosis and interceptive treatment. Open Dent J. 2011;5:39–47.
3. Cardaropoli D, Debernardi C, Cardaropoli G. Immediate placement of implant into impacted maxillary canine extraction socket. Int J Periodontics Restorative Dent. 2007;27:71–7.
4. Spiechowicz E, Piekarczyk J, Gawor E, Stendera P, Ciechowicz B, Mierzwinska-Nastalska E. Reimplantation, bone augmentation, and implantation procedures for impacted maxillary canines: a clinical report. J Prosthet Dent. 2004;91:223–7.
5. Ru N. Canine autotransplantation: effect of extraction site preservation with a titanium prosthesis and a bioresorbable membrane. Am J Orthod Dentofacial Orthop. 2013;143:724–34.
6. Garcia B, Boronat A, Larrazabal C, Penarrocha M, Penarrocha M. Immediate implants after the removal of maxillary impacted canines: a clinical series of nine patients. Int J Oral Maxillofac Implants. 2009;24:348–52.
7. Almpani K. Autotransplantation of teeth in humans: a systematic review and meta-analysis. Clin Oral Investig. 2015. doi: 10.1007/s00784-015-1473-9.
8. Nimcenko T. Tooth auto-transplantation as an alternative treatment option: a literature review. Dent Res J. 2013;10:1–6.
9. Alqerban A. Radiographic predictors for maxillary canine impaction. Am J Orthod Dentofacial Orthop. 2015;147:345–54.
10. D'Amato S, Redemagni M. Immediate postextraction implantation with provisionalization of two primary canines and related impacted permanent canines: a case report. Int J Periodontics Restorative Dent. 2014;34:251–6.
11. De Bruyn H, Raes S, Ostman PO, Cosyn J. Immediate loading in partially and completely edentulous jaws: a review of the literature with clinical guidelines. Periodontol 2000. 2014;66:153–87.
12. Slagter KW, den Hartog L, Bakker NA, Vissink A, Meijer HJ, Raghoebar GM. Immediate placement of dental implants in the esthetic zone: a systematic review and pooled analysis. J Periodontol. 2014;85:e241–50.
13. Hof M, Pommer B, Ambros H, Jesch P, Vogl S, Zechner W. Does Timing of implant placement affect implant therapy outcome in the aesthetic zone? A clinical, radiological, aesthetic, and patient-based evaluation. Clin Implant Dent Relat Res. 2014. doi: 10.1111/cid.12212.
14. den Hartog L, Slater JJ, Vissink A, Meijer HJ, Raghoebar GM. Treatment outcome of immediate, early and conventional single-tooth implants in the aesthetic zone: a systematic review to survival, bone level, soft-tissue, aesthetics and patient satisfaction. J Clin Periodontol. 2008;35:1073–86.
15. De Rouck T, Collys K, Cosyn J. Single-tooth replacement in the anterior maxilla by means of immediate implantation and provisionalization: a review. Int J Oral Maxillofac Implants. 2008;23:897–904.
16. Cosyn J, Hooghe N, De Bruyn H. A systematic review on the frequency of advanced recession following single immediate implant treatment. J Clin Periodontol. 2012;39:582–9.
17. Kan JY, Rungcharassaeng K, Lozada JL, Zimmerman G. Facial gingival tissue stability following immediate placement and provisionalization of maxillary anterior single implants: a 2- to 8-year follow-up. Int J Oral Maxillofac Implants. 2011;26:179–87.
18. Kan Joseph YKJY. Effects of the facial osseous defect morphology on gingival dynamics after immediate tooth replacement and guided bone regeneration: 1-year results. J Oral Maxillofac Surg. 2007;65:13–9.
19. Bell C. Immediate restoration of NobelActive implants placed into fresh extraction sites in the anterior maxilla. J Oral Implantol. 2014;40:455–8.
20. Moretto DD. Immediate loading: a new implant technique with immediate loading and aesthetics: Nobel Active. Oral Implantol. 2008;1:50–5.
21. De Rouck T, Collys K, Wyn I, Cosyn J. Instant provisionalization of immediate single-tooth implants is essential to optimize esthetic treatment outcome. Clin Oral Implants Res. 2009;20:566–70.
22. Cosyn J, De Bruyn H, Cleymaet R. Soft tissue preservation and pink aesthetics around single immediate implant restorations: a 1-year prospective study. Clin Implant Dent Relat Res. 2013;15:847–57.
23. Cardaropoli D. Soft tissue contour changes at immediate postextraction single-tooth implants with immediate restoration: a 12-month prospective cohort study. Int J Periodontics Restorative Dent. 2015;35:191–8.
24. Del Fabbro M. Immediate loading of postextraction implants in the esthetic area: systematic review of the literature. Clin Implant Dent Relat Res. 2015;17:52–70.

# A biomechanical investigation of mandibular molar implants: reproducibility and validity of a finite element analysis model

Miyuki Omori*, Yuji Sato, Noboru Kitagawa, Yuta Shimura and Manabu Ito

## Abstract

**Background:** Three-dimensional finite element analysis (FEA) is effective in analyzing stress distributions around dental implants. However, FEA of living tissue involves many conditions, and the structures and behaviors are complex; thus, it is difficult to ensure the validity of the results. To verify reproducibility and validity, we embedded implants in experimental models and constructed FEA models; implant displacements were compared under various loading conditions.

**Methods:** Implants were embedded in the molar regions of artificial mandibles to fabricate three experimental models. A titanium superstructure was fabricated and three loading points (buccal, central, and lingual) were placed on a first molar. A vertical load of 100 N was applied to each loading point and implant displacements were measured. Next, the experimental models were scanned on micro-computed tomography (CT) and three-dimensional FEA software was used to construct two model types. A model where a contact condition was assumed for the implant and artificial mandible (a contact model) was constructed, as was a model where a fixation condition was assumed (a fixation model). The FEA models were analyzed under similar conditions as the experimental models; implant displacements under loading conditions were compared between the experimental and FEA models. Reproducibility of the models was assessed using the coefficient of variation (CV), and validity was assessed using a correlation coefficient.

**Results:** The CV of implant displacement was 5% to 10% in the experimental and FEA models under loading conditions. Absolute values of implant displacement under loading were smaller in FEA models than the experimental model, but the displacement tendency at each loading site was similar. The correlation coefficient between the experimental and contact models for implant displacement under loading was 0.925 ($p < 0.01$). The CVs of equivalent stress values in the FEA models were 0.52% to 45.99%.

**Conclusions:** Three-dimensional FEA models were reflective of experimental model displacements and produced highly valid results. Three-dimensional FEA is effective for investigating the behavioral tendencies of implants under loading conditions. However, the validity of the absolute values was low and the reproducibility of the equivalent stresses was inferior; thus, the results should be interpreted with caution.

**Keywords:** Three-dimensional finite element analysis; FEA; Displacement; Stress distribution; Reproducibility; Validity

* Correspondence: m-omori@dent.showa-u.ac.jp
Department of Geriatric Dentistry, Showa University, School of Dentistry, 2-1-1 Kitasenzoku, Ota-ku, Tokyo 145-8515, Japan

## Background

Bone remodeling to maintain osseointegration between bone and implant is absolutely essential to ensure favorable results and long-term stability in implant treatment [1,2]. Bone remodeling requires that various stresses generated around the bone caused by the occlusal load applied to the implant be within an appropriate range. Concentrations of stress at the bone-implant interface, which are caused by overloading, have been reported to result in bone resorption [3-5]. However, much remains to be understood about the relationship between mechanical stimulation of the bone and bone dynamics. It is therefore very important to shed light on how peri-implant bone is affected under various conditions, such as the positioning of the implant, placement angle, and bone quality. In recent years, a number of studies using biomechanical investigations have been performed to explore these clinical issues [6-10]. Photoelastic tests, strain gauge method, and three-dimensional finite element analyses (FEAs) have been used in typical biomechanical investigations. In experimental analyses, the photoelastic test and strain gauge method have the advantage of measuring the actual implant. However, the photoelastic test has the disadvantage that model fabrication is complicated. A disadvantage of the strain gauge method is that it is not possible to measure the subject's entire stress. On the other hand, it is possible to use an FEA to ascertain the stress distributions of a subject's interior, which are difficult to measure in an experimental analysis. To extract various physical data such as stress, strain, and displacement, conditions can be set more easily than in other biomechanical investigations [11]. This is the reason why FEAs have been studied in typical biomechanical investigations in recent years.

However, three-dimensional FEA of living tissue entails some disadvantages, including the large number of condition settings and assumptions often included and the complexity of internal structures and behaviors. Moreover, there are lingering questions about the reliability of results produced from a stress analysis, and it is difficult to ensure the validity of the results. One method to verify the validity of three-dimensional FEA models is to carry out experimental analyses in parallel to confirm the extent to which actual behaviors are reproduced and to determine the consistency in displacement between the two models [12-15]. In the future, it appears necessary to fabricate a three-dimensional FEA model that is reproducible and valid to continue revealing problems that arise when actual implant treatments are performed.

With the purpose of verifying the reproducibility and validity of a three-dimensional finite element model, the displacements of implants embedded in an experimental model and in three-dimensional FEA models constructed from the experimental model were compared under various loading conditions.

## Methods

### Fabrication of the experimental model

#### *Artificial mandibular bone*

An artificial mandibular bone (P9-X.1135, Nissin Dental Products, Kyoto, Japan) with free-end edentulism of the left mandibular first premolar (no. 34), second premolar (no. 35), and first molar (no. 36) was used (Figure 1). The model is composed of a two-layer structure of artificial cortical bone (urethane resin) and artificial cancellous bone (urethane resin foam).

#### *Implant placement*

Using the anatomical crown width diameter as a reference [16], we embedded three implants. The distance between the second premolar and mandibular first premolar implants was 8 mm. The distance between the first molar and second premolar implants was 10 mm.

An implant placement guide (Landmark Guide™, iCAT, Osaka, Japan) was fabricated to precisely embed the implants in the artificial mandible. A drilling machine (Enkoh's, Enshu Industrial, Shizuoka, Japan) and implant placement guide were used to embed the implants perpendicular to the bottom surface of the artificial mandible. A drill to form implant cavities (Brånemark System® Twist

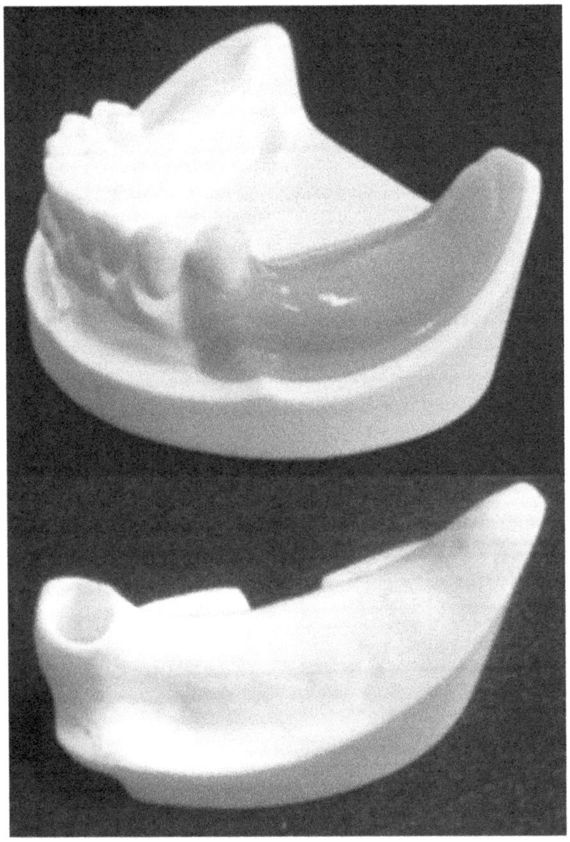

**Figure 1** An artificial mandible.

Drills, Nobel Biocare, Göteborg, Sweden) was mounted onto the drilling machine, and three implant cavities 3.0 mm in diameter and 10 mm in depth were formed. Then, in each of the implant cavities, an implant 3.75 mm in diameter and 10 mm in length (Brånemark System® Mk III, Nobel Biocare, Göteborg, Sweden) was embedded using 40 N · cm of torque (Figure 2).

#### *Preparation of the superstructure*

Using the anatomical crown width as a reference [16], it was determined that the occlusal surface view of the superstructure would be trapezoidal with a 7-mm buccolingual width in the mesial first premolar section, a 10-mm buccolingual width in the distal first molar section, and a 26-mm mesiodistal width (Figure 3). The vertical dimension was 8 mm; the upper 4 mm was the thickness of the superstructure and the lower 4 mm was the abutment connection. Three loading points 2 mm in diameter and 0.2 mm in depth were applied to the occlusal surface of the first molar; these formed the buccal loading point (Figure 3a), central loading point (Figure 3b), and lingual loading point (Figure 3c). The superstructure was made of titanium (ISUS, DENTSPLY Sankin, Tokyo, Japan) and fabricated using computer-aided design/computer-aided manufacturing (CAD/CAM). Three experimental models were fabricated where the superstructure was mounted onto an implant-embedded artificial mandible.

### Construction of three-dimensional FEA models

The experimental models were fixed in a micro-CT scanner (inspeXio SMX-90CT, SHIMADZU, Kyoto, Japan) and scanned under the following imaging conditions: tube voltage, 90 kV; tube current, 109 nA; and slice thickness, 100 μm. FEA software (Mechanical Finder®, Research Center of Computational Mechanics, Tokyo, Japan) was used to construct three-dimensional FEA models from the resulting computed tomography (CT) data. The mesh was constructed of tetrahedral elements, and the total numbers of nodes and elements were approximately 270,000 and 1,500,000, respectively. For the Young's modulus and Poisson ratio of each element, the artificial mandible manufacturer's publicly disclosed values were used so that they would be similar to the physical properties of the experimental model. They were 628 MPa and 0.3 for artificial cancellous bone, 1,372 MPa and 0.3 for artificial cortical bone, and 100,800 MPa and 0.3 for the implant and superstructure (Table 1). The implant, abutment, and superstructure were assumed to be a continuous structure made of titanium; no intervening conditions were set between the implant and abutment, nor between the abutment and superstructure. The artificial cortical bone, artificial cancellous bone, implant, and superstructure were assumed to be homogeneous, isotropic, and linearly elastic.

To better understand how peri-implant bone is affected by differences in boundary conditions, two different kinds

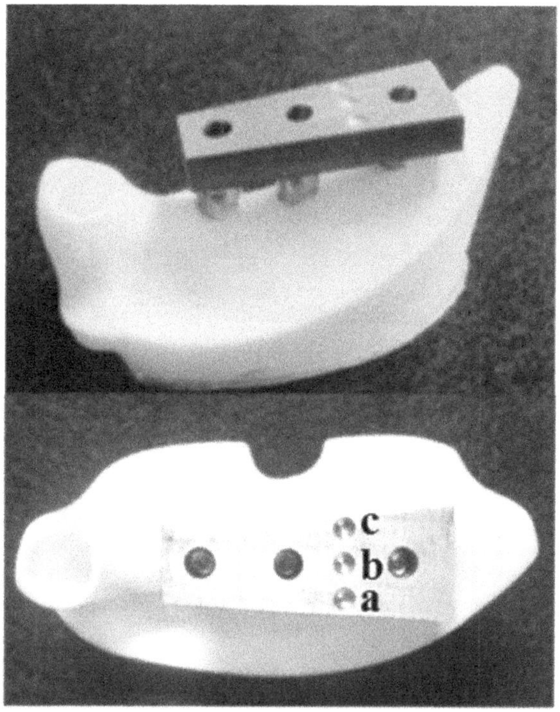


**Figure 3** An experimental model. **(a)** Buccal loading, **(b)** central loading, and **(c)** lingual loading are shown.

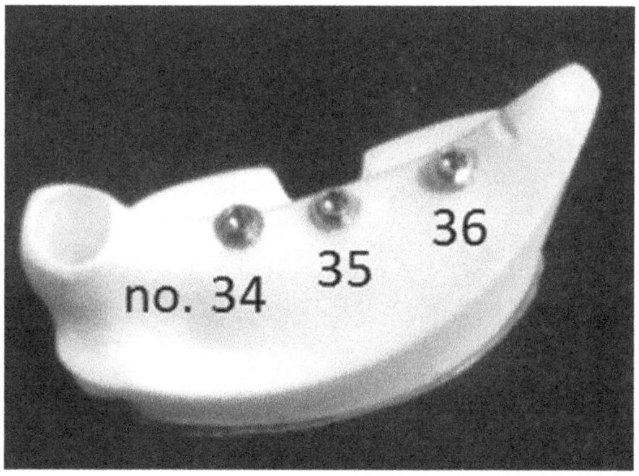


**Figure 2** Three implants were embedded in an artificial mandible.

**Table 1 Mechanical properties of the materials used in the FEA**

| Material | Young's modulus (MPa) | Poisson ratio |
|---|---|---|
| Artificial cancellous bone | 628 | 0.3 |
| Artificial cortical bone | 1,373 | 0.3 |
| Implant and superstructure | 100,600 | 0.3 |

*FEA* finite element analysis.

of models were fabricated by changing the boundary conditions between the implant and artificial mandibular bone. One was called a 'contact model,' in which the artificial mandible and implant were in complete contact. The coefficient of friction of the interface between the implants and artificial mandibular bones was set to zero. The boundary conditions of the experimental model were reproduced by the contact model of FEA. Immediate loading was assumed in this model, because a state of contact was reproduced between the implant and artificial mandibular bone. The other was called a 'fixation model,' in which the artificial mandible and implant were completely bonded together. Delayed loading after the acquisition of osseointegration was assumed in this model. Fixation models were constructed by changing the boundary conditions of the contact model.

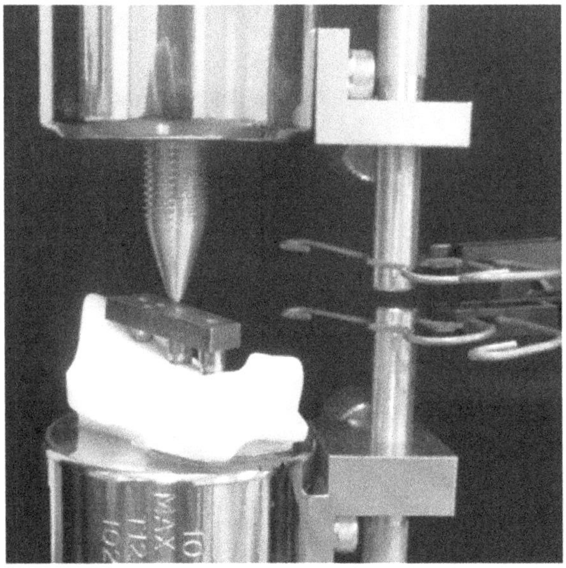

**Figure 4** An experimental model loading test.

### Displacement measurements

#### *Implant displacement measurements under loading conditions in the experimental model*

Implant displacement measurements under loading conditions were measured using an Instron-type universal testing machine (Instron-5500R®, Instron Japan, Kanagawa, Japan) for the experimental model. The experimental models were placed on the worktable of an Instron-type universal testing machine, and compression tests were performed using a conical jig. A vertical load was applied at a rate of 0.5 mm/s to the three loading points. Using a report [17] stating that the maximum occlusal force applied to an implant superstructure in the molar region is 200 N as a reference, we selected 100 N for loading, assuming the forces used during mastication, which are not excessive occlusal forces. A strain gauge (2630-100, Instron Japan, Kanagawa, Japan) was attached between the worktable and jig, and the change in the distance between the worktable and jig was measured under the assumption that it would be the same as the implant displacements under loading conditions (Figure 4). Measurements were taken five times at each loading site, and the mean of the five measurements was taken as the representative value of the loading site in that model.

#### *Implant displacement measurements under loading conditions in the FEA models*

All nodes at the bottom of the artificial mandible were completely restrained, 100 N of vertical load was applied to the three loading points, and an elastic analysis was performed. The vertical displacement of the loading points was assumed to be the displacement of the implants under loading conditions, and analyses were performed for the three loading sites (Figure 5).

#### *Measurements of three-dimensional displacement in the FEA models*

We analyzed the three-dimensional displacements of the three implants when 100 N of vertical load was applied. The assessment sites were the neck and tip of the

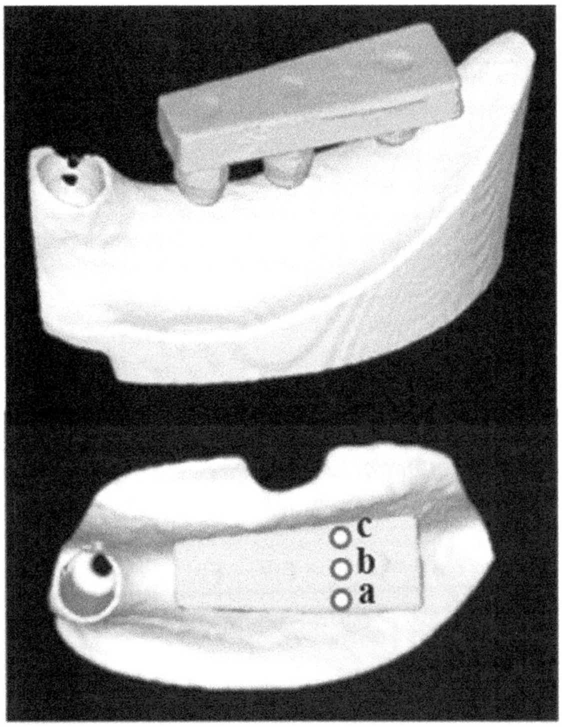


**Figure 5** An FEA model. **(a)** Buccal loading, **(b)** central loading, and **(c)** lingual loading are shown.

implant, and the displacements of the implants under loading were analyzed with respect to the buccolingual direction ($x$-axis), the mesiodistal direction ($y$-axis), and the inferior-superior direction ($z$-axis).

### Assessments of stress distributions and values in the FEA models

The stress distribution (equivalent stress) generated in the interior of the artificial mandible under loading conditions was assessed. We also compared the equivalent stress values of each of loading point at the bone surrounding the necks and tips of the three implants.

### Statistical analysis

Regarding displacement under loading, a one-way analysis of variance (ANOVA) was used to investigate statistically significant differences between the loading sites. A three-way ANOVA was used to investigate statistically significant differences in three-dimensional implant displacements under loading conditions. The assessment site, dental formula, and loading point were used as intra-subject parameters.

Additionally, a three-way ANOVA was used to investigate statistically significant differences in equivalent stress values. The boundary conditions, dental formula, and loading point were used as intra-subject parameters.

To assess the reproducibility of each of the models, the coefficient of variation (CV) was calculated for implant displacement under loading conditions and the equivalent stress values from each of the three experimental and FEA models. To assess the validity of the FEA models, Pearson's correlation coefficient was calculated for implant displacement under loading conditions in the experimental model and the contact model. Statistical processing was performed using PASW Statistics 18 (SPSS, Tokyo, Japan).

## Results

### Implant displacement under loading conditions

Figure 6 and Table 2 show the results for implant displacement under 100 N of vertical loading at each loading point and in each model.

The implant displacement under loading conditions in the experimental model and the two FEA models showed a tendency to exhibit the smallest values under central loading; substantially similar values were exhibited in buccal and lingual loading. Buccal loading ($p < 0.05$) in the experimental model and buccal ($p < 0.01$) and lingual loading ($p < 0.05$) values in the FEA models were significantly greater than the values obtained from central loading. The implant displacement under loading conditions in the FEA models showed lower values than in the

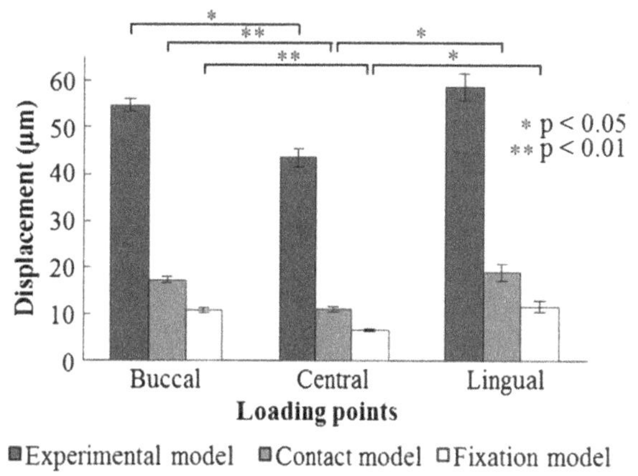


**Figure 6** Implant displacement under loading conditions.

experimental model at all loading points, but aspects of implant displacement under loading caused by differences in the loading point showed a similar tendency. The correlation coefficient between the experimental model and the contact model was 0.925, representing a significant and strong correlation ($p < 0.01$). The maximum CV value was 4.90% in the experimental model, 9.64% in the contact model, and 9.26% in the fixation model (Table 2).

### Three-dimensional displacements in the FEA models

Figure 7 shows the results of three-dimensional implant displacement for each loading point under 100 N of vertical loading.

#### *Three-dimensional displacement in the buccolingual direction (x-axis)*

Under buccal and lingual loading conditions, displacement involving rotation inclined towards the loaded side was exhibited; the displacements were substantially equal (Figure 8). Central loading resulted in the smallest displacement, and almost no displacement was observed. The fixation model had less displacement than the contact model. With regard to the aspects of displacement, similar tendencies were shown in both the contact model and the

**Table 2 Coefficients of variation in implant displacement under loading conditions**

| Model | Loading | | | Average |
|---|---|---|---|---|
| | Buccal loading | Central loading | Lingual loading | |
| Experimental model | 2.49 | 4.76 | 4.90 | 4.05 |
| Contact model | 4.55 | 4.48 | 9.64 | 6.22 |
| Fixation model | 5.26 | 4.85 | 9.26 | 6.45 |

Coefficient of variation (%) = (S.D.)/(mean).

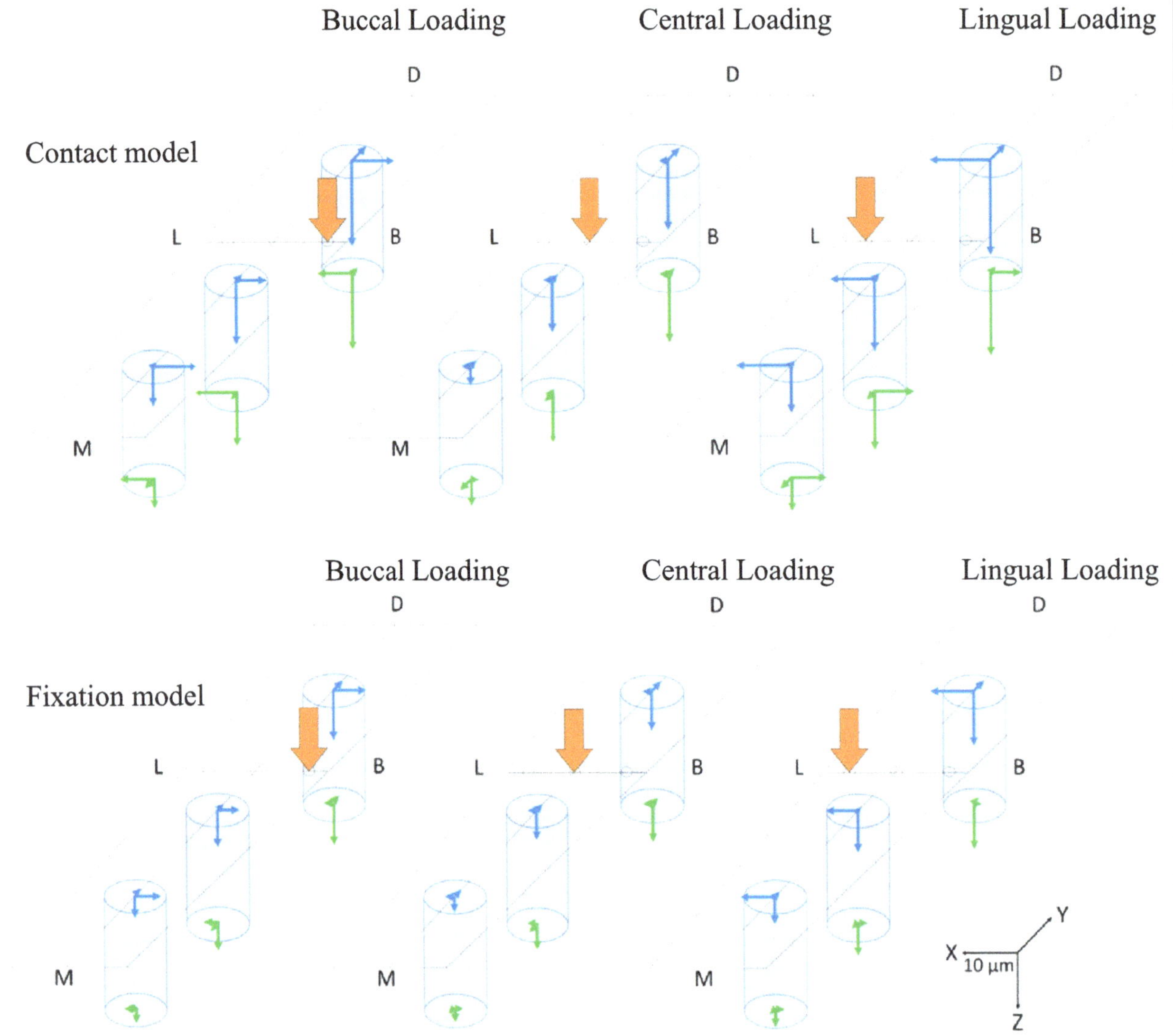


**Figure 7** The displacement of the three implants. (M) Mesial side, (D) Distal side, (B) Buccal side, and (L) Lingual side are shown.

fixation model. The results of the ANOVA showed that for both the contact and fixation models, the loading site was a significant factor in the three-dimensional displacement ($p < 0.01$) (Table 3).

***Three-dimensional displacement in the mesiodistal direction (y-axis)***

At all three loading points, no. 34 and no. 35 showed displacements that were rotated and inclined towards the distal direction; in contrast, no. 36 showed a displacement that moved parallel to the distal direction (Figure 9). Compared with the contact model, the fixation model had less displacement, but aspects of the displacements showed similar tendencies. The results of the ANOVA showed that significant factors for three-dimensional displacement were assessment site, dental formula, and loading point in the contact model, and assessment site and dental formula in the fixation model ($p < 0.05$) (Table 4).

***Three-dimensional displacement in the inferior-superior direction (z-axis)***

At all three loading sites, no. 36 had the greatest displacement; the more mesial the implant, the less the displacement, and the distal portions showed a sinking displacement (Figure 10). Central loading resulted in the least displacement; buccal and lingual loading showed substantially similar displacements. Compared with the contact model, the fixation model demonstrated less displacement, but aspects of the displacements showed similar tendencies. The results of the ANOVA showed that significant factors for the three-dimensional displacement were assessment site, dental formula, and loading point in both the contact and fixation models ($p < 0.05$) (Table 5).

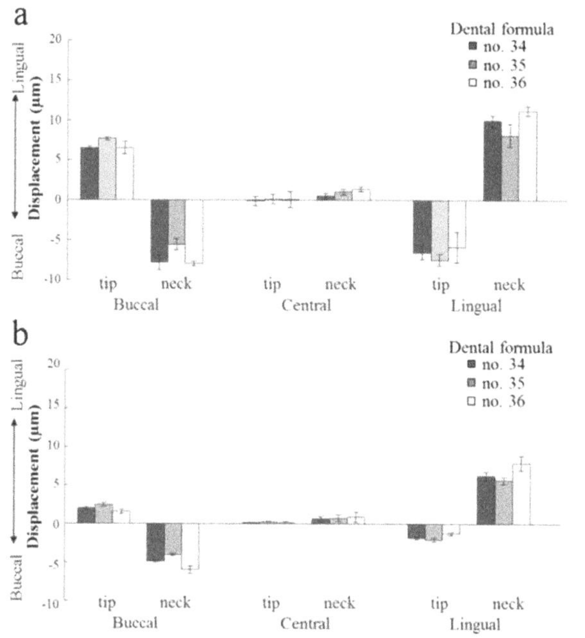


**Figure 8** Displacement in the buccolingual direction (*x*-axis). **(a)** The contact model and **(b)** the fixation model.

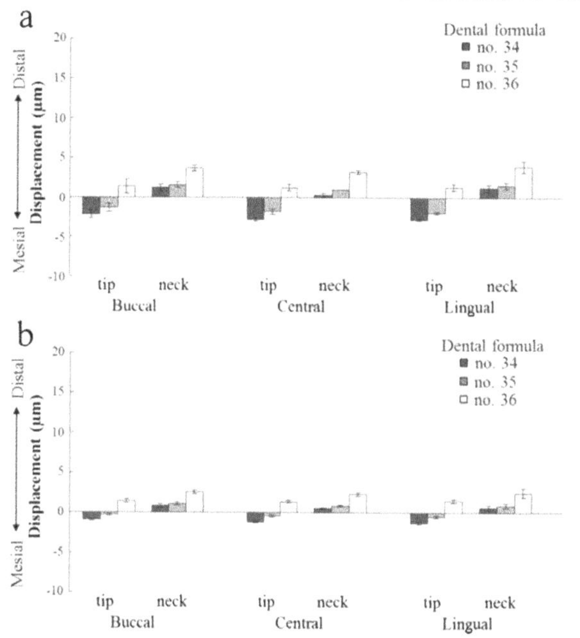


**Figure 9** Displacement in the mesiodistal direction (*y*-axis). **(a)** The contact model and **(b)** the fixation model.

## Equivalent stress in the FEA models

### *Stress distribution*

Figure 11 shows the equivalent stress distribution for each loading point in the first molar implant section under 100 N of vertical loading. The concentrated site of equivalent stress generated in the artificial mandibular bone in the contact and fixation models was on the buccal side of the bone surrounding the implant neck during buccal loading, the lingual side during lingual loading, and the distal center during central loading. This means that a stress concentration was observed in the bone surrounding the implant neck on the loading side. A minute amount of stress generation was observed at the implant tip and threads as well. The contact model had a larger stress concentration range than the fixation model.

### *Equivalent stress values*

Figure 12, Table 6, and Table 7 show the results for the equivalent stress values of the implants at each loading point under 100 N of vertical loading.

**Equivalent stress values in the bone surrounding the implant neck** The equivalent stress values of the fixation model were lower at all loading sites than the contact model (Figure 12a). The value was smallest under central loading; buccal loading and lingual loading showed

**Table 3 Three-way ANOVA (displacement in the buccolingual direction [*x*-axis])**

| Source | Sum of squares | *df* | Mean squared | *F* value | *p* value |
|---|---|---|---|---|---|
| Contact model | | | | | |
| A: Observed area | 16.346 | 1 | 16.346 | 4.362 | 0.172 |
| B: Dental formula | 2.106 | 2 | 1.053 | 5.019 | 0.081 |
| C: Loading points | 25.372 | 2 | 12.686 | 109.445 | 0.000** |
| Fixation model | | | | | |
| A: Observed area | 5.568 | 1.000 | 5.568 | 9.006 | 0.095 |
| B: Dental formula | 0.294 | 2.000 | 0.147 | 5.323 | 0.075 |
| C: Loading points | 139.681 | 1.106 | 126.319 | 308.735 | 0.002** |

**$p < 0.01$.

**Table 4 Three-way ANOVA (displacement in the mesiodistal direction [*y*-axis])**

| Source | Sum of squares | *df* | Mean squared | *F* value | *p* value |
|---|---|---|---|---|---|
| Contact model | | | | | |
| A: Observed area | 116.630 | 1 | 116.630 | 197.889 | 0.005** |
| B: Dental formula | 109.456 | 2 | 54.728 | 171.628 | 0.000** |
| C: Loading points | 2.544 | 2 | 1.272 | 10.139 | 0.027* |
| Fixation model | | | | | |
| A: Observed area | 26.825 | 1 | 26.825 | 695.121 | 0.001** |
| B: Dental formula | 48.534 | 2 | 24.267 | 323.554 | 0.000** |
| C: Loading points | 0.406 | 2 | 0.203 | 1.945 | 0.257 |

*$p < 0.05$, **$p < 0.01$.

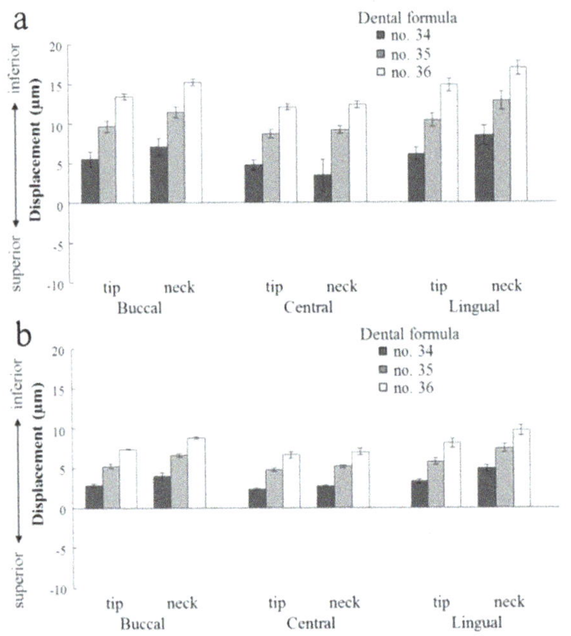


**Figure 10** Displacement in the inferior-superior direction (*z*-axis). **(a)** The contact model and **(b)** the fixation model.

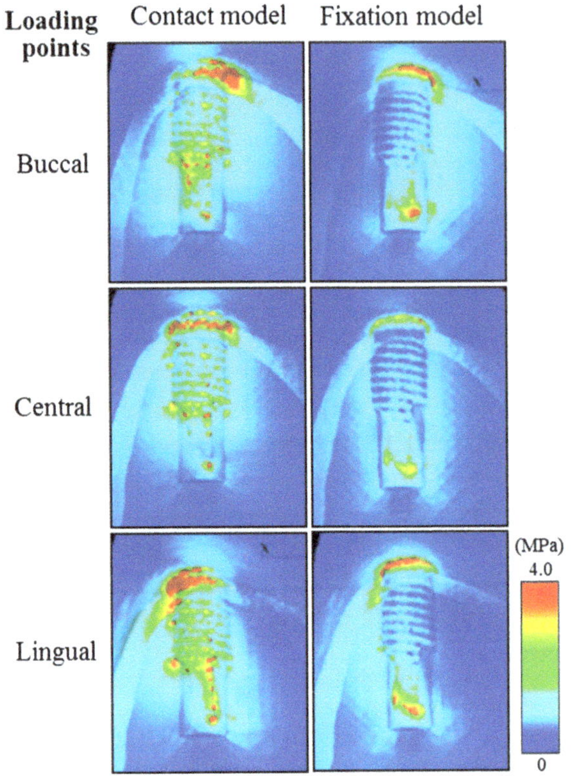


**Figure 11** The distribution of equivalent stress (MPa) around the first molar.

equivalent values. For more distal implants, greater stress values were exhibited. The results of the ANOVA showed that in bone surrounding the implant neck, significant factors for the equivalent stress value were boundary conditions, dental formula, and loading point ($p < 0.01$) (Table 6). The maximum CV was 16.75% in the contact model and 7.03% in the fixation model (Table 7).

**Equivalent stress values in the bone surrounding the implant tip** Central loading resulted in the lowest equivalent stress value, while buccal and lingual loading showed substantially similar values (Figure 12b). In the bone surrounding the implant tip, the loading point was

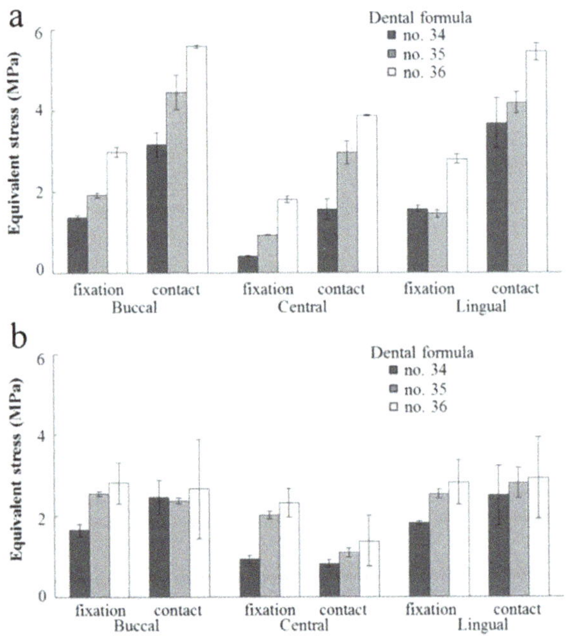


**Figure 12** Equivalent stresses at **(a)** the neck and **(b)** the tip of the implant.

**Table 5 Three-way ANOVA (displacement in the inferior-superior direction [*z*-axis])**

| Source | Sum of squares | *df* | Mean squared | *F* value | *p* value |
|---|---|---|---|---|---|
| Contact model | | | | | |
| A: Observed area | 22.324 | 1 | 22.324 | 68.424 | 0.014* |
| B: Dental formula | 610.338 | 2 | 305.169 | 915.448 | 0.000** |
| C: Loading points | 92.755 | 2 | 46.377 | 22.619 | 0.007** |
| Fixation model | | | | | |
| A: Observed area | 16.600 | 1 | 16.600 | 360.045 | 0.003** |
| B: Dental formula | 190.012 | 2 | 95.006 | 2641.293 | 0.000** |
| C: Loading points | 27.806 | 2 | 13.903 | 78.581 | 0.001** |

$^*p < 0.05$, $^{**}p < 0.01$.

**Table 6 Three-way ANOVA (equivalent stress)**

| Source | Sum of squares | *df* | Mean squared | *F* value | *p* value |
|---|---|---|---|---|---|
| The neck of the implant | | | | | |
| A: Boundary conditions | 64.725 | 1 | 64.725 | 230.721 | 0.004** |
| B: Dental formula | 29.391 | 2 | 14.695 | 365.583 | 0.000** |
| C: Loading points | 20.123 | 2 | 10.062 | 140.179 | 0.000** |
| The tip of the implant | | | | | |
| A: Boundary conditions | 0.037 | 1 | 0.037 | 0.044 | 0.854 |
| B: Dental formula | 5.941 | 2 | 2.971 | 2.684 | 0.182 |
| C: Loading points | 14.050 | 2 | 7.025 | 39.959 | 0.002** |

**$p < 0.01$.

a significant factor for the equivalent stress value ($p < 0.01$) (Table 6). The maximum CV was 45.99% in the contact model and 19.79% in the fixation model (Table 7).

## Discussion

### Experimental methods

#### *Experimental model*

When a three-dimensional FEA is used to analyze the mechanics of peri-implant bone, it is ideal to construct an FEA model that approximates the material properties and structures of an actual mandible. Moreover, the results should be compared with the behavior of an implant in an actual mandible. However, in an actual oral cavity, individual differences exist resulting from bone morphology and physical properties; therefore, it is difficult to conduct experiments under constant conditions and to obtain results that can be applied to all individuals. In other words, to systematically analyze the mechanics of peri-implant bone, an artificial bone model in which individual differences can be eliminated is regarded as valid. The artificial mandibular bone used in this study was regarded as type II in the Lekholm and Zarb classification [18] and had been fabricated on the assumptions of having adequate bone quality, internal structure, and morphology for clinically valid implant therapy. It is difficult to say whether the experimental model was an ideal model because the experimental model has different material properties from those of an actual mandible. However, the purpose of this study was not to compare it with the behavior of an implant in an actual oral cavity; the purpose was to perform a comparison between an experimental model and FEA model to verify the reproducibility and validity of a three-dimensional finite element model. Therefore, we used artificial mandibular bone in the experimental model rather than an actual mandible.

**Table 7 Coefficients of variation for equivalent stresses**

| Model | Loading points | | | |
|---|---|---|---|---|
| | Buccal loading | Central loading | Lingual loading | Average |
| The neck of the implant | | | | |
| Contact model | | | | |
| No. 34 | 9.62 | 16.43 | 16.75 | 14.27 |
| No. 35 | 9.39 | 9.81 | 6.43 | 8.54 |
| No. 36 | 0.72 | 0.52 | 4.04 | 1.76 |
| Fixation model | | | | |
| No. 34 | 3.36 | 3.24 | 5.69 | 4.10 |
| No. 35 | 3.04 | 0.54 | 7.03 | 3.53 |
| No. 36 | 4.03 | 4.44 | 3.91 | 4.13 |
| The tip of the implant | | | | |
| Contact model | | | | |
| No. 34 | 17.31 | 11.83 | 29.53 | 19.55 |
| No. 35 | 2.83 | 10.34 | 13.62 | 8.93 |
| No. 36 | 45.69 | 45.99 | 34.13 | 41.94 |
| Fixation model | | | | |
| No. 34 | 9.67 | 10.44 | 2.22 | 7.45 |
| No. 35 | 2.33 | 4.53 | 4.43 | 3.76 |
| No. 36 | 18.09 | 15.09 | 19.79 | 17.65 |

Coefficient of variation (%) = (S.D.)/(mean).

#### *FEA models*

In many reports on the three-dimensional FEA of implants, loading was carried out using a simplified FEA model in which the cancellous bone interior was regarded as a homogeneous body [19-23]. This is partly because X-ray CT imaging does not provide adequate resolution, and it is difficult for CT to accurately reflect the state of contact between the trabecular structure and the implant [24]. Therefore, it is inevitable that loading will be performed using a simplified FEA model in which the cancellous bone interior is regarded as being a homogeneous body, as was the case in the present experiment. FEA in industry has been utilized as a 'rough analysis' (first-order analysis) tool by simplifying the details in order to ascertain an overall tendency in the first stages of structural design [25]. Therefore, in the present study, a 'first-order analysis' was utilized to ascertain the behavioral tendencies of the implants as a first step before proceeding with an analysis of implant mechanics using a three-dimensional FEA. As has been performed in many reports on the FEA of implants, we verified the validity of the FEA models by studying the extent to which the actual behaviors were reproduced when the trabecular structure in the FEA models was simplified and compared with the experimental model.

### Experimental results

#### *Implant displacement under loading conditions*

In the experimental model, an implant cavity 3.0 mm in diameter was formed prior to embedding an implant 3.75 mm in diameter. In theory, the threads were completely mechanically fitted to the artificial mandibular bone. It does not osseointegrate, but does represent the circumstances of immediate loading in a state of full contact with the bone. The contact model reproduced the state of contact between the bone and implant in the experimental model; theoretically, displacements under loading conditions should show values equivalent to those in the experimental model. Nonetheless, the displacement under loading conditions in the contact model had values 1/3 to 1/4 of those observed in the experimental model. There are three conceivable possibilities. One is that it is possible that consecutive loading of the superstructure on the buccal and lingual sides causes implant loosening. In such a case, displacement under loading conditions would be larger than in the experimental model. Sato et al. [26] reported that the yield tensile load of a screw was 656 N. The fatigue limit causing screw loosening or fracture is half of the yield tensile load, or 328 N. Using a geometric analysis, the largest tensile force in the gold screw after a buccal loading of 100 N was 73 N. In this reported case, if more than 450 N was applied to the loading point, the screw will loosen or fracture. Therefore, 100 N of consecutive superstructure loading on the buccal and lingual sides was not a cause of implant loosening. Furthermore, it is not a reason for displacement under loading conditions in the experimental model to be greater. The second reason is that the experimental model was simply placed on the worktable. Therefore, there is the possibility that minute movements occurred during the vertical loading process. Additionally, measured implant displacement under loading may have overestimated the actual displacement. In order to reproduce complete constraint conditions in FEA models under loading conditions, the bottom surface of the artificial mandibular bone should be adhered completely to the worktable with adhesive; this should stabilize the experimental model and minimize minute movements during the loading process. The third reason is that it is thought that the Young's modulus assigned to the FEA models was different from the actual Young's modulus of artificial mandibular bone. In an FEA, the physical properties assigned to elements reportedly have a major impact on the analysis results [27,28]. Nomura et al. [29] reported that displacement under loading conditions increases when the Young's moduli of the cortical and cancellous bone are reduced. We used the manufacturer's publicly disclosed values for the Young's modulus of the artificial mandibular bone, but it is not clear how these values were measured. In particular, with respect to artificial cancellous bone, the interior has become a foam state and it is thought that the Young's modulus is smaller than the publicly disclosed value. In such a case, displacement under loading conditions would be greater than measured in this study's FEA models and would be nearer to the displacement under loading conditions in the experimental model. An accurate method for measuring the Young's modulus also requires future study.

In the experimental and contact models, the absolute values of displacement under loading were different, but aspects of the displacement under loading conditions caused by differences in the loading points were similar and showed similar tendencies. The correlation coefficient of the two was 0.925, representing a significant and strong correlation ($p < 0.01$). This shows that the behavioral tendencies of the contact model are reflective of those in the experimental model and that the results obtained had high validity. The CV of the displacement under loading conditions was calculated as about 10% in some areas of the FEA models, but the mean was about 5% for all three models, representing a relatively low value. This suggests that all models had highly reproducible displacements under loading and that the results obtained had high validity. Although there are limitations to the reproducible range, it appears possible to infer phenomena to an extent if the properties are understood and the limitations are known. Analysis by three-dimensional finite element models has been shown to be an effective means for studying the behavioral tendencies of implants under loading conditions.

#### *Three-dimensional displacement in the FEA models*

**Directions of implant displacement** Hotta et al. [30] measured the amount of displacement under the loading of implants placed in human mandibles. When a load is applied at a location that deviates from the long-axial direction of implant more buccally and lingually, the forces from rotation and inclination are propagated to the implant as an eccentric axial load. The implant displacement of eccentric axial loading has been reported to be larger than that during long-axial direction loading. Awazawa et al. [31] measured displacements under the loading of implants placed in canine mandibles and reported no substantial difference in displacement based on whether the loading direction was towards the buccal or lingual side during buccolingual loading. These reports are consistent with the results of $x$-axis displacement in this study and support the clinical validity of the constructed FEA models.

**Impacts of different boundary conditions on displacement** It has been reported that when micromovement of an implant occurs, an ingrowth of soft tissue occurs after the implant is embedded; therefore, it is difficult to achieve osseointegration [32-34]. Brunski et al. [35] reported that when immediate loading or early loading is carried out, micromovements of the implant should be controlled to 100 μm or less and excessive movement of the implant not only impairs osseointegration but also encourages the growth of connective tissue. In the experimental results of the present study, the displacement of the contact model, which assumed immediate loading, showed greater values than the fixation model, which assumed delayed loading. That is to say, in the FEA models constructed in the present study, the results support the notion that micromovements are likely to occur during immediate loading and that suppressing these as much as possible is necessary for successful osseointegration.

#### *Equivalent stress values and their occurrence sites*

When assessing stress values of FEA models, it is desirable to do so after confirmation of the validity of the models [11]. Therefore, we first confirmed the validity of the FEA models from comparisons of the correlation coefficients of the displacements under loading conditions in the experimental and contact models. Then, the equivalent stress values and their sites of occurrence were assessed to examine how peri-implant bone is impacted by differences in boundary conditions and loading points.

**Impacts from differences in loading sites** The equivalent stress values in both the contact and fixation models were smallest for central loading, while buccal and lingual loading showed substantially equivalent values greater than that of central loading. Equivalent stress occurrence sites were observed to be high in bone surrounding the implant neck on the loading side, similar to previous reports [36,37]. Hobo et al. [38] stated that while implants were resistant to vertical pressure, horizontal pressure (bending movements) generated torque in the implants and had more harmful effects; therefore, it would be wise to limit the occlusal contact of the superstructure to vertical pressure and avoid horizontal pressure as much as possible. This was also consistent with reports that lateral loading generated more stress than vertical loading, as is also found in Sato et al.'s report using a geometric analysis [39], and supports the existing clinical concept that a lateral force applied to an implant greatly increases the stress in the surrounding bone.

**Impacts of differences in boundary conditions** The equivalent stress values of the contact model were higher at the implant neck than the tip, and the stress generation range was also broader. However, in the fixation model, the implant neck and tip had substantially equivalent values and the stress generation range was also narrower than that of the contact model. This shows that under immediate loading conditions, there is a high likelihood that loading applied to the superstructure is also supported by cancellous bone at the implant threads and tip, but the majority is supported by cortical bone at the implant neck. That is, under immediate loading conditions, it is believed there is a need to be mindful of the stress concentration at the implant neck. The material properties of the FEA models constructed in the present study cannot not be compared to actual oral cavity stress values because they differ significantly from an actual bone. However, when regarding how peri-implant bone is impacted by contact between the implant and bone, it is considered sufficiently useful in predicting tendencies.

**Reproducibility of the equivalent stress values in the FEA models** The CV of the equivalent stress values was calculated to assess the reproducibility of the contact and fixation models. The CV ranged from 0.52 to 45.99, showing a tendency for higher overall values compared with the CV for displacement under loading. The reproducibility of the equivalent stress values had considerable variance from model to model in some regions. In particular, the contact model showed a higher CV at both the neck and tip. In an analysis of contact conditions, moving the nodes also dramatically changed the stress and strain occurring at the interface; a stress concentration was also generated depending on the shape of the model [40]. Though the FEA models were fabricated under similar conditions, it appears that a minute error in shape caused in the element divisions appeared in the form of a large error in equivalent stress values. It is necessary to verify whether the numerical stress values obtained from the FEA have validity by attaching a strain gauge to an experimental model and observing correlations in stress values between the experimental and FEA models.

## Conclusions

With the objective of verifying the reproducibility and validity of three-dimensional finite element models, we fabricated finite element models and multiple models in which implants were embedded in artificial mandibles and compared implant displacements under various loading conditions; the results obtained produced the following conclusions:

1. The CVs as calculated from the amount of displacement under loading in the experimental, contact, and fixation models were about 5% to 10%, and all models had high reproducibility with respect to implant displacement under loading.
2. If three loading points were applied in the experimental and FEA models, the aspects of vertical implant displacement were similar in both.
3. The correlation coefficient of implant displacement under loading conditions in the experimental and contact models was 0.925, representing a high correlation, and the validity of the displacement under loading was high in the contact model.

4. The CV as calculated from equivalent stress values in the contact and fixation models ranged from 0.52% to 45.99%, and the reproducibility of the equivalent stress values showed considerable variance from model to model.

The above results show that the three-dimensional finite element models were reflective of displacement tendencies in the experimental model, and the results obtained had high reproducibility and validity. However, it was shown that when the validity of the absolute value of displacement was low, the reproducibility of the equivalent stress values was also inferior. Three-dimensional FEA was observed to be an effective means for investigating the behavioral tendencies of implants under loading conditions. Although there are limitations to the reproducible range, it is possible to infer phenomena to an extent if the properties are understood and the limitations are known. However, the results need to be interpreted cautiously, with a full understanding that FEA methods are purely numerical data that are mathematically enumerated.

**Abbreviations**

FEA: finite element analysis; CT: computed tomography; CV: coefficient of variation; CAD/CAM: computer-aided design/computer-aided manufacturing; ANOVA: analysis of variance.

**Competing interests**

Miyuki Omori, Yuji Sato, Noboru Kitagawa, Yuta Shimura and Manabu Ito declare that they have no competing interests.

**Authors' contributions**

MO drafted the manuscript. YS contributed advice regarding the manuscript. All authors have read and approved the final manuscript.

**Acknowledgements**

The authors would like to express their deep appreciation to the teaching staff of the Geriatric Dentistry course at Showa University Dental Hospital for their help and cooperation. This study was supported by a Grant-in-Aid for Scientific Research from the Ministry of Education, Culture, Sports, Science, and Technology (Showa University Grant-in-Aid for Scientific Research (C)) (Grant Number 25463016). A partial summary of this thesis was presented at the 43rd Annual Meeting of the Japanese Society of Oral Implantology in Fukuoka, Japan, in September 2013.

**References**

1. Frost HM. Wolff's Law and bone's structural adaptations to mechanical usage: an overview for clinicians. Angle Orthod. 1994;64:175–88.
2. Duyck J, Rønold HJ, Van Oosterwyck H, Naert I, Vander Sloten J, Ellingsen JE. The influence of static and dynamic loading on marginal bone reactions around osseointegrated implants: an animal experimental study. Clin Oral Implants Res. 2001;12:207–18.
3. Quirynen M, Naert I, van Steenberghe D. Fixture design and overload influence marginal bone loss and fixture success in the Brånemark system. Clin Oral Implants Res. 1992;3:104–11.
4. Hoshaw SJ, Brunski JB, Cochran GVB. Mechanical loading of Brånemark implants affects interfacial bone modelling and remodeling. Int J Oral Maxillofac Implants. 1994;9:345–60.
5. Isidor F. Loss of osseointegration caused by occlusal load of oral implants. A clinical and radiographic study in monkeys. Clin Oral Implants Res. 1996;7:143–52.
6. Kitagawa T, Tanimoto Y, Nemoto K, Aida M. Influence of cortical bone quality on stress distribution in bone around dental implant. Dent Mater. 2005;24:219–24.
7. Limbert G, van Lierde C, Muraru OL, Walboomers XF, Frank M, Hansson S, et al. Trabecular bone strains around a dental implant and associated micromotions. A micro-CT-based three-dimensional finite element study. J Biomech. 2010;43:1251–61.
8. Matsunaga S, Naito H, Tamatsu Y, Takano N, Abe S, Ide Y. Consideration of shear modulus in biomechanical analysis of peri-implant jaw bone: accuracy verification using image-based multi-scale simulation. Dent Mater. 2013;32:425–32.
9. de Vasconcellos LG, Nishioka RS, de Vasconcellos LM, Balducci I, Kojima AN. Microstrain around dental implants supporting fixed partial prostheses under axial and non-axial loading conditions, in vitro strain gauge analysis. J Craniofac Surg. 2013;24:546–51.
10. Menani LR, Tiossi R, de Torres ÉM, Ribeiro RF, de Almeida RP. Photoelastic stress analysis of different designs of cement-retained fixed partial dentures on Morse taper oral implants. J Craniofac Surg. 2011;22:674–8.
11. Korioth TW, Versluis A. Modeling the mechanical behavior of the jaws and their related structures by finite element (FE) analysis. Crit Rev Oral Biol Med. 1997;8:90–104.
12. Morita Y, Qian L, Todo M, Matsushita Y, Arakawa K, Koyano K. Stress and strain distribution analyses of porcine mandibular periodontium by experimental mechanics and finite element analysis. Jpn J Clin Biomech. 2009;30:7–13 [in Japanese].
13. Taira S. Modern material mechanics. Tokyo: Ohmsha; 2011. p. 235–8 [in Japanese].
14. Morita Y. Experimental study on displacement and strain distributions around dental implant using digital image correlation method. J Jpn Soc Oral Implant. 2012;25:488–95 [in Japanese].
15. Wakabayashi N. Advanced applications of finite element method in dental research: recent progress in non-linear analysis. J Dent Mater. 2013;32:226–39 [in Japanese].
16. Kraus BS, Jordan RE, Abrams L. Dental anatomy and occlusion: a study of the masticatory system. Baltimore: Williams and Wilkins; 1969.
17. Regina M, Patrick A, Ernö M, Walter B. Occlusal force and oral tactile sensibility measured in partially edentulous patients with ITI implants. Int J Oral Maxillofac Implants. 1995;10:345–54.
18. Lekholm U, Zarb GA. Patient selection and preparation. In: Zarb GA, Albrektsson T, editors. Tissue-integrated prostheses. Osseointegration in clinical dentistry. Chicago: Quintessence; 1985. p. 199–209.
19. Eraslan O, Inan O, Secilmis A. The effect of framework design on stress distribution in implant-supported FPDs: a 3-D FEM study. Eur J Dent. 2010;4:374–82.
20. Sugiura T, Yamamoto K, Fujimoto M, Murakami K, Horita S, Kirita T, et al. Effect of initial loading time and bone quality on stress distribution in bone around dental implant. Jpn J Clin Biomech. 2011;32:27–32 [in Japanese].
21. Ausiello P, Franciosa P, Martorelli M, Watts DC. Effects of thread features in osseo-integrated titanium implants using a statistics-based finite element method. Dent Mater. 2012;28:919–27.
22. Yamanishi Y, Yamaguchi S, Imazato S, Nakano T, Yatani H. Influences of implant neck design and implant-abutment joint type on peri-implant bone stress and abutment micromovement. Dent Mater. 2012;28:1126–33.
23. Bahrami B, Shahrbaf S, Mirzakouchaki B, Ghalichi F, Ashtiani M, Martin N. Effect of surface treatment on stress distribution in immediately loaded dental implants. A 3D finite element analysis. Dent Mater. 2014;30:89–97.
24. Matsunaga S, Ide Y. Morphological characteristics of peri-implant trabecular bone using μ-CT and its mechanical evaluation. BONE. 2009;23:289–92 [in Japanese].
25. Yokoyama M. Modeling techniques and stress analysis in finite element methods. Tokyo: Yokendo; 2007. p. 1–22 [in Japanese].
26. Sato Y, Shindoi N, Hosokawa R, Tsuga K, Akagawa Y. A biomechanical effect of wide implant placement and offset placement of three implants in the posterior partially edentulous region. J Oral Rehabil. 2000;27:15–21.
27. Anderson JD. Three dimensional finite element analysis of osseointegration at implant/bone interface under occlusal force. Problems associated with edentulous and partially edentulous cases. J Jpn Soc Oral Implant. 1992;5:337–47.
28. Koretake K. Development of a three-dimensional finite element model with elastic moduli of bone microstructures around an osseointegrated implant. J Hiroshima Univ Dent Soc. 2001;33:31–46 [in Japanese].

29. Nomura T. An experimental study on the influence of the stiffness of mandibular bone surrounding fixture on the displaceability of osseointegrated implant under horizontal loading. J Tokyo Dent Coll Soc. 1995;95:633–52 [in Japanese].
30. Hotta H. Experimental study on the displaceability of fixture under pressure in osseointegrated implant of mandible. J Tokyo Dent Coll Soc. 1992;92:1–65 [in Japanese].
31. Awazawa S. An experimental study on the load supporting mechanism of bone tissues surrounding fixture in the osseointegrated implant applied to jaw bone of dog. J Tokyo Dent Coll Soc. 1995;95:687–728 [in Japanese].
32. Brunski JB. Biomechanical factors affecting the bone-dental implant interface. Clin Mater. 1992;10:153–201.
33. Pilliar RM. Quantitative evaluation of the effect of movement at porous coated implant-bone interface. In: Davies EJ, editor. The bone biomaterial interface. 3rd ed. Toronto: University of Toronto Press; 1995. p. 380–7.
34. Szmukler-Moncler S, Salama H, Reingewirtz Y, Dubruille JH. Timing of loading and effect of micromotion on bone-dental implant interface: review of experimental literature. J Biomed Mater Res. 1998;43:192–203.
35. Brunski JB. In vivo bone response to biomechanical loading at the bone/dental-implant interface. Adv Dent Res. 1999;13:99–119.
36. Tada S, Stegaroiu R, Kitamura E, Miyakawa O, Kusakari H. Influence of implant design and bone quality on stress/strain distribution in bone around implants: a 3-dimensional finite element analysis. Int J Oral Maxillofac Implants. 2003;18:357–68.
37. Sevimay M, Turhan F, Kilicarslan MA, Eskitascioglu G. Three-dimensional finite element analysis of the effect of different bone quality on stress distribution in an implant-supported crown. J Prosthet Dent. 2005;93:227–33.
38. Hobo S, Hosoyama H. Occlusion for implant. Tokyo: Quintessence; 2006. p. 89–95 [in Japanese].
39. Sato Y, Shindoi N, Hosokawa R, Tsuga K, Akagawa Y. Biomechanical effects of double or wide implants for single molar replacement in the posterior mandibular region. J Oral Rehabil. 2000;27:842–45.
40. Kishi M. Practical handbook of finite element methods for structural analysis. Tokyo: Morikita Publishing; 2008. p. 108–17 [in Japanese].

# 11

# Genomic analyses of early peri-implant bone healing in humans: a systematic review

Siddharth Shanbhag[1,2], Vivek Shanbhag[2] and Andreas Stavropoulos[1*]

**Abstract**

**Objective:** The objective of the study was to systematically review the literature for studies reporting gene expression analyses (GEA) of the biological processes involved in early human peri-implant bone healing.

**Methods:** Electronic databases (MEDLINE, EMBASE) were searched in duplicate. Controlled and uncontrolled studies reporting GEA of human peri-implant tissues - including ≥5 patients and ≥2 time points - during the first 4 weeks of healing were eligible for inclusion. Methodological quality and risk of bias were also assessed.

**Results:** Four exploratory studies were included in reporting GEA of either tissues attached to SLA or SLActive implants after 4 to 14 days or cells attached to TiOBlast or Osseospeed implants after 3 to 7 days. A total of 111 implants from 43 patients were analyzed using validated array methods; however, considerable heterogeneity and risk of bias were detected. A consistent overall pattern of gene expression was observed; genes representing an immuno-inflammatory response were overexpressed at days 3 to 4, followed by genes representing osteogenic processes at day 7. Genes representing bone remodeling, angiogenesis, and neurogenesis were expressed concomitantly with osteogenesis. Several regulators of these processes, such as cytokines, growth factors, transcription factors, and signaling pathways, were identified. Implant surface properties seemed to influence the healing processes at various stages via differential gene expression.

**Conclusion:** Limited evidence from gene expression studies in humans indicates that osteogenic processes commence within the first post-operative week and they appear influenced at various stages by implant surface properties.

**Keywords:** Dental implant; Osseointegration; Gene expression; Molecular assessment

## Review

### Introduction

Osseointegrated oral implants are an integral part of modern reconstructive dentistry and are associated with favorable long-term therapeutic outcomes [1]. Osseointegration was originally defined as the direct contact between vital bone and a load-bearing implant observed at the light microscopic, i.e., histological, level [2]. Morphogenesis of implant osseointegration has been assessed in several preclinical *in vivo* and clinical histological studies [3-6], providing the basis for understanding the biological process.

The biological events during the early phase of osseointegration are directly influenced by the osseous microenvironment (i.e., cells, signaling molecules, and matrix) into which the implant is placed and have many similarities with general wound healing mechanisms [7]. Implant surgery induces trauma, resulting in bleeding and fibrin clot formation and an inflammatory reaction that dominate the events of the first post-operative week. The deposition of vital new bone on the implant surface by osteoblasts (osteogenesis), a fundamental requirement for osseointegration, occurs via secretion of a complex extracellular matrix (ECM) of proteins, which subsequently undergoes mineralization to form bone [8,9]. Primary (woven) bone lined by osteoblasts can indeed be observed on the implant surface already after 1 week [3,5]. In parallel, removal of the created bone debris and remodeling of necrotized bone (due to the pressure exerted by the implant) is underway. Replacement of woven bone by organized and mechanically superior lamellar

* Correspondence: andreas.stavropoulos@mah.se
[1]Department of Periodontology, Faculty of Odontology, Malmö University, Carl Gustafs väg 34, 214 21 Malmö, Sweden
Full list of author information is available at the end of the article

bone can be observed from the second to fourth week (depending on the species) and progressively increases until woven bone is almost entirely replaced (8 to 12 weeks). These events, including the nutrition of the newly formed tissue, are sustained through concomitantly occurring angiogenesis, i.e., formation of new blood vessels from existing ones [10,11]. Thus, osseointegration is a dynamic process whereby bone formation and remodeling occur in parallel around the implant [4,6].

Morphogenesis of osseointegration and assessment of the degree of bone-to-implant contact is usually performed by means of histological evaluation [12], while the underlying molecular processes may be more precisely evaluated at genetic level [13,14]. Data from gene expression analyses of fracture healing provide the basis for understanding these processes [15]. These studies have identified the cells, signals, and interactions governing the key processes of bone regeneration. Bone-forming osteoblasts are primarily derived from marrow-resident multipotent progenitor cells (mesenchymal stem cells (MSCs)), which are recruited to the regeneration site. This process of MSC recruitment and differentiation along the osteogenic lineage is termed as osteoinduction and is controlled primarily by various pro/anti-inflammatory cytokines (CKs) and by growth factors (GFs) secreted by inflammatory cells and/or osteoblasts or by GF resident within the extracellular matrix (e.g., bone morphogenetic proteins (BMPs)) in response to injury [16-18]. Moreover, CKs and GFs act as signaling molecules via specific signaling pathways and guide the process of cell differentiation in the proper temporal sequence [19,20]. Intermediaries in this process are various bone-specific transcription factors (TFs), which act as 'molecular switches' during cell differentiation and are targets of CKs and GFs [21]. TFs facilitate bone-specific gene transcription and ultimately gene expression by which MSCs undergo differentiation and acquire the osteoblastic phenotype [22]. While GFs regulate mainly osteoinduction and osteogenesis, pro-inflammatory CKs regulate the antagonist process of bone resorption by inducing the differentiation of hematopoietic stem cells (HSCs) into osteoclasts and macrophages [23], contributing to the dynamic nature of bone regeneration and remodeling.

Recent *in vitro* [24] and preclinical *in vivo* [25] studies have focused on the early molecular biological responses to various titanium implant surfaces. Understanding these early responses is essential for efforts aiming to accelerate and enhance the process of osseointegration [26]. Upregulation or downregulation of specific genes in peri-implant tissues identified by analyses of genetic material (DNA, RNA) reflects the nature and timing of the various healing processes, which in turn could be potential 'molecular targets' for enhancing osseointegration [27,28]. The aim of the present study was to systematically review the available literature on gene expression analyses of the biological processes involved in early human peri-implant bone healing.

## Methods

### Study design

A study protocol for a systematic qualitative literature review was developed based on recommended methods [29]. The focused question was 'what biological processes are reflected by gene expression analyses in peri-implant tissues of humans during the early stages (up to 4 weeks) of healing?'

### Inclusion and exclusion criteria

All studies, controlled (using different implants) or uncontrolled, reporting gene expression analyses of peri-implant tissues harvested from ≥5 human patients at ≥2 time points during the first 4 weeks of healing, were eligible for inclusion. Studies reporting the use of either 'experimental' (micro) or standard implants with clear description of implant surface properties, placed in the maxilla or mandible and retrieved at a later time point, were eligible for inclusion. Studies reporting (1) analyses of peri-implant mucosa or sulcular fluid or peri-implant tissues of failing or infected implants (peri-implantitis), (2) only histological or immunohistochemical analyses without gene expression of harvested tissues, and (3) *in vitro* and preclinical *in vivo* studies were excluded. Primary outcome of interest was the biological process (or processes) reflected by gene expression at a particular time point of peri-implant tissue healing.

### Search strategy

Electronic databases of MEDLINE (via PubMed) and EMBASE were searched by one author (SS) for relevant English-language literature up to and including June 2014. The search strategy used for MEDLINE was ((((("gene expression" OR transcriptome OR transcriptional OR molecular OR microarray))) AND ((osseointegration OR healing OR "peri implant"))) AND implants) AND ((human OR humans OR patients OR subjects)). Unpublished literature was searched via the Google and Google Scholar search engines. Additionally, the bibliographies of all relevant studies and review articles were searched.

### Study selection

Titles and abstracts of the search identified studies were screened by two authors (SS and VS) based on the inclusion criteria, and full texts of all eligible studies were obtained. Differences in assessment of eligibility were resolved by discussion with the third author (AS). Full texts were independently reviewed by both reviewers, and final inclusion was based on the aforementioned inclusion criteria.

### Data extraction

Both reviewers independently extracted data from the full texts of included articles using specially designed forms. Data on author(s), study design, implant type/surface, any additional procedures performed, number of patients (in each group), presence of a control group, procedure and time of implant retrieval, methods of gene expression analysis, and main results, were extracted. Descriptive summaries of the studies were entered into tables, and a qualitative synthesis of evidence was planned. Any disagreement between the reviewers regarding data extraction was resolved by discussion.

### Assessment of methodology and risk of bias

Assessment of the methodological validity of the included studies was performed using criteria adapted from previous reports [30,31]. Aspects of study design, genotyping methods, and data analyses were considered using nine criteria (Table 1).

The risk of bias in the included studies was assessed using an adaptation of published guidelines for reporting systematic reviews of periodontal genetic association studies [32]. Mainly, aspects of study design and methodological validity were assessed using 15 criteria and scored as 'yes,' 'no,' or 'unclear' based on the information provided in the study manuscript (Table 2). Moreover, published guidance [33] regarding the qualitative and quantitative syntheses of results from genetic association studies was consulted, and heterogeneity across the included studies was assessed to explore the possibility of a meta-analysis.

## Results and discussion

The included studies basically report on commercially available implants from two major manufacturers and involve comparisons of different implant surface technologies in regard with topography and/or chemistry modifications within each implant system. Various analyses were performed in the included studies; however, an attempt has been made to synthesize the various findings and discuss them herein irrespective of the specific implant systems, based on the assumption that basic biological mechanisms of peri-implant bone wound healing are largely implant system independent.

### Search results and study characteristics

Of the 242 search identified studies, only four studies were finally included in the review, all focusing on the impact of implant surface on early human peri-implant bone healing (Figure 1; Table 3). Genetic analyses of total RNA isolated from either newly formed peri-implant bone harvested by trephination [34,35] or from cells adherent to implants retrieved by reverse threading [36,37] were

**Table 1 Assessment of the genotyping methodology in the included studies**

| Methodology | Ivanovski et al. [34] | Donos et al. [35] | Bryington et al. [36] | Thalji et al. [37] |
|---|---|---|---|---|
| Tissue harvesting | Tissue attached to implant carefully removed with a curette, preexisting hard tissue discarded | Tissue attached to implant carefully removed with a curette and homogenized | Implants removed by reverse threading and homogenized; cell lysates isolated | Implants removed by reverse threading and homogenized; cell lysates isolated |
| Sample preparation | Total RNA isolation, purification, quantity/ quality analysis and biotin-labeling | Total RNA isolation, purification, quantity/ quality analysis and biotin-labeling | Total RNA isolation, quantification | Total RNA isolation, purification, quantity/quality analysis and biotin-labeling |
| Array technique | Microarray hybridization (Human WG-6 V3) | Microarray hybridization (Human WG-6 V3) | RT-PCR (custom RT-PCR array for osteogenesis genes; human inflammatory cytokines and receptors PCR array) | Microarray hybridization (Affymetrix Human Gene 1.1 ST) |
| Scanning, data preparation | Bead Station 500/Bead Studio v3 software, raw probe expression values extracted | Bead Station 500/ Bead Studio v3 software, raw probe expression values extracted | $RT^2$ SYBR Green qPCR Master Mix/7500 Real-Time PCR system | Affymetrix Gene Chip Scanner |
| Processing | Noisy data discarded | Noisy data discarded | Normalization of osteogenesis and cytokine array | Unclear |
| Clustering | GO categories (DAVID tool) | GO categories (DAVID tool) | Osteogenesis genes; cytokine-related genes | GO categories (Gene Spring) |
| Statistical analysis | Gene Spring software | Gene Spring software | $RT^2$ Profiler software | Gene Spring software |
| Comparisons | Pair-wise comparisons between three time points (4 vs. 7 days, 7 vs. 14 days, and 4 vs. 14 days) | Pair-wise comparisons at each time point (4, 7, and 14 days) between SLA and SLActive surfaces | T-test to evaluate differences between each implant surface per time point | Two-way ANOVAs to determine differences between implant surface type and time points; pair-wise comparisons of each implant surface independently at different time points (day 7 vs. day 3) |

GO, gene ontology; DAVID, Database for Annotation, Visualization and Integrated Discovery.

**Table 2 Assessment of risk of bias and heterogeneity within and across the included studies**

| Category | Ivanovski et al. [34] | Donos et al. 2011 [35] | Bryington et al. [36] | Thalji et al. [37] |
|---|---|---|---|---|
| Study design | | | | |
| Comparison | None (only SLActive) | SLA vs. SLActive | TiOBlast vs. Osseospeed | TiOBlast vs. Osseospeed |
| Setting | University | University | University | University |
| Population, inclusion criteria | 9 healthy volunteers with no mandibular third molars, no contraindications for oral surgery; age 21 to 48, median 29 years | 9 healthy volunteers with no mandibular third molars; age 21 to 48, median 29 years | 6 women, 4 men; implant patients, systemically healthy (no HTN, diabetes, CVD); age 25 to 58, mean 36.2 years | 9 women, 2 men; implant patients, systemically healthy; age 47 to 69, mean 60.2 years |
| Exclusion criteria | Smokers | Smokers | Smokers, pregnancy, periodontal/periapical disease, subjects taking bisphosphonates, hormone replacement therapy, corticosteroids | Smokers, uncontrolled diabetes, history of head/neck radiotherapy, taking corticosteroids, bisphosphonates |
| Comparability of groups | Unclear | Unclear | Unclear | Unclear |
| Potential confounders, e.g., post-op medication | Unclear | Unclear | Unclear | Unclear |
| Power calculation | No | No | No | No |
| Statistical correction | For multiple sampling | For multiple sampling | Unclear | For multiple sampling |
| Methods | | | | |
| Tissue analyzed | Peri-implant tissue | Peri-implant tissue | Implant-adherent cells | Implant-adherent cells |
| Genetic material analyzed | Total RNA | Total RNA | Total RNA | Total RNA |
| Success rate | Unclear | 16/18 samples (88.8%) | 7/10 subject samples (70%) | Unclear |
| Genotyping method | Microarray | Microarray | RT-PCR | Whole-genome microarray |
| Genotype counts | Yes | Yes | Yes | Yes |
| Blinding | Unclear | Unclear | Yes | Unclear |
| Reproducibility, validated genotyping accuracy | No | No | No | No |

All studies were judged to be at a high risk of bias with substantial heterogeneity across studies.

performed. In total, 111 implants from 43 patients were analyzed. All four studies reported the use of commercially existing implant surfaces, i.e., either a chemically modified, hydrophilic, sand-blasted, acid-etched surface (SLActive®, Institute Straumann AG, Basel, Switzerland); or a hydrophilic (SLActive®) versus a hydrophobic unmodified SLA® (Institute Straumann AG, Basel, Switzerland) surface; or a micro-topographic titanium-oxide grit-blasted surface (TiOBlast®, AstraTech, Molndal, Sweden) versus a chemically modified nano-topographic grit-blasted

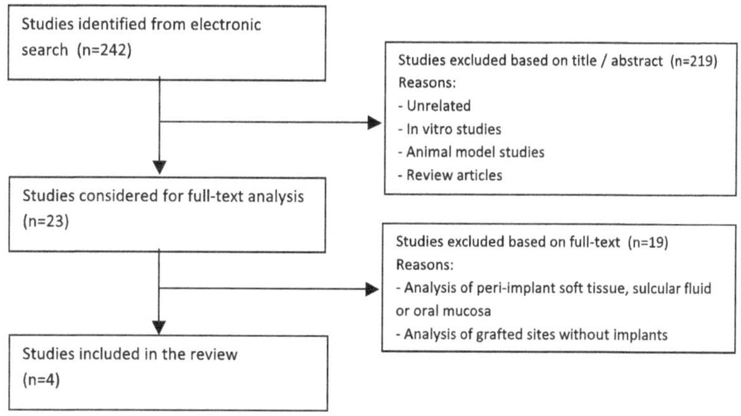


**Figure 1** Flowchart for study selection (*n* = number of studies).

**Table 3 Summary of findings from the included studies ($n = 4$)**

| Study | Ivanovski et al. [34] | Donos et al. [35] | Bryington et al. [36] | Thalji et al. [37] |
|---|---|---|---|---|
| Design | 9 patients; 9 implants placed | 18 patients; 18 implants placed | 10 patients; 60 implants placed | 11 patients; 44 implants placed |
| | Total RNA extracted from peri-implant tissue (trephine) | 16 samples analyzed | 42 samples analyzed | Total RNA extracted from implant adherent cells (reverse thread) |
| | | Total RNA extracted from peri-implant tissue (trephine) | Total RNA extracted from implant adherent cells (reverse thread) | |
| Surface | SLActive | SLA vs. SLActive | TiOBlast vs. Osseospeed | TiOBlast vs. Osseospeed |
| GE day 3/4 | Upregulated | Upregulated on SLA | Upregulated on both surfaces | No significant differences between surfaces at any time point ($P > 0.05$) |
| | CKs (TNF-a, IL-6, IL-2) | Neurogenesis | Osteogenesis (Runx2, Osx, BMP6, OPN) | Results presented as GE at day 7 vs. day 3 for each surface |
| | Immune-inflammatory cells (LC, MP) | Collagen organization | Inflammatory CKs (IL-1A,B, TNF) | |
| | Inflammatory NF-kB p/w | Upregulated on SLActive | MP activity | |
| | | Ras protein p/w | Upregulated on Osseospeed | |
| | | Collagen organization | Chemotaxis (CCL18, CXCL10, CXCL14) | |
| | | CK response | Anti-inflammatory CKs (TOLLIP, IL9, IL22) | |
| GE day **7** | Upregulated | Upregulated on both surfaces | Upregulated on both surfaces | Upregulated on both surfaces |
| | MSC genes (HOX, Sp3) | Inflammatory CKs (IL1, IL2, IL6, TNFS) | Osteogenesis (Runx2, Osx*, OCN*, OPN, BMP6, BSP) | ECM (Coll, GPs, PGs) |
| | GF (TGF-B receptor) | Neurogenesis | [* Osseo > TiOB; $P < 0.05$] | Collagen organization (PLODs, LOX, PCOLCE) |
| | VEGF sig. (vs. day 14) | Upregulated on SLActive | | Angiogenesis/VEGF sig. (ANXA, EPAS1) |
| | Wnt p/w | Neurogenesis (BDNF, NTF3) | | Ossification |
| | Downregulated | ECM (OPN) | | Remodeling (MMPs, TIMPs) |
| | Inflammatory NF-kB p/w (vs. day 4) | BMP p/w (BMP4, BMP2K) | | Osteoclastic (CTSK, ACP5) |
| | | MAPK sig. | | Chemotaxis (CKs, MP activity) |
| | | Mineralization | | Anti-inflammatory CKs (CCL22, CCL18) |
| | | Focal adhesion (integrins) | | Downregulated on both surfaces |
| | | Angiogenesis (VEGF sig., P13-Akt p/w) | | Inflammatory CKs (IL1A, IL1B) |
| | | Downregulated on SLActive | | |
| | | Inflammatory cells (LC) | | |
| GE day 14 | Upregulated | Upregulated on both surfaces | - | |
| | ECM (Coll, OC, ON, ALP) | BMP p/w (BMP4, BMP2K) | | |
| | TFs (Osx, Dlx5, Twist1, Smad6) | Downregulated on both surfaces | | |
| | Remodeling (MMP, CTSK) | Inflammatory cells (LC) | | |
| | GFs (BMP, GDF) | | | |
| | Angiogenesis (VEGF sig.) | | | |
| | Neurogenesis | | | |

**Table 3 Summary of findings from the included studies (*n* = 4)** *(Continued)*

| |
|---|
| TGF-b/BMP, Notch p/w |
| Ras protein p/w |
| Wnt-receptor genes |
| Notch genes (up/down) |
| Downregulated |
| Inflammatory response (vs. day 7) |

GE, gene expression; CKs, cytokines; p/w, pathway; MSC, mesenchymal stem cells; GF, growth factors; sig., signaling; ECM, extracellular matrix; TFs, transcription factors; MP, macrophage; LC, lymphocytes; GPs, glycoproteins; PGs, proteoglycans.

surface (Osseospeed®, AstraTech, Molndal, Sweden). Implant retrieval times were at 3 or 4 days and 7 days in all studies and additionally at 14 days in two studies [34,35].

### Assessment of methodology and risk of bias

All studies used validated methods for gene expression analysis; genetic data was analyzed using microarray (three studies) or real-time PCR (RT-PCR) (one study) methods (Table 1). Total RNA was isolated from lysates of either trephined peri-implant tissues or implant-adherent cells, and subjected to microarray processing or RT-PCR. Although moderate-to-good agreement has been reported between the two methods, validation of DNA microarray results by the more sensitive PCR array is generally recommended [38]. None of the microarray studies identified have validated their results using RT-PCR. Genotyping data (gene lists) were imported and analyzed using computer software and further condensed into functionally and biologically relevant categories. Nevertheless, differential gene expression in relation to a particular cell type or region of tissue analyzed was not performed [35]. Gene 'upregulation' was reported when genes were expressed at a higher level on one implant surface in comparison to another; in context, differentiation between gene expression and overexpression may be difficult to define. Statistical methods were used to compare differences in gene expression between different time points and/or implant surfaces ($P < 0.05$ significance level), while correcting for possible errors, i.e., false gene discovery rate due to multiple sampling [39]. There was considerable heterogeneity across the included studies in terms of study design, population, implant surface technology, genotyping methods, and data analyses (Table 2). Therefore, no meta-analysis of association between gene expression and implant surface properties was relevant.

Thus, high risk of bias should be considered when interpreting the results, due to the above methodological limitations and the overall limited information (four studies) available.

### Biological processes identified through gene expression in peri-implant tissues

Conventional implant surgery involves osteotomy preparation and insertion of the implant into the alveolar bone. The immediate local effects of this procedure, functionally relevant to subsequent healing processes, are (1) bone trauma, (2) formation of bone debris, (3) hemostasis and clot formation, and (4) hypoxia. These effects involve the release of specific CKs and GFs within the local environment [7], resulting in recruitment of two primary cell types to the site, inflammatory cells and progenitor cells (MSCs and HSCs) [19], which in turn regulate the subsequent healing processes. A summary of differentially regulated genes relating to the involved biological processes is presented in Table 4, while Figure 2 represents an evidence-based illustrative model summarizing these processes.

### Inflammation

All studies reported a significant upregulation of genes associated with inflammation during the first time point of observation (day 3 or 4) regardless of the implant surface. Specifically, upregulation regarded pro-inflammatory cytokines of the interleukin (IL), tumor necrosis factor (TNF), and interferon (IFN) families, as well as genes associated with proliferation of lymphocytes and macrophages (MPs). Previous *in vitro* [40,41] and animal [42] studies have reported the significance of MPs at the bone-implant interface and identified favorable MP activity in relation to modified rough surfaces as demonstrated by *in vitro* gene expression that was associated with increased *in vivo* bone formation. Also, the nuclear factor-kB (NF-kB) inflammatory pathway was upregulated at day 4 [34], while macrophage activity and chemokines of the CCL and CXL families in the peri-implant tissues continued to remain prominent at day 7.

However, this inflammatory response was generally downregulated at later time points (day 7 or 14). For example, in one study, genes associated with pro-inflammatory cytokines (IL-1B, IL-1A, IL-1R2) and chemokines (CCL22, CCL18) were downregulated and upregulated, respectively, on day 7,

**Table 4 Summary of biological processes and associated genes reported in the included studies**

| Process | Upregulated genes<br>Category (gene code) |
|---|---|
| Inflammation/immune response | |
| Pro-inflammatory cytokines | Tumor necrosis factor (TNF-a, TNFSF9) |
| | Interleukin (IL-6, IL-2, IL-1 F9, IL-23A, IL-6ST) |
| | Interferon (IFNA2) |
| | Nuclear factor-kB (I-kB kinase/NF-kB) |
| Anti-inflammatory cytokines | Interleukin (IL-22, IL-9) |
| | Toll interacting protein (TOLLIP) |
| Cells | Lymphocyte, macrophage negative proliferation (BTLA, LST1) |
| | Macrophage scavenger receptor (MSR1) |
| Chemotaxis | Chemokines (CCR8, CCL18, CCL22, CXCL10, CXCL14) |
| Osteoinduction/osteogenesis | |
| Growth factors (GF)/ signaling pathways | Insulin-like GF (IGF1) |
| | Transforming GF (TGF-b, TGF-b receptor 1, 2 and 3, TGF-a) |
| | Platelet-derived GF (PDGF receptor) |
| | Bone morphogenetic proteins (BMP4, BMP6, BMP receptor 1A, BMP2-K) |
| | Growth and differentiation factor (GDF10) |
| | Wnt frizzled receptor (FZD3, FZD8, FRZB) |
| | Notch (NOTCH2) |
| | Ras-protein signal transduction (RAP1B, RAP1A, RASGRP4) |
| | Mitogen activated protein kinase (MAP3K7IP2, MAPK9, MAP2K3, MAP3K2) |
| Transcription factors | 'Master switches' [RUNX2, SP7 (OSX)] |
| | Homeobox (DLX1, DLX5, HOXD12, MSX1, HOXA5, HOXB1, HOXB6, HOXC6) |
| | SP [SP1, SP3, SP7 (Osx)] |
| | Twist (TWIST 1-receptor) |
| ECM deposition/ organization | Collagen (Col1A1, Col12A1, Col6A3, Col3A1, Col6A1, Col11A1, Col11A2, Col13A1, Col5A2) |
| | Non-collagen proteins [BGLAP (OC), SPARC (ON), SPP1 (OP), BSP, IBSP, POSTN, ECM1] |
| | Small leucine-rich proteoglycans (SLRP) (DCN, BGN, LUM) |
| | Heat-shock protein 47 (HSP47) |
| | Alkaline phosphatase (ALPL) |
| | Cadherin (CDH11) |
| | Integrin (ITGB4, ITGB5) |
| | Laminin (LAMA2, LAMA3) |
| | Pro-collagen lysyl-hydroxylase (PLOD1, PLOD2, PLOD3) |
| | Pro-collagen C-endopeptidase enhancer (PCOLCE) |
| | Lysyl-oxidase (LOX) |

**Table 4 Summary of biological processes and associated genes reported in the included studies** *(Continued)*

| | |
|---|---|
| Osteoclast activity/ remodeling | Cathepsin K (CTSK, CTSK-receptor) |
| | Tartarate-resistant acid phosphatase (TRAP/ACP5) |
| | Matrix metallopeptidase (MMP2, MMP12, MMP9, MMP7, MMP13) |
| | Tissue inhibitor metallopeptidase (TIMP2, TIMP3) |
| Angiogenesis | Vascular endothelial GF-signaling (EPAS1, ANXA2, EGR1-binding protein) |
| | Phosphatidyl-inositol 3-kinase (PI3K)-Akt signaling |
| Neurogenesis | Brain-derived neurotrophic factor (BDNF) |
| | Neurotrophin 3 (NTF3) |
| | NK2 homeobox 2(NKX2-2) |
| | Tubby-like protein 3 (TULP3) |

at both implant surface technologies examined (Osseospeed and TiOBlast) [37]. Moreover, the anti-inflammatory response seemed to be modulated by surface properties. In one study, genes related to anti-inflammatory cytokines such as IL-9, IL-22, toll-like receptor inhibitor protein (TOLLIP), and several key chemokines (CCL18, CXCL10, CXCL18) were significantly upregulated on Osseospeed surfaces but not TiOBlast, at day 3 [36]. In another study, genes associated with inflammatory cell proliferation were significantly downregulated earlier on SLActive surfaces compared to the SLA, i.e., at day 7 instead of day 14 [35]. Therefore, the initial inflammatory response seems to be important for the recruitment of cells that govern subsequent healing processes and is regulated by a natural biological immune response which may be further modified by implant surface properties.

### Osteogenic differentiation

Cells along the osteogenic differentiation pathway may be artificially categorized as (1) undifferentiated MSCs, (2) osteo-chondro-progenitor cells, (3) pre-osteoblasts, and (4) osteoblasts; although in reality, a developmental continuum without distinct boundaries may exist [43]. While pre-differentiated osteoblasts in the marrow compartment only play a minor role in bone wound healing, a more prominent role is that of undifferentiated MSCs which are recruited to the regeneration site where they differentiate into osteoblasts [16]. The recruitment and differentiation of MSCs is regulated by CKs and GFs [17,19]. The GFs most commonly implicated in bone wound healing are BMPs, members of the TGF-$\beta$ family, PDGF, and IGF-1 [19,20]. Moreover, the bone debris created during implant surgery, the peri-implant blood clot (i.e., platelets) and the differentiating MSCs themselves further contribute to release of GFs at the site [44,45].

All studies reported some evidence of osteogenic differentiation at an early time point (day 3 or 4) via

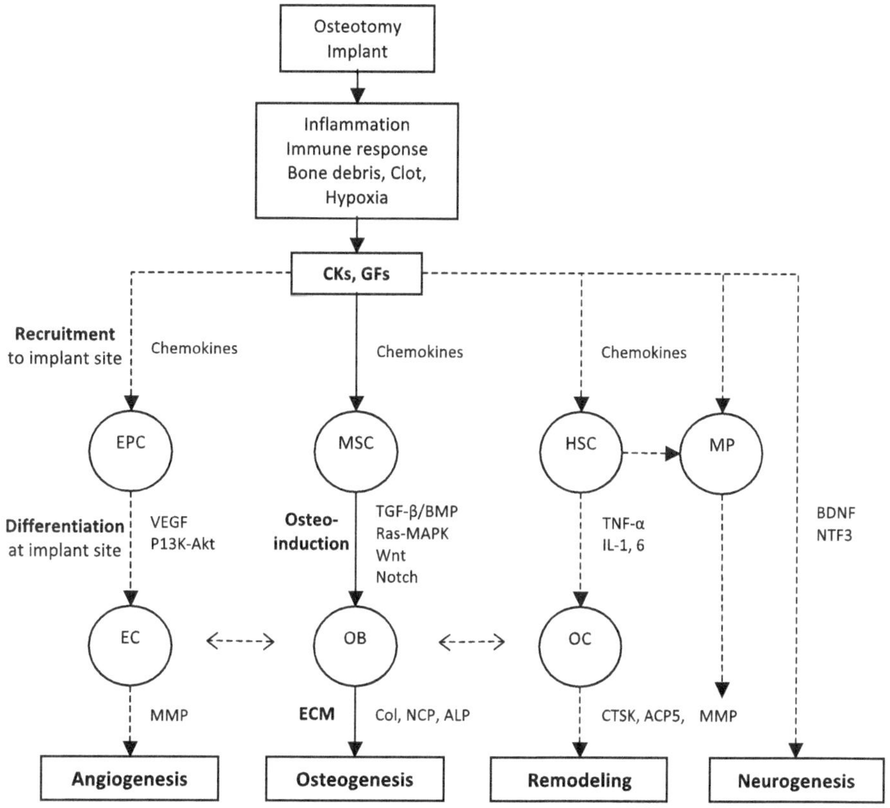


**Figure 2 Summary of biological processes identified via gene expression during early peri-implant bone healing.** CKs, cytokines; GFs, growth factors; EPC, endothelial progenitor cells; EC, endothelial cells; MSC, mesenchymal stem cells; OB, osteoblasts; ECM, extracellular matrix; HSC, haematopoietic stem cells; MP, macrophages; OC, osteoclasts.

expression of genes associated with key growth factors (bone morphogenetic proteins (BMP4, BMP6, BMP2-kinase), growth and differentiation factor-10 (GDF10), transforming growth factors (TGF-α, TGF-β), platelet-derived growth factor (PDGF), and insulin-like growth factor-1 (IGF1)), transcription factors (Runx2, Osx, Dlx3, Dlx5, Msx1, HOX genes, Sp1, Sp3), and/or osteogenic signaling pathways (TGF-β/BMP signaling, Wnt-receptors, Ras-protein/mitogen-activated protein kinase (Ras/MAPK) signal transduction). In all studies, these genes were further upregulated at day 7. Upregulation of osteogenic factors seemed regulated by implant surface. The key transcription factor osterix (Osx) was upregulated on the Osseospeed surface, but not TiOBlast at day 7 [36], while tissues adjacent to SLActive surfaces demonstrated comparatively greater BMP and Ras/MAPK expression compared to SLA surfaces at day 7 [35]. Previous *in vivo* animal studies have reported correlations between upregulated osteogenic gene expression in peri-implant tissues and enhanced histological and biomechanical measures of osseointegration during early (1- to 4-week) healing times [27,46]; nevertheless, it is unclear whether upregulation and/or overexpression of genes at a specific time point directly correlates to increased protein production *in vivo*.

The key signaling pathways, via which GFs guide osteogenic cell differentiation, are the TGF-β/BMP- and Wnt-mediated pathways [19,47]. While the BMP pathway ensures differentiation of MSCs into osteo-chondro-progenitors (OCPs), the Wnt pathway is essential for subsequent osteoblastic commitment, i.e., Wnt acts 'downstream' of BMP to ensure that OCPs differentiate into osteoblasts and not chondroblasts [47]. Genes associated with both TGF-β/BMP and Wnt pathway (Wnt receptors) were upregulated at day 7 [34,35] and day 14 [34] on SLA and SLActive surfaces, suggesting the occurrence of osteogenic differentiation at these time points.

GF-regulated signaling pathways exert their effects on differentiating cells via activation of TFs. The TFs Runx2 and Osx are considered as 'master switches' and absolute requirements for osteoblast differentiation [21] - while Runx2 is essential for MSC differentiation, Osx acting 'downstream' of Runx2 controls osteoblastic fate determination [48,49]. An upregulation of these genes was observed in relation to the TiOBlast, Osseospeed, and SLActive surfaces in the present review. However, at day 7, expression of Osx was significantly greater on Osseospeed than TiOBlast surfaces. This finding is consistent with previous animal [50,51] and human studies

[52] where superior *in vivo* osseointegration (i.e., larger amount of bone-to-implant contact occurring earlier) of Osseospeed versus TiOBlast implants was reported. Thus, it appears that implant surface topography and/or chemistry influence peri-implant bone healing in humans both at the signaling pathway and transcription factor level.

### ECM production

Deposition of new bone on the implant surface involves the secretion of a complex ECM (scaffold) of proteins by osteoblasts, which subsequently undergoes mineralization [9]. Expression of ECM proteins is a reliable indicator of early osteogenic activity [19] and was identified in all four studies at days 7 and 14. All studies reported some evidence of ECM production and/or organization at days 7 and 14. Upregulated genes associated with ECM deposition included various collagens (Col 1 to 11), non-collagen proteins (osteopontin (OPN), osteonectin (ON), osteocalcin (OCN), bone sialoprotein (IBSP), periostin (POSTN), and ECM protein-1), alkaline phosphatase (ALP), and bone-specific adhesion proteins (integrins (ITGB4, ITGB5), laminins (LAMA2, LAMA3), and cadherins (CDH11)). Osteocalcin, the most bone-specific ECM protein and a late marker of osteogenic differentiation [19], was significantly upregulated on Osseospeed (versus TiOBlast) surfaces at day 7 [36]. Osteopontin, an ECM protein essential for mineralization [53], was significantly upregulated on SLActive comparing to SLA surfaces at day 7 [35]. The possibility that implant surface features enhance osteogenic differentiation of MSCs via upregulation of specific genes (e.g., SLActive versus SLA in regard with BMP and Wnt signaling) has been demonstrated *in vitro* [54].

Furthermore, genes associated with collagen fibril formation/organization (heat-shock protein-47 (HSP-47), pro-collagen C-endopeptidase enhancer (PCOLCE), small leucine-rich proteoglycans (SLRP)) and post-translational modification (pro-collagen lysyl-hydroxylases (PLOD1, PLOD2, PLOD3) and lysyl-oxidase (LOX)) were upregulated on Osseospeed and TiOBlast surfaces [37]. Collagen comprises approximately 90% of the ECM and collagen fibrillogenesis and organization directly determine the biomechanical properties of bone [55,56]. Genes associated with collagen fibril formation, maturation, and post-translational modification expressed by osteoblasts [57,58] were upregulated on TiOBlast and Osseospeed implants, representing early ECM organization at the bone-implant interface. These modifications determine the pattern of collagen cross-linking which in turn influences tissue organization, mineralization, and ultimately mechanical bone strength [56], and in the case of osseointegration, the integrity of the bone-implant interface [37].

### Osteoclastic activity and remodeling

While GFs regulate osteogenesis, pro-inflammatory CKs (e.g., IL-1, IL-6, TNF-α) simultaneously regulate the antagonist process of bone resorption via osteoclasts [23]. Moreover, osteoblasts themselves stimulate osteoclastogenesis via macrophage colony stimulating factor (M-CSF) and receptor activator of NF-kB ligand (RANKL) genes but also closely regulate this process via osteoprotegerin (OPG), an inhibitor of RANKL [59].

Two studies reported expression of genes associated with osteoclastic activity and ECM degradation (cathepsin-K (CTSK), tartarate-resistant acid phosphatase (ACP5), and/or matrix metalloproteinases (MMPs)), on Osseospeed and TiOBlast surfaces at day 7 [37], and SLActive surfaces at day 14. However, upregulation of MMP inhibitors (TIMP-2, -3) was also reported on TiOBlast and Osseospeed surfaces suggesting a control of the resorption process. Although no studies reported differential RANKL/OPG expression, a previous *in vitro* study [60] reported significant downregulation of osteoclastogenic genes on SLActive surfaces. Collectively, these data reaffirm the dynamic nature of bone formation and resorption at the implant-bone interface, even in early healing stages, and suggest the possibility for implant surface technology modulation of bone remodeling.

### Angiogenesis

Angiogenesis is closely related to osteogenesis and occurs simultaneously during bone regeneration [11]. Physiological oxygen tensions in bone are about 12.5% $O_2$ but fall to 1% $O_2$ in regeneration sites due to disruption of the local vasculature as a result of injury and/or surgery [61,62]. A key event that stimulates angiogenesis (and osteogenesis) at regeneration sites is hypoxia, via the hypoxia inducible (transcription) factor-1 (HIF-1) that regulates expression of angiogenic genes [63]. The key cells involved in angiogenesis are macrophages, which in response to hypoxia and inflammation release chemotactic and angiogenic growth factors (e.g., VEGF) [40,64], and endothelial progenitor cells (EPCs) which differentiate into endothelial cell lining blood vessels [65]. VEGF is the single most important regulator of EPC differentiation and vessel formation [66]. Moreover, a role for VEGF in osteogenic differentiation has also been suggested mainly via interaction with the BMP signaling pathway [67].

In the present review, a significant simultaneous upregulation of several angiogenesis-related genes was identified at day 7 in all included studies. Pro-angiogenic factors (ANXA2, EPAS-1) were upregulated at TiOBlast and Osseospeed surfaces at day 7 [37]. Genes associated with VEGF and P13K-AKT signaling pathways were upregulated at SLActive (but not SLA) surfaces on day 7 and continued to be upregulated on day 14 [35]. The P13K-AKT pathway is reported to be important for endothelial cell survival, migration, and vessel formation, in addition to aiding VEGF-mediated angiogenesis [68]. Previous *in vitro* studies have reported the pro-angiogenic effects of SLActive surfaces by promoting VEGF expression in EPCs and osteoblasts [65,69], while enhanced histological osseointegration of SLActive implants has been directly correlated with increased angiogenesis in a dog model [70,71]. Thus, implant surface technology appears to have the possibility to also influence angiogenesis at early stages of wound healing.

### Neurogenesis

Bone innervation includes both myelinated and unmyelinated nerve fibers located in the periosteum, bone cortex, Haversian systems, Volkmann's canals, and the marrow spaces [72]. An interesting finding in the present review was the significant upregulation of genes associated with neurogenesis, more than any other biological process, on SLActive and SLA surfaces at all time points [34,35]. Specific processes represented were axon formation, growth and differentiation, and the neural signaling pathway. This is consistent with previous *in vivo* reports of murine fracture healing [73] and calvarial defect regeneration in relation to SLA surfaces [74,75]. Key neurotrophic factors (brain-derived neurotrophic factor (BDNF) and neurotrophin 3 (NTF3)), essential for neuronal survival and differentiation during development [76], were significantly upregulated on SLActive versus SLA surfaces at day 7 suggesting an effect of surface modulation. The P13K-AKT pathway, upregulated on SLActive surfaces (in relation to angiogenesis), has also been implicated in neuronal survival and subsequent neural development [77,78] and could have contributed to upregulation of neurogenic genes at these surfaces. Indeed, previous histologic reports have described changes in bone innervation after implant placement (and loading) and the presence of nerve fibers within the peri-implant bone, in animals and humans [79-81].

It can be hypothesized that peri-implant neurogenesis is one of the underlying mechanisms governing the phenomenon of osseoperception, defined as the tactile sensibility of osseointegrated implants to occlusal forces induced via activation of nerve endings and/or receptors in the peri-implant environment [82,83]. Moreover, recent evidence suggests that implant surface properties may influence the degree of osseoperception in humans [84], which can be correlated with the genomic evidence for implant surface modulation of neurogenesis during osseointegration.

Finally, the present review findings are consistent with a recent gene expression study of healing extraction sockets in humans [85]. This study reported an initial upregulation of pro-inflammatory cytokines (IL-1, IL-6) at day 1, but by day 7, genes suggestive of immune response (IL-10), osteogenesis (TGF, BMP4, BMP7, OCN and ALP), and angiogenesis (VEGF) were upregulated, continuing until day 14, suggesting that the basic biological processes governing alveolar wound healing and osseointegration are the same.

## Conclusions

Based on limited evidence of gene expression data from four studies involving 43 patients, the following remarks can be made:

1. Early peri-implant healing (2 weeks) involves a sequence of biological events which are similar to those observed in other bone wound healing scenarios (fractures, extraction-sockets).
2. Osseointegration depends on osteogenesis at the implant interface, but other simultaneously occurring processes such as inflammation, bone resorption, angiogenesis and neurogenesis also play an important role, as evidenced by consistent and concomitant gene expression.
3. Several genes associated with key regulators of biological processes, such as cells, cytokines, growth factors, transcription factors, signaling pathways, and secretory products, were shown to be differentially regulated during peri-implant healing in a manner that was largely consistent - in terms of nature and timing - with previous *in vitro* and preclinical *in vivo* histological studies of osseointegration.
4. Implant surface technology can influence osseointegration, at every step of the early wound healing process, i.e., anti-inflammatory response, progenitor cell recruitment, osteoinduction, growth factor/transcription factor expression, signaling pathway regulation, and extracellular matrix production. However, the relevance of those observations is questionable; no distinct differences have been demonstrated in terms of histological outcomes at later time points or short- and long-term clinical performance among the various implant surface technologies discussed herein.

**Competing interests**
The authors declare that they have no competing interests.

**Authors' contributions**
SS conceived and carried out the study and drafted the manuscript. VS and AS participated in carrying out the study and drafting the manuscript. All authors read and approved the final manuscript.

**Author details**
[1]Department of Periodontology, Faculty of Odontology, Malmö University, Carl Gustafs väg 34, 214 21 Malmö, Sweden. [2]Centre for Oral Rehabilitation & Implant Dentistry, 1 Laxmi Niwas, 87 Bajaj Road, Vile Parle West, Mumbai 400056, India.

## References


1. Setzer FC, Kim S. Comparison of long-term survival of implants and endodontically treated teeth. J Dent Res. 2014;93(1):19–26. doi:10.1177/0022034513504782.
2. Albrektsson T, Brånemark PI, Hansson HA, Lindström J. Osseointegrated titanium implants. Requirements for ensuring a long-lasting, direct bone-to-implant anchorage in man. Acta Orthop Scand. 1981;52(2):155–70.
3. Berglundh T, Abrahamsson I, Lang NP, Lindhe J. De novo alveolar bone formation adjacent to endosseous implants. Clin Oral Implants Res. 2003;14(3):251–62. doi:972.
4. Abrahamsson I, Berglundh T, Linder E, Lang NP, Lindhe J. Early bone formation adjacent to rough and turned endosseous implant surfaces. An experimental study in the dog. Clin Oral Implants Res. 2004;15(4):381–92. doi: 10.1111/j.1600-0501.2004.01082.x.
5. Lang NP, Salvi GE, Huynh-Ba G, Ivanovski S, Donos N, Bosshardt DD. Early osseointegration to hydrophilic and hydrophobic implant surfaces in humans. Clin Oral Implants Res. 2011;22(4):349–56. doi:10.1111/j.1600-0501.2011.02172.x.
6. Bosshardt DD, Salvi GE, Huynh-Ba G, Ivanovski S, Donos N, Lang NP. The role of bone debris in early healing adjacent to hydrophilic and hydrophobic implant surfaces in man. Clin Oral Implants Res. 2011;22(4):357–64. doi:10.1111/j.1600-0501.2010.02107.x.
7. Terheyden H, Lang NP, Bierbaum S, Stadlinger B. Osseointegration - communication of cells. Clin Oral Implants Res. 2012;23(10):1127–35. doi:10.1111/j.1600-0501.2011.02327.x.
8. Marco F, Milena F, Gianluca G, Vittoria O. Peri-implant osteogenesis in health and osteoporosis. Micron. 2005;36(7–8):630–44. doi:10.1016/j.micron.2005.07.008.
9. Sela J, Gross UM, Kohavi D, Shani J, Dean DD, Boyan BD, et al. Primary mineralization at the surfaces of implants. Crit Rev Oral Biol Med. 2000;11(4):423–36.
10. Raghavendra S, Wood MC, Taylor TD. Early wound healing around endosseous implants: a review of the literature. Int J Oral Maxillofac Implants. 2005;20(3):425–31.
11. Kanczler JM, Oreffo RO. Osteogenesis and angiogenesis: the potential for engineering bone. Eur Cell Mater. 2008;15:100–14.
12. Sağirkaya E, Kucukekenci AS, Karasoy D, Akça K, Eckert SE, Çehreli MC. Comparative assessments, meta-analysis, and recommended guidelines for reporting studies on histomorphometric bone-implant contact in humans. Int J Oral Maxillofac Implants. 2013;28(5):1243–53.
13. Kojima N, Ozawa S, Miyata Y, Hasegawa H, Tanaka Y, Ogawa T. High-throughput gene expression analysis in bone healing around titanium implants by DNA microarray. Clin Oral Implants Res. 2008;19(2):173–81. doi:10.1111/j.1600-0501.2007.01432.x.
14. Lin Z, Rios HF, Volk SL, Sugai JV, Jin Q, Giannobile WV. Gene expression dynamics during bone healing and osseointegration. J Periodontol. 2011;82(7):1007–17. doi:10.1902/jop.2010.100577.
15. Ai-Aql ZS, Alagl AS, Graves DT, Gerstenfeld LC, Einhorn TA. Molecular mechanisms controlling bone formation during fracture healing and distraction osteogenesis. J Dent Res. 2008;87(2):107–18.
16. Albrektsson T, Johansson C. Osteoinduction, osteoconduction and osseointegration. Eur Spine J. 2001;10 Suppl 2:S96–101. doi:10.1007/s005860100282.
17. Miron RJ, Zhang YF. Osteoinduction: a review of old concepts with new standards. J Dent Res. 2012;91(8):736–44. doi:10.1177/0022034511435260.
18. Ito H. Chemokines in mesenchymal stem cell therapy for bone repair: a novel concept of recruiting mesenchymal stem cells and the possible cell sources. Mod Rheumatol. 2011;21(2):113–21. doi:10.1007/s10165-010-0357-8.
19. Hughes FJ, Turner W, Belibasakis G, Martuscelli G. Effects of growth factors and cytokines on osteoblast differentiation. Periodontol 2000. 2006;41:48–72. doi:10.1111/j.1600-0757.2006.00161.x.
20. Scheller EL, Krebsbach PH. The use of soluble signals to harness the power of the bone microenvironment for implant therapeutics. Int J Oral Maxillofac Implants. 2011;26(Suppl):70–9. discussion 80–4.
21. Marie PJ. Transcription factors controlling osteoblastogenesis. Arch Biochem Biophys. 2008;473(2):98–105. doi:10.1016/j.abb.2008.02.030.
22. Fakhry M, Hamade E, Badran B, Buchet R, Magne D. Molecular mechanisms of mesenchymal stem cell differentiation towards osteoblasts. World J Stem Cells. 2013;5(4):136–48. doi: 10.4252/wjsc.v5.i4.136.
23. Minkin C, Marinho VC. Role of the osteoclast at the bone-implant interface. Adv Dent Res. 1999;13:49–56.
24. Thalji G, Cooper L. Molecular assessment of osseointegration in vitro: a review of the current literature. Oral & Craniofacial Tissue Engineering. 2012;2(3):221–49.
25. Thalji G, Cooper LF. Molecular assessment of osseointegration in vivo: a review of the current literature. Int J Oral Maxillofac Implants. 2013;28(6):e521–34.
26. Cooper LF. Biologic determinants of bone formation for osseointegration: clues for future clinical improvements. J Prosthet Dent. 1998;80(4):439–49.
27. Omar OM, Lennerås ME, Suska F, Emanuelsson L, Hall JM, Palmquist A, et al. The correlation between gene expression of proinflammatory markers and bone formation during osseointegration with titanium implants. Biomaterials. 2011;32(2):374–86. doi:10.1016/j.biomaterials.2010.09.011.
28. Nishimura I. Genetic networks in osseointegration. J Dent Res. 2013;92(12 Suppl):109S–18. doi:10.1177/0022034513504928.
29. Higgins JPT, Green S, editors. *Cochrane Handbook for Systematic Reviews of Interventions* Version 5.1.0 [updated March 2011]. The Cochrane Collaboration, 2011. Available from www.cochrane-handbook.org; 2011.
30. Tarca AL, Romero R, Draghici S. Analysis of microarray experiments of gene expression profiling. Am J Obstet Gynecol. 2006;195(2):373–88. doi:10.1016/j.ajog.2006.07.001.
31. Slonim DK, Yanai I. Getting started in gene expression microarray analysis. PLoS Comput Biol. 2009;5(10):e1000543. doi:10.1371/journal.pcbi.1000543.
32. Nibali L. Suggested guidelines for systematic reviews of periodontal genetic association studies. J Clin Periodontol. 2013;40(8):753–6. doi:10.1111/jcpe.12128.
33. Little J, Higgins JP, Ioannidis JP, Moher D, Gagnon F, von Elm E, et al. Strengthening the reporting of genetic association studies (STREGA): an extension of the STROBE statement. PLoS Med. 2009;6(2):e22. doi:10.1371/journal.pmed.1000022.
34. Ivanovski S, Hamlet S, Salvi GE, Huynh-Ba G, Bosshardt DD, Lang NP, et al. Transcriptional profiling of osseointegration in humans. Clin Oral Implants Res. 2011;22(4):373–81. doi:10.1111/j.1600-0501.2010.02112.x.
35. Donos N, Hamlet S, Lang NP, Salvi GE, Huynh-Ba G, Bosshardt DD, et al. Gene expression profile of osseointegration of a hydrophilic compared with a hydrophobic microrough implant surface. Clin Oral Implants Res. 2011;22(4):365–72. doi:10.1111/j.1600-0501.2010.02113.x.
36. Bryington M, Mendonça G, Nares S, Cooper LF. Osteoblastic and cytokine gene expression of implant-adherent cells in humans. Clin Oral Implants Res. 2012; doi:10.1111/clr.12054.
37. Thalji GN, Nares S, Cooper LF. Early molecular assessment of osseointegration in humans. Clin Oral Implants Res. 2013; doi:10.1111/clr.12266.
38. Morey JS, Ryan JC, Van Dolah FM. Microarray validation: factors influencing correlation between oligonucleotide microarrays and real-time PCR. Biol Proced Online. 2006;8:175–93. doi:10.1251/bpo126.
39. Benjamini Y, Drai D, Elmer G, Kafkafi N, Golani I. Controlling the false discovery rate in behavior genetics research. Behav Brain Res. 2001;125(1–2):279–84.
40. Alfarsi MA, Hamlet SM, Ivanovski S. Titanium surface hydrophilicity modulates the human macrophage inflammatory cytokine response. J Biomed Mater Res A. 2013; doi:10.1002/jbm.a.34666.
41. Pajarinen J, Kouri VP, Jämsen E, Li TF, Mandelin J, Konttinen YT. The response of macrophages to titanium particles is determined by macrophage polarization. Acta Biomater. 2013;9(11):9229–40. doi:10.1016/j.actbio.2013.06.027.
42. Chehroudi B, Ghrebi S, Murakami H, Waterfield JD, Owen G, Brunette DM. Bone formation on rough, but not polished, subcutaneously implanted Ti surfaces is preceded by macrophage accumulation. J Biomed Mater Res A. 2010;93(2):724–37. doi:10.1002/jbm.a.32587.
43. Heng BC, Cao T, Stanton LW, Robson P, Olsen B. Strategies for directing the differentiation of stem cells into the osteogenic lineage in vitro. J Bone Miner Res. 2004;19(9):1379–94. doi:10.1359/JBMR.040714.
44. Dhore CR, Snel SJ, Jacques SV, Naert IE, Walboomers XF, Jansen JA. In vitro osteogenic potential of bone debris resulting from placement of titanium screw-type implants. Clin Oral Implants Res. 2008;19(6):606–11. doi:10.1111/j.1600-0501.2007.01519.x.
45. Kim DH, Yoo KH, Choi KS, Choi J, Choi SY, Yang SE, et al. Gene expression profile of cytokine and growth factor during differentiation of bone marrow-derived mesenchymal stem cell. Cytokine. 2005;31(2):119–26. doi:10.1016/j.cyto.2005.04.004.
46. Omar O, Svensson S, Zoric N, Lenneras M, Suska F, Wigren S, et al. In vivo gene expression in response to anodically oxidized versus machined titanium implants. J Biomed Mater Res A. 2010;92(4):1552–66. doi:10.1002/jbm.a.32475.

47. Marcellini S, Henriquez JP, Bertin A. Control of osteogenesis by the canonical Wnt and BMP pathways in vivo: cooperation and antagonism between the canonical Wnt and BMP pathways as cells differentiate from osteochondroprogenitors to osteoblasts and osteocytes. Bioessays. 2012;34(11):953–62. doi:10.1002/bies.201200061.
48. Nakashima K, Zhou X, Kunkel G, Zhang Z, Deng JM, Behringer RR, et al. The novel zinc finger-containing transcription factor osterix is required for osteoblast differentiation and bone formation. Cell. 2002;108(1):17–29.
49. Komori T. Regulation of osteoblast differentiation by Runx2. Adv Exp Med Biol. 2010;658:43–9. doi:10.1007/978-1-4419-1050-9_5.
50. Guo J, Padilla RJ, Ambrose W, De Kok IJ, Cooper LF. The effect of hydrofluoric acid treatment of TiO2 grit blasted titanium implants on adherent osteoblast gene expression in vitro and in vivo. Biomaterials. 2007;28(36):5418–25. doi:10.1016/j.biomaterials.2007.08.032.
51. Mendonça G, Mendonça DB, Simões LG, Araújo AL, Leite ER, Duarte WR, et al. Nanostructured alumina-coated implant surface: effect on osteoblast-related gene expression and bone-to-implant contact in vivo. Int J Oral Maxillofac Implants. 2009;24(2):205–15.
52. Rocci M, Rocci A, Martignoni M, Albrektsson T, Barlattani A, Gargari M. Comparing the TiOblast and Osseospeed surfaces. Histomorphometric and histological analysis in humans. Oral Implantol (Rome). 2008;1(1):34–42.
53. Qin C, Baba O, Butler WT. Post-translational modifications of sibling proteins and their roles in osteogenesis and dentinogenesis. Crit Rev Oral Biol Med. 2004;15(3):126–36.
54. Vlacic-Zischke J, Hamlet SM, Friis T, Tonetti MS, Ivanovski S. The influence of surface microroughness and hydrophilicity of titanium on the up-regulation of TGFβ/BMP signalling in osteoblasts. Biomaterials. 2011;32(3):665–71. doi:10.1016/j.biomaterials.2010.09.025.
55. Viguet-Carrin S, Garnero P, Delmas PD. The role of collagen in bone strength. Osteoporos Int. 2006;17(3):319–36. doi:10.1007/s00198-005-2035-9.
56. Saito M, Marumo K. Collagen cross-links as a determinant of bone quality: a possible explanation for bone fragility in aging, osteoporosis, and diabetes mellitus. Osteoporos Int. 2010;21(2):195–214. doi:10.1007/s00198-009-1066-z.
57. Pornprasertsuk S, Duarte WR, Mochida Y, Yamauchi M. Lysyl hydroxylase-2b directs collagen cross-linking pathways in MC3T3-E1 cells. J Bone Miner Res. 2004;19(8):1349–55. doi:10.1359/JBMR.040323.
58. Kaku M, Mochida Y, Atsawasuwan P, Parisuthiman D, Yamauchi M. Post-translational modifications of collagen upon BMP-induced osteoblast differentiation. Biochem Biophys Res Commun. 2007;359(3):463–8. doi:10.1016/j.bbrc.2007.05.109.
59. Boyce BF. Advances in the regulation of osteoclasts and osteoclast functions. J Dent Res. 2013;92(10):860–7. doi:10.1177/0022034513500306.
60. Mamalis AA, Markopoulou C, Vrotsos I, Koutsilirieris M. Chemical modification of an implant surface increases osteogenesis and simultaneously reduces osteoclastogenesis: an in vitro study. Clin Oral Implants Res. 2011;22(6):619–26. doi:10.1111/j.1600-0501.2010.02027.x.
61. Heppenstall RB, Grislis G, Hunt TK. Tissue gas tensions and oxygen consumption in healing bone defects. Clin Orthop Relat Res. 1975;106:357–65.
62. Potier E, Ferreira E, Andriamanalijaona R, Pujol JP, Oudina K, Logeart-Avramoglou D, et al. Hypoxia affects mesenchymal stromal cell osteogenic differentiation and angiogenic factor expression. Bone. 2007;40(4):1078–87. doi:10.1016/j.bone.2006.11.024.
63. Mamalis AA, Cochran DL. The role of hypoxia in the regulation of osteogenesis and angiogenesis coupling in intraoral regenerative procedures: a review of the literature. Int J Periodontics Restorative Dent. 2013. doi:10.11607/prd.0868.
64. Nucera S, Biziato D, De Palma M. The interplay between macrophages and angiogenesis in development, tissue injury and regeneration. Int J Dev Biol. 2011;55(4–5):495–503. doi:10.1387/ijdb.103227sn.
65. Ziebart T, Schnell A, Walter C, Kämmerer PW, Pabst A, Lehmann KM, et al. Interactions between endothelial progenitor cells (EPC) and titanium implant surfaces. Clin Oral Investig. 2013;17(1):301–9. doi:10.1007/s00784-012-0691-7.
66. Clarkin CE, Gerstenfeld LC. VEGF and bone cell signalling: an essential vessel for communication? Cell Biochem Funct. 2013;31(1):1–11. doi:10.1002/cbf.2911.
67. Zhang F, Qiu T, Wu X, Wan C, Shi W, Wang Y, et al. Sustained BMP signaling in osteoblasts stimulates bone formation by promoting angiogenesis and osteoblast differentiation. J Bone Miner Res. 2009;24(7):1224–33. doi:10.1359/jbmr.090204.
68. Shiojima I, Walsh K. Role of Akt signaling in vascular homeostasis and angiogenesis. Circ Res. 2002;90(12):1243–50.
69. Raines AL, Olivares-Navarrete R, Wieland M, Cochran DL, Schwartz Z, Boyan BD. Regulation of angiogenesis during osseointegration by titanium surface microstructure and energy. Biomaterials. 2010;31(18):4909–17. doi:10.1016/j.biomaterials.2010.02.071.
70. Schwarz F, Ferrari D, Herten M, Mihatovic I, Wieland M, Sager M, et al. Effects of surface hydrophilicity and microtopography on early stages of soft and hard tissue integration at non-submerged titanium implants: an immunohistochemical study in dogs. J Periodontol. 2007;78(11):2171–84. doi:10.1902/jop.2007.070157.
71. Schwarz F, Herten M, Sager M, Wieland M, Dard M, Becker J. Histological and immunohistochemical analysis of initial and early osseous integration at chemically modified and conventional SLA titanium implants: preliminary results of a pilot study in dogs. Clin Oral Implants Res. 2007;18(4):481–8. doi:10.1111/j.1600-0501.2007.01341.x.
72. Lambrichts I. Histological and ultrastructural aspects of bone innervation. In: Jacobs R, editor. Osseoperception. Leuven, Belgium: UZ Leuven; 1998. p. 13–20.
73. Bais M, McLean J, Sebastiani P, Young M, Wigner N, Smith T, et al. Transcriptional analysis of fracture healing and the induction of embryonic stem cell-related genes. PLoS One. 2009;4(5):e5393. doi:10.1371/journal.pone.0005393.
74. Ivanovski S, Hamlet S, Retzepi M, Wall I, Donos N. Transcriptional profiling of "guided bone regeneration" in a critical-size calvarial defect. Clin Oral Implants Res. 2011;22(4):382–9. doi:10.1111/j.1600-0501.2010.02104.x.
75. Donos N, Retzepi M, Wall I, Hamlet S, Ivanovski S. In vivo gene expression profile of guided bone regeneration associated with a microrough titanium surface. Clin Oral Implants Res. 2011;22(4):390–8. doi:10.1111/j.1600-0501.2010.02105.x.
76. Skaper SD. The neurotrophin family of neurotrophic factors: an overview. Methods Mol Biol. 2012;846:1–12. doi:10.1007/978-1-61779-536-7_1.
77. Vaillant AR, Mazzoni I, Tudan C, Boudreau M, Kaplan DR, Miller FD. Depolarization and neurotrophins converge on the phosphatidylinositol 3-kinase-Akt pathway to synergistically regulate neuronal survival. J Cell Biol. 1999;146(5):955–66.
78. Wilkins A, Kemp K, Ginty M, Hares K, Mallam E, Scolding N. Human bone marrow-derived mesenchymal stem cells secrete brain-derived neurotrophic factor which promotes neuronal survival in vitro. Stem Cell Res. 2009;3(1):63–70. doi:10.1016/j.scr.2009.02.006.
79. Buma P, Elmans L, Oestreicher AB. Changes in innervation of long bones after insertion of an implant: immunocytochemical study in goats with antibodies to calcitonin gene-related peptide and B-50/GAP-43. J Orthop Res. 1995;13(4):570–7. doi:10.1002/jor.1100130412.
80. Corpas Dos Santos L, Lambrichts I, Quirynen M, Collaert B, Politis C, Vrielinck L, et al. Peri-implant bone innervation: histological findings in humans. Eur J Oral Implantol. 2014;7(3):283–92.
81. Huang Y, Jacobs R, Van Dessel J, Bornstein MM, Lambrichts I, Politis C. A systematic review on the innervation of peri-implant tissues with special emphasis on the influence of implant placement and loading protocols. Clin Oral Implants Res. 2014; doi:10.1111/clr.12344.
82. Abarca M, Van Steenberghe D, Malevez C, Jacobs R. The neurophysiology of osseointegrated oral implants. A clinically underestimated aspect. J Oral Rehabil. 2006;33(3):161–9. doi:10.1111/j.1365-2842.2005.01556.x.
83. Klineberg I, Calford MB, Dreher B, Henry P, Macefield V, Miles T, et al. A consensus statement on osseoperception. Clin Exp Pharmacol Physiol. 2005;32(1–2):145–6. doi:10.1111/j.1440-1681.2005.04144.x.
84. Enkling N, Utz KH, Bayer S, Stern RM. Osseoperception: active tactile sensibility of osseointegrated dental implants. Int J Oral Maxillofac Implants. 2010;25(6):1159–67.
85. Canuto RA, Pol R, Martinasso G, Muzio G, Gallesio G, Mozzati M. Hydroxyapatite paste Ostim, without elevation of full-thickness flaps, improves alveolar healing stimulating BMP- and VEGF-mediated signal pathways: an experimental study in humans. Clin Oral Implants Res. 2013;24 Suppl A100:42–8. doi:10.1111/j.1600-0501.2011.02363.x.

# 12

# A piezo surgery with corticotomies and implant placement as part of a multidisciplinary approach to treat malocclusion disorder in an adult patient: clinical report

Federico Gelpi[1*], Daniele De Santis[2], Simone Marconcini[3], Francesco Briguglio[4] and Marco Finotti[5]

**Abstract**

This clinical report illustrates a multidisciplinary approach for the rehabilitation of a young adult patient affected by a bilateral edentulous space and an anterior deep bite. The patient required orthodontics and surgical corticotomy and implantology (both performed with a piezo device). A multidisciplinary planning approach, including orthodontics, oral and periodontic surgery, and restorative dentistry, has an important role in the final outcome of treatment. In fact a dental class I occlusion has been established only on the right side. The left side could not be restored to an ideal class I relationship due to the pontic prosthesis. The original collapsed right posterior occlusion was corrected. A stable posterior occlusion was established, and the balancing interference was eliminated. Centric relation and centric occlusion were established at the same vertical dimension of occlusion. The cephalometric analysis and clinical aspect at the end of treatment showed that the patient had improvements in overbite and overjet.

Multidisciplinary management, including endodontic and restorative dentistry, periodontics, corticotomy-assisted orthodontics, implants, and prosthetics, was used for a young female patient with multiple missing teeth, anterior deep bite, and a malocclusion with cant of the occlusal plane. The interaction of interdisciplinary specialties and careful treatment planning were required. The patient also benefited esthetically from our effort.

**Keywords:** Multidisciplinary approach; Oral implantology; Piezo device; Corticotomies

## Background

In the adult patient, the loss of teeth or periodontal support can cause pathologic migration of a single tooth or group of teeth. This can result in the development of median diastema or general spacing of the teeth with or without incisor inclination, rotation, or tipping of the premolars and molars and consequently collapse of the posterior occlusion with decreasing vertical dimension [1].

Regaining the lost interocclusal space is a requirement for successful treatment in these cases. A multidisciplinary approach such as reduction of the overerupted teeth, which may require a combination of endodontic treatment, periodontal surgery, and a fixed prosthesis afterwards; extraction of the overerupted teeth; surgical reconstruction of the edentulous space; and orthodontic intrusion of the extruded teeth has been suggested for regaining the original space [2–5].

Intrusion of the extrusive opposing teeth orthodontically is the most conservative but also the most difficult and long-acting treatment option [5, 6].

The maxillary corticotomy is another available and suggested technique that facilitates orthodontic intrusion.

This clinical report illustrates a multidisciplinary approach for the rehabilitation of a young adult patient affected by a bilateral edentulous space. The patient required orthodontics and surgical corticotomy and implantology (both performed with a piezo device).

* Correspondence: federico.gelpi@libero.it
[1]Via delle Mimose, 8 Colognola ai Colli, 37030 Verona, Italy
Full list of author information is available at the end of the article

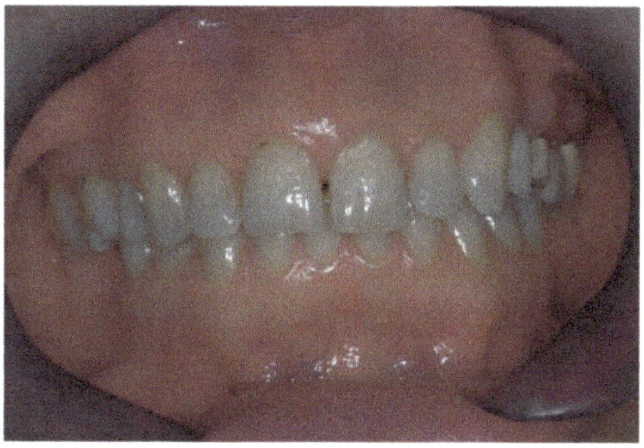

**Fig. 1** Initial frontal intraoral aspect

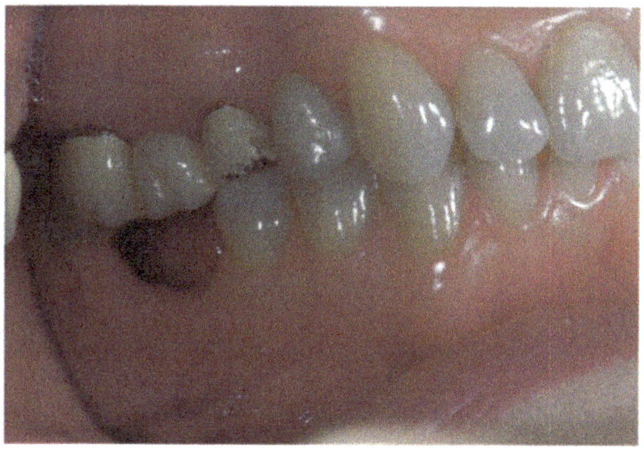

**Fig. 3** Some metal ceramic crowns in the upper left maxillary arch with a very poor esthetic appearance

## Case presentation

### Diagnosis and etiology

A young female patient was referred to our dental clinic to resolve a malocclusion disorder due to missing teeth. She was unsatisfied with the functional aspect of her dentition. She had a second upper right molar very damaged by caries (17) (Figs. 1 and 2); it was also extruded due to missing antagonist teeth (I and II lower right molars 46–47) (Fig. 3). The first upper molar was medially oriented due to a II premolar agenesis. There were some metal ceramic crowns in her upper left maxillary arch with a very poor esthetic appearance. A thorough examination, which included mounted diagnostic casts, was performed.

Clinical examination, panoramic radiography, mounted diagnostic casts, and cephalometric analysis revealed a partially edentulous mandible, and the diagnosis was established: anterior deep bite, a I skeletal class and a III dental class, supraeruption, and drifting and rotation of elements 16 and 17 (Figs. 4 and 5).

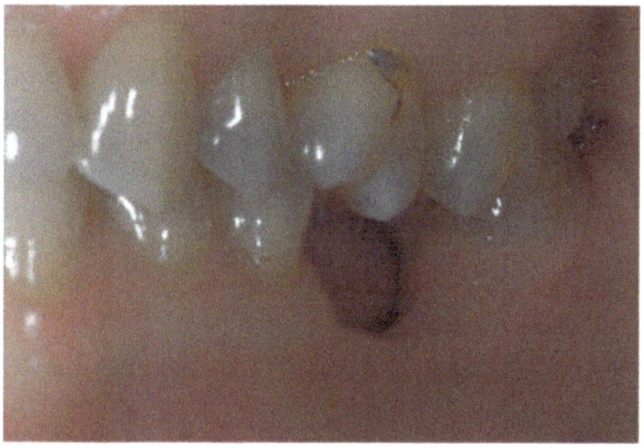

**Fig. 2** Initial lateral intraoral aspect

Because of her youth, esthetic requirements, and economic opportunities, the patient was advised she could be treated with a multidisciplinary approach to achieve a satisfactory esthetic and functional rehabilitation with restored occlusion.

### Treatment objectives

The following treatment objectives were established for this patient: (1) conservative and endodontic treatment in the teeth damaged by caries; (2) reestablishment of the correct occlusal plane; (3) corticotomy surgery (performed with a piezo device) to accelerate orthodontic-assisted tooth intrusion, alignment, and tipping; and (4) improvement of mouth posterior function through implant surgery to replace missing teeth (performed with a piezo device).

### Treatment progress

After the diagnostic workup was completed, a treatment plan was developed using a specialist team approach involving endodontic, orthodontic, oral surgery, and prosthodontic specialists. The proposed treatments included

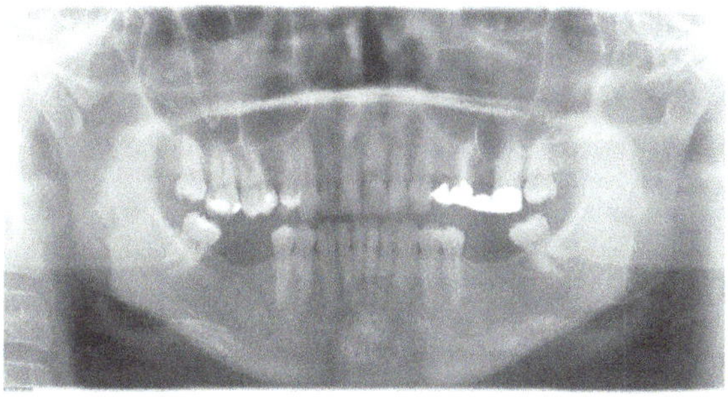

**Fig. 4** The panoramic radiography and cephalometric analysis revealed a partially edentulous mandible

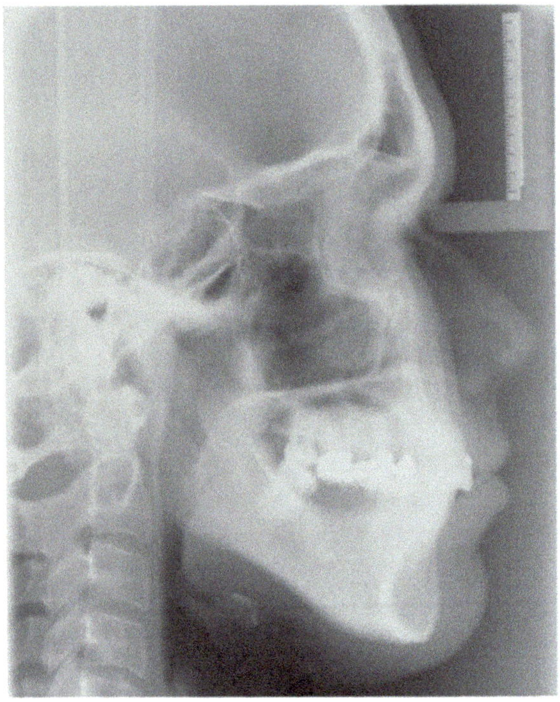

**Fig. 5** The panoramic radiography and cephalometric analysis revealed a partially edentulous mandible

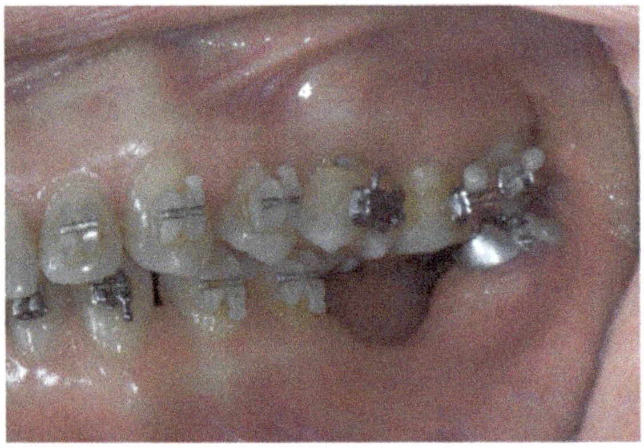

**Fig. 7** Ortodontic bracket placement: right side view

orthodontic intrusion and tipping of the I and II upper right molars (16 and 17) and uprighting of the lower wisdom teeth and dental alignment.

The first step consisted of endodontic treatment of element 17 and subsequent fiber post buildup and esthetic restoration on elements 11 and 21.

After that, the 26 pontic removal was planned, and subsequently, orthodontic brackets were placed (Figs. 6, 7, and 8).

This was a preliminary stage before the first surgical corticotomy (performed with a piezo device).

A microsurgical corticotomy was mandatory to assist orthodontic tipping and intrusion of elements 16 and 17. This surgical procedure was performed by a piezo approach (Fig. 9).

A total width flap was elevated to make the cortical subapical and longitudinal bone cut possible. The surgeon had to respect a minimum of 3-mm distance from the apex and 1 mm from the periodontal ligament. A triangular-shaped corticotomy was performed with inserts OT7 0.55 mm and OT7 special 0.35 mm to accelerate orthodontic tooth movements (Fig. 10). The bone cut design was conceived to surgically reduce the amount of bone among root surfaces and assist orthodontic tooth movement.

Moreover, a mesiobuccal root surface exposure of element 16 due to a bone defect was evident. It required bone regeneration through Bio Oss and bone chip application (Figs. 11 and 12).

Orthodontic therapy involved immediate application of strong intrusive forces (>250 g) after corticotomy surgery. A NiTi $18 \times 22$ diameter archwire was applied to

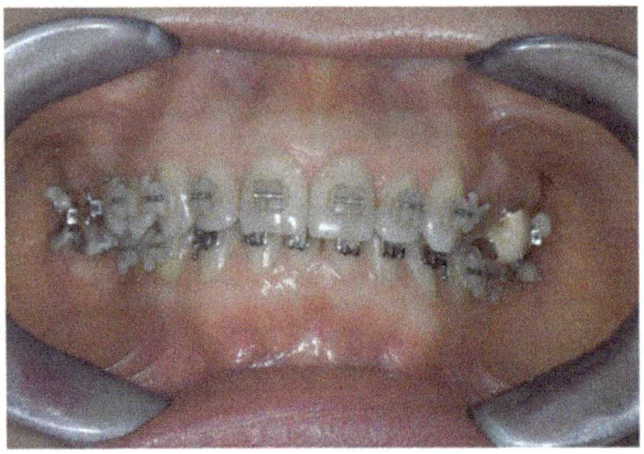

**Fig. 6** Orthodontic bracket placement: frontal view

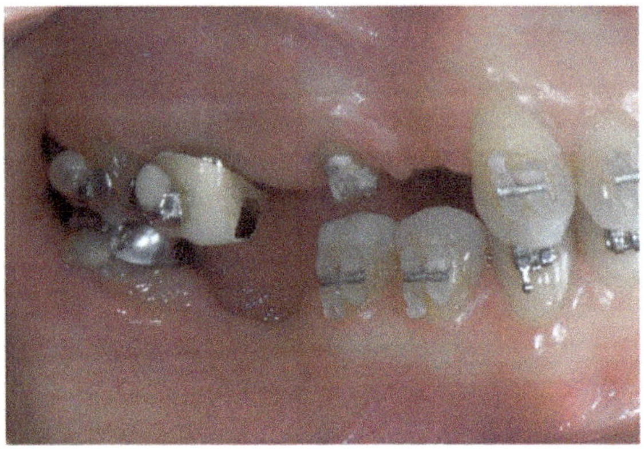

**Fig. 8** Orthodontic bracket placement: left side view

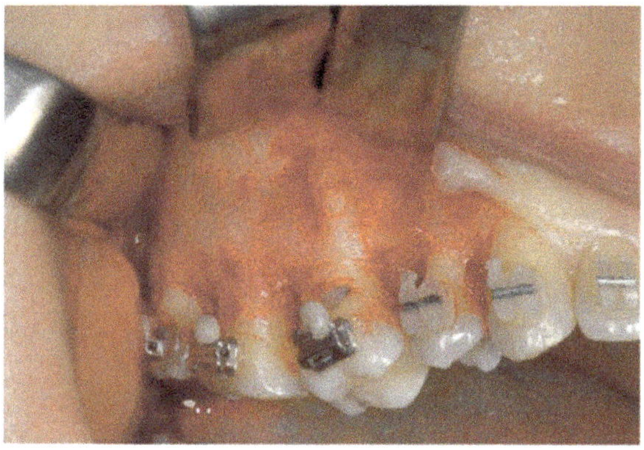

**Fig. 9** A microsurgical corticotomy was mandatory to assist orthodontic tipping and intrusion of elements 16 and 17

the brackets. It ensured mobilization of the bone maxillary block. The tipping movement of elements 16 and 17 took approximately 12 weeks. The patient was controlled weekly for the first 2 months and twice in the third month. No complications involving the periodontal

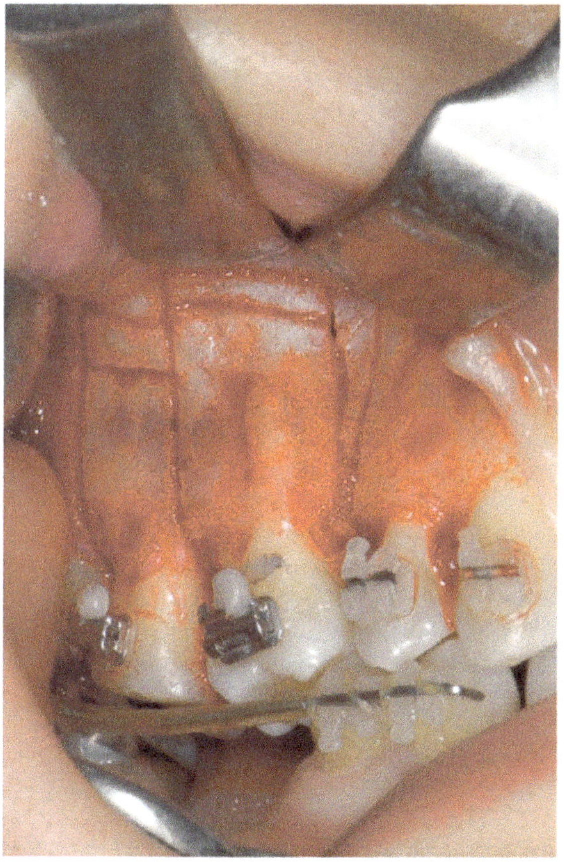

**Fig. 10** A triangular-shaped corticotomy was performed with inserts OT7 0.55 mm and OT7 special 0.35 mm to accelerate orthodontic tooth movements

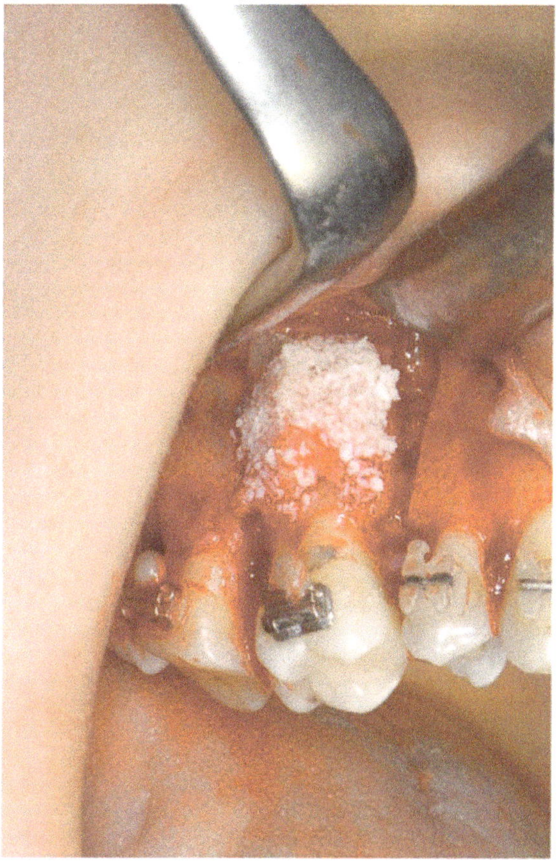

**Fig. 11** A mesiobuccal root surface exposure of element 16 required bone regeneration through Bio Oss and bone chip application

ligaments or endodontic vessels were observed in the weekly follow-ups.

After 7 months, a secondary surgical phase was planned: five Camlog Screw (Line Promote Plus) implants were placed with a minimum 35 N torque in 24 (4.3 mm × 13 mm), 36 (3.8 mm × 13 mm), 37 (3.8 mm × 13 mm), 46 (3.8 mm × 13 mm), and 47 (3.8 mm × 11 mm) sites. This feasible technique provided dedicated inserts for implant site preparation: OP5, IM2, OT4, and IM3 (correctly in sequence) (Figs. 13 and 14) and ensured minimally invasive and stressed implant site preparation. All implants received immediate healing screws (Fig. 15).

The orthodontic treatment took approximately 16 months. After that, the prosthodontic phase took place (Fig. 16). When tooth alignment was completed, all brackets were removed and the definitive restorations were placed. Implants were used for implant-retained prostheses (abutment-cemented crowns), and a three-unit fixed partial denture pontic (crowns 25–27) was placed (Figs. 17 and 18).

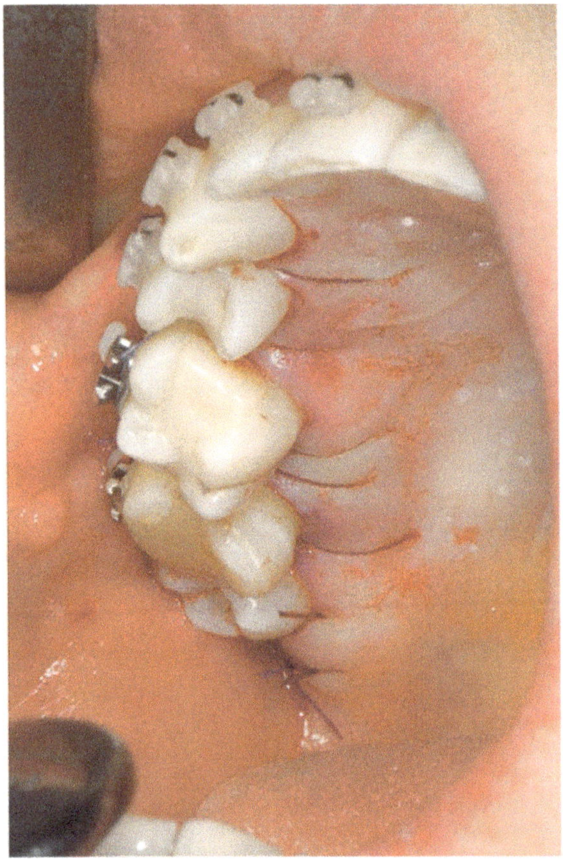

**Fig. 12** The total width flap was sutured

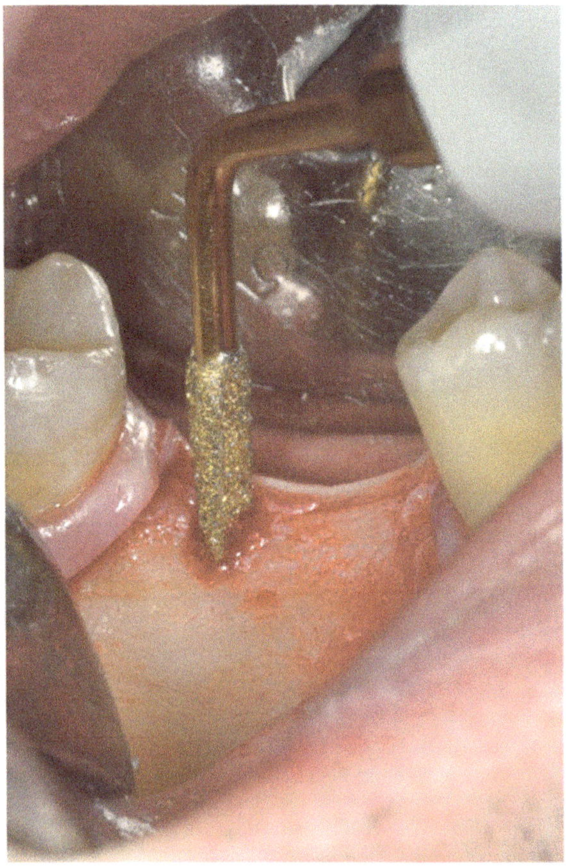

**Fig. 13** Implant site preparation: OP5, IM2, OT4, and IM3 (correctly in sequence)

### Treatment results

The left side could not be restored to an ideal class I relationship due to the pontic prosthesis (Figs. 19 and 20). A dental class I occlusion was established only on the right side (Fig. 21). The original collapsed right posterior occlusion was corrected. A stable posterior occlusion was established, and the balancing interference was eliminated. Centric relation and centric occlusion were established at the same vertical dimension of occlusion. The cephalometric analysis and clinical aspect at the end of treatment showed that the patient had improvements in overbite and overjet.

### Discussion

The management of an anterior deep bite requires adequate treatment planning, especially if the clinical condition is associated with posterior DVO (vertical occlusion dimension) reduction due to multiple missing teeth. A multidisciplinary planning approach, including orthodontics, oral and periodontic surgery, and restorative dentistry, has an important role in the final outcome of treatment [7].

In this case, before orthodontic alignment, we decided to intrude elements 16 and 17 (supraeruption and rotation) with a local corticotomy associated with intrusive orthodontic movement. The feasibility of this minimally invasive surgery is strictly linked to the use of a piezo surgery device to perform latero-posterior segmental maxillary osteotomy. Ultrasonic bone-cutting surgery has recently been introduced as a feasible alternative to the conventional tools of cranio-maxillo-facial surgery, due to its technical characteristics of precision and safety.

In fact, it is possible to perform a linear, clean, and thin osteotomic bone cut with maintenance of the integrity of the vascular network. This particular aspect avoids damage of the palatal mucosa and spares use of the chisel to complete the corticotomy. Many studies indicate that conventional cutting tools can produce impairment of pulp blood flow and loss of tooth vitality [8]. Furthermore, vascular compromise can occur due to direct or heat-induced injury to the soft tissue pedicles. To prevent such complications, we support the use of piezoelectric surgery in this critical multipiece surgery, as reported in the literature [9].

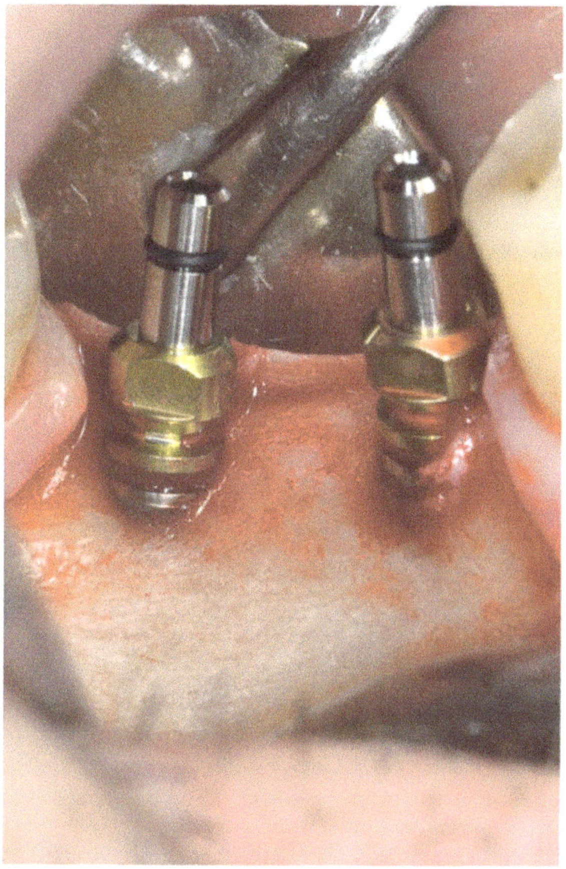

**Fig. 14** Implants placement after site preparation

In these anatomically difficult conditions, a piezo surgery device provides good intraoperative visibility and a safe and precise osteotomy due to its micrometric characteristics and selective cut [9].

The piezo device offers many versatile inserts; inserts for implant site preparation appear to be particularly useful and versatile. We believe that the piezo surgery device offers many intra- and postoperative advantages and provides desirable clinical outcomes such as a favorable implant success rate, as reported in the literature [10].

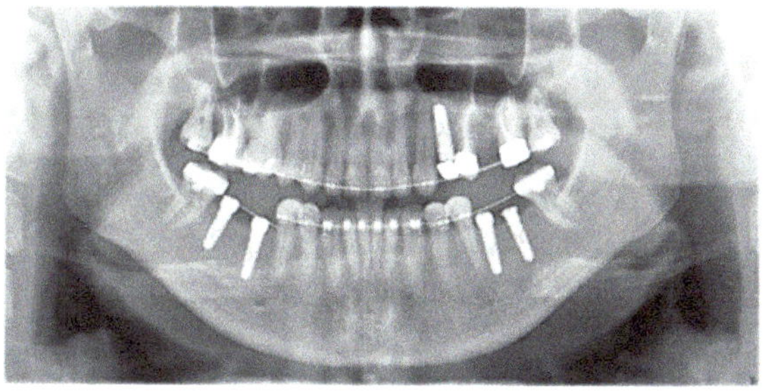

**Fig. 15** All implants received immediate healing screws

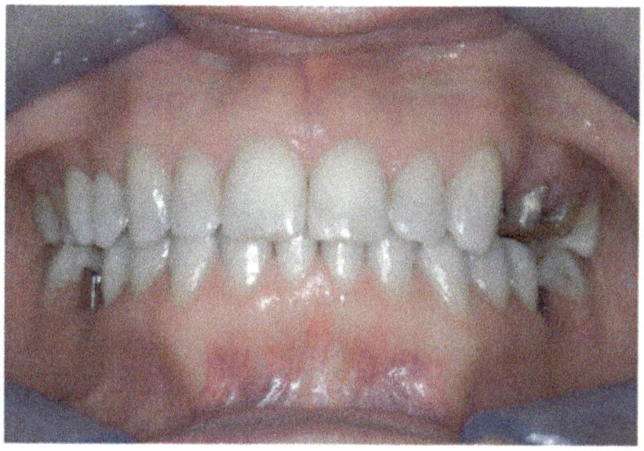

**Fig. 16** After orthodontic treatment was completed, the prosthodontic phase took place

In a multidisciplinary treatment approach, a multi-use specific tool such as a piezo device allows simplification of each surgical step within very difficult and complex management planning. In fact, it is possible to reduce intra- and postoperative complications (damage to soft tissues such as nerves, the blood vessel network, and dental pulp), to assist and accelerate intrusive and tipping orthodontic movement of migrated teeth, and to perform safe oral surgery [9].

Moreover, intrusion can be a reliable therapeutic treatment in patients with a healthy periodontal status because it does not result in a decrease of marginal bone level [11].

The best results are obtained when tooth intrusion is performed with light forces (5–15 g) and the line of action of the force passes close to the center of resistance. However, in our clinical report, after corticotomy surgery, tooth intrusion was performed with very high forces (>250 g) to mobilize the bone block, but the final

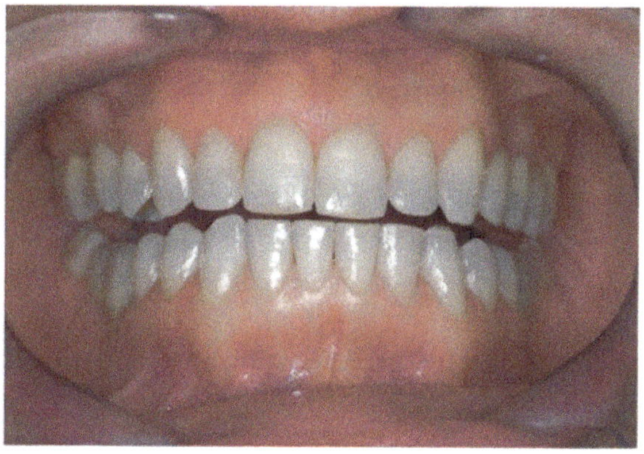

**Fig. 17** Implants were used for implant-retained prostheses (abutment-cemented crowns), and a three-unit fixed partial denture pontic (crowns 25–27) was placed

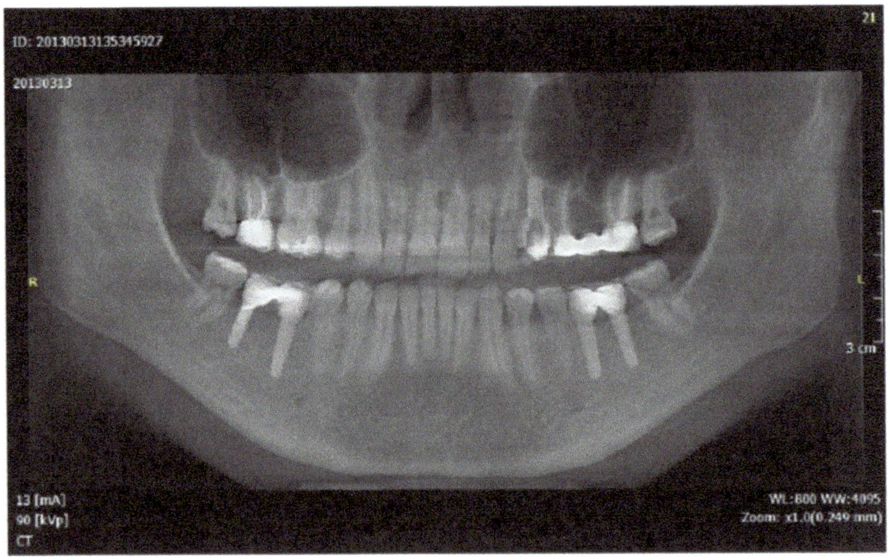


**Fig. 18** OPT after prosthodontic finalization

clinical outcomes and periodontal status were satisfactory anyway. In this case, forces did not act on the tooth ligament but on the corticotomized bone: if forces were long-term and intensive on the ligament, hypoxia, root resorption, and vascular damage might occur.

A number of reports have indicated that orthodontic treatment can improve the periodontal situation in patients with pathologic migration by providing good function and improved esthetics after realignment.

It is generally recommended that orthodontic treatment should be preceded by periodontal therapy. In fact, orthodontic treatment when there is an inflammation/periodontal defect can lead to irreversible breakdown of the periodontal system [1].

According to this principle, we decided to cover the root exposure on element 16. Obviously, the corticotomized area was also covered by Bio Oss and bone chips.

This corrective phase was completed before the orthodontic treatment.

Finally, the implant surgery using the piezo device took place. Dental implants have become predictable and reliable adjuncts for oral rehabilitation [12–14].

In this case, no GBR or other sensitive surgical techniques were necessary before or during implant placement.

In our opinion, the piezo device's versatility offers advantages in implant surgery [9] and improves implant prognosis [10].

A multidisciplinary therapy is usually an expensive and long-term treatment. In this case, the corticotomy

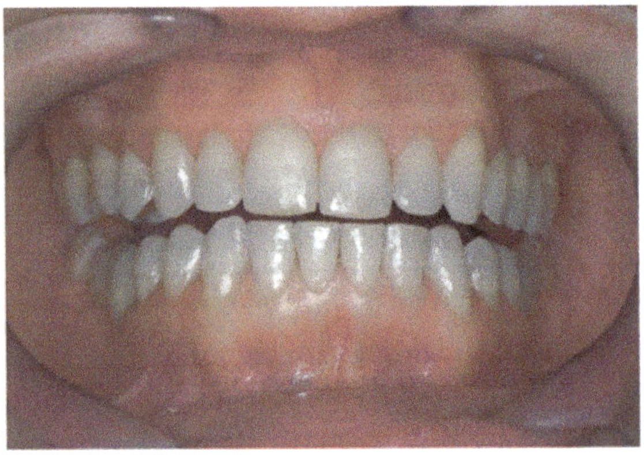

**Fig. 19** A full-mouth frontal aspect

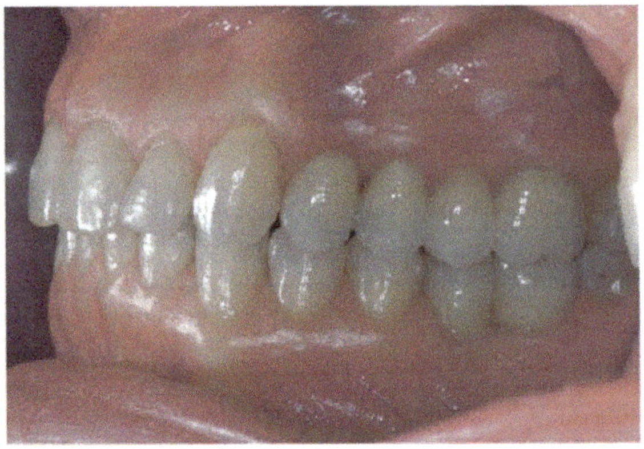

**Fig. 20** The left side could not be restored to an ideal class I relationship from the original class II due to the pontic prosthesis

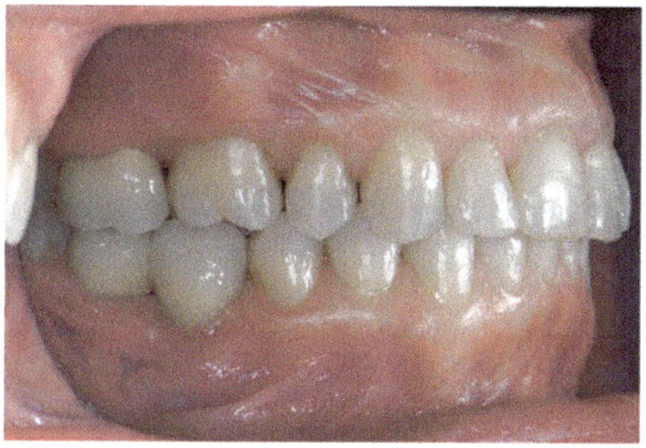

**Fig. 21** A dental class I occlusion was established only on the right side (lateral aspect)

performed by the piezo device, as well as precise and flowable planning without any clinical complications, allowed treatment acceleration so it could be tolerated more easily by the patient.

## Conclusions

Multidisciplinary management, including endodontic and restorative dentistry, periodontics, corticotomy-assisted orthodontics, implants, and prosthetics, was used for a young female patient with multiple missing teeth, anterior deep bite, and a malocclusion with cant of the occlusal plane. The interaction of interdisciplinary specialties and careful treatment planning were required. The patient also benefited esthetically from our effort.

The English in this document has been checked by at least two professional editors, both native speakers of English. For a certificate, please see http://www.textcheck.com/certificate/Ml6kvQ.

## Consent

Written informed consent was obtained from the patient for publication of this case report and any accompanying images. A copy of the written consent is available for review by the Editor-in-Chief of this journal.

#### Competing interests

Federico Gelpi, Daniele De Santis, Simone Marconcini, Francesco Briguglio, and Marco Finotti declare that they have no competing interests.

#### Authors' contributions

FG and SM wrote the manuscript. FB took intra- and postoperative pictures of the case. Finally, DDS and MF treated surgically and orthodontically the patient. All authors read and approved the final manuscript.

#### Acknowledgements

A special acknowledgement goes to Dr Giovanni Rigoni who tragically died some days ago.

#### Disclaimer

The authors certify that the research is original, and it has never been published nor it is presently under consideration for publication elsewhere. The final manuscript has been seen and approved by all the authors; they have taken due care to ensure the integrity of the work. The authors of the manuscript have no conflicts and no financial interests in the products and devices used in the current work.

#### Author details

[1]Via delle Mimose, 8 Colognola ai Colli, 37030 Verona, Italy. [2]Dental and Maxillofacial Department, University of Verona, Verona, Italy. [3]Department of surgery, University of Pisa Ist. Stomatologico, Tirreno, Italy. [4]Messina, Italy. [5]Padova, Italy.

#### References

1. Ong MA, Wang HL, Smith FN. Interrelationship between periodontics and adult orthodontics. J Clin Periodontol. 1998;25(4):271–7.
2. Mopsik ER, Buck RP, Connors JO. Surgical intervention to reestablish adequate intermaxillary space before fixed or removable prosthodontics. J Am Dent Assoc. 1977;95:957–60.
3. Chun YS, Row J, Yang SJ. Management of extruded maxillary molars to accommodate a mandibular restoration: a clinical report. J Prosthet Dent. 2000;83:604–6.
4. Chen CM, Tseng YC, Huang IY. Interdisciplinary management of dental implant patient: a case report. J Med Sci. 2004;20:415–8.
5. Bonetti GA, Giunta D. Molar intrusion with a removable appliance. J Clin Orthod. 1996;30:434–7.
6. Melsen B, Fiorelli G. Upper molar intrusion. J Clin Orthod. 1996;30:91–6.
7. Kelly Jr JT. A multidisciplinary approach to restoring posterior bite collapse. Compend Contin Educ Dent. 1997;18(5):483–5. 488–9; quiz 490.
8. Scheideman G, Kawamura H, Finn R, Bell W. Wound healing after anterior and posterior subapical osteotomy. J Oral Maxillofac. 1985;43:408–16.
9. Robiony M, Polini F, Costa F, Vercellotti T, Politi M. Piezoelectric bone cutting in multipiece maxillary osteotomies. J Oral Maxillofac Surg. 2004;62:759–61.
10. Danza M, Guidi R, Carinci F. Comparison between implants inserted into piezo split and unsplit alveolar crests. J Oral Maxillofac Surg. 2009;67(11):2460–5.
11. Melsen B, Agerbaek N, Markenstam G. Intrusion of incisors in adult patients with marginal bone loss. Am J Orthod Dentofacial Orthop. 1989;96(3):232–41.
12. Wehrbein H. Endosseous titanium implants as orthodontic anchoring elements. Experimental studies and clinical application. Fortschr Kieferorthop. 1994;55:236–50.
13. Wehrbein H, Diedrich P. Endosseous titanium implants during and after orthodontic load—an experimental study in the dog. Clin Oral Implants Res. 1993;4:76–82.
14. Wehrbein H, Merz BR, Diedrich P, Glatzmaier J. The use of palatal implants for orthodontic anchorage. Design and clinical application of the orthosystem. Clin Oral Implants Res. 1996;7:410–6.

# 13

# Evaluation of the maxillary sinus in panoramic radiography—a comparative study

Johann Malina-Altzinger[1*], Georg Damerau[2], Klaus W Grätz[3] and PD Bernd Stadlinger[2]

## Abstract

**Background:** The aim of this study was to evaluate the validity and the inter- and intra-examiner reliability of panoramic-radiograph-driven findings of different maxillary sinus anatomic variations and pathologies, which had initially been prediagnosed by cone beam computed tomography (CBCT).

**Methods:** After pairs of two-dimensional (2D) panoramic and three-dimensional (3D) CBCT images of patients having received treatment at the outpatient department had been screened, the predefinition of 54 selected maxillary sinus conditions was initially performed on CBCT images by two blinded consultants individually using a questionnaire that defined ten different clinically relevant findings. Using the identic questionnaire, these consultants performed the evaluation of the panoramic radiographs at a later time point. The results were analyzed for inter-imaging differences in the evaluation of the maxillary sinus between 2D and 3D imaging methods. Additionally, two resident groups (first year and last year of training) performed two diagnostic runs of the panoramic radiographs and results were analyzed for inter- and intra-observer reliability.

**Results:** There is a moderate risk for false diagnosis of findings of the maxillary sinus if only panoramic radiography is used. Based on the ten predefined conditions, solely maxillary bone cysts penetrating into the sinus were frequently detected differently comparing 2D to 3D diagnostics. Additionally, on panoramic radiographs, the inter-observer comparison demonstrated that basal septa were significantly often rated differently and the intra-observer comparison showed a significant lack in reliability in detecting maxillary bone cysts penetrating into the sinus.

**Conclusions:** Panoramic radiography provides the most information on the maxillary sinus, and it may be an adequate imaging method. However, particular findings of the maxillary sinus in panoramic imaging may be based on a rather examiner-dependent assessment. Therefore, a persistent and precise evaluation of specific conditions of the maxillary sinus may only be possible using CBCT because it provides additional information compared to panoramic radiography. This might be relevant for consecutive surgical procedures; consequently, we recommend CBCT if a precise preoperative evaluation is mandatory. However, higher radiation dose and costs of 3D imaging need to be considered.

**Keywords:** Panoramic radiography; Cone beam computed tomography; Maxillary sinus; Inter-imaging method differences; Inter-examiner reliability; Intra-examiner reliability

## Background

The development of two-dimensional (2D) panoramic imaging techniques began in the first half of the 20th century, but the first device applying this technology was only described in 1959 [1]. Since then, this radiographic technique has steadily been improved and has become a standard diagnostic tool in a clinician's daily practice. In parallel, cone beam computed tomography (CBCT), first described in 1982 [2], was introduced as a tool for dental and maxillofacial diagnostics.

The advantages of three-dimensional (3D) CBCT over 2D conventional panoramic tomography include an excellent imaging quality of high-contrast structures like the maxillofacial bone anatomy, no geometric distortion, and no superimposition of surrounding anatomic structures [3]. The advantages of panoramic radiography, on the other hand, are comparatively low-radiation doses, its general availability, and the comparatively low costs. Further, it is especially useful in the initial diagnostic

* Correspondence: Johann.malina-altzinger@insel.ch
[1]Clinic of Cranio-Maxillofacial Surgery, University Hospital of Bern, Freiburgstrasse 4, 3010 Bern, Switzerland
Full list of author information is available at the end of the article

phase of implant planning because it relates information on both dental arches, the inferior alveolar canals, and the maxillary sinuses to its pathologic conditions [4]. However, limitations include the lack of visualization of structures like the bucco-lingual ridge pattern and the visual loss of cortical plates or undulating concavities [5]; moreover, the fact that more than 80 % of measurements from the crest of the residual alveolar ridge to the inferior alveolar canal have errors of more than 1 mm renders panoramic radiography unsuitable as a single imaging source for dental-implant site assessment [4]. Furthermore, it is well known that an average magnification factor of 1.25 can be expected in panoramic radiographs. This demands calibration of the image with the help of a defined reference device when determining the appropriate implant size [6].

Precise assessment of the maxillary sinus is mandatory when planning a lateral or internal sinus floor elevation [7, 8]. It has been claimed that, besides clinical examination, evaluation of the maxillary sinuses is possible by panoramic radiography [9] and CBCT [7, 10]. Though it is known that millions of sinus lift operations were performed with panoramic radiographs without any problems, especially due to the superimposition of different structures, precise assessment of a maxillary sinus finding is difficult in 2D panoramic radiography [11]. This difficulty implies that, as a clinical consequence, patients are often referred to specialists on the basis of a suspected maxillary pathology visualized on a panoramic image. This further requires a CBCT, and the question arises whether a primary CBCT should be performed in cases of maxillary sinus diagnostics instead of an initial panoramic radiography. Moreover, the inter- and intra-examiner variation in the interpretation of 2D radiographs may exceed the variation in imaging techniques and diagnostic yield [12], leading to a rather examiner-dependent assessment of panoramic images.

Therefore, the present study had three aims: the evaluation of the validity (1), the inter- (2), and the intra-examiner (3) reliability of panoramic-radiograph-driven findings of different maxillary sinus conditions which had initially been prediagnosed in CBCT images.

## Methods

The study protocol was approved by the Eidgenössische Expertenkommission für das Berufsgeheimnis in der medizinischen Forschung (Federal expert committee for professional confidentiality in medical research, BAG 035.0001-125/196). All patients have consented to provide their data for research and publication. Prior to this study, a statistical study design was performed, and in a retrospective approach, radiographic images of patients having received treatment at the outpatient department of the Clinic of Cranio-Maxillofacial and Oral Surgery at the University of Zurich were screened. Inclusion criteria were patients having received 2D panoramic radiographs (Cranex, Soredex, Tuusula, Finland) and 3D CBCT (KaVo 3D eXam, Biberach, Germany) showing the maxillary sinus without any surgical procedure in between the two examinations (mean 8.6 days, SD 21 days). Subsequently, possible clinically relevant anatomic variations and pathologies of the maxillary sinus were predefined (nine findings, one unimpaired condition) (Table 1) from a surgical point of view. Twenty-eight patients were selected (63 % males, 37 % females, mean age 47.8 years, range: 20–85 years) according to the conditions shown in Table 1, corresponding to a total amount of 56 maxillary sinuses (one per side).

All radiographic images were anonymized and analyzed using the OsiriX Imaging software (version 5.0.2) and a monitor with a display resolution of 1680 × 1050 pixel. Image manipulation through change of brightness, zoom in and out, and rotation was used when needed. No time limit was appropriated, and all observations were performed in the same room under comparable light conditions. Findings of the maxillary sinus were purely based on radiographic appearance without using any other additional clinical or histological information. A questionnaire served for recording the diagnoses (Table 1).

The predefinition of maxillary sinus conditions was initially performed on 3D CBCT images by two consultants in a separate evaluation using the questionnaire. The following reconstruction parameters in all three dimensions (sagittal, coronal, axial) were used: voxel edge length 0.4 × 0.4 × 0.4 mm, slice thickness 1 mm. The two assessors were blinded—disagreement was solved by discussion.

### Evaluation of inter-imaging technique differences

The CBCT assessment served as a reference group for later 2D panoramic image diagnostics which were performed separately by the same two consultants more

**Table 1** Predefined findings of the maxillary sinus

| | |
|---|---|
| 1. | Complete opacity |
| 2. | Basal opacity |
| 3. | Foreign body |
| 4. | Oro-antral communication |
| 5. | Basal septum |
| 6. | Polypoid mucosal thickening |
| 7. | Maxillary bone cyst penetrating into the sinus |
| 8. | Fluid level |
| 9. | Status post sinus lift |
| 10. | No finding |

than 6 months after predefinition on CBCT images. An identical questionnaire was used for both 3D and later 2D diagnostics. Inter-imaging technique differences in evaluating the maxillary sinus with 2D or 3D imaging method were analyzed with regard to false-positive and false-negative decisions.

### Evaluation of the inter-observer reliability

Using the same questionnaire, four blinded residents separately performed the evaluation of the 2D panoramic radiographs—two in the first year and two in the last year of training. Agreement between these two rating groups in detecting findings in the maxillary sinus was analyzed for calculating inter-observer reliability.

### Evaluation of the intra-observer reliability

After more than 4 weeks, the same residents newly evaluated all maxillary sinuses on 2D panoramic images. Reassessment served for the calculation of the intra-observer reliability, which means individual agreement between the two elevation runs.

The results were further evaluated with regard to the prevalence of radiographic findings in the maxillary sinus.

### Data analyses and statistical methods

Data was recorded using Excel 2013 (Microsoft) and analyzed using IBM SPSS Statistics for Macintosh, Verion 22.0 (Armonk, NY: IBM Corp.). Collected data was analyzed to demonstrate degree of agreement using the following statistical tests: logistic regression was used to estimate odds ratios. $p$ values were calculated using a chi-squared test. Kappa coefficient and McNemar's test were used for evaluating the reliability between the two consultants analyzing the CBCT scans. Calculated $p$ values were considered significant for values <0.05. Descriptive statistics computed means and standard deviation for quantitative variables as well as absolute and relative frequencies for qualitative variables.

## Results

This study analyzed comparative and descriptive data for the evaluation of the maxillary sinus. Significant differences in the detection of ten predefined findings between 2D and 3D imaging methods were calculated. Furthermore, the degree of agreement in detecting the ten conditions on the panoramic radiographs was measured between different observers and within the same observer. The radiographic images of 28 patients (56 maxillary sinuses, 1 per side) were examined. One patient had to be excluded from the study as the radiographic finding on the CBCT did not clearly match any of the predefined ten conditions.

### Differences between CBCT- and panoramic-radiograph-driven evaluations of the maxillary sinus

As illustrated by Table 2, the results of the present study demonstrate that in panoramic-radiograph-driven diagnosis a "no finding" was selected in a quite similar way as if CBCT was used ($p = 0.803$, odds ratio (OR) = 1.220). The difference between the two imaging methods was significant solely for maxillary bone cyst penetrating into the sinus ($p = 0.032$). The estimated OR of this specific finding was significantly lower than 1 (OR = 0.275). No significant differences between 2D and 3D imaging methods were found for the detection of a complete opacity ($p = 0.998$), a basal opacity ($p = 0.714$), a foreign body ($p = 0.571$), an oro-antral communication ($p = 0.998$), a basal septum ($p = 0.911$), a polypoid mucosal thickening (0.123), a fluid level ($p = 0.253$), and a status post sinus lift ($p = 0.998$) (Table 2; Fig. 1).

### Inter-observer differences

Good inter-observer reliability [13] between the two consultants analyzing the CBCT scans was confirmed by Kappa coefficient (0.7) and McNemar's test ($p > 0.05$).

The comparison of the two resident groups (first-year, last-year) examining 2D panoramic images showed that basal septa were significantly often rated differently by these two groups ($p = 0.004$, OR = 0.542). Further, it was shown that there is a significant good inter-observer agreement in detecting complete opacities ($p < 0.001$, OR = 6.133) (Table 3; Fig. 2).

### Intra-observer reliability

The intra-observer comparison showed that assessors of panoramic radiographs were largely reliable considering

**Table 2** Comparison of panoramic radiography and CBCT in detecting ten different conditions of maxillary sinus

| | $p$ | OR |
|---|---|---|
| Complete shadow | 0.998 | [a] |
| Basal shadow | 0.714 | 0.822 |
| Foreign body | 0.571 | 1.831 |
| Oro-antral communication | 0.998 | [a] |
| Basal septum | 0.911 | 0.945 |
| Polypoid mucosal thickening | 0.123 | 0.376 |
| Maxillary bone cyst penetrating into the sinus | 0.032* | 0.275 |
| Fluid level | 0.253 | 0.238 |
| Status post sinus lift | 0.998 | [a] |
| No finding | 0.803 | 1.22 |

Shown $p$ values define the degree of agreement
[a]Describes an odds ratio close to zero or infinity due to numerical problems
* $p < 0.05$

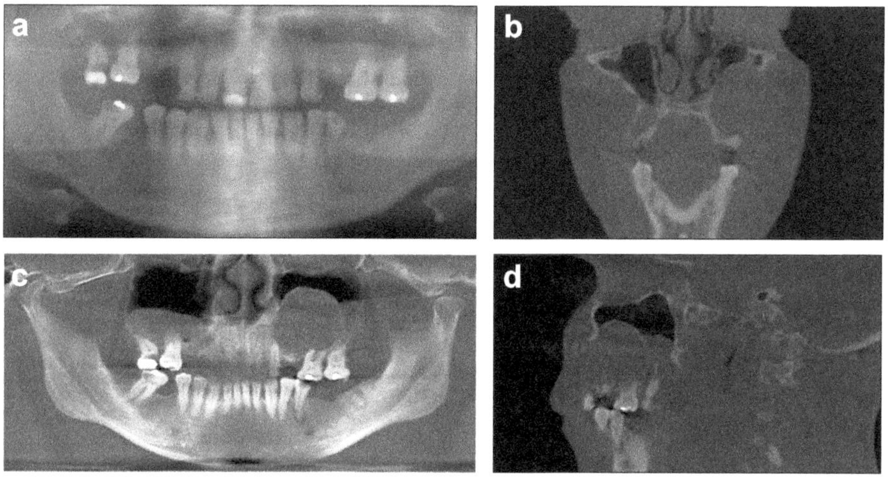

**Fig. 1** Radiographic findings of patient 26: basal opacity, maxillary bone cyst penetrating into the sinus; **a** panoramic radiography (Soredex, Cranex); **b–d** CBCT images (KaVo 3D eXam): coronal plane (**b**); panoramic reconstruction view (**c**); CBCT sagittal plane, left sinus (**d**)

the two evaluation runs of the same 2D panoramic images with a 4-week interval in between. The analysis indicated a significant lack of reliability ($p = 0.044$, OR = 0.331) in diagnosing maxillary bone cysts penetrating into the sinus (Table 3).

### Prevalence of findings

On the basis of 54 evaluated maxillary sinuses, the most frequent radiographic findings in CBCT were basal septa (54 %), followed by basal opacities (43 %), and foreign bodies (15 %) (Fig. 3).

**Table 3** Agreement in evaluating the maxillary sinus on panoramic images

| | Inter-examiner | | Intra-examiner | |
|---|---|---|---|---|
| | *p* | OR | *p* | OR |
| Complete shadow | <0.001* | 6.133 | 0.549 | 1.387 |
| Basal shadow | 0.441 | 1.186 | 0.621 | 0.806 |
| Foreign body | 0.596 | 1.207 | 0.991 | 0.993 |
| Oro-antral communication | 0.842 | 1.083 | 0.432 | 0.547 |
| Basal septum | 0.004* | 0.542 | 0.375 | 0.704 |
| Polypoid mucosal thickening | 0.052 | 1.748 | 0.060 | 0.404 |
| Maxillary bone cyst penetrating into the sinus | 0.628 | 0.855 | 0.044* | 0.331 |
| Fluid level | 0.653 | 1.515 | 0.999 | 0.000 |
| Status post sinus lift | 1.000 | 1.000 | 0.696 | 0.765 |
| No finding | 0.511 | 0.866 | 0.280 | 0.562 |

Inter-examiner describes agreement between two rating groups (first-year and last-year residents) and intra-examiner describes individual agreement between two evaluation runs. Shown *p* values define the degree of agreement
* $p < 0.05$

## Discussion

The purpose of this study was to analyze the validity of different anatomic variations and pathologies of the maxillary sinus found in 2D panoramic radiography by comparing them to those initially detected on CBCT images. Additional aims were the evaluation of inter- and intra-examiner differences on panoramic-radiograph-driven evaluation of the maxillary sinus.

### Differences between CBCT- and panoramic-radiograph-driven evaluations of the maxillary sinus

There is a moderate risk for false diagnosis of the maxillary sinus if only panoramic radiography rather than CBCT is used. In the present study, comparing 2D to 3D imaging, solely maxillary bone cysts penetrating into the sinus were frequently detected differently. Maestre-Ferrin et al. compared the efficacy of panoramic radiography, computed tomography (CT), and 3D CT in the diagnosis of mucosal thickening, mucous cysts, or complete opacity when using implant-planning software and showed that panoramic radiography was comparatively inferior [14]. Maestre-Ferrin et al. [14, 15] also showed that panoramic radiography led to false-positive and false-negative findings in the visualization of maxillary sinus septa in almost half of their cases, and Krenmair et al. [16] observed the same inaccuracy of panoramic radiography in detecting antral sinus septa in 13 out of 61 cases. Our study demonstrated no significant differences between 2D and 3D imaging methods in the detection of basal septa.

### Inter-observer reliability

The inter-observer disagreement between the two resident groups (first-year vs. last-year residents) examining

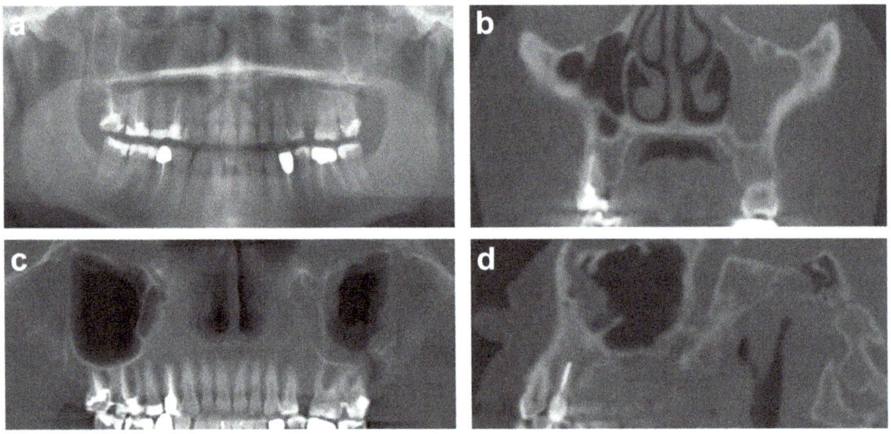


**Fig. 2** Radiographic findings of patient 19: oro-antral communication, basal opacity, basal septa; **a** panoramic radiography (Soredex, Cranex); **b–d** CBCT images (KaVo 3D eXam): coronal plane (**b**); panoramic reconstruction view (**c**); CBCT sagittal plane, right sinus (**d**)

2D panoramic images was significant in the detection of the basal septa. As mentioned above, Maestre-Ferrin et al. have already indicated that panoramic radiography is insufficient for the detection of sinus septa [15], which complements to Shahbazian et al.'s finding that even though panoramic radiography provides a broad view of the sinus floor, it is unsuitable for detecting small lesions, due to low spatial resolution [11]. A similar observation was obtained by Dreiseidler et al. who confirmed superior visualization of all important high-contrast structures for CBCT compared to panoramic radiography with a focus on presurgical implant planning [17].

### Intra-observer reliability

There was only little intra-observer variation. The literature shows that the intra- and inter-examiner variation in the interpretation of radiographs may exceed the variation of imaging techniques and diagnostic yield [12, 18, 19]. That some variations may not be eliminated despite observer training has already been indicated by Kullman et al. [20]. Their study analyzed inter- and intra-observer differences in assessing panoramic radiographs with regard to radiographic bone height at two assessments several weeks apart. Both outcomes of two observers were described as reliable but not excellent though both raters were experienced.

One limitation of the latter and also of the present study may be the relatively small number of raters. Another limitation of this study may be the prevalence imbalance of different findings in the maxillary sinus resulting in a negative impact on our statistical calculation. This might include not only the low prevalence of maxillary bone cysts penetrating into the sinus but also the high prevalence of basal septa, an imbalance former studies have already demonstrated [15, 21, 22].

An explanation for our reported findings may be that, due to the superimposition of different structures, low spatial resolution and visual loss of cortical plates or

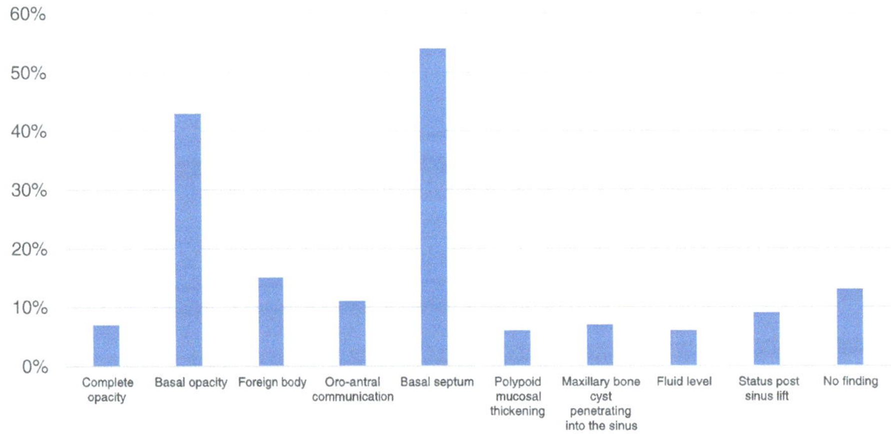


**Fig. 3** Descriptive illustration of 54 evaluated maxillary sinuses

undulating concavities, precise evaluation of a maxillary sinus finding is difficult in 2D panoramic radiography [5, 11]. Moreover, this difficulty might express that, as a consequence, the shown inter- and intra-observer variation in the interpretation of 2D radiographs may exceed the diagnostic yield [12].

Undiagnosed sinus conditions may be associated with chronic orofacial pain that is one of the most common reasons why patients consult physicians [23]. Moreover, precise assessment of the maxillary sinus by obtaining information on bone characteristics, on condition of Schneiderian membrane, on the presence of septa, and on the lateral sinus wall is mandatory prior to any lateral or internal sinus floor elevation [7, 8]. Currently, different radiographic means are used for preoperative tooth and bone-site and implant-site assessment. Clinicians commonly use 2D or 3D radiography. Both options imply advantages and disadvantages [4]. CBCT is used primarily to evaluate bony anatomy and to screen for overt pathology of the maxillary sinuses prior to dental implant treatment [24, 25]. However, prior to any radiographic imaging, especially for young patients, its benefit must be to weigh against its risk, with highest attention to the ALARA principle (*a*s *l*ow *a*s *r*easonably *a*chievable) [8]. This study indicates that panoramic radiography provides a sufficient view of the maxillary sinus for basic diagnostics, and it may be an adequate imaging method especially in the initial diagnostic phase. A precise assessment of different conditions of the maxillary sinus may only be possible using CBCT.

## Conclusions

The results of this study emphasize that panoramic radiography visualizes relevant findings of the maxillary sinus. In comparison to panoramic radiography, CBCT facilitates diagnosis of special conditions like penetrating cysts. The inter-observer comparison on panoramic radiographs demonstrated that basal septa were significantly often rated differently, and panoramic imaging may be based on a rather examiner-dependent assessment. Supplementary, the detection of maxillary bone cysts penetrating into the sinus with panoramic radiography showed a significant lack in reliability in the intra-observer comparison. Therefore, precise preoperative evaluation of the maxillary sinus on panoramic radiographs may be difficult. This could be relevant for consecutive surgical procedures; however, higher radiation dose and costs of three-dimensional imaging need to be considered.

#### Competing interest

Johann Malina-Altzinger, Georg Damerau, Klaus W. Grätz and Bernd Stadlinger declare that they have no competing interests.

#### Authors' contributions

JMA selected the patients, performed the statistical analysis in conjunction with the institute of statistics, and drafted the manuscript. GD participated in the evaluation of CBCT and in the design of the study. KWG helped to conceive and coordinate the study and edited the manuscript. BS conceived and coordinated the study and helped to draft and edit the manuscript. All authors read and approved the final manuscript.

#### Acknowledgements

We would like to thank Dominique Bichsel, Martin Bigler, Johanna Jauernik, Margrit Roos, Silvio Valdec, and Marius Wolf for their help.

#### Author details

[1]Clinic of Cranio-Maxillofacial Surgery, University Hospital of Bern, Freiburgstrasse 4, 3010 Bern, Switzerland. [2]Clinic of Oral Surgery, Center of Dental Medicine, University of Zurich, Plattenstrasse 11, 8032 Zurich, Switzerland. [3]Former Head of the Department of Cranio-Maxillofacial and Oral Surgery, University of Zurich, Plattenstrasse 11, 8032 Zurich, Switzerland.

#### References

1. PAATERO YV. Orthoradial jaw pantomography. Ann Med Intern Fenn Suppl. 1959;48(Supp 28):222–7.
2. Robb RA. The dynamic spatial reconstructor: an X-Ray video-fluoroscopic CT scanner for dynamic volume imaging of moving organs. IEEE Trans Med Imaging. 1982;1(1):22–33.
3. Price JB, Thaw KL, Tyndall DA, Ludlow JB, Padilla RJ. Incidental findings from cone beam computed tomography of the maxillofacial region: a descriptive retrospective study. Clin Oral Implants Res. 2012;23(11):1261–8.
4. Tyndall DA, Price JB, Tetradis S, Ganz SD, Hildebolt C, Scarfe WC, et al. Position statement of the American academy of oral and maxillofacial radiology on selection criteria for the use of radiology in dental implantology with emphasis on cone beam computed tomography. Oral Surg Oral Med Oral Pathol Oral Radiol. 2012;113(6):817–26.
5. Jaju PP, Jaju SP. Clinical utility of dental cone-beam computed tomography: current perspectives. Clin Cosmet Investig Dent. 2014;6:29–43.
6. Schropp L, Stavropoulos A, Gotfredsen E, Wenzel A. Calibration of radiographs by a reference metal ball affects preoperative selection of implant size. Clin Oral Investig. 2009;13(4):375–81.
7. Bornstein MM, Scarfe WC, Vaughn VM, Jacobs R. Cone beam computed tomography in implant dentistry: a systematic review focusing on guidelines, indications, and radiation dose risks. Int J Oral Maxillofac Implants. 2014;29 Suppl:55–77.
8. Dula K, Bornstein M, Buser D, Dagassan-Berndt D, Ettlin D, Fillipi A, et al.(2014) SADMFR Guidelines for the use of cone-beam computed tomography/digital volume tomography. Swiss Dent J. 2014;124:1170–1183.
9. Mathew AL, Pai KM, Sholapurkar AA. Maxillary sinus findings in the elderly: a panoramic radiographic study. J Contemp Dent Pract. 2009;10(6):E041–8.
10. Neugebauer J, Ritter L, Mischkowski RA, Dreiseidler T, Scherer P, Ketterle M, et al. Evaluation of maxillary sinus anatomy by cone-beam CT prior to sinus floor elevation. Int J Oral Maxillofac Implants. 2010;25(2):258–65.
11. Shahbazian M, Vandewoude C, Wyatt J, Jacobs R. Comparative assessment of panoramic radiography and CBCT imaging for radiodiagnostics in the posterior maxilla. Clin Oral Investig. 2014;18(1):293–300.
12. Helminen SE, Vehkalahti M, Wolf J, Murtomaa H. Quality evaluation of young adults' radiographs in Finnish public oral health service. J Dent. 2000;28(8):549–55.
13. Altmann DG: Practical statistics for medical research (1990) London: Chapman & Hall. 1991.
14. Maestre-Ferrín L, Galán-Gil S, Carrillo-García C, Peñarrocha-Diago M. Radiographic findings in the maxillary sinus: comparison of panoramic radiography with computed tomography. Int J Oral Maxillofac Implants. 2011;26(2):341–6.
15. Maestre-Ferrín L, Carrillo-García C, Galán-Gil S, Peñarrocha-Diago M. Prevalence, location, and size of maxillary sinus septa: panoramic radiograph versus computed tomography scan. J Oral Maxillofac Surg. 2011;69(2):507–11.
16. Krennmair G, Ulm CW, Lugmayr H, Solar P. The incidence, location, and height of maxillary sinus septa in the edentulous and dentate maxilla. J Oral Maxillofac Surg. 1999;57(6):667–71. discussion 671–662.

17. Dreiseidler T, Mischkowski RA, Neugebauer J, Ritter L, Zöller JE. Comparison of cone-beam imaging with orthopantomography and computerized tomography for assessment in presurgical implant dentistry. Int J Oral Maxillofac Implants. 2009;24(2):216–25.
18. Reit C, Hollender L. Radiographic evaluation of endodontic therapy and the influence of observer variation. Scand J Dent Res. 1983;91(3):205–12.
19. Pliskin JS, Shwartz M, Gröndahl HG, Boffa J. Reliability of coding depth of approximal carious lesions from non-independent interpretation of serial bitewing radiographs. Community Dent Oral Epidemiol. 1984;12(6):366–70.
20. Kullman L, Al-Asfour A, Zetterqvist L, Andersson L. Comparison of radiographic bone height assessments in panoramic and intraoral radiographs of implant patients. Int J Oral Maxillofac Implants. 2007;22(1):96–100.
21. Lana JP, Carneiro PM, Machado VC, de Souza PE, Manzi FR, Horta MC. Anatomic variations and lesions of the maxillary sinus detected in cone beam computed tomography for dental implants. Clin Oral Implants Res. 2012;23(12):1398–403.
22. Underwood AS. An inquiry into the anatomy and pathology of the maxillary sinus. J Anat Physiol. 1910;44(Pt 4):354–69.
23. Brüllmann DD, Schmidtmann I, Hornstein S, Schulze RK. Correlation of cone beam computed tomography (CBCT) findings in the maxillary sinus with dental diagnoses: a retrospective cross-sectional study. Clin Oral Investig. 2012;16(4):1023–9.
24. Vogiatzi T, Kloukos D, Scarfe WC, Bornstein MM. Incidence of anatomical variations and disease of the maxillary sinuses as identified by cone beam computed tomography: a systematic review. Int J Oral Maxillofac Implants. 2014;29(6):1301–14.
25. Ritter L, Lutz J, Neugebauer J, Scheer M, Dreiseidler T, Zinser MJ, et al. Prevalence of pathologic findings in the maxillary sinus in cone-beam computerized tomography. Oral Surg Oral Med Oral Pathol Oral Radiol Endod. 2011;111(5):634–40.

# 14

# Effect of bite force in occlusal adjustment of dental implants on the distribution of occlusal pressure: comparison among three bite forces in occlusal adjustment

Sho Kayumi[1,2], Yoshiyuki Takayama[1*], Atsuro Yokoyama[2] and Nana Ueda[1]

**Abstract**

**Background:** The purpose of this study was to investigate the influence of occlusal forces (the contractile force of masticatory muscles) exerted during occlusal adjustment on the distribution of the forces among teeth, implants, and temporomandibular joints (TMJs) in intercuspal clenching in cases with bilateral missing molars and premolars by using finite element analysis.

**Methods:** A three-dimensional finite element model of the mandible with eight implants in the premolar and molar regions was constructed. Linearly elastic material properties were defined for all elements except the periodontal ligament, which was defined as nonlinearly elastic. The TMJs and antagonists were simplified and replaced with nonlinear springs. Antagonists were assumed to be natural teeth or implants and had two- or three-stage displaceability. We constructed finite element (FE) models in which occlusal adjustment with three kinds of occlusal force (40 N as a light bite, 200 N as a hard bite, and 400 N as a maximum biting force) was performed. The clearance by occlusal adjustment was decided beforehand with a trial-and-error method so that the occlusal forces were distributed similarly to the distribution of the natural dentition. Each model was evaluated under loads of 40, 100, 200, 400, and 800 N to determine the distribution of occlusal forces on the teeth and implants.

**Results:** The occlusal forces were concentrated on the most posterior implants while the load was larger, and the percentage of bearing force at the TMJ was small, and vice versa.

**Conclusions:** Maximum biting force was better for occlusal adjustment to prevent overloading of the most posterior implant.

**Keywords:** Implants; Occlusal adjustment; Nonlinear finite element analysis

## Background

Dental implants have been widely used to restore or maintain occlusion, function, and esthetics and are particularly effective for partially edentulous jaws [1]. However, the difference of the displaceability of the implants and natural teeth with periodontal ligaments (PDLs) [2] may cause a problem in an arch that includes both implants and teeth. There is controversy about whether this difference should be considered in occlusal adjustment. Misch [3] stated that a clearance equivalent to the displaceability of the PDL should be allowed for the occlusal surfaces of implant-retained prostheses to prevent stress concentration. Contrastingly, Miyata et al. [4] stated that occlusal contact in implants should be equal to that of natural teeth to maintain the stomatognathic system. Kasai et al. [5] reported that hard biting appeared to be better for occlusal adjustment to avoid overloading of the most posterior implant in unilateral distal extension. However, when the occlusal load is mainly supported by implants, it has not been clarified whether the occlusal adjustment of the implants should be done as in the case of natural dentition. Moreover, in such cases, it is also necessary to

* Correspondence: takayama@den.hokudai.ac.jp
[1]Removable Prosthodontics, Hokkaido University Hospital, Hokkaido University, Kita-14, Nishi-5, Kita-Ku, Sapporo 060-8648, Japan
Full list of author information is available at the end of the article

consider the far lower displaceability of implants than that of temporomandibular joints (TMJs) in the stomatognathic system.

The purpose of this study was, therefore, to investigate the influence of occlusal forces (the contractile force of masticatory muscles) exerted during occlusal adjustment on the distribution of forces among teeth, implants, and TMJs during intercuspal clenching in cases with bilateral missing molars and premolars by using finite element analysis.

## Methods

### Finite element model

Three-dimensional finite element (FE) models were based on those reported by Kasai et al. [5] and consisted of a mandible, natural teeth with periodontal ligaments, and titanium implants with superstructures. All elements were homogenous and isotropic. In the models, eight implants replaced all of the premolars and molars (Fig. 1).

The mass/volume and the shape of the mandible were assumed to be 2 and B, respectively, according to the classification of Lekholm and Zarb [6]. The implant fixtures were 3.75 mm in diameter and 10 mm in length [7]. The dimensions of the natural teeth and periodontal ligaments were based on the literature [8–10]. The surface area of the periodontal ligament (PDL) corresponded to the anatomical value [10], and its thickness was 0.25 mm at all sites. The occlusal surfaces of the implants and the teeth were simplified and flattened in agreement with Monson's sphere. The FE model consisted of approximately 42,000 nodes and 210,000 tetrahedral elements.

The properties of the materials, except for the PDL, were based on previous studies [11–15] (Table 1). The biphasic properties for the PDL were determined according to the literature [2, 3, 16, 17]. The PDL was assigned two-phase properties. Young's modulus and Poisson's ratio were 0.33 MPa and 0.3 for phase 1, respectively. For phase 2, they were 16 MPa and 0.45, respectively. Phase 2 was applied when the von Mises stress exceeded 0.025 MPa. The load-displacement curve of the teeth was verified with the analysis described below (Fig. 2a).

### Boundary conditions of the model and simulation of occlusal adjustment

The boundary conditions used to verify the displaceability of teeth and analyze the distribution of occlusal forces are shown in Fig. 2a, b, respectively. In the former model, a vertical load was applied to the left canine with the restriction of nodes on the bottom of the mandible (Fig. 2a). FE analysis was performed under various loads following the construction of a load-displacement curve. In the FE models used to analyze the distribution of occlusal force, TMJs, maxillary teeth, and maxillary implants were replaced with appropriate springs to simplify the model (Fig. 2b).

The antagonists of the mandibular anterior teeth were assumed to be natural teeth, and those of mandibular implants were assumed to be either teeth or implants.

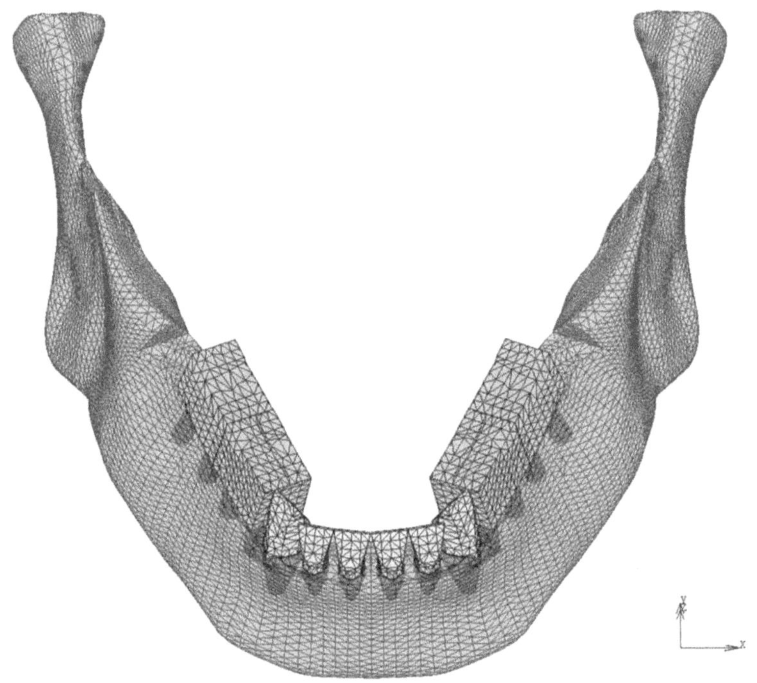


**Fig. 1** Finite element models (model-I and model-T). The tooth roots and the implant bodies are displayed with permeability

**Table 1** Material properties

| Materials | Modulus of elasticity (MPa) | Poisson ratio |
|---|---|---|
| Enamel | 80,000 | 0.3 |
| Dentin | 17,600 | 0.25 |
| Inplant (titanium) | 117,000 | 0.32 |
| Superstructure (gold alloy) | 94,000 | 0.3 |
| Cortical bone | 14,000 | 0.3 |
| Cancellous bone | 7,900 | 0.3 |

According to the condition of the antagonists of the mandibular implants, the models with opposing natural teeth and implants were designated model-T and model-I, respectively.

The springs for the maxillary teeth or implants, except for the anterior teeth, were directed perpendicular to the occlusal plane. Each of those springs linked an external restricted node to the node corresponding to the occlusal central pit on a mandibular tooth, which allowed displacement perpendicular to the occlusal plane. The springs for temporomandibular joints linked an external restricted node to the top of the mandibular condyle. Nonlinear characteristics according to the load-displacement curves of the teeth [2, 3, 16, 17] and cartilage [18] were given to the springs of the opposing teeth and TMJs, respectively. The springs for maxillary implants had linear compression characteristics. The springs for antagonists had little resistance under tension to simulate detachment. The properties of these springs were confirmed by load-displacement curves (Fig. 3) obtained using a simple FE model consisting of an element and a spring.

Occlusal adjustment was simulated by means of altering the load-displacement curves of the springs on the implants. The load-displacement curve was shifted so that the spring provided little resistance to compressive forces until the gap that was assumed to be made by occlusal adjustment closed (Figs. 3, 4, and 5). The size of each gap was decided by trial and error (Table 2) so that the occlusal force, i.e., the reaction force of the springs on the occlusal surface, was similar to that calculated with the FE model with natural dentition (model-N, Fig. 6).

### Loading conditions

The loading conditions assumed intercuspal clenching. On the assumption that occlusal force was generated by the contractile force of four bilateral masticatory muscles, the masseter, temporalis, mesial, and lateral pterygoid muscles, the loading points and the directions of the loads were determined based on the report by Korioth and Hannam [11] and anatomical findings [8–10]. The amount of the load was represented by the summation of the reaction forces at the occlusal surfaces of teeth in model-N. For example, the load condition that resulted in a total reaction force of 100 N in model-N was defined as Load100N.

### Procedure for analysis

The load conditions used during occlusal adjustment were Load40N, as a light bite (Adj40N), Load200N, as a hard bite (Adj200N), and Load400N, as the maximum biting force (Adj400N). Occlusal adjustment was performed through trial and error with reference to the distribution of the occlusal force calculated by FE analysis. When the similarities of the distribution of the reaction force on the superstructures to that on the natural teeth in model-N were confirmed, the occlusal adjustment was completed. Thereafter, the FE analysis was performed again under the load conditions of Load40N, Load100N, Load200N, Load400N, and Load800N using the FEA software package MSC.Marc2010 (MSC Software). The distributions of the reaction forces on the occlusal surface and on the mandibular condyle, which were regarded as the occlusal force and the load on the TMJ, respectively, were evaluated.

## Results

### Displaceability of teeth

The load-displacement curve of the left canine under vertical load indicated two-phase displacement as shown in Fig. 7.

### Model-T

The results of model-T are shown in Fig. 8. Adj40N resulted in the concentration of approximately 25 % of the occlusal force at the most posteriorly located implant on each side. In other words, about half of the total occlusal force occurred at these implants under Load100N, Load200N, Load400N, and Load800N. At the premolar site implants, 6.9 and 4.8 % of the occlusal force was distributed under Load100N and Load200N, respectively. However, under Load400N and Load800N, occlusal force scarcely occurred there. The percentage of the total occlusal force (hereinafter abbreviated as POF) borne by the TMJ was smaller than that in model-N under all loading conditions.

Adj200N resulted in a smaller POF than in model-N at the implants in molar sites under Load40N and Load100N, which were conditions with less load than that exerted during occlusal adjustment. On the other hand, under these conditions, the occlusal force was larger than in model-N at the most anteriorly located implant. The POF in the TMJ was slightly larger than in model-N. Under Load400N, when the load was larger than that exerted during occlusal adjustment, 35.9 % of the occlusal force was concentrated at the molar site implants. Under Load800N, when the load was larger than that exerted during occlusal adjustment, 37.7 % of the

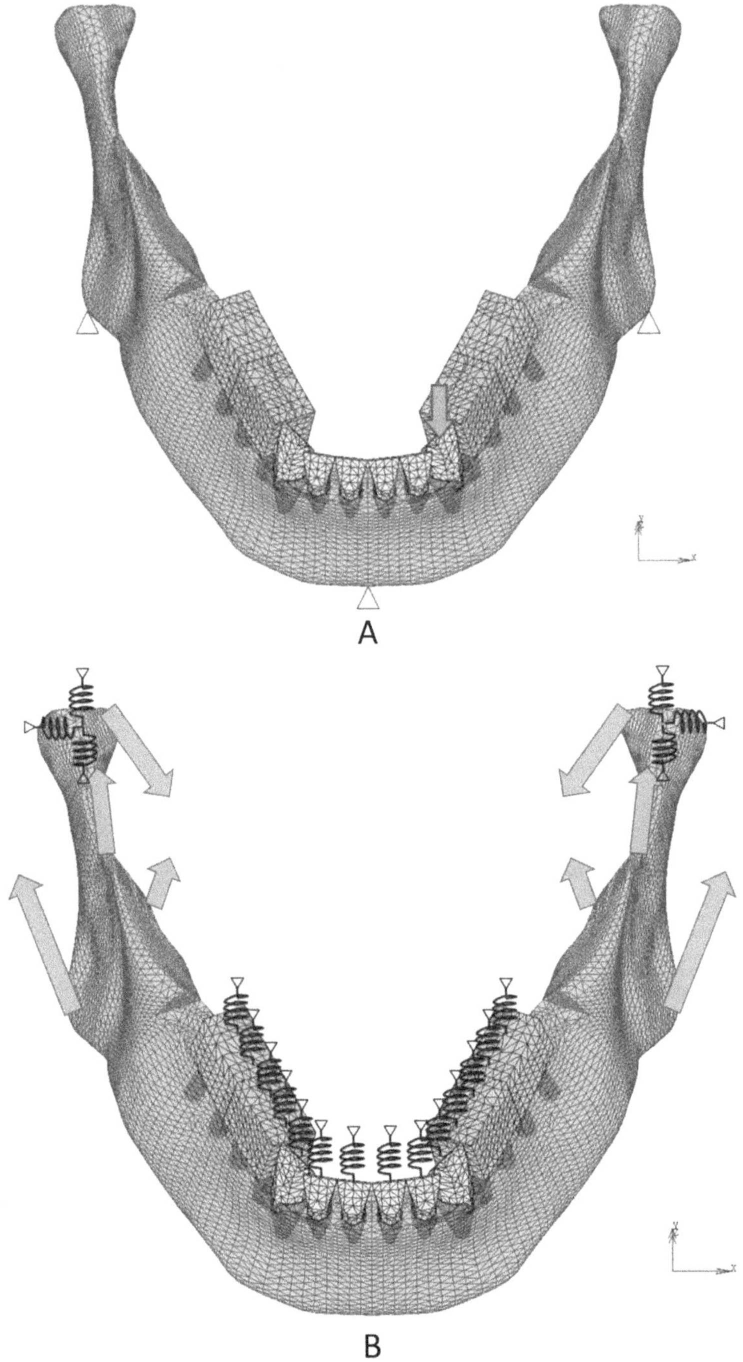


**Fig. 2** Boundary conditions to verify the displaceability of teeth (**a**) and analyze the distribution of occlusal forces (**b**). *Arrows*: loads, *triangles*: restricted nodes, *zigzags*: springs

occlusal force was concentrated at the molar site implants. In contrast, little or no occlusal force occurred at the premolar site implants. The POF in the TMJ was 12.1 % under Load400N and 11.7 % under Load800N.

Adj400N resulted in the reduction of POF at the molar site implants to half of the POF in model-N under Load40N and Load100N. On the other hand, 19.1 and 17.9 % of the occlusal force was distributed at the premolar site implants under Load40N and Load100N, respectively. The POF in the TMJ was 16.1 and 17.0 % under Load40N and Load100N, respectively. Under Load200N, 20.3 % of the occlusal force was distributed at the molar site implants and 14.0 % of the occlusal force was distributed at the premolar site implants. The

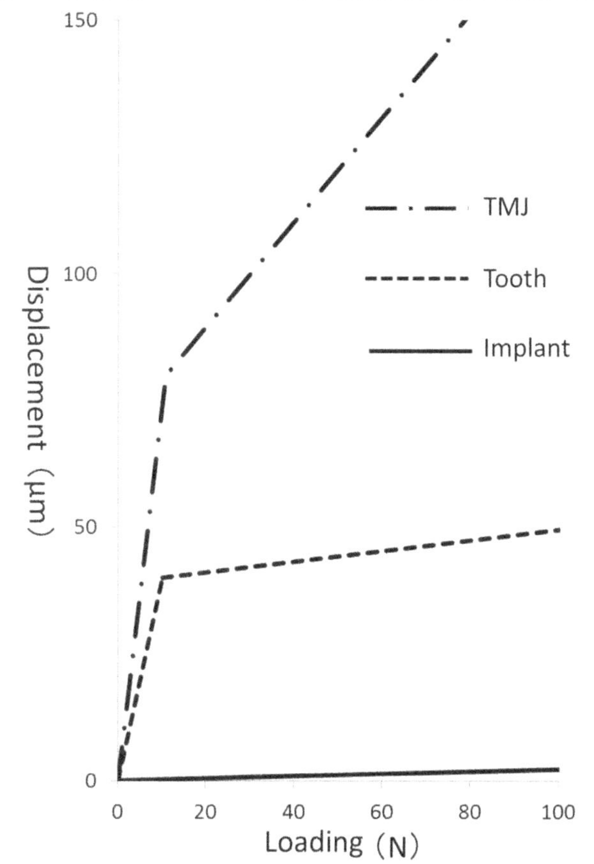


**Fig. 3** Load-displacement curves of the springs

POF in the TMJ was larger than that in model-N. Under Load800N, the POF at the molar site implants was 36.3 %. However, almost no occlusal force occurred at the premolar site implants and anterior teeth. The POF in the TMJ was almost the same as in model-N.

#### Model-I

The results of model-I are shown in Fig. 8. Adj40N resulted in the concentration of approximately 40 % of the occlusal force at the most posteriorly located implant on each side under all loading conditions. In other words, about 80 % of the total occlusal force occurred at these implants. However, the occlusal force scarcely occurred at the premolar site implants and natural teeth. Around 10 % of the occlusal force was distributed at the TMJ. The POF was smaller than that in model-N.

Adj200N resulted in the concentration of the occlusal force at the most anterior implant under Load40N and Load100N. The POF in the anterior teeth and the TMJs was larger than that in model-N under Load40N and Load100N. Under Load400N, 38.0 % of the occlusal force was concentrated at the molar site implants. Under Load800N, 39.2 % of the occlusal force was concentrated at the molar site implants. Little occlusal force was present at the premolar site implants and natural teeth. At the TMJs, the POF was smaller than in model-N under Load400N and Load800N. Adj400N resulted in a concentration of occlusal force ten times larger at the most anterior implant than in model-N under Load40N, Load100N, and Load200N. The POF at the anterior teeth increased as the total occlusal load decreased. While the load was less than that exerted during occlusal adjustment, the POF at the most posterior implant was smaller than that in model-N. Under Load800N, 30.0 % of the occlusal force was concentrated at the most posterior implant. The POF in the TMJ was 23.3, 22.5, and 20.1 % under Load40N, Load100N, and Load200N, respectively.

## Discussion

### FE models

The FE models in this study were based on those reported by Kasai et al. [5]. The material properties of the soft tissues such as the PDL and the TMJ, which were mainly deformed in the analysis, were considered to be crucial, because the aim of this study was to investigate the distribution of occlusal forces on the teeth, implants, and TMJs. In Figs. 3 and 8, the PDLs of anterior teeth and the springs corresponding to opposing teeth show two-stage displaceability as reported previously [16, 17] and were considered to be appropriate. The load-displacement curve of the springs corresponding to TMJs was assumed to be similar to that of the cartilage [18] because of its far smaller elastic modulus than that of the TMJ disc [19, 20]. Therefore, the elastic modulus of the springs corresponding to TMJs was determined based on the thicknesses of the TMJ disc [21] and articular cartilage [19], the stress-strain curve of the intervertebral discs [18], and the displacement of the condyle [22, 23] in intercuspal clenching by indirect measurement. Although the material properties of human body depend on the individual, the models in this study were therefore considered to be appropriate to investigate the distribution of occlusal forces on the teeth, implants, and TMJs.

### The meaning of "occlusal adjustment" in this study

In the FE model before loading, there is no stress or deformation anywhere in the model with perfect even occlusal contact. However, this situation cannot really occur because of the existence of some occlusal load in the intercuspal position (ICP). Since the displaceability of dental implants is quite different from that of the natural teeth and TMJ, the distribution of the occlusal force exerted on the occlusal surface of natural teeth and superstructures depends on the amount of the occlusal load, i.e., the contractile force of the musculature. Thus, the "occlusal adjustment" performed on the FE models in this study was not a clinical procedure itself but a procedure

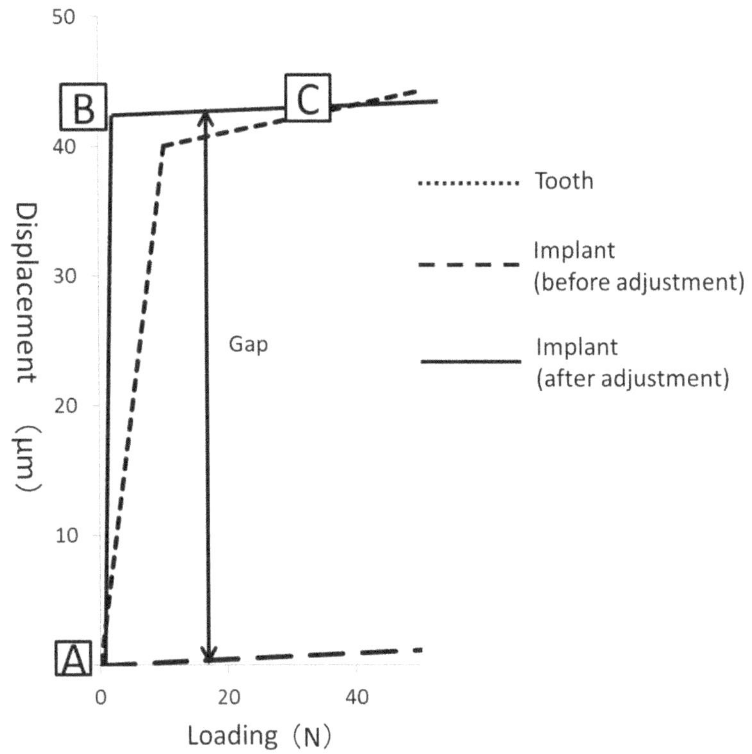


**Fig. 4** Occlusal adjustment was simulated by altering the load-displacement curves of the springs

to set the models in the state of the ICP under various occlusal loads. This problem can be clarified by the definition of the ICP itself. Although load and deformation of the bone, joints, periodontal ligaments, and teeth in the ICP depend on the amount of the occlusal load, its definition does not include how much occlusal load is appropriate to determine that a mandible is in the ICP [24]. The problem of occlusal adjustment of the superstructures on dental implants is, in a sense, deeply related to the definition of the ICP.

#### Loading conditions

In this study, we selected the loading conditions assuming intercuspal clenching, because the effect of occlusal adjustment was considered to appear clearly. Based on the literature [25, 26], occlusal loading of 200 N was considered to correspond with a hard bite. The value for the "light bite" (40 N) was chosen so that the load intruded on all of the posterior teeth with a displacement corresponding to the midpoint of the first phase in the stress-displacement curve. This study was performed on

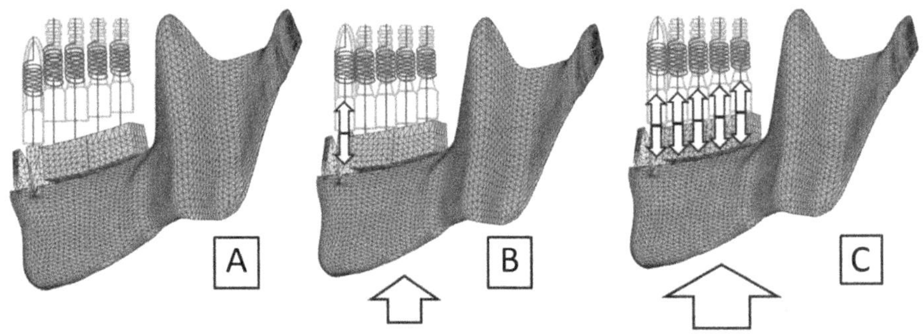


**Fig. 5** Schematic diagram for each phase of the load-displacement curve after occlusal adjustment of implants. **a**: Before loading, only anterior natural teeth were in contact with opposing teeth. Occlusal forces were not yet exerted anywhere. **b**: When a slight load caused the displacement of the mandible upward by the distance corresponding to the gap, i.e., the quantity of occlusal adjustment, the anterior teeth displaced into the socket and the implants were in contact with antagonists. Occlusal force was exerted only on anterior teeth. **c**: If the gaps were determined such that occlusal adjustment was completed, occlusal forces were distributed among natural teeth and implants under certain amounts of load

**Table 2** Size of each gap

| Occlusal adjustment (model) | 4 | 5 | 6 | 7 |
|---|---|---|---|---|
| Adj40N (model-T) | 25.0 | 26.0 | 13.0 | 12.0 |
| Adj200N (model-T) | 30.0 | 37.0 | 23.5 | 24.0 |
| Adj40N (model-I) | 39.4 | 41.0 | 42.8 | 43.5 |
| Adj200N (model-I) | 70.9 | 75.4 | 79.9 | 81.6 |

the assumption that the maximum functional force was 400 N. Calculations were also performed under a load of 800 N, which was assumed to be the maximum nonfunctional occlusal force, such as that exerted in nocturnal bruxism. Because of the difficulty to control nocturnal bruxism, this value was considered to be sufficient to include the condition under the maximum force [27] as the load in bruxism.

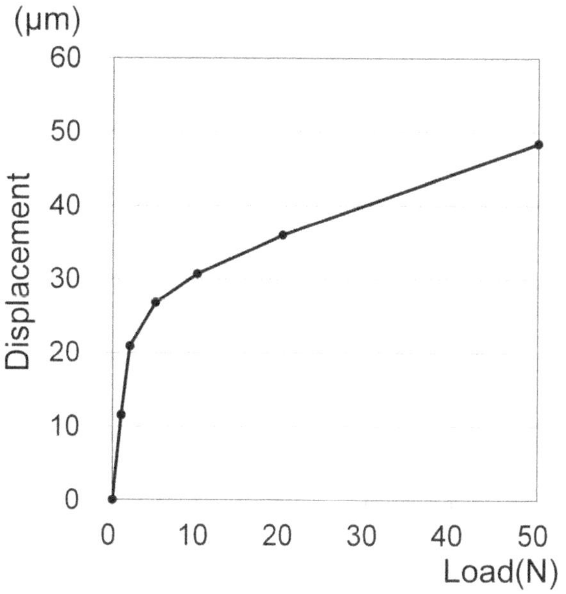


**Fig. 7** Load-displacement curve of the left canine

### Effect of occlusal loading in occlusal adjustment and antagonists of implants

The occlusal force was concentrated on the most posterior implants while the load was larger under all loading conditions. This concentration of the occlusal force could be explained by the displaceability of TMJs. Since it was far larger than that of the teeth and implants (Fig. 3), the TMJs and ramus of the mandible were displaced upward and the most posterior implants became fulcrums of the rotation of the mandible. On the other hand, posterior implants were considered to be separated from opposing teeth and implants when the load was less than that exerted during occlusal adjustment. However, because of the smaller load itself, the actual occlusal force on the anterior implants was considered

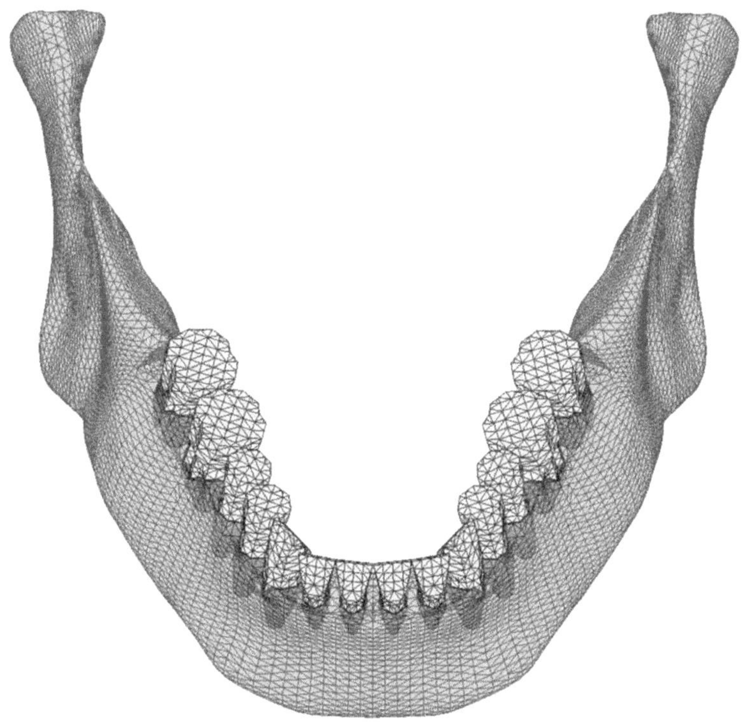

**Fig. 6** FE model with natural dentition (model-N). Tooth root is displayed with permeability

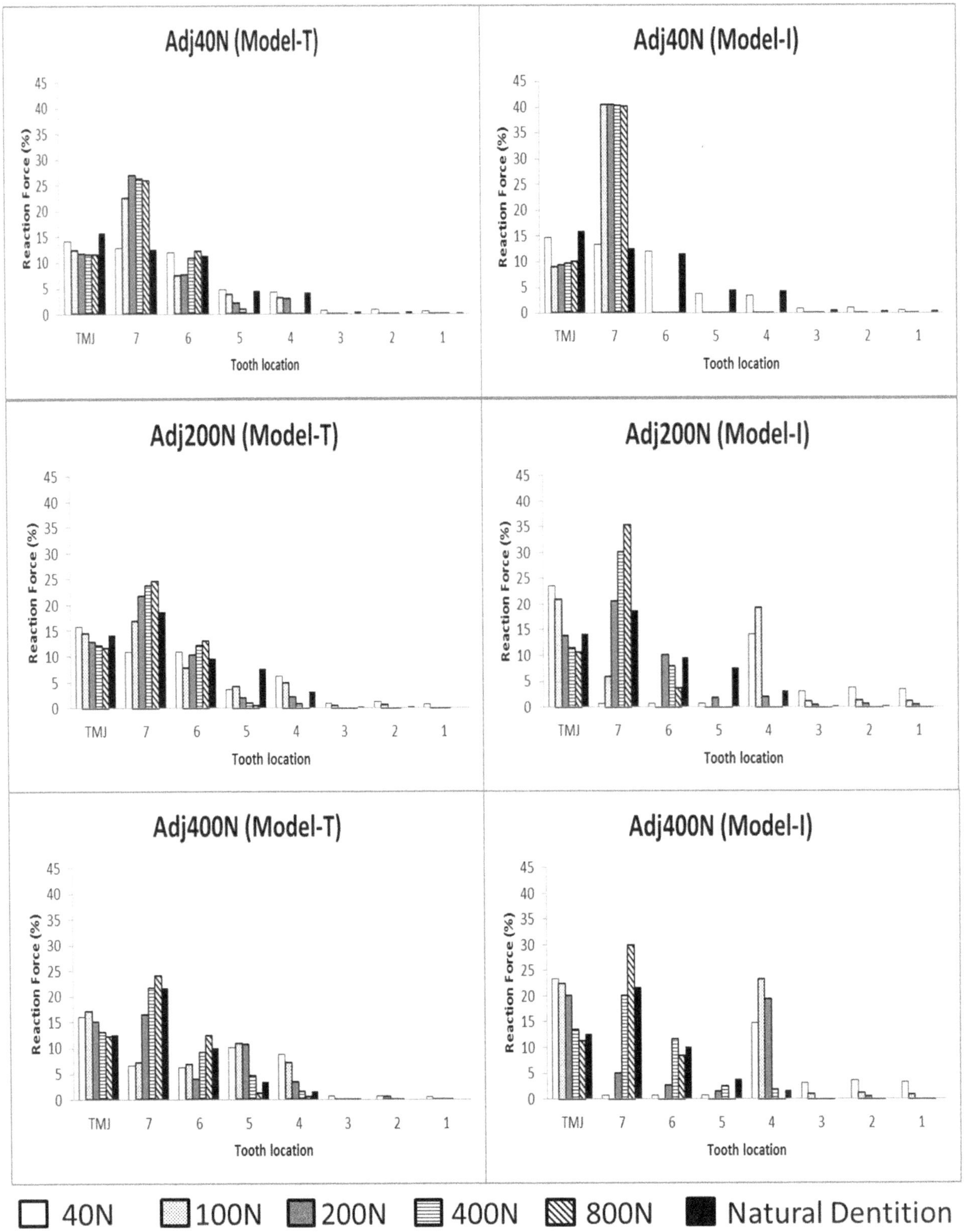


**Fig. 8** Distribution of the occlusal forces. *Left column*: model-T, *right column*: model-I, "Natural dentition" indicates the results in model-N under the load during occlusal adjustment

to be less harmful. The concentration of occlusal force was more marked in model-I than in model-T. This suggested the need for more careful occlusal adjustment in the case of opposing implants in both jaws because of the absence of the buffering effect of periodontal ligaments.

### Load bearing on TMJs

The percentage of bearing force at the TMJ was larger while the load was less than that exerted during occlusal adjustment, and vice versa. However, when the percentage of bearing force at the TMJ was large, the absolute force was not larger than in model-N under the load during occlusal adjustment, because the load itself was small. Therefore, the load borne by the TMJ was not considered to be harmful in any case of occlusal adjustment or load because the occlusal force itself was kept comparatively small even if the percentage of the bearing load increased.

### Suggestion of a clinical procedure for occlusal adjustment

In this study, when the load was larger than that exerted during occlusal adjustment, the concentration of the occlusal force in the molar region was considered to be harmful. However, since the occlusal force concentrated in the premolar region was relatively low when the load was less than that in occlusal adjustment, it was considered to be less harmful than in the former case. Therefore, according to our results, occlusal adjustment under maximum biting force was considered to be better to avoid the concentration of occlusal force on both implants and TMJs in Kennedy class I cases.

### Limitations of this study

It should be noted that these results were obtained under conditions of vertical loading by bilaterally balanced muscle activity with tight intercuspation in the correct mandibular position because the horizontal displacement of the premolars and molars was restrained. The actual distribution of occlusal forces may be different from the results of this study because there are individual differences in the material properties of the soft tissue. The lateral load, which may occur in lateral movement of the mandible during mastication, was not considered. These are problems that remain to be clarified in future research.

## Conclusions

Within the limitations of this study, it was concluded that the maximum biting force was better for occlusal adjustment with intercuspal clenching in bilateral distal extension of the superstructures on dental implants to prevent overloading of both TMJs and of the most posterior implants, especially in the case of opposing implants.

**Competing interests**
Sho Kayumi, Yoshiyuki Takayama, Atsuro Yokoyama, and Nana Ueda declare that there are no competing interests.

**Authors' contributions**
SK participated in the design of the study and the construction of FE models, and carried out the final calculation. YT participated in the construction of the FE models and programming for non-linear FE analysis. AY participated in the construction of FE models. NU participated in the construction of the FE models. All authors read and approved the final manuscript.

**Author details**
[1]Removable Prosthodontics, Hokkaido University Hospital, Hokkaido University, Kita-14, Nishi-5, Kita-Ku, Sapporo 060-8648, Japan. [2]Department of Oral Functional Prosthodontics, Division of Oral Functional Science, Graduate School of Dental Medicine, Hokkaido University, Kita-13, Nishi-7, Kita-Ku, Sapporo 060-8648, Japan.

### References

1. Isidor F. Loss of osseointegration caused by occlusal load of oral implants. A clinical and radiographic study in monkeys. Clin Oral Implants Res. 1996;7:143–52.
2. Kim Y, Oh T, Misch CE, Wang H. Occlusal considerations in implant therapy: clinical guidelines with biomechanical rationale. Clin Oral Implants Res. 2005;16:26–35.
3. Misch CE. Occlusal considerations for implant-supported prostheses: implant protective occlusion and occlusal materials. In: Misch CE, Bidez M, editors. Contemporary implant dentistry. 2nd ed. St. Louis: Mosby; 1999. p. 609–28.
4. Miyata T, Kobayashi Y, Araki H, et al. The influence of controlled occlusal overload on peri-implant tissue. Part 3: a histologic study in monkeys. Int J Oral Maxillofac Implants. 2000;5:425–43.
5. Kasai K, Takayama Y, Yokoyama A: Distribution of occlusal forces during occlusal adjustment of dental implant prostheses: a nonlinear finite element analysis considering the capacity for displacement of opposing teeth and implants. J Oral Maxillofac Implants, 2012;27: 329–335
6. Zarb GA, Bolender CL. Implant prosthodontics for edentulous patients: current and future directions. In: Elsubeihi ES, Attard N, Zarb GA, editors. Prosthodontic treatment for edentulous patients: complete denture and implant-supported prostheses. 12th ed. St. Louis: Mosby; 2004. p. 532–4.
7. Gross MD. Occlusion in implant dentistry. A review of the literature of prosthetic determinants and current concepts. Australian Dental Journal. 2008;53 Suppl 1:S60–8.
8. Sicher H, DuBrul EL. The musculature. The dentition and occlusion. In: Sicher H, DuBrul EL, editors. Sicher and DuBrul's Oral Anatomy. 8th ed. St. Louis; Tokyo: Ishiyaku EuroAmerica; 1988. p. 89–95. 33–146.
9. Schroeder HE. Development, structure, and function of periodontal tissues. In: Schroeder HE, editor. The periodontium. Berlin; New York: Springer; 1986. p. 23–6.
10. Schroeder HE. Development, structure, and function of periodontal tissues. In: Schroeder HE, editor. The periodontium. Berlin: Springer; 1986. p. 182–5.
11. Korioth TWP, Hannam AG. Deformation of the human mandible during simulated tooth clenching. J Dent Res. 1994;73:56–66.
12. Kunavisarut C, Lisa AL, Stoner BR, Felton DA. Finite element analysis on dental implant-supported prostheses without passive fit. J Prosthodont. 2002;11:30–40.
13. Van Zyl PP, Grundling NL, Jooste CH, Terblanche E. Three-dimensional finite element model of a human mandible incorporating six osseointegrated implants for stress analysis of mandibular cantilever prostheses. Int J Oral Maxillofac Implants. 1995;10:51–7.
14. Kitamura E, Stegaroiu R, Nomura S, Miyakawa O. Influence of marginal bone resorption on stress around an implant—a three-dimensional finite element analysis. J Oral Rehabil. 2005;32:279–86.
15. Kobayashi K, Yorimoto T, Hikita K, Maida T. Abutment forms and restorative materials in adhesive prosthesis: a finite element analysis. Dent Mater J. 2004;23:75–80.
16. Perfitt GJ. Measurement of the physiological mobility of individual teeth in an axial direction. J Dent Res. 1960;39:608–18.

17. Miura H, Hasegawa S, Okada D, Ishihara H. The measurement of physiological tooth displacement in function. J Med Dent Sci. 1998;45:103–5.
18. Martinez JB, Oloyede VOA, Broom ND. Biomechanics of load-bearing of the intervertebral disc: an experimental and finite element model. Med Eng Phys. 1997;19:145–56.
19. Singh M, Detamore MS. Biomechanical properties of the mandibular condylar cartilage and their relevance to the TMJ disc. J Biomech. 2009;42:405–17.
20. Tanaka E, Eijden T. Biomechanical behavior of the temporomandibular joint disc. Crit Rev Oral Biol Med. 2003;14:138–50.
21. Hansson T, Nordström B. Thickness of the soft tissue layers and articular disk in temporomandibular joints with deviations in form. Acta Odontol Scand. 1977;35:281–8.
22. Minagi S, Ohmori T, Sato T, Matsunaga T, Akamatsu Y. Effect of eccentric clenching on mandibular deviation in the vicinity of mandibular rest position. J Oral Rehabil. 2000;27:174–8.
23. Yamazaki M, Yugami K, Baba K, Ohyama T. Effect of clenching level on mandibular displacement in Kennedy class II partially edentulous patients. Int J Prosthodont. 2003;16:183–8.
24. The Academy of Prosthodontics. The glossary of prosthodontic terms (GPT-8). J Prosthet Dent 2005; 94: 10–92.
25. Gibbs CH, Mahan PE, Lundeen HC, Brehnan K, Walsh EK, Holbrook WB. Occlusal forces during chewing and swallowing as measured by sound transmission. J Prosthet Dent. 1981;46:443–9.
26. Kumagai H, Suzuki T, Hamada T, Sondang P, Fujitani M, Nikawa H. Occlusal force distribution on the dental arch during various levels of clenching. J Oral Rehabil. 1999;26:932–5.
27. Nishigawa K, Bando E, Nakano M. Quantitative study of bite force during sleep associated bruxism. J Oral Rehabil. 2001;28:485–91.

# Occlusal status of implant superstructures at mandibular first molar immediately after setting

Yukihiko Okada*, Yuji Sato, Noboru Kitagawa, Keiichiro Uchida, Tokiko Osawa, Yoshiki Imamura and Mayumi Terazawa

**Abstract**

**Background:** Occlusal contact on the implant superstructures is important for successful treatment. The purpose of this study was to investigate the occlusal contact of single implant superstructures at the mandibular first molar immediately after seating from weak to strong clenching.

**Methods:** Subjects were nine patients who had just been fitted with an implant prosthesis in the mandibular first molar region, with no missing teeth other than in the implant region. First, while masseter muscle activity was monitored, maximum clenching strength (100 % maximum voluntary contraction (MVC)) was determined with an electromyogram. Next, occlusal load and occlusal contact area were measured three times at clenching intensities of 40, 60, 80, and 100 % MVC by the use of pressure-sensitive film for occlusal force diagnostic and Occluzer for occlusal force measurement. Finally, the occlusal contact area was measured once each at 20, 40, and 60 % MVC using a silicone testing material and BiteEye for occlusal contact measurement. A two-way analysis of variance (ANOVA) was used to determine occlusal loading and occlusal area as dependent variables, and clenching strength and presence or absence of implant as between-subject factors. A multiple comparison test was performed using the Bonferroni method.

**Results:** The occlusal contact area and occlusal load of the implant prosthesis increased with clenching strength, and the increases in occlusal contact area and occlusal load of the implant prosthesis were less than those of the contralateral tooth at high clenching strength. However, significant difference was not observed when compared with both sides of the molar region regardless of clenching strength.

**Conclusions:** The occlusal contact area of the implant had a tendency to be adjusted smaller than the natural tooth by a dental technician and a dentist. On the other hand, despite the small tissue displaceability of the implant, occlusal load on the implant prosthesis was smaller than on the natural tooth at high clenching strength.

**Keywords:** Occlusal load; Occlusal contact area; Implant; Clenching strength; Occluzer; BiteEye

## Background

Implants maintain osseointegration with the inside of the bone over long periods of time, and mechanical factors are important for retaining function [1]. Particularly, when natural teeth and implants are present together, differences in tissue displaceability when they are subjected to occlusal force may cause dynamic imbalance from strong to weak clenching [2–4].

Therefore, there is a school of thought that prosthetic implants should be given a lower occlusion than natural teeth [5–7]. On the other hand, from the perspective of jaw function, it is also argued that prosthetic implants should be given the same occlusion as intact natural teeth neighboring the implant [8]. In a study using two-dimensional finite element analysis, Maezawa et al. [9] suggested that, even if the occlusal surface of the prosthetic implant is made lower than the occlusal plane, high clenching intensity can result in an excessive occlusal load on the prosthetic implant. In addition, Koyama et al. [10] found no significant differences in occlusal contact point between prosthetic implants and natural teeth, even if clenching intensity varies. From these studies, it appears that the occlusal contact of implant

* Correspondence: okada.yuki@dent.showa-u.ac.jp
Department of Geriatric Dentistry, School of Dentistry Showa University, 2-1-1 Kitasenzoku, Ota Ward, Tokyo 145-8515, Japan

prostheses is the same level on natural teeth, regardless of clenching strength, and that occlusal load on implant prosthesis increases more than contralateral natural teeth as clenching strength increases. Methods of quantitative evaluation used to clarify mechanical factors of implant prostheses include pressure-sensitive films for occlusal force diagnostic use and silicone testing materials, but few studies have examined the occlusal contact from weak to strong clenching strength under the same conditions.

In this department to date, Okuyama et al. [11] used a pressure-sensitive film to examine the occlusal contact and to calculate the mean occlusal gap and occlusal load of implants that had progressed satisfactorily, as well as natural teeth. Imamura et al. [12] used a new silicone test material and a pressure-sensitive film to develop a method for investigating changes in occlusal contact from weak to strong clenching intensity in subjects with natural dentition.

Occlusal contact is a reflection of the degree of functional recovery and measurement of factors such as number of occlusal contact points, contact area, and distribution. Occlusal center is advisable before and after treatment [13]. Therefore, the purpose of this study was to investigate the occlusal contact of single implant superstructures at the mandibular first molar immediately after seating by using two different materials with an electromyogram. Ultimately, we aimed to obtain clinical suggestions for the occlusion that should be given to prosthetic implants through a longitudinal follow-up study.

## Methods

### Subjects and dentition

Subjects were nine outpatients (5 male, 4 female) attending Showa University Dental Hospital, aged 35–69 years (mean age, 49 ± 12 years) (Table 1). All subjects were cases of single implants placed at the mandibular first molar deficit, on the day of implant prosthesis setting and occlusal adjustment. The criteria for subject selection were no inflammatory symptoms (redness, swelling) in the implantation area [14, 15], no implant mobility, no subjective symptoms, and no noticeable resorption on X-ray photographs.

**Table 1** Site of implants

| No. | Sex | Age | Implant system | Implant site |
|---|---|---|---|---|
| 1 | F | 35 | Straumann | Right |
| 2 | F | 39 | Brånemark | Left |
| 3 | F | 47 | Brånemark | Left |
| 4 | F | 49 | Brånemark | Left |
| 5 | M | 43 | Straumann | Right |
| 6 | M | 46 | Straumann | Right |
| 7 | M | 69 | Straumann | Right |
| 8 | M | 48 | Brånemark | Left |
| 9 | M | 67 | Brånemark | Right |

The requirements for dentition were that other than the implant, which was the tooth to be studied, all teeth were natural; 28 teeth were present from the central incisors to the second molars, which includes the implant area; there were no mobile teeth; a basic periodontal test showed no pockets of 4 mm or more; there was no history of orthodontic therapy; and there was no oromandibular dysfunction such as temporomandibular disorder, masticatory muscle pain, or mandibular movement abnormality. In addition, occlusal adjustment was performed by a doctor in attendance. The implant prosthesis had one or more occlusal contact points at maximum clenching strength. Moreover, it has been adjusted as not to interfere with existing guide during lateral movement. Fourteen patients were selected based on these conditions, and consent was obtained from the doctor in charge of the 12 patients. Of these, nine patients consented to take part and acted as subjects.

The study was approved by Showa University Ethics Committee and was carried out after all subjects received a full explanation of the aims and methods of the study and gave their consent to participate (approval no. 2012-020).

### Electromyograph attachment

Masseter muscle activity was measured using an electromyograph (PowerLab; ADInstruments, Nagoya, Japan). Silver disk electrodes of 10 mm in diameter with bipolar leads (Duotrode; Morita Corp., Osaka, Japan) were adhered on both sides of the central part of the masseter muscle. The distance between electrodes was 21 mm, and the electrodes were placed parallel to the direction in which the masseter muscle fibers run.

The activity of the masseter muscle, when subjects clenched their teeth at full strength with nothing interposed between the upper and lower teeth, was defined at 100 % maximum voluntary contraction (MVC), and subjects were able to see the amount of muscle force displayed in numerical values through visual feedback.

### Measurement and analysis of subject dentition

#### *Measurement of occlusal loading and occlusal contact area using Occluzer*

Pressure-sensitive film (Dental Prescale 50H type R; Fuji Photo Film Co., Tokyo, Japan) for occlusal force diagnostic use was used to examine the occlusal contact area and occlusal load in the intercuspal position together. Masseter muscle activity (clenching strength) was set at 40, 60, 80, and 100 % MVC, and subjects were measured three times at each of these clenching intensities using visual feedback. Subjects remained in a seated position, and the head on the headrest of the dental unit with the occlusal plane is parallel to the floor.

Subjects were instructed to open their mouths one finger width and the Prescale was inserted, and subjects were then instructed to slowly close their mouths and clench their teeth. The Prescale was interposed between the full dentition between the second molars on either side, and subjects were instructed to bite in the intercuspal position. Clenching on the Prescale was carried out for 3 s, and considering the content of muscle fatigue, measurements were taken at 5-min intervals.

The Prescale was kept in a cool, dark place for 24 h; after which, the colored parts, their surface area, and their color density were analyzed using a dedicated analyzer (Occluzer FPD707®; Fuji Photo Film Co., Tokyo, Japan). Occlusal force was analyzed by a software (DePROS-PC; GC, Tokyo, Japan), and these data were converted to pressure values. The occlusal loading and occlusal contact area for molars were then calculated.

### *Measurement of occlusal contact area using BiteEye*

A material for checking accuracy of fit (Blue Silicone®; GC, Tokyo, Japan) was used to examine the occlusal contact in the intercuspal position. The occlusal contact area was measured once at each clenching strength (20, 40, and 60 % MVC) using visual feedback. Subject posture was the same as during Prescale measurement. Subjects were instructed to open their mouths one finger width and Blue Silicon was inserted above the lower row of teeth, and subjects were then instructed to keep it in the mouth for 15 s. Subjects were instructed to keep the clenching strength of provisions while displaying the strength clenching on the monitor. Subjects clenched their teeth at the required strength for 30 s and kept the Blue Silicone in their mouths for a further 30 s until it hardened. Taking muscle fatigue into account, measurements were taken at 5-min intervals.

Thus, the Blue Silicone impressions obtained were examined using a BiteEye occlusal contact analyzer (BiteEye-I®; GC, Tokyo, Japan). The thickness of the Blue Silicone film at the points of occlusal contact was set at 10, 20, and 30 μm, and the occlusal contact area was calculated. When the thickness of the Blue Silicone film at the points of occlusal contact was set at 10 μm, Dental Prescale and Blue Silicone approximate in the occlusal contact area in the natural dentition [12].

While there have been studies in which the occlusal contact area was calculated from the silicone method, the thickness of silicone (μm) that is defined as occlusion has not been quantitatively clarified. Okada et al. [16] found functional occlusal contacts can be recorded at the silicone thickness 30 μm. From the above sentence, the thickness of the Blue Silicone film at the points of occlusal contact was set at 10–30 μm.

### *Analysis of the results from Occluzer and BiteEye*

The following calculations were performed:

1. Comparison of Occluzer and BiteEye in the occlusal contact area
2. Comparison of the occlusal contact area and occlusal load between the implant and same number of natural teeth on the contralateral side
3. Comparison of the occlusal contact area and occlusal load between molar areas of the implant side and contralateral side
4. Comparison of the occlusal contact area and occlusal load between molar areas of the implant side and contralateral side excluding the first molar
5. Comparison of the proportion of the occlusal contact area and occlusal load on the molar region accounted for by the prosthetic implant and contralateral tooth

Analysis of results from Occluzer and BiteEye was performed by two-way ANOVA with occlusal loading and occlusal area as dependent variables, and clenching strength and presence or absence of implant as between-subject factors. The level of significance for multiple comparison tests was set at 5 %.

In addition, multiple comparison test was performed using the Bonferroni method. PASW Statistics 18 was used for all statistical calculations (SPSS, Tokyo, Japan).

## Results

### Comparison of occlusal contact areas evaluated using Occluzer and BiteEye

Occlusal contact area values obtained with BiteEye and Occluzer at clenching intensities from 20 to 100 % MVC were compared (Fig. 1). At different clenching intensities, the contact area values of BiteEye with silicone thickness of 10 μm (BE 10 μm) were the most similar to the contact area values of Occluzer. Thus, comparisons

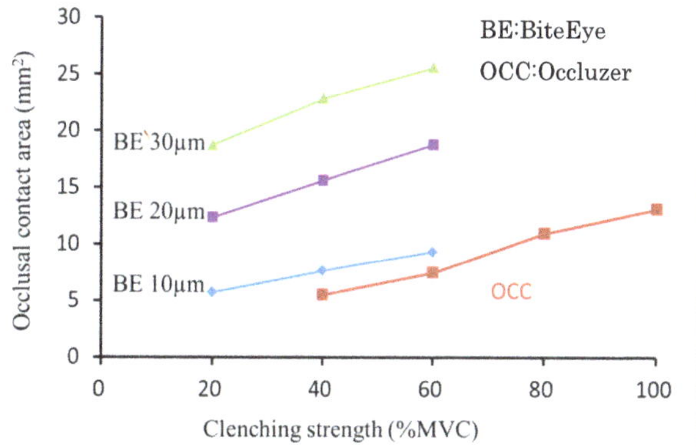


**Fig. 1** Comparison of the occlusal contact area between Occluzer and BiteEye

of occlusal contact area values between Occluzer and BiteEye were carried out with a silicone thickness of 10 μm.

### Comparison of implant region and contralateral tooth

#### *Comparison of occlusal contact area*

The occlusal contact area of implant prostheses increased with clenching strength and was always less than that of the contralateral tooth (Fig. 2). ANOVA results (Table 2) show a significant difference between implants and natural teeth with BiteEye ($P < 0.05$). Multiple comparison test showed that the occlusal contact area of implants was significantly smaller than the occlusal contact area of contralateral teeth with BiteEye at clenching intensities of 40 and 60 % MVC and Occluzer at clenching intensities of 80 and 100 % MVC ($P < 0.05$).

#### *Comparison of occlusal load*

Occlusal load on implant prostheses increased with clenching strength and was always less than that on the contralateral teeth (Fig. 2). At 100 % MVC, the occlusal load on the implant prosthesis was 47.7 ± 39.0 N and that on the contralateral tooth was 81.4 ± 41.1 N. ANOVA results (Table 3) showed a significant interaction in the difference in occlusal load between implants and natural teeth, and clenching strength ($P < 0.05$). Multiple comparison test showed that the occlusal load was significantly smaller on the implant prostheses than on the contralateral teeth at clenching intensities of 80 and 100 % MVC ($P < 0.05$).

The rate of increase in occlusal load from 40 to 100 % MVC was 106.1 % for the implant prosthesis and 127.4 % for the contralateral tooth.

### Comparison of implant side and contralateral side molar regions

#### *Comparison of occlusal contact area in the molar region*

The occlusal contact area in the molar region on the implant and contralateral sides increased with clenching strength and, at clenching intensity of 60 % MVC or above, was less on the implant side molar region (Fig. 3). ANOVA results (Table 4) showed no significant differences in occlusal contact area between the implant side molar region and the contralateral side molar region with BiteEye ($P = 0.092$). Multiple comparison tests showed no significant differences in the occlusal contact area between the molar region on the implant side and the molar region on the contralateral side at any clenching intensity with either BiteEye or Occluzer ($P > 0.05$).

#### *Comparison of occlusal load on the molar region*

Occlusal load on the implant side molar region and the contralateral side molar region increased with clenching strength and, at clenching intensity of 80 % MVC and above, was less on the implant side molar region (Fig. 3). At 100 % MVC, the occlusal force on the implant side molar region was 212.7 ± 57.6 N and on the contralateral side molar region was 274.4 ± 111.5 N. ANOVA results (Table 5) showed no significant differences in occlusal load between the implant side molar region and the contralateral side molar region ($P = 0.278$). Multiple comparison test showed no significant differences in occlusal load between the molar region on the implant side and the molar region on the contralateral side at any clenching intensity ($P > 0.05$).

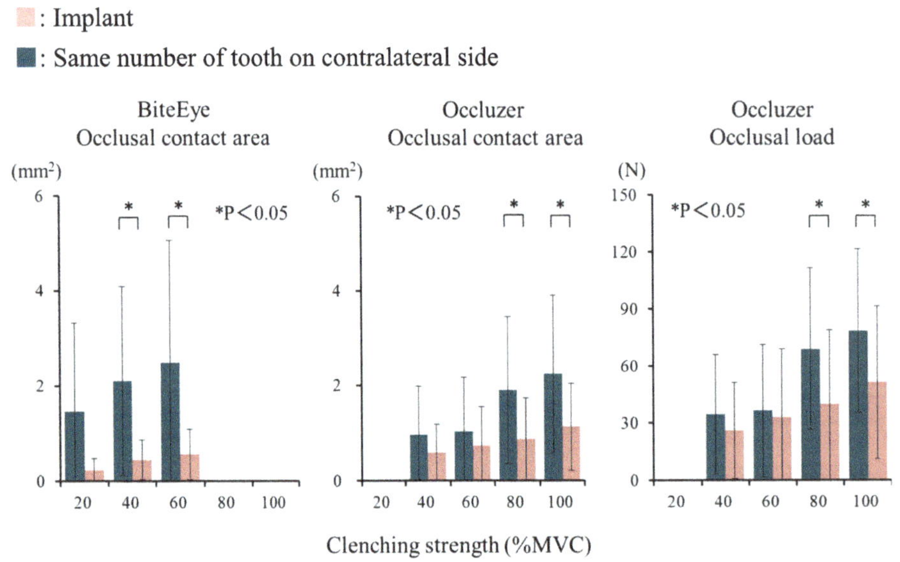


**Fig. 2** Comparison of occlusal contact area and occlusal load between implant and contralateral tooth

**Table 2** Two-way ANOVA of the occlusal contact area of the implant prosthesis and contralateral tooth

| | Source | Sum of square | *df* | Mean square | *F* value | *P* value |
|---|---|---|---|---|---|---|
| Occluzer | Implant or natural tooth | 1941.060 | 1 | 1941.060 | 1.074 | 0.333 |
| | MVC | 424.098 | 3 | 141.336 | 1.958 | 0.147 |
| | Interaction | 262.581 | 3 | 87.527 | 1.345 | 0.283 |
| BiteEye | Implant or natural tooth | 28.022 | 1 | 28.022 | 6.892 | 0.030 |
| | MVC | 3.374 | 2 | 1.687 | 1.927 | 0.178 |
| | Interaction | 0.916 | 2 | 0.458 | 0.827 | 0.455 |

#### Comparison of implant side and contralateral side molar regions excluding the first molar

##### *Comparison of occlusal contact area in the molar region excluding the first molar*

The occlusal contact area in the molar region excluding the first molar on the implant and contralateral sides increased with clenching strength (Fig. 4). ANOVA results (Table 6) showed no significant differences in the occlusal contact area between the implant side molar region and the contralateral side molar region with BiteEye ($P = 0.400$). Multiple comparison tests showed no significant differences in the occlusal contact area between the molar region excluding the first molar on the implant side and the molar region on the contralateral side at any clenching intensity with either BiteEye or Occluzer ($P > 0.05$).

##### *Comparison of occlusal load on the molar region excluding the first molar*

Occlusal load on the implant side molar region and the contralateral side molar region excluding the first molar increased with clenching strength (Fig. 4). At 100 % MVC, the occlusal force on the implant side molar region was 165.0 ± 45.8 N and on the contralateral side molar region was 193.3 ± 85.8 N. ANOVA results (Table 7) showed no significant differences in occlusal load between the implant side molar region and the contralateral side molar region ($P = 0.990$). Multiple comparison test showed no significant differences in occlusal load between the molar region excluding the first molar on the implant side and the molar region on the contralateral side at any clenching intensity ($P > 0.05$).

**Table 3** Two-way ANOVA of occlusal load of implant prosthesis and contralateral tooth

| Source | Sum of square | *df* | Mean square | *F* value | *P* value |
|---|---|---|---|---|---|
| Implant or natural tooth | 8732.252 | 1 | 8732.252 | 13.299 | 0.007 |
| MVC | 14,619.565 | 3 | 4872.855 | 16.724 | 0.001 |
| Interaction | 2200.789 | 3 | 733.596 | 8.442 | 0.001 |

#### Comparison of proportion of occlusal contact area and occlusal load on the molar region accounted for by prosthetic implant and contralateral tooth

With both BiteEye and Occluzer, the proportion of the occlusal contact area on the molar region overall accounted for by the prosthetic implant was less than the proportion accounted for by the contralateral natural tooth, and ANOVA showed this difference to be significant ($P < 0.05$) (Fig. 5, Table 8). Multiple comparison test also showed that the prosthetic implant accounted for a significantly smaller proportion of occlusal contact area at all clenching intensities other than 40 and 60 % MVC with Occluzer ($P < 0.05$). With occlusal load as well, the prosthetic implant accounted for a significantly smaller proportion than the contralateral tooth, and at 100 % MVC, the occlusal load on the prosthetic implant was 9.1 % of the load on the molar region while the occlusal load on the contralateral tooth was 16.3 %. Multiple comparison test showed that the proportion of occlusal load on the molar region accounted for by the prosthetic implant was significantly smaller than that accounted for by the contralateral tooth at clenching intensities other than 40 and 60 % ($P < 0.05$).

No significant differences in the proportion of occlusal area or occlusal load on the molar region attributable to clenching strength were found with the prosthetic implant or the contralateral tooth with either BiteEye or Occluzer ($P > 0.05$) (Table 8).

## Discussion

#### Subjects and dentition

Males outnumbered females in the present study, but there have been no reports of differences in mean occlusal load between males and females in the 50–54 age group [17]. While there have been reports that in healthy, dentulous subjects, the total occlusal force in the molar region on one side is approximately 400 N at maximum clenching strength [18], in the present study, the mean occlusal force on the natural tooth side at 100 % MVC was 274.4 ± 111.5 N. However, considering the subjects in the present study were of middle and old age, with mean age 49 years, the results probably have a certain validity [17–19].

Occlusal force is often measured across the whole jaw [20, 21]. The Dental Prescale used for occlusal force measurement has a thickness of approximately 100 μm, and concern has been raised that this thickness might affect the results of occlusal force distribution measurement. However, as good reproducibility of results from the molar region has been reported, in the present study, the molar region from the first premolar to the second molar on both sides was examined [11, 12, 22].

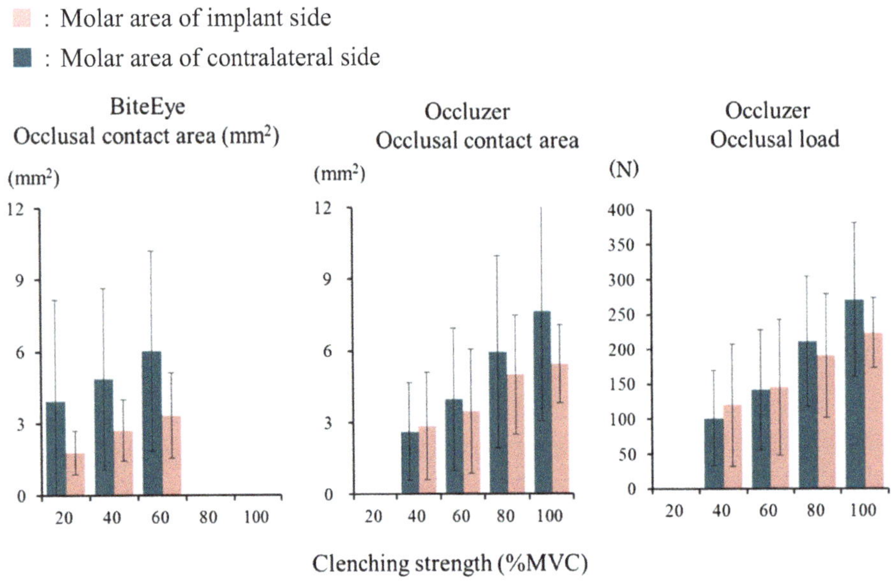


**Fig. 3** Comparison of the occlusal contact area and occlusal load between the implant side molar region and contralateral side molar region

## Study methods

### *Examination of occlusal contact*

Materials such as wax, occlusal registration paper, and pressure-sensitive paper are used to examine occlusal contact. The present study utilized an examination method using silicone [11, 12, 16]. The Blue Silicone used in the present study is a cartridge type, which allows a nearly constant mixing ratio to be maintained, it has low viscosity and thus flows well, and it shows little dimensional change over time. It therefore fully met the requirements for a material for registration of occlusal contact status.

A prior study reported low reproducibility when using Dental Prescale at low clenching strength [22]. In addition, the use of Blue Silicone to take impressions at high clenching intensities of 80 and 100 % MVC places a burden on subjects, as Blue Silicone takes a long time to harden. For these reasons, when measurements from low to high clenching strength were made in the present study, Blue Silicone was used at clenching intensities of 20, 40, and 60 % MVC, and Dental Prescale was used at 40, 60, 80, and 100 % MVC.

**Table 4** Two-way ANOVA of the occlusal contact area of the implant side molar region and contralateral side molar region

| | Source | Sum of square | *df* | Mean square | *F* value | *P* value |
|---|---|---|---|---|---|---|
| Occluzer | Implant side and contralateral side | 24.453 | 1 | 24.453 | 2.334 | 0.165 |
| | MVC | 159.749 | 3 | 53.253 | 26.918 | 0.000 |
| | Interaction | 16.135 | 3 | 5.378 | 3.786 | 0.024 |
| BiteEye | Implant side and contralateral side | 51.431 | 1 | 51.431 | 3.674 | 0.092 |
| | MVC | 32.471 | 2 | 16.236 | 8.125 | 0.004 |
| | Interaction | 0.236 | 2 | 0.118 | 0.072 | 0.931 |

### *Measurement of occlusal load*

Occlusal load was measured with Dental Prescale and analyzed with Occluzer. The Dental Prescale system allows occlusal contact pressure to be measured quickly and easily across the dentition, and it is of enormous clinical utility because its accuracy and reproducibility in the molar region have been confirmed [16, 20, 22]. The technique using this sequence and also the method of cross-checking occlusal contact points using silicone and Dental Prescale are clinically useful and have been widely studied and reported [16, 20].

## Comparison of occlusal contact areas evaluated using Occluzer and BiteEye

Blue Silicone with a thickness of 10 μm and Dental Prescale gave similar values for the occlusal contact area at 40 and 60 % MVC. These results probably have more validity than those reported by Imamura et al. [12].

**Table 5** Two-way ANOVA of occlusal load of the implant side molar region and contralateral side molar region

| Source | Sum of square | *df* | Mean square | *F* value | *P* value |
|---|---|---|---|---|---|
| Implant side and contralateral side | 8578.099 | 1 | 8578.099 | 1.354 | 0.278 |
| MVC | 193,888.518 | 3 | 64,629.506 | 36.593 | 0.000 |
| Interaction | 30,575.358 | 3 | 4016.245 | 3.153 | 0.430 |

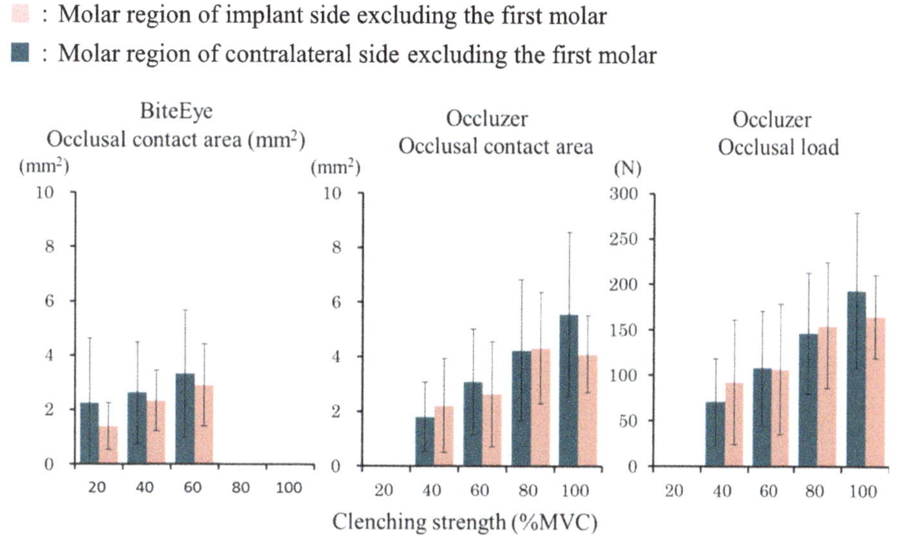


**Fig. 4** Comparison of the first molar-eliminated occlusal contact area and load between the implant side molar region and contralateral side molar region

## Analysis of implant region

### *Occlusal load on implant region*

An occlusal load of approximately 130 N on the first molar has been reported at maximum clenching strength in healthy, dentulous subjects [18]. In the present study, occlusal load on the mandibular first molar was somewhat less, at 81.2 ± 41.1 N. However, bearing in mind that the subjects in the prior study were in their 20 s whereas those in the present study were of middle to old age, with a mean age of 49 years, the present results are probably somewhat valid. Implant prostheses probably have greater occlusal load than natural teeth at higher clenching intensities because they lack the mechanical buffering function of the periodontal membrane. A study using two-dimensional finite element analysis on the mandibular first molar by Maezawa et al. [9] suggests that even if the occlusal surface of the prosthesis is made lower than the occlusal plane, the implant area may still be subjected to excess occlusal load with increased clenching strength.

In the present study, however, the occlusal load on the implant prosthesis tended not to increase as much as the load on the contralateral tooth when the clenching strength was higher. A possible reason is that the dentists adjusted the implant prostheses with pressure displacement in mind, giving a smaller occlusal contact area so that there were fewer loading points than in the contralateral tooth [4, 21, 22].

When considering the balance of occlusal load in the molar region, it is better to give the same occlusal load on both molar regions at 100 % MVC [12, 16]. However, in this study, the occlusal load was significantly smaller on the implant prosthesis than on the contralateral tooth at 100 % MVC.

### *Measurement of occlusal contact area of implant prosthesis*

Dental Prescale has a thickness of approximately 100 μm, whereas Blue Silicone has less thickness and is therefore likely to give more accurate measurements of the occlusal contact area [12, 23]. In addition, when the occlusal contact areas of implant prostheses and their contralateral

**Table 6** Two-way ANOVA of the occlusal contact area of the implant side molar region and contralateral side molar region excluding the first molar

| | Source | Sum of square | *df* | Mean square | *F* value | *P* value |
|---|---|---|---|---|---|---|
| Occluzer | Implant side and contralateral side | 2.177 | 1 | 2.177 | 0.383 | 0.165 |
| | MVC | 90.753 | 3 | 30.251 | 25.800 | 0.553 |
| | Interaction | 9.011 | 3 | 3.004 | 2.209 | 0.113 |
| BiteEye | Implant side and contralateral side | 3.527 | 1 | 3.527 | 0.789 | 0.400 |
| | MVC | 15.013 | 2 | 7.541 | 10.636 | 0.001 |
| | Interaction | 0.790 | 2 | 0.395 | 0.661 | 0.530 |

**Table 7** Two-way ANOVA of occlusal load of the implant side molar region and contralateral side molar region excluding the first molar

| Source | Sum of square | *df* | Mean square | *F* value | *P* value |
|---|---|---|---|---|---|
| Implant side and contralateral side | 0.690 | 1 | 0.690 | 0.000 | 0.990 |
| MVC | 102,482.810 | 3 | 34,160.937 | 30.344 | 0.000 |
| Interaction | 6049.786 | 3 | 2016.595 | 1.336 | 0.286 |

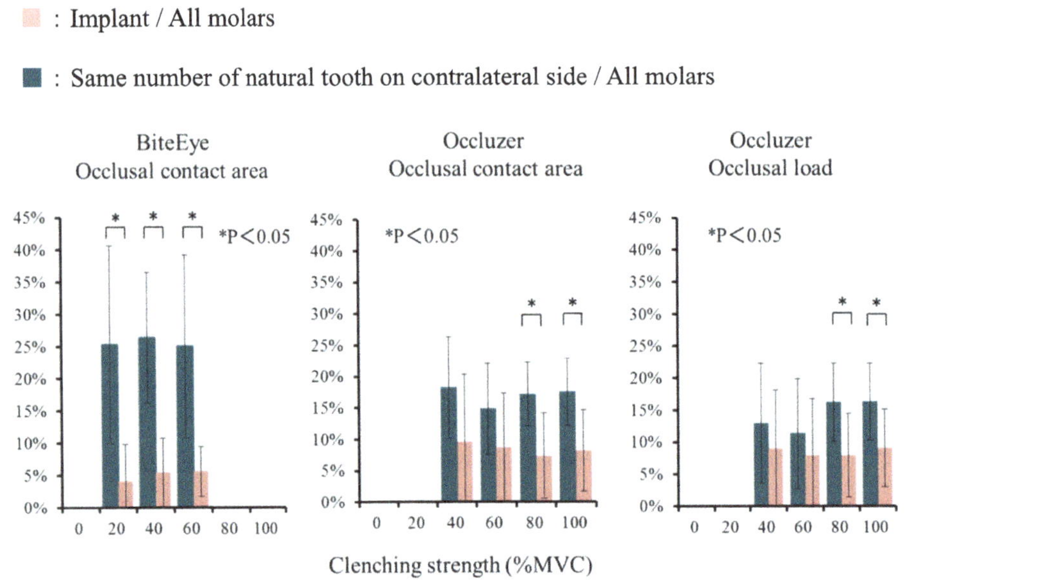


**Fig. 5** Proportion of the occlusal contact area and occlusal load of the whole molar region accounted for by the implant prosthesis and by the contralateral tooth

teeth were compared, the occlusal contact area of the contralateral teeth was significantly greater at higher clenching strength. This is probably because occlusion between natural teeth results in greater displacement due to the presence of a periodontal membrane on both teeth. In addition, Koyama et al. [10] reported no significant differences between the molar region on the implant side and on the contralateral side, even when clenching strength varied. Similarly, when clenching strength varied in this study, the occlusal contact area of the implant prosthesis did not increase than the contralateral tooth.

**Table 8** Two-way ANOVA of the proportion of occlusal load and contact area for implants and first molars based on molar area

| | | Source | Sum of square | *df* | Mean square | *F* value | *P* value |
|---|---|---|---|---|---|---|---|
| Occlusal load | | | | | | | |
| | Occluzer | Implant or natural tooth | 585.390 | 1 | 585.390 | 9.870 | 0.014 |
| | | MVC | 53.901 | 3 | 53.901 | 1.768 | 0.220 |
| | | Interaction | 46.872 | 3 | 46.872 | 3.791 | 0.870 |
| Occlusal contact area | | | | | | | |
| | Occluzer | Implant or natural tooth | 0.087 | 1 | 0.087 | 11.101 | 0.010 |
| | | MVC | 0.003 | 3 | 0.003 | 1.202 | 0.305 |
| | | Interaction | 0.004 | 3 | 0.004 | 2.178 | 0.178 |
| | BiteEye | Implant or natural tooth | 0.291 | 1 | 0.291 | 12.210 | 0.008 |
| | | MVC | 0.040 | 2 | 0.040 | 1.287 | 0.290 |
| | | Interaction | 0.000 | 2 | 0.000 | 0.070 | 0.798 |

#### *Comparison of proportion of occlusal contact area and occlusal load in all teeth accounted for by prosthetic implant and contralateral tooth*

The proportion of occlusal force on the molar region of healthy dentition accounted for by the mandibular first molar on one side has previously been reported as 16 % [20]. In the present study, however, the implant prosthesis accounted for a lower proportion of 9 % of the occlusal force on the molar region. No significant differences in occlusal load were observed between sides, but the proportion of occlusal load on all teeth borne by the implant prosthesis was less than that borne by the contralateral tooth. However, there was no significant difference in occlusal load between both molar regions. It suggested that occlusal loading on both molar regions have been balanced.

### Future research

The present study examined implant prostheses immediately after setting, but the occlusal contact of implant prostheses is believed to change over time as a result of factors such as extrusion of opposing teeth, abrasion from neighboring surfaces, and tooth attrition. In the future, we intend to use the results of the present study to carry out a prospective study that will survey the period of 1 year from immediately after setting, which is when problems are most common. This future study will have a greater number of subjects and will evaluate parameters such as mastication function. This study will aim to clarify how the occlusal contact of the implant prosthesis changes within the dentition and to draw up guidelines on this basis.

## Conclusions

The results suggest that the occlusal contact of implant prostheses can be evaluated from low to high clenching intensities using Blue Silicone and Dental Prescale. There was a trend for implant prostheses to be adjusted such that immediately after setting the occlusal contact area, the occlusal load of the implant superstructure was less than that of the contralateral tooth. This is likely to be due to dentists taking into account the small tissue displaceability of implants.

The occlusal load on implant prostheses in a single intermediary mandibular first molar deficit tended to increase less with clenching strength than the load on the contralateral tooth. In addition, the proportion of the occlusal load on the whole dentition accounted for by the implant prosthesis was less than the proportion accounted for by the contralateral tooth. However, there was no significant difference in occlusal load between both molar regions. It suggested that occlusal loading on both molar regions has been balanced. The adequate occlusion on implant prosthesis has not been clear. However, we will be able to obtain clinical suggestions for the occlusion that should be given to prosthetic implants through a longitudinal follow-up study.

### Abbreviations

MVC: maximum voluntary contraction; Prescale: Dental Prescale 50H type R; Occluzer: Occluzer FPD707; BiteEye: BiteEye-I; ANOVA: analysis of variance.

### Competing interests

Yukihiko Okada, Yuji Sato, Noboru Kitagawa, Keiichiro Uchida, Tokiko Osawa, Yoshiki Imamura, and Mayumi Terazawa declare that they have no competing interests.

### Authors' contributions

YO drafted the manuscript. YS contributed advice regarding the manuscript. NK, KU, TO, YI, and MT checked and improved the manuscript. All authors read and approved the final manuscript.

### Acknowledgements

The authors would like to express their deep appreciation to the staff of Implant Center at Showa University Dental Hospital for their help and cooperation. This study was supported by a Grant-in-Aid for Scientific Research from the Ministry of Education, Culture, Science, and Technology (Showa University Grant-in-Aid for Scientific Research (C)) (Grant Number 25463016). A partial summary of this thesis was presented at the 44th Annual Meeting of the Japanese Society of Oral Implantology in Tokyo, Japan in September 2014.

### References

1. Hobo S, Hosoyama H. Occlusion for implant. Tokyo: Quintessence; 2006. p. 89–95 [in Japanese].
2. Schulte W. Implants and the periodontium. Int Dent J. 1995;45:16–26.
3. Miura H. Occlusal function and periodontal tissue. J Stomatol Soc Jpn. 2000;67:1–10 [in Japanese].
4. Morikawa O. Influence of occlusal contacts of implant on adjacent teeth and antagonists displacements. J Stomatol Soc Jpn. 2003;70:224–33 [in Japanese].
5. DARIO LJ. How occlusal forces change in implant patients: a clinical research report. J Am Dent Assoc. 1995;126:1130–3.
6. RANGERT BR, SULIIVAN RM, JEMET TM. Load factor control for implants in the posterior partially edentulous segment. Int J Oral Maxillofac Implnts. 1997;12:360–70.
7. Kim Y, Oh TJ, Misch CE, Wang HL. Occlusal considerations in implant therapy: clinical guidelines with biomechanical rationale. Clin Oral Implants Res. 2005;16:26–35.
8. Doi N, Inoue M, Inai T, Watanabe M, Sasaki K. Occlusal force on the dental arch in patients with dental implants at the free-end edentulous area. J Japanese Soc Oral Implantol. 2006;19:466–77.
9. Maezawa N, Wakabayashi N, Yokoyama S, Shiota M, Suzuki T. Influence of intensity of occlusal contact in implant-retained single restoration on stress distributions of crown surface and supporting bone. J Japan Prosthodontic Soc. 2007;51:582–91 [in Japanese].
10. Koyama K, Kusumoto T, Kawazoe T. Occlusal contacts in intercuspal position of prostheses without stress absorbing elements on osseointegrated implants. J Japanese Soc Oral Implantol. 2005;18:563–71.
11. Okuyama T, Sato Y, Ozawa K, Kitagawa N, Uchida K. Occlusion of prostheses supported by an implant for a single intermediate missing posterior tooth with satisfactory prognosis. J Japanese Soc Oral Implantol. 2010;23:209–19 [in Japanese].
12. Imamura Y, Sato Y, Kitagawa N, Uchida K, Osawa T, Omori M, Okada Y. Influence of occlusal loading force on occlusal contacts in natural dentition. J Prosthodont Res. 2015;59:113–120.
13. Kohno S, Shiva H, Nakano M, Furuya R, Mayanagi A, Minagi S, Kobayashi H. A guideline of three dentistry area disorders. J Japan Prosthodontic Soc. 2002;46:577–627 [in Japanese].
14. Smith DE, Zarb GA. Criteria for success of osseointegrated endosseous implant. J Prosthet Dent. 1989;62:567–72.
15. Albrektsson R, Zarb GA. Current interpretations of the osseointegrated response: clinical significance. Int J Prosthodont. 1993;6:95–105.
16. Daizo O. Teeth displacements and occlusal contacts depending on clenching force. J Jpn Prosthodont Soc. 1998;42:1013–23.
17. Kurosawa M. Studies on human biting force gender differences and lateral dominance with development and growth. J Japanese Academy Occlusion Health. 2002;8:8–16 [in Japanese].
18. Tanaka M, Johnston EL. The prediction of the size of unerupted canines and premolars in a contemporary orthodontic population. J Am Dent Assoc. 1974;88:798–801.
19. Hidaka O, Iwasaki M, Saito M. Influence of clenching intensity on bite pressure. J Dent Res. 1999;78:1336–44.
20. Hattori Y, Satoh C, Watanabe M. Bite force distribution on dental arch during clenching. J Japanese Soc Stomatognathic Function. 1996;2:111–17 [in Japanese].
21. Suzuki T, Kumagai H, Yoshitomi N. Clinical evaluation of measuring system of occlusal force. J Stomatol Soc Jpn. 1994;61:437–45 [in Japanese].
22. Yamaguchi T, Hisatsune Y, Kimura T. Examination of occlusal contacts by using "Dental Prescale" special reference to the rate of detected occlusal contacts in the intercuspal position. J Prosthodont Res. 1995;39:1113–20 [in Japanese].
23. Baba K, Tsukiyama Y, Clark GT. Reliability, validity, and utility of various occlusal measurement methods and techniques. J Prosthet Dent. 2000;83:83–9.

# 16

# The relationship between the bone characters obtained by CBCT and primary stability of the implants

Masahiro Wada*, Yasutane Tsuiki, Tohru Suganami, Kazunori Ikebe, Motofumi Sogo, Ikuhisa Okuno and Yoshinobu Maeda

**Abstract**

**Background:** The aim of this study is to investigate the correlation between the thickness of the cortical bone or the voxel values that are obtained by cone beam CT (CBCT) and the insertion torque values (ITVs) or the implant stability quotient (ISQ) values.

**Methods:** A pig's ilium was used as the implant placement site. The implants used in this study were two kinds of diameters (3.8 mm, 5.0 mm) and two kinds of lengths (7.0 mm, 12.0 mm) having a general threadlike shape with a mechanically polished surface. To measure the bone density and the cortical thickness around the implants accurately, the CBCT scanning was performed immediately just after the formation of the implant cavity. The initial stabilities were evaluated by the ITVs and the ISQ values. The bone density and cortical thickness around the implants were measured by an implant simulation software (Landmarker ver. 5.0 with special specifications for this study). The relationships of the thickness of the cortical bone and the voxel values with the ITVs and the ISQ values were analyzed using Pearson's correlation coefficient. To evaluate the influence on the ITVs and the ISQ values among multiple factors, multiple regression analysis was performed. $P < 0.05$ was considered statistically significant.

**Results:** A significant positive correlation was found between the thickness of the cortical bone and the ITVs or the ISQ values in all kinds of implants. In addition, a significant positive correlation was also found between the voxel values and the ITVs. From the multiple regression analysis, the thickness of the cortical bone and the voxel values had a positive influence on the ITVs and the ISQ values. In addition, the length of the implant had a positive influence on the ISQ values at the 3.8-mm-diameter implant.

**Conclusions:** In this limited study, there were correlations between the thickness of the cortical bone or the voxel values obtained from the CBCT scanning and the implant stabilities. Besides, it was confirmed that the thickness of the cortical bone, the voxel value, and the implant length had positive correlations with the ITVs and the ISQ values.

**Keywords:** Primary stability; CBCT; Voxel value

## Background

The primary stability of an implant at the time of placement is considered as one of the key factors for clinical success of implant treatment [1-6]. Orenstein et al. reported that implants that were appropriately stabilized without any mobility at the time of placement had a significantly high survival rate compared with those that were not [7].

The evaluation of the primary implant stability is usually performed after placement. Some of the main methods include mobility test, resonance frequency analysis, and the measurements of the removal torque values and the insertion torque values (ITVs). In particular, the measurement of the removal torque values is an objective evaluation method, but its clinical application is difficult because it is an irreversible and invasive method. Mobility test is useful for the evaluation of an implant whose osseointegration was surely obtained, but there is a possibility that the primary stability could decrease by the impact of the tapping head. On the other

* Correspondence: masahiro@dent.osaka-u.ac.jp
Department of Prosthodontics, Gerodontology and Oral Rehabilitation, Osaka University Graduate School of Dentistry, 1-8 Yamadaoka, Suita, Osaka 565-0871, Japan

hand, the measurement of ITVs and the measurement of implant stability quotient (ISQ) values by using a resonance frequency analyzer are non-invasive, convenient, and objective evaluation methods. Therefore, these methods are used for evaluation in various researches investigating the primary stability including immediate loading implants [8-11].

The primary stability is significantly affected by bone quality. Herrmann conducted a study of the prognosis for as long as more than 5 years and reported that poor bone quality and quantity had a major impact on the long-term failure rate of implants [12]. Jaffin observed the prognosis of implants for 5 years after providing the final restoration [13]. As a result, the failure rate of the implants was 3% when the implant was placed in the alveolar bone having a thick cortical bone or otherwise a dense spongy bone even if the cortical bone was thin, whereas it was 35% when the implant was placed in the alveolar bone having both a thin cortical bone and a sparse spongy bone.

Some of the methods to evaluate the bone quality that influences the primary implant stability have already been applied in a clinical practice. Lekholm and Zarb classified bone density into four types in terms of radiography, with the thickness of the cortical bone and the density of the spongy bone as the indexes [14]. This classification method is accepted most commonly at present but is problematic with accuracy and reproducibility because it is a subjective evaluation. On the other hand, Misch classified CT values (Hounsfield unit) into five steps (D1: >1,250 HU; D2: 850 to 1,250 HU; D3: 350 to 850 HU; D4: 150 to 350 HU; D5: <150 HU) to evaluate the bone quality [15]. The CT value is the value obtained by multi-detector CT (MDCT) and is defined as the relative value of the X-ray attenuation coefficient of the object for water, with the X-ray attenuation by water defined as zero. Today, this classification has been used for the evaluation of the bone quality because it is an objective method compared with that of Lekholm and Zarb.

Turkyilmaz et al. placed 24 implants in human dry bones and calculated CT values using MDCT images before surgery to examine correlations with the ITVs and the ISQ values [16]. They reported that there were significant correlations of CT values with both ITVs and ISQ values and that bone density (CT value) was one of the factors that had an influence on the primary implant stability.

In recent years, cone beam CT (CBCT) has been used for preoperative diagnosis in implant treatment. CBCT is superior for its high definition, reduction of the exposure dose, low cost, and usability compared with MDCT [17-21]. However, CBCT does not have a linear relationship compared with the CT values obtained by MDCT, and therefore, it is considered difficult to evaluate bone density quantitatively [22-24]. The major causes arise from the lack of calibration of X-rays, the localized imaging area that allows various external anatomical structures, and too many scattered radiations.

It is therefore considered that MDCT is appropriate for the precise evaluation of bone density. However, since the use of CBCT is spreading rapidly among general practitioners, it is clinically of great significance to predict the primary stability after implant placement using the information obtained by CBCT. In addition, in late years, CBCT or the calibration software which can convert the voxel values into CT values is developed.

We therefore investigated in this study the correlation between the thickness of the cortical bone or the voxel values that are obtained by CBCT and the ITVs or the ISQ values.

## Methods

### Bone models

A flat part of a pig's ilium was used as the implant placement site to secure as vertical implant placement and an equal depth of insertion to the bone surface as possible (Figure 1).

### CBCT scan

GXCB-500® (GENDEX, Des Plaines, IL, USA) was used as the CBCT device to obtain almost identical voxel values to the CT values that could be obtained from MDCT. Scanning conditions were as follows: the tube current, 5 mA; the tube voltage, 120 kV; the field of view (FOV), 85-mm diameter to secure a complete size for

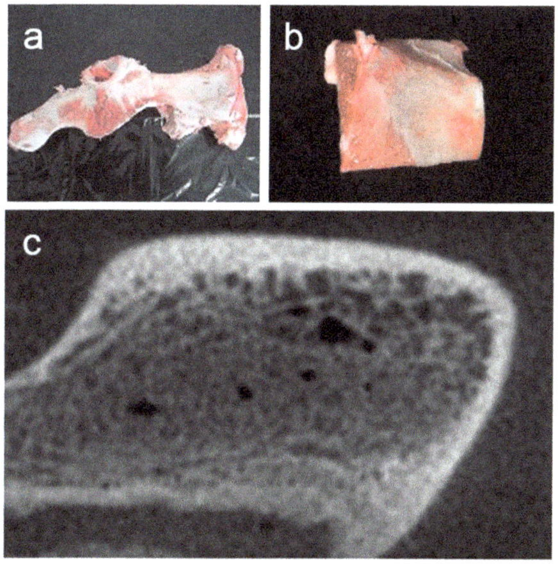


**Figure 1 The bone model in this study (a pig's ilium). (a)** The whole picture of the ilium. **(b)** The flat part of the posterior margin of the ilium. **(c)** The CT image of the ilium.

scanning; and the voxel size, 0.1 $mm^3$. In addition, the scanning was performed by immersing the samples in a polypropylene container with water in it to create as similar scanning environment as possible to the one that had soft tissues around the bone model. Of note, the scanning was performed immediately just after the formation of the implant cavity to accurately measure the voxel values around the inserted implants.

#### Implants

External Hex Implants for laboratory use (SETiO®, GC Company, Tokyo, Japan) having a general threadlike shape with a mechanically polished surface were used. They were two kinds of diameters (3.8 mm, 5.0 mm) and two kinds of lengths (7.0 mm, 12.0 mm) consisting a total of four groups, and 25 pieces of implants were used in each group (Figure 2).

#### Formation of the implant cavities

When forming an implant cavity, it is necessary to move the drill back and forth along the insertion direction. This process is usually done by an operator with freehand, but it is likely to cause unevenness in the diameter of the implant cavity. Therefore, an implant cavity-forming device was used to prevent this in our experiment (Figure 3). This device is able to adjust the up-and-down movement speed and the rotation speed of the drill. In this study, the implant cavity was constructed at a moving speed of 5 mm/s that was close to the actual up-and-down movement speed obtained from the preliminary experiment and at 800 rpm according to the manufacturer's protocol. It was also confirmed in the preliminary experiment that using this device would significantly reduce the unevenness of the diameter of the implant cavity.

All the procedures of forming an implant cavity were unified as follows according to protocols. Firstly, the implant cavity was constructed by using a 2.0-mm-depth drill after marking the implant site using a guide drill. Secondly, a 3.1-mm pilot drill and a 3.1-mm twist drill were used to form a cavity for an implant with 3.8-mm diameter, and a 4.3-mm pilot drill and a 4.3-mm twist drill were used to form a cavity for an implant with 5.0-mm diameter. Of note, this experiment was performed under a non-irrigation environment because the rise of temperature would not be problematic.

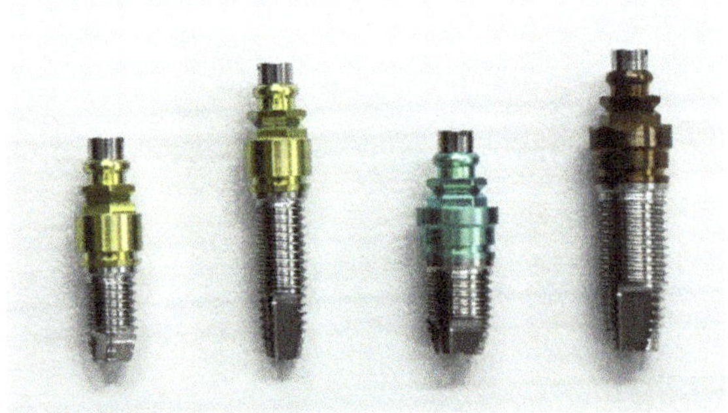

**Figure 2 The implants in this study.** Two kinds of diameters (3.8 mm, 5.0 mm) and two kinds of lengths (7.0 mm, 12.0 mm) having a general threadlike shape with a mechanically polished surface.

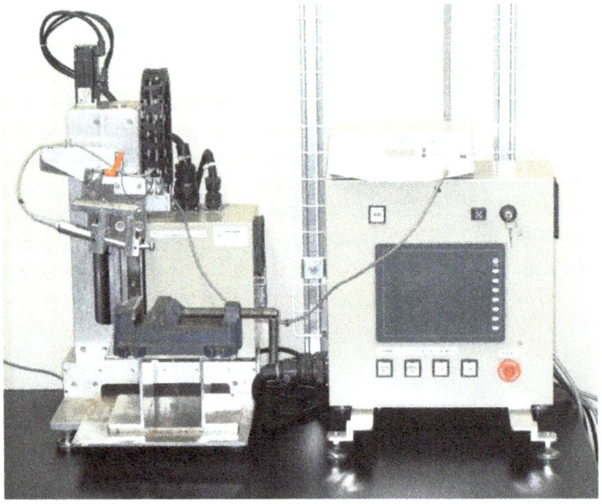

**Figure 3 The special implant cavity-forming device.** This device is able to adjust the up-and-down movement speed and the rotation speed of the drill.

#### Placement of an implant and the measurement of the implant stabilities

Handy Type Torque Meter (HTG2-200NC, IMADA-SS Corp, Aichi, Japan) was used for the placement of an implant, and the maximum torque values were measured. The specifications of the Handy Type Torque Meter were as follows: the measurement unit, Ncm; the accuracy, within ±0.5% FS; the measurement maximum torque, 200 Ncm; and the minimum resolution function, 0.1 Ncm. Thus, the device had enough coverage of the torque measurement in this study (96.0 Ncm at maximum).

Osstell Mentor® (Integration Diagnostics AB, Gôteborg, Sweden) was used as a resonance frequency analysis device to measure the ISQ values. The accompanying smart peg (type 1) was attached to the implant for the measurement at every 90°, and the average value was calculated.

#### Measurement of the voxel values and the thickness of the cortical bone around implants

An implant simulation software (Landmarker ver. 5.0 with special specifications for study purposes, iCAT, Osaka, Japan) was used for analysis. The evaluation site was selected on the smallest area that was as adjacent to the implant as possible so as not to include the area that was immune to the primary stability. Specifically, the width of the measurement site was defined as 0.50 mm, i.e., from 0.25 mm inside (the to-be-compressed area at the time of placement) to 0.25 mm outside of the virtual implant. The area adjacent to the bottom of the implant was excluded from the measurement site because the maximum torque value and the ISQ value were both subject to the lateral force a great deal (Figures 4 and 5). Then, the voxel values of the measurement site were extracted into the comma-separated values (CSV) files. Subsequently, the average of the voxel values of the measurement site was calculated and defined as the voxel value of the whole bone around the implant. Additionally, the average of the voxel values was calculated at every 0.1-mm depth from the surface of the bone to determine the thickness of the cortical bone from the voxel values. The threshold of the voxel value for the border of the cortical bone and the spongy bone was decided to be 350, which had a strong correlation (Pearson's correlation coefficient, 0.897) with the actual measurement in the preliminary examination.

### Statistical analysis

The relationships of the thickness of the cortical bone and the voxel values with the ITVs and the ISQ values were analyzed using Pearson's correlation coefficient. Then, multiple regression analysis was performed using the ITVs or the ISQ values as the dependent variable and using the thickness of the cortical bone, the voxel value, and the length of the implant as the independent variables to evaluate the influence on the ITVs and the ISQ values among multiple factors. The statistical analyses were performed using the SPSS ver. 22 software (SPSS Co., Chicago, IL, USA). $P < 0.05$ was considered statistically significant.

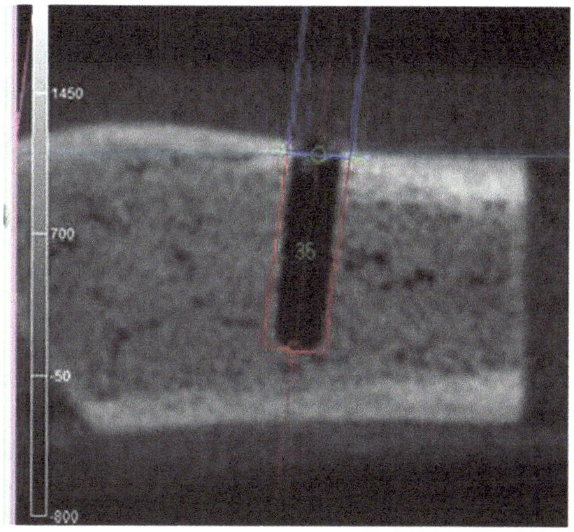


**Figure 4 Setting the evaluation site.** An implant placement simulation software (Osaka Landmarker ver. 5.0 with special specifications for study purposes, iCAT, Osaka, Japan) was used as the image analysis software. The virtual implant was placed in the implant cavity by simulation.

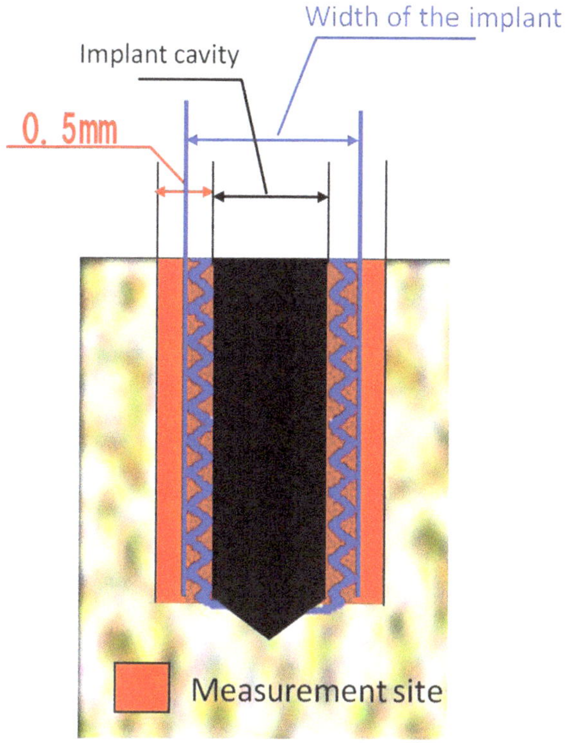


**Figure 5 Measurement site of the voxel values.** The width of the measurement site was defined as 0.50 mm, i.e., from 0.25 mm inside (the to-be-compressed area at the time of placement) to 0.25 mm outside (the same width of the aforementioned) of the virtual implant.

## Results

### Relationship between the thickness of the cortical bone and voxel values with implant stabilities

A significant positive correlation was found between the thickness of the cortical bone and ITVs or ISQ values in all kinds of implants. In addition, a significant positive correlation was also found between the voxel values and ITVs. On the other hand, in the relationship between the voxel values and ISQ values, we cannot confirm a correlation of the implant of 5.0 mm in width and 12.0 mm in length (Table 1).

### Influence of the implant of 3.8 mm in width on the ITVs and the ISQ values of each factor

Multiple regression analysis was performed using the ITVs or the ISQ values as the dependent variable and using the thickness of the cortical bone, the voxel value, and the length of the implant as the independent variables. The standardized partial regression coefficients of the thickness of the cortical bone and the voxel value were 0.400 and 0.459, respectively, which turned out to be significant explanatory variables. However, that of the

**Table 1 Correlation between bone factors and stability factors**

| Bone factors/stability factors | Diameter (mm) | Length (mm) | *r* | *P* | *n* |
|---|---|---|---|---|---|
| Thickness of the cortical bone/ITVs | 3.8 | 7 | 0.744** | <0.001 | 24 |
| | | 12 | 0.560** | 0.005 | 23 |
| | 5 | 7 | 0.815** | <0.001 | 25 |
| | | 12 | 0.760** | <0.001 | 24 |
| Thickness of the cortical bone/ISQ | 3.8 | 7 | 0.831** | <0.001 | 24 |
| | | 12 | 0.409 | 0.052 | 23 |
| | 5 | 7 | 0.707** | <0.001 | 25 |
| | | 12 | 0.426* | 0.038 | 24 |
| Voxel values/ITVs | 3.8 | 7 | 0.601** | 0.002 | 24 |
| | | 12 | 0.745** | <0.001 | 23 |
| | 5 | 7 | 0.850** | <0.001 | 25 |
| | | 12 | 0.667** | <0.001 | 24 |
| Voxel values/ISQ | 3.8 | 7 | 0.684** | <0.001 | 24 |
| | | 12 | 0.447* | 0.032 | 23 |
| | 5 | 7 | 0.695** | <0.001 | 25 |
| | | 12 | 0.270 | 0.202 | 24 |

ITVs, insertion torque values. $^{**}P < 0.01$; $^{*}P < 0.05$.

length of the implant did not become an explanatory variable. When using the ISQ values as the independent variable, the standardized partial regression coefficients of the thickness of the cortical bone, the voxel value, and the length of the implant were 0.326, 0.304, and 0.420, respectively, all of which became significant explanatory variables. From these results, it was confirmed that the thickness of the cortical bone and the voxel values had a positive influence on ITVs, while the thickness of the cortical bone, the voxel value, and the length of the implant had a positive influence on the ISQ values (Table 2).

**Table 2 Statistical analysis of the results of the multiple regression analysis of the 3.8-mm-width implant**

| | |
|---|---|
| Dependent variable = ITVs | ($n = 47$) |
| Independent variables | Standardized partial regression coefficient (*P* value) |
| Thickness of the cortical bone | 0.400 (=0.02) |
| Voxel value | 0.459 (<0.01) |
| Length of the implant | 0.005 (=0.97) |
| | $R^2 = 0.633$ |
| Dependent variable = ISQ values | ($n = 47$) |
| Independent variables | Standardized partial regression coefficient (*P* value) |
| Thickness of the cortical bone | 0.326 (=0.04) |
| Voxel value | 0.304 (<0.01) |
| Length of the implant | 0.420 (<0.01) |
| | $R^2 = 0.593$ |

#### Influence of each factor of the implant of 5.0 mm in width on ITVs and the ISQ values

The standardized partial regression coefficients of ITVs for the thickness of the cortical bone and the length of the implant were 0.408 and 0.526, respectively, which became significant explanatory variables. In addition, those of the ISQ values for the thickness of the cortical bone and the length of the implant were 0.440 and 0.750, respectively, which also became significant explanatory variables. From these results, it was confirmed that the thickness of the cortical bone and the length of the implant had a positive influence on ITVs and the ISQ values. However, the voxel value of ITVs and that of the ISQ values failed to become explanatory variables (Table 3).

## Discussion

### Measurement of the cortical bone thickness and the voxel values

Ikumi used a MDCT scan for actual patients to calculate the CT values of the 1-mm surrounding area of the planned implant placement site using implant simulation software [25]. However, it is likely that the precise measurement cannot be performed in the case where the actual implant cavity was formed off the planned implant site because the density of the bone around the planned implant site was evaluated by preoperative simulation.

Therefore, we evaluated the bone quality 0.5 mm surrounding the implant, which was thought to have a strong effect on the primary stabilities, by CBCT scanning after forming the implant cavities.

**Table 3 Statistical analysis of the results of the multiple regression analysis of the 5.0-mm-width implant**

| | |
|---|---|
| Dependent variable = ITVs | ($n$ = 49) |
| Independent variables | Standardized partial regression coefficient ($P$ value) |
| Thickness of the cortical bone | 0.408 (=0.04) |
| Voxel value | 0.365 (=0.10) |
| Length of the implant | 0.526 (<0.01) |
| | $R^2$ = 0.638 |
| Dependent variable = ISQ values | ($n$ = 49) |
| Independent variables | Standardized partial regression coefficient ($P$ value) |
| Thickness of the cortical bone | 0.440 (=0.02) |
| Voxel value | −0.060 (=0.98) |
| Length of the implant | 0.750 (<0.01) |
| | $R^2$ = 0.836 |

Nkenke used an axial image to define the thickness of the cortical bone from the average thickness of the cortical bone around the implant measured by eye estimation and then evaluated its relationship with ITVs [26]. Whereas in this study, we measured the thickness of the cortical bone by setting the threshold for the voxel values around the implant for the purpose of securing reproducibility of the measurement of the thickness of the cortical bone. The threshold that we set was determined in the preliminary experiment so that it would highly correlate with the measurement values of the thickness of the cortical bone measured by eye estimation. Conversely, the limitation of this study is that the CBCT device is lacking some precision for estimation of bone density compared to quantitative computed tomography.

### Relationship between the thickness of the cortical bone and the voxel values measured by CBCT and the primary stability of the implant

To date, there are several studies that investigated the relationship between the thickness of the cortical bone and the primary stability of the implant. Motoyoshi placed a total of 87 mini-implants, which were used as anchors for orthodontic treatment, in the buccal alveolar bone in the molar region of actual patients [27]. As a result, they reported that they found a positive significant correlation between the thickness of the cortical bone measured by using medical CT images and the torque value at the time of placement. Roze measured the thickness of the cortical bone of the jawbones in three human bodies using μCT and placed a total of 22 implants [28]. According to this report, there was a significant correlation between the thickness of the cortical bone and the ISQ values measured immediately after the implant placement. Furthermore, Isoda reported a significant correlation between the bone quality around the implants and the implant stabilities.

Although this study is different from the previous studies in that the thickness of the cortical bone and bone density were determined from the voxel values calculated by CBCT, a significantly positive correlation of the thickness of the cortical bone and the voxel values with ITVs and ISQ values was confirmed as in the previous studies. Furthermore, the multiple regression analysis with the ITVs and the ISQ values as the dependent variables showed that the thickness of the cortical bone as well as the voxel values had a positive influence.

Based on these results, it was revealed that the thickness of the cortical bone obtained from CBCT had a correlation with the ITVs and the ISQ values which are the indexes of the primary stability of the implant. It was also revealed that the voxel values correlated with ITVs and ISQ values. It is desirable to be able to infer the primary stability at the time of implant placement not only from the thickness of the cortical bone but also from the voxel values, if the cortical bone cannot be observed on the CT images of the extraction socket immediately after or at a certain period of time after the tooth extraction (until the maturation of the bone). Conversely, there was no statistical correlation between the voxel values and ISQ values among 5-mm-diameter, 12-mm-length implants. These ISQ values were high enough regardless of bone densities, and this caused that the correlation did not confirm between voxel values and ISQ values.

In addition, these results were confirmed by using mechanically polished surface implants. Therefore, it is thought that primary stability becomes more stable by using rough-surface implants.

## Conclusions

In this limited study, there was a correlation between the thickness of the cortical bone or the voxel values obtained from the CBCT scanning images prior to the implant placement and the implant stabilities. Besides, it was confirmed that the thickness of the cortical bone, the voxel value, and the length of the implant had positive correlations with the ITVs and that the thickness and length had positive correlations with the ISQ values.

#### Competing interests

Masahiro Wada, Yasutane Tsuiki, Tohru Suganami, Kazunori Ikebe, Motofumi Sogo, Ikuhisa Okuno and Yoshinobu Maeda declare that they have no competing interests.

#### Authors' contributions

MW drafted the article and collected the data. YT and TS collected the data. KI performed the data analysis and statistical analysis. MS interpreted the data. IO analyzed the data. YM designed the research and approved the article. All authors read and approved the final manuscript.

#### Acknowledgements

This study was partially supported by GC Company.

**References**

1. Ottoni JM, Oliveira ZF, Mansini R, Cabral AM. Correlation between placement torque and survival of single-tooth implants. *Int J Oral Maxillofac Implants.* 2005; **20**:769–76.
2. Beer A, Gahleitner A, Holm A, Tschabitscher M, Homolka P. Correlation of insertion torques with bone mineral density from dental quantitative CT in the mandible. *Clin Oral Implants Res.* 2003; **14(5)**:616–20.
3. Meredith N. Assessment of implant stability as a prognostic determinant. *Int J Prosthodont.* 1998; **11(5)**:491–501.
4. Martinez H1, Davarpanah M, Missika P, Celletti R, Lazzara R. Optimal implant stabilization in low density bone. *Clin Oral Implants Res.* 2001; **12(5)**:423–32.
5. Lioubavina-Hack N, Lang NP, Karring T. Significance of primary stability for osseointegration of dental implants. *Clin Oral Implants Res.* 2006; **17(3)**:244–50.
6. Molly L. Bone density and primary stability in implant therapy. *Clin Oral Implants Res.* 2006; **17(Suppl 2)**:124–35.
7. Orenstein IH, Tarnow DP, Morris HF. Three-year post-placement survival of implants mobile at placement. *Ann Periodontol.* 2000; **5**:32–41.
8. Turkyilmaz I, Company AM. Sensitivity of resonance frequency analysis method to assess implant stability. *NY State Dent J.* 2011; **77(5)**:44–9.
9. Su YY, Wilmes B, Hönscheid R, Drescher D. Application of a wireless resonance frequency transducer to assess primary stability of orthodontic mini-implants. An in vitro study in pig ilia. *Int J Oral Maxillofac Implants.* 2009; **24(4)**:647–54.
10. Ohta K, Takechi M, Minami M, Shigeishi H, Hiraoka M, Nishimura M, Kamata N. Influence of factors related to implant stability detected by wireless resonance frequency analysis device. *J Oral Rehabil.* 2010; **37(2)**:131–7.
11. Turkyilmaz I. A comparison between insertion torque and resonance frequency in the assessment of torque capacity and primary stability of Brånemark system implants. *J Oral Rehabil.* 2006; **33(10)**:754–59.
12. Herrmann I, Lekholm U, Holm S, Kultje C. Evaluation of patient and implant characteristics as potential prognostic factors for oral implant failures. *Int J Oral Maxillofac Implants.* 2005; **20**:220–30.
13. Jaffin RA, Berman CL. The excessive loss of Branemark fixtures in type IV bone: a 5-year analysis. *J Periodontol.* 1991; **62**:2–4.
14. Lekholm U, Zarb G. Patient selection and preparation. In: *Osseointegration in Clinical Dentistry.* Chicago: Quintessence Publishing Co, Inc. 1985; p. 199–209
15. Misch CE. *Contemporary Implant Dentistry.* St. Louis: Mosby, 1993; p. 469–85.
16. Turkyilmaz I, Sennerby L, McGlumphy EA, Tozum TF. Biomechanical aspects of primary implant stability: a human cadaver study. *Clin Implant Dent Relat Res.* 2009; **11**:113–9.
17. Kobayashi K, Shimoda S, Nakagawa Y, Yamamoto A. Accuracy in measurement of distance using limited cone-beam computerized tomography. *Int J Oral Maxillofac Implants.* 2004; **19**:228–31.
18. Loubele M, Maes F, Schutyser F, Marchal G, Jacobs R, Suetens P. Assessment of bone segmentation quality of cone-beam CT versus multislice spiral CT: a pilot study. *Oral Surg Oral Med Oral Pathol Oral Radiol Endod.* 2006; **102**:225–34.
19. Schulze D, Heiland M, Thurmann H, Adam G. Radiation exposure during midfacial imaging using 4- and 16-slice computed tomography, cone beam computed tomography systems and conventional radiography. *Dentomaxillofac Radiol.* 2004; **33**:83–8.
20. De Vos W, Casselman J, Swennen GR. Cone-beam computerized tomography (CBCT) imaging of the oral and maxillofacial region: a systematic review of the literature. *Int J Oral Maxillofac Surg.* 2009; **38**:609–25.
21. KI H, Kawashima S, Araki M, Iwai K, Sawada K, Akiyama Y. Comparison of image performance between cone-beam computed tomography for dental use and four-row multidetector helical CT. *J Oral Sci.* 2006; **48(1)**:27–34.
22. Araki K, Okano T. The effect of surrounding conditions on pixel value of cone beam computed tomography. *Clin Oral Implants Res.* 2013; **24(8)**:862–5.
23. Eskandarloo A, Abdinian M, Salemi F, Hashemzadeh Z, Safaei M. Effect of object location on the density measurement in cone beam computed tomography versus multislice computed tomography. *Dent Res J (Isfahan).* 2012; **9(Suppl 1)**:S81–7.
24. Nackaerts O, Maes F, Yan H, Couto Souza P, Pauwels R, Jacobs R. Analysis of intensity variability in multislice and cone beam computed tomography. *Clin Oral Implants Res.* 2011; **22(8)**:873–9.
25. Ikumi N, Tsutsumi S. Assessment of correlation between computerized tomography values of the bone and cutting torque values at implant placement: a clinical study. *Int J Oral Maxillofac Implants.* 2005; **20**:253–60.
26. Nkenke E, Hahn M, Weinzierl K, Radespiel-Troger M, Neukam FW, Engelke K. Implant stability and histomorphometry: a correlation study in human cadavers using stepped cylinder implants. *Clin Oral Implants Res.* 2003; **14**:601–9.
27. Motoyoshi M, Yoshida T, Ono A, Shimizu N. Effect of cortical bone thickness and implant placement torque on stability of orthodontic mini-implants. *Int J Oral Maxillofac Implants.* 2007; **22**:779–84.
28. Roze J, Babu S, Saffarzadeh A, Gayet-Delacroix M, Hoomaert A, Layrolle P. Correlating implants stability to bone structure. *Clin Oral Implants Res.* 2009; **20**:1140–45.

# 17

# Peri-implant mucosal dehiscence coverage with a modified semilunar coronary positioned flap in posterior maxilla: a case report

Daisuke Ueno[1*], Jayanetti Asiri Jayawardena[2] and Takashi Kurokawa[3]

**Abstract**

Soft tissue dehiscence around dental implant has frequently been observed and it may lead to poor oral hygiene, especially around crowns that exhibit contours with prominent convexity. The present case demonstrates a peri-implant mucosal dehiscence coverage with modified semilunar coronary positioned flap (CPF) in #15 and 16. A semilunar partial-thickness incision was performed 7–10 mm apical from the facial gingival margin. Then, intrasulcular partial-thickness incision was tunneled to the semilunar incision. The tunnel preparation was extended interproximally under each papilla due to improvement of flap extension. Then, the tunneled flap was coronary positioned with a coronary-anchored suturing technique. Sub-epithelial connective tissue graft (SCTG) from the palate was inserted from the semilunar incision to the inside of the coronary positioned flap and sutured to stabilize the SCTG and supplemental site. Significant mucosal gain was achieved without any complication. The soft tissue volume was maintained at 9 months post-surgery, and the cleanability was improved. This technique has the potential in improving the graft survival and mucosa gain around implants.

**Keywords:** Coronary positioned flap; Connective tissue graft; Dental implant; Dehiscence coverage

## Introduction

Mucosal dehiscence around dental implants has frequently been observed. This phenomenon not only causes an esthetic disturbance in the anterior region but it may also lead to poor oral hygiene in the posterior region, because molar teeth exhibit contours with prominent convexities leading to accumulation of plaque. A few clinical articles on mucosal dehiscence coverage around dental implant have been published [1, 2]. Of these, only one study has been randomized controlled [3], whereas the other has been either a small a series of cases or a case report related to recession around a single implant. A literature review and a conference paper cited that dehiscence coverage around dental implant is technique-sensitive [1, 2]. Although no recommendation can be made to support the selection of one technique over another [1, 2], coronary positioned flap (CPF) with sub-epithelial connective tissue graft (SCTG) is considered to be a major treatment option. The present case report demonstrates a peri-implant mucosal dehiscence coverage technique with modified semilunar CPF in the posterior zone. This favorable result may be attributed to improved peri-operative usability and post-operative stability of the conventional technique.

## Case report

Two implants with simultaneous GBR in #15 and 16 were placed in a 65-year-old male patient in Tsurumi University Dental Hospital on September 2013 (Fig. 1a). At 5 months after implant placement, the successfully integrated implants were restored by provisional prosthesis. Since the implant-abutment connection was 1 mm supragingival and the crown contours exhibited prominent convexity, it became increasingly difficult to clean adequately around the implants (Fig. 1b). To

* Correspondence: ueno@kdu.ac.jp
[1]Department of Implantology and Periodontology, Graduate School of Dentistry, Kanagawa Dental University, 3-31-6 Tsuruya-cho, Kanagawa-ku, Yokohama, Japan
Full list of author information is available at the end of the article

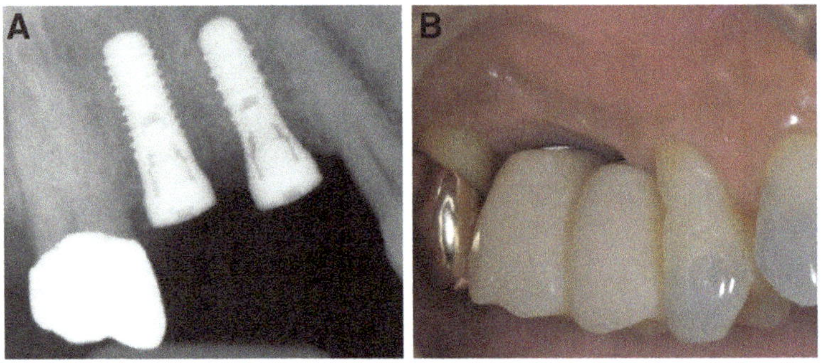


**Fig. 1** Preoperative dental X-ray (**a**) and preoperative intraoral view (**b**)

improve the cleanability, soft tissue augmentation was carried out around the implants.

Following local anesthesia, a semilunar partial-thickness incision was made 7–10 mm apical from the facial gingival margin using a #15C blade (Fig. 2a). Furthermore, intrasulcular partial-thickness incision was tunneled to the semilunar incision using a mini-crescent knife[1] (Fig. 3). The partial-thickness tunnel was extended interproximally under each papilla. After confirmation of flap extension (Fig. 2b), the 25-mm wide × 15-mm high tunneled flap was coronary positioned with a coronary-anchored suturing technique using 5.0 nylon sutures. The coronary-anchored suture was suspended and tied on a groove which was created in the coupling portion of the connecting provisional crown. A 18 × 10-mm-size SCTG was harvested from the palate in the right canine to the second molar region. The graft tissue was trimmed to fit the formerly prepared recipient bed. Then, the SCTG was inserted from the semilunar incision to the inside of the CPF (Fig. 2c) and sutured with 5.0 nylon to stabilize the SCTG and supplemental site (Fig. 2d). Suture at the access incision was removed after 2 weeks. The coronary-anchored suture was removed 2 weeks post-

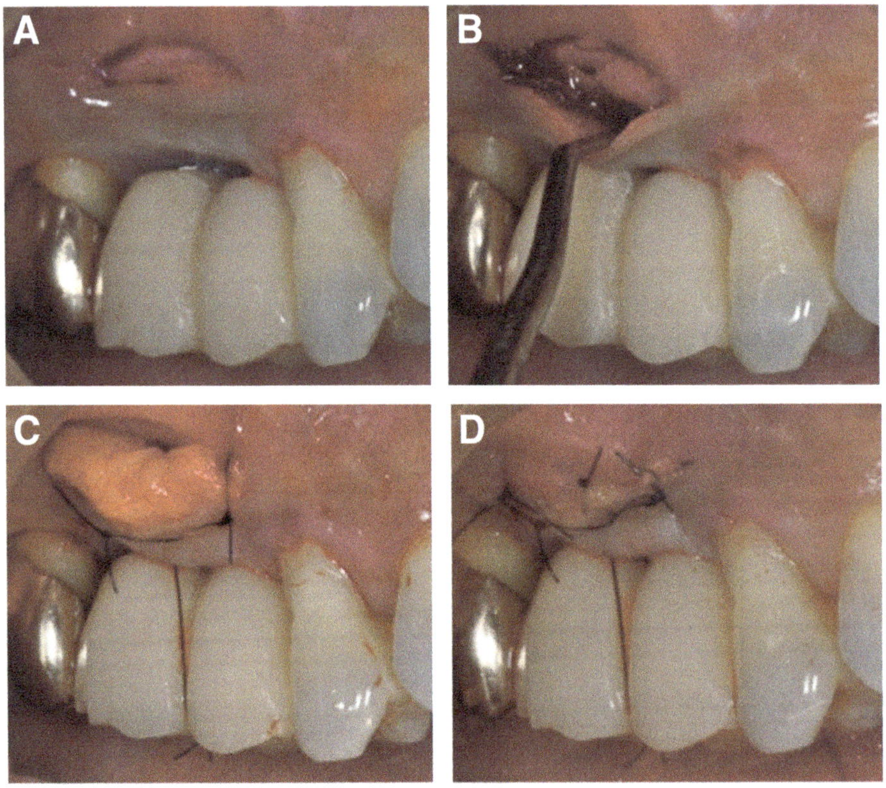


**Fig. 2 a**–**d** Surgical steps of a modified semilunar coronary positioned flap (CPF) with sub-epithelial connective tissue graft (SCTG)

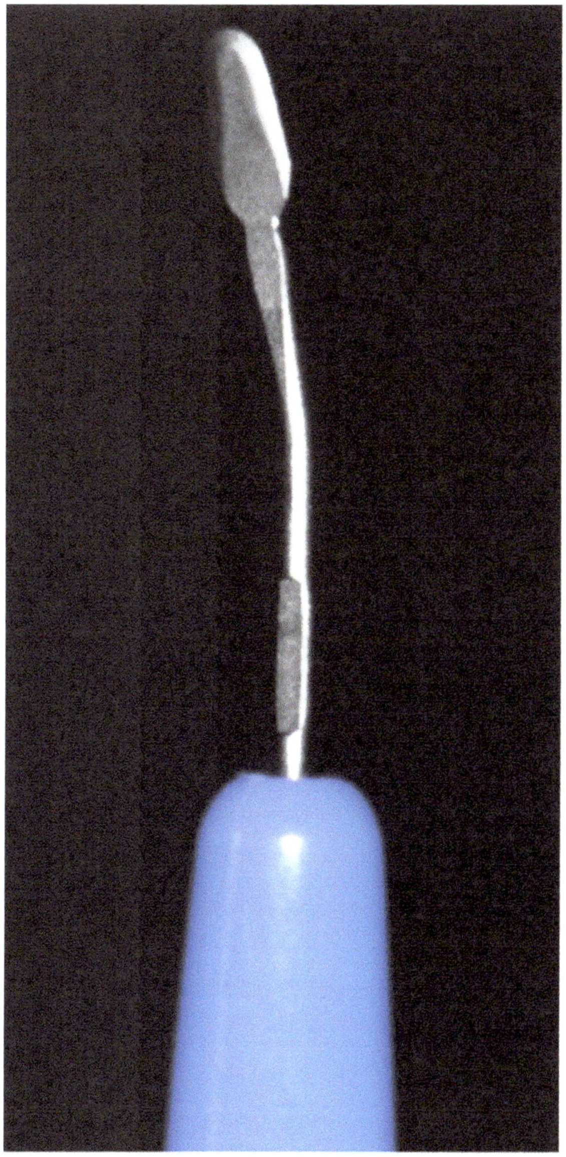

**Fig. 3** Mini-crescent knife

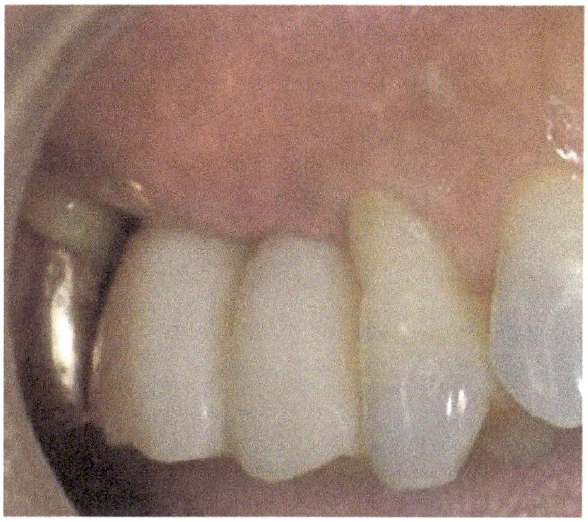

**Fig. 4** Intraoral appearance at 3 months post-surgery

surgery. No complications had arisen within 3 months post-surgery.

Since adequate vertical and horizontal mucosal volume was gained at 3 months after the grafting (Fig. 4), the provisional prosthesis was replaced by a cement-retained metal-ceramic crown. The dehiscence sites #15 and 16 were covered successfully with regenerated mucosa. The vertical mucosal gain was 2 mm in #15 and 3 mm in #16. The horizontal mucosal gain was 2 mm in #15 and 3 mm in #16. The gain of width of keratinized mucosa was 2 mm (#15) and 2 mm (#16), respectively. At 9 months after the SCTG, the soft tissue volume was maintained, and the cleanability was improved (Fig. 5).

## Discussion

In this case, a modified semilunar CPF with SCTG successfully filled the mucogingival defect around implants. Previously, several techniques such as the rotational flap procedures (laterally sliding flap, double papilla flap, oblique rotated flap), advanced flap procedures (CPF, semilunar CPF), and regenerative procedures (with barrier membrane or application of enamel matrix proteins) have been introduced for root coverage [4]. Although all root coverage procedures can provide significant reduction in recession depth and clinical attachment (CAL) gain in Miller [5] class I and class II gingival recession, CPF in combination with SCTG is more effective than CPF in achieving root coverage and gain of keratinized mucosa [6, 7].

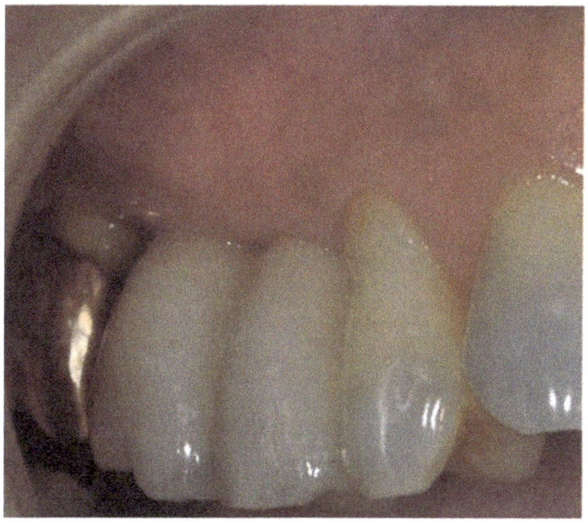

**Fig. 5** Intraoral appearance at 9 months post-surgery

Only a limited number of articles have been published in peri-implant dehiscence coverage [1, 2]. Most of the cases involved autogenous mucosal graft. A conventional CPF using vertical releasing incisions (VRIs) in combination with SCTG has been considered to be a major treatment option in peri-implant dehiscence coverage. However, VRIs have risks with esthetic disturbance and post-operative course. Therefore, we previously reported a technique with coronary positioned envelope flap using SCTG [8]. The CPF with envelope technique has the advantages of increasing keratinized mucosa, a better post-operative course, and a more positive esthetic evaluation such as scars after healing than CPF with VRIs [9]. In contrast, coronary positioning of flap is difficult in cases with scarring recipient mucosa and multi-implant recession due to less flap mobility. In such cases, additional semilunar incision is useful in improving the flap mobility. Coronary-anchored suture (CAS) facilitates to make space for insertion of connective tissue and to fix the position of CPF. Since reduction of micromotion during healing period influences graft survival, CAS may be useful in envelope and tunneling techniques. Further studies are needed to evaluate the usefulness of this technique.

## Endnote

[1]Mini-crescent angled knife (size 1.25 mm), Sharpoint™, PA, USA

### Competing interests

Daisuke Ueno, Jayanetti Asiri Jayawardena, and Takashi Kurokawa declare that they have no competing interests.

### Authors' contributions

DU designed and performed the surgery and wrote the paper; AJ wrote and compiled the paper; TK assisted in the surgery and wrote the paper. All authors read and approved the final manuscript.

### Authors' information

DU is the Senior Assistant Professor, Department of Implantology and Periodontology, Kanagawa Dental University, Graduate School of Stomatology, Yokohama, Japan. JAJ is an Assistant Professor, Department of General Education, Tsurumi University, School of Dental Medicine. TK is a Clinical Research Associate, Unit of Oral and Maxillofacial Implantology, Tsurumi University Dental Hospital, Yokohama, Japan.

### Acknowledgements

The authors report no acknowledgement related to this report.

### Author details

[1]Department of Implantology and Periodontology, Graduate School of Dentistry, Kanagawa Dental University, 3-31-6 Tsuruya-cho, Kanagawa-ku, Yokohama, Japan. [2]Department of General Education, School of Dental Medicine, Tsurumi University, Yokohama, Japan. [3]Unit of Oral and Maxillofacial Implantology, Tsurumi University Dental Hospital, Yokohama, Japan.

### References

1. Levine R, Huynh-Ba G, Cochran DL. Soft tissue augmentation procedures for mucogingival defects in esthetic sites. Int J Oral Maxillofac Implants. 2014;29:155–85.
2. Tonetti MS, Jepsen S. Clinical efficacy of periodontal plastic surgery procedures: consensus report of Group 2 of the 10th European Workshop on Periodontology. J Clin Periodontol. 2014;41:S36–43.
3. Basegmez C, Ersanli S, Demirel K, Bölükbasi N, Yalcin S. The comparison of two techniques to increase the amount of peri-implant attached mucosa: free gingival grafts versus vestibuloplasty. One-year results from a randomized controlled trial. Eur J Oral Implantol. 2012;5:139–45.
4. Zucchellu G, Mounssif I. Periodontal plastic surgery. Periodontol. 2015;68:333–68.
5. Miller Jr PD. A classification of marginal tissue recession. Int J Periodontics Restorative Dent. 1985;5:8–13.
6. Cairo F, Nieri M, Pagliaro U. Efficacy of periodontal plastic surgery procedures in the treatment of localized facial gingival recessions. A systematic review. J Clin Periodontol. 2014;41:S44–62.
7. Chambrone L, Tatakis D. Periodontal soft tissue root coverage procedures: a systematic review from the AAP regeneration workshop. J Periodontol. 2015;86:S8–S51.
8. Hidaka T, Ueno D. Mucosal dehiscence coverage for dental implant using split pouch technique: a two-stage approach. J Periodontal & Implant Science. 2012;42:105–9.
9. Zucchelli G, Mele M, Mazzotti C, Marzadori M, Montebugnoli L, De Sanctis M. Coronally advanced flap with and without vertical releasing incisions for the treatment of multiple gingival recessions: a comparative controlled randomized clinical trial. J Periodontol. 2009;80:1083–94.

# 18

# Case presentation of two patients using diagonal platform-switched double implants for maxillary single-first-molar replacement as the alternative of a single-tooth implant

Yasunori Hotta*, Koji Ito, Shinichi Komatsu and Takashi Saito

**Abstract**

A single-tooth implant restoration is generally performed for maxillary single-first-molar replacement. If the interdental space between the second premolar and the second molar is large enough, a double-implant placement can be performed to avoid creating mesiodistal cantilever and to distribute occlusal loading forces.

If there is not adequate space for a double-implant placement to be performed mesiodistally along the crest of the alveolar ridge line, they should be placed along a diagonal line offset lingually to increase the space. This procedure has two primary advantages. First, greater stability is provided by a double-implant placement. Resistance to lateral forces (palatal-buccal) is much stronger than two implants placed along the alveolar crest ridge line. Residual palatal and buccal bone can provide support against occlusal forces, provided that there is adequate residual bone in these regions.

If anatomical conditions are favorable, the placement of two diagonal implants in the palatal and buccal residual bones can be a rational procedure.

We report on two typical patients. The progress of these patients was followed using computed tomography for 7 and 6 years, respectively.

**Keywords:** Implant, Double implants, Maxillary single-first-molar replacement, Diagonal implant placement, Platform-switched implant

## Background

We report on two patients who were missing a maxillary first molar. In general clinical practice, only a single-tooth implant seems to be used as a prosthesis in patients with a missing maxillary molar tooth [1]. In addition, if there is insufficient residual bone between the bottom of the sinus and the crest of the alveolar ridge, GBR (guided bone regeneration) technique [2] or sinus elevation [3] surgery is required. Even though these procedures can promote osteogenesis, whether the quality of newly formed bone is similar to that of the existing residual bone remains unclear [4–8]. If there is enough residual D2 or D3 bone (Misch Bone Density Classification) [9] for implant placement, the use of such bone is recommended whenever possible. If we accept the above, a double-implant placement [10, 11] inserted in the buccal and palatal sides, not the center of the alveolar ridge, may be a reasonable option for maxillary-first-molar replacement because these regions sometimes retain more bone volume than the center of defects.

## Case presentation

### Patient 1

The patient was a 51-year-old man who was a non-smoker. He was referred to my clinic in April 2004. The #26 tooth had already been extracted because of severe periodontitis. He returned to my clinic in March 2006 to

* Correspondence: hotta-dc@ff.iij4u.or.jp
Aichi Implant Center, Hotta Dental Clinic, 13, Morimaki-cho, Moriyama-ku, Nagoya 463-0073, Japan

receive implant treatment (Fig. 1). The medical history was unremarkable. A hematological analysis was performed to assess his overall medical status. The #26 tooth was confirmed to be missing, and there was severe bone resorption around the buccal roots of #27, associated with an apical lesion (Fig. 2).

In May of the same year, double implants (Ankylos implants [12]; diameter, 3.5 mm; length, 9.5 mm; DENTSPLY, made in Germany) were placed diagonally in the defect with sinus elevation (crestal approach) (Fig. 3). In addition, Emdogain (enamel matrix protein) [13–15] was applied to the root surface of #27. Then, endodontic treatment of #27 was performed (Fig. 4d). Six months after implant surgery, the screw-retained superstructure was seated (Fig. 4).

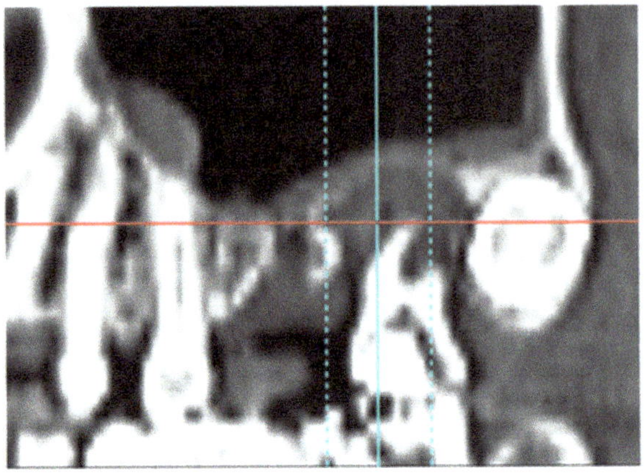
**Fig. 2** Case 1. May 2006. Preoperative panoramic slice of MDCT scan. There was severe bone resorption in the region of #26 and lesions around the root apexes of #27

#### Patient 2

Similar to the first patient, our second patient was a nonsmoking man, 43 years of age. He was referred to my clinic by another dentist in January 2008 and was first examined at that time. He complained of pain due to serious periodontitis in #26. The medical history was unremarkable. He was examined in a similar manner as patient 1.

In the same month, #26 was extracted. After extraction, bone resorption including the buccal cortical plate occurred more severely than in most patients (Figs. 5 and 6). Two months after extraction, only GBR was performed to repair the bone defect. Double implants (Ankylos implants; diameter, 3.5 mm; length, 9.5 and 11 mm) were placed diagonally in the missing region 3 months after GBR (Fig. 7). In November of the same year, a screw-retained superstructure was seated (Fig. 8).

#### Treatment results

The patients' clinical progress has been good as of 7 years and 5 months in patient 1 (Figs. 9 and 10) and 6 years and 7 months in patient 2 (Fig. 11). Computed tomographic (CT) scans showed that both patients' implants were inserted at appropriate positions, as planned before surgery (Figs. 12 and 13).

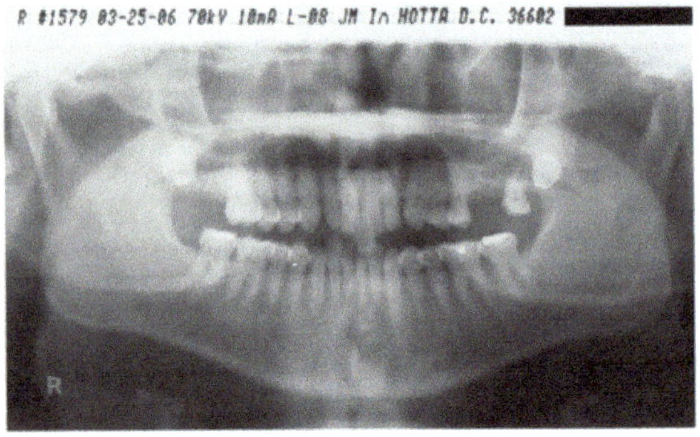
**Fig. 1** Case 1. March 2006. A panoramic X-ray film obtained before treatment

#### Discussion

Insertion of a single implant for single molar replacement is established practice. Levin et al. reported that a single implant can serve as a good long-term and predictable treatment modality to replace a single molar with low complication and failure rates [16].

However, weak points of single-first-molar replacement were reported.

Mazor et al. reported that 33 patients received 66 narrow double implants of 3 mm replacing 33 missing first molars. All implants survived the follow-up time of 10 to 18 months. Wide-diameter implants are a suitable alternative for replacing a missing molar in some cases, but there has been a greater incidence of screw loosening, resulting in a higher failure rate. However, the use of a double-implant placement has been successfully demonstrated to be a functional and more biomechanically sound method of molar replacement. He concluded that replacing a single missing molar with two narrow dental implants might serve as a viable treatment option providing good and predictable long-term results [17].

Sullivan reported that when using standard-diameter 3.75-mm titanium screw implants in molar regions, up to 14 % of single-tooth, molar implants could fracture, so there remains an unacceptable risk of implant fracture [18].

In addition, a double-implant placement has been reported to be superior to a single stand implant. The advantages and disadvantages of a single standard implant, a wide-diameter implant, and double implants for single-molar replacement have been debated with biomechanics [10, 11, 19–21].

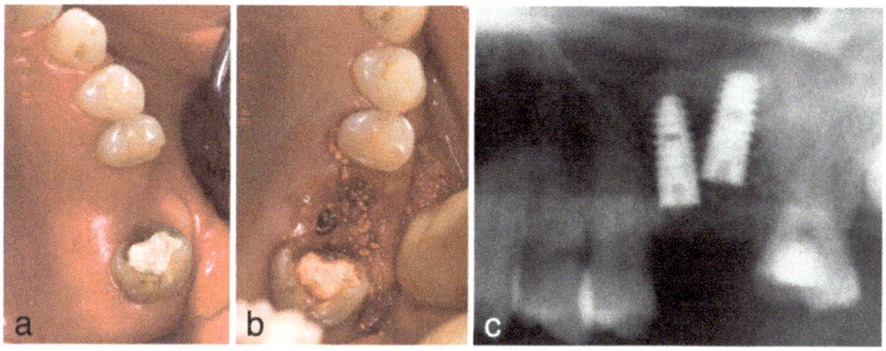


**Fig. 3** Case 1. May 2006. **a** Before implant surgery. **b** Double implants were placed diagonally in the missing area. **c** Magnified panoramic X-ray film obtained immediately after insertion of double implants

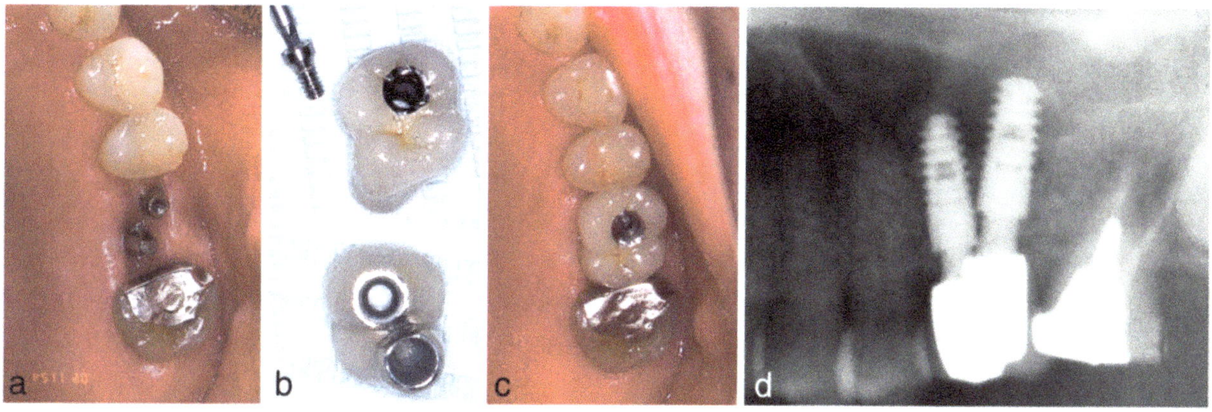


**Fig. 4** Case 1. November 2006. Six months after implant insertion. **a**–**c** The superstructure was attached with a screw. **d** Magnified panoramic X-ray film obtained immediately after superstructure placement

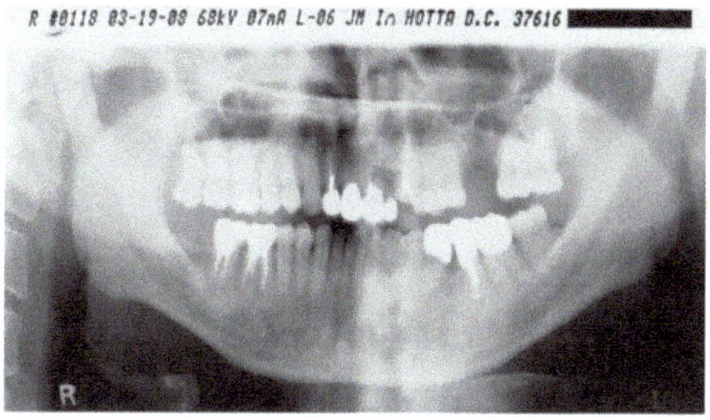


**Fig. 5** Case 2. March 2008. Panoramic X-ray film taken before #26 GBR

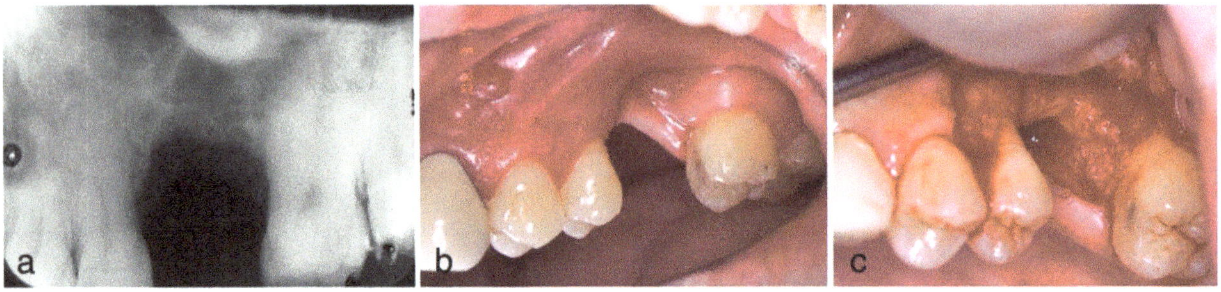


**Fig. 6** Case 2. March 2008. Two months after extraction of #26. **a** Periapical X-ray film of #26 before surgery. **b**, **c** Oral view shows very severe bone resorption, especially vertically

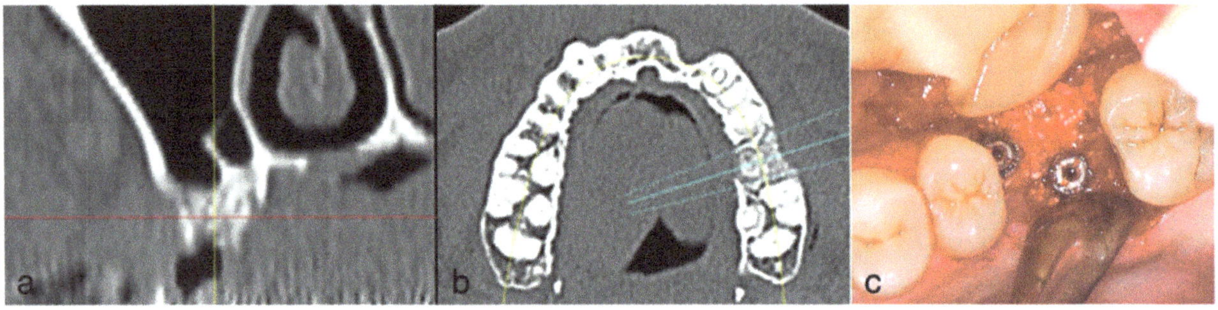


**Fig. 7** Case 2. June 2008. **a**, **b** 3 months after GBR without implant insertion, MDCT was performed to evaluate. **c** Double implants were placed diagonally

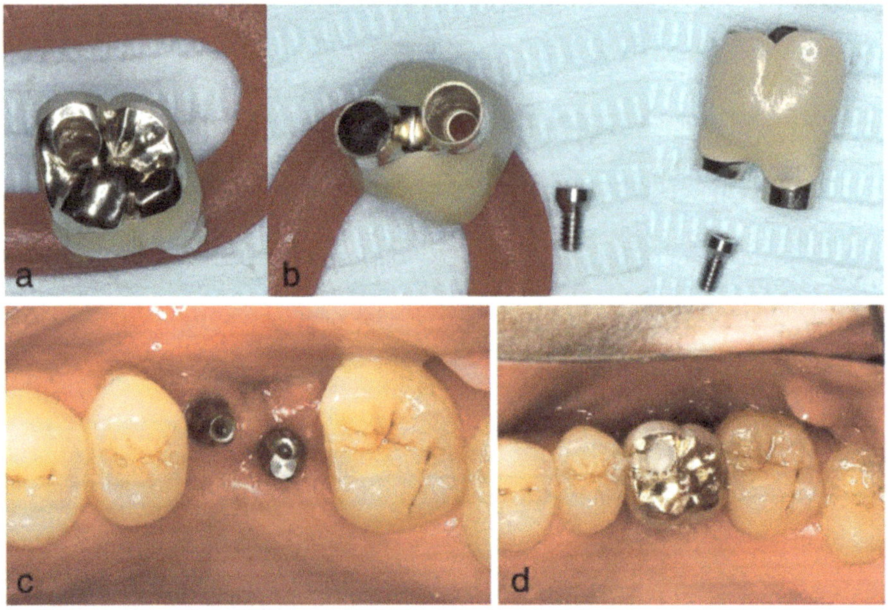


**Fig. 8** Case 2. November 2008. Five months after implant insertion. **a** A fitted superstructure was made. **b** Before the placement of the superstructure. The double implants were placed diagonally. **c** The superstructure was attached with a screw as in case 1.**d** After placement of superstructure

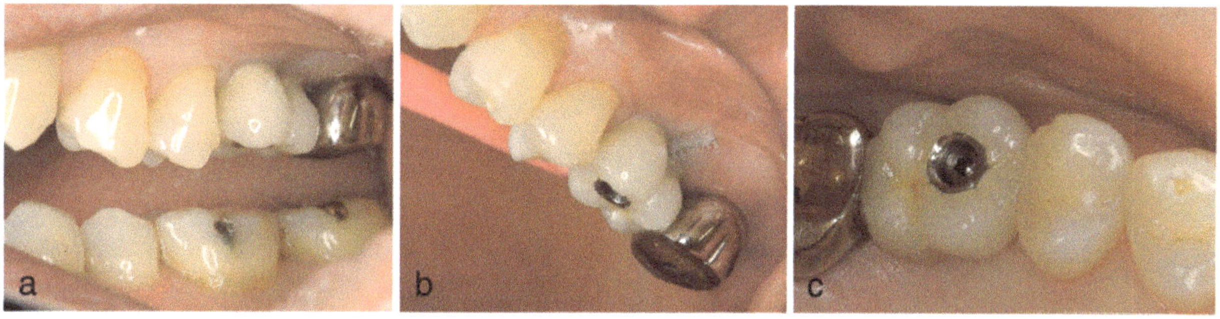


**Fig. 9** Case 1. April 2013. Six years and 5 months after superstructure placement. **a** The buccal oral view of the superstructure. **b** An interdental brush can easily clean the interimplant space. **c** April 2014, 7 years and 5 months after superstructure placement

If there is 13 mm between the maxillary second premolar and the second molar, a double-implant placement can be performed in the crest of the alveolar ridge line. When 3.5-mm diameter implants are used, there should be a minimum space of 3 mm between implants [22] and 1.5 mm between the implants and adjacent teeth [23] ($1.5 + 3.5 + 3 + 3.5 + 1.5 = 13$ mm). However, the average Japanese mesiodistal dimension of the maxillary first molar is between 10 and 11 mm [24]. Therefore, if a double-implant placement is used, it has to be placed diagonally to create a larger inter-implant space and accommodate international implant sizing [1].

As for the vertical bone dimension, if there is insufficient residual bone volume between the bottom of the sinus and the crest of the alveolar ridge, GBR or sinus elevation surgery is required for all implants. If there is sufficient existing residual D2 or D3 bone near the buccal and palatal cortical plates, the use of such bone is recommended whenever possible. If double implants can engage these cortical plates, greater support can be obtained with diagonal double implants than with a single stand implant.

In both patients, we used Ankylos implants, which have a medialized step between the implant body and abutment. Therefore, Ankylos is a platform-switched implant. The benefits of this shape have been reported. With platform-switched implants, the shape affects the cortical bone more than the trabecular bone [25], which contributes to the maintenance of inter-implant bone height and soft tissue level [26] and reduces bone loss [27]. The horizontal discrepancy between the outer edge of the implant platform and the implant-abutment interface influences post-restorative biologic processes [28]. This horizontal discrepancy may reduce bone resorption around the implant neck because it horizontally offsets the bone away from the microgap that exists between the implant and abutment. This increased distance is thought to attenuate the loss of crestal bone height [29].

Effects of the inter-implant distance between platform-switched implants have been reported. Even when the

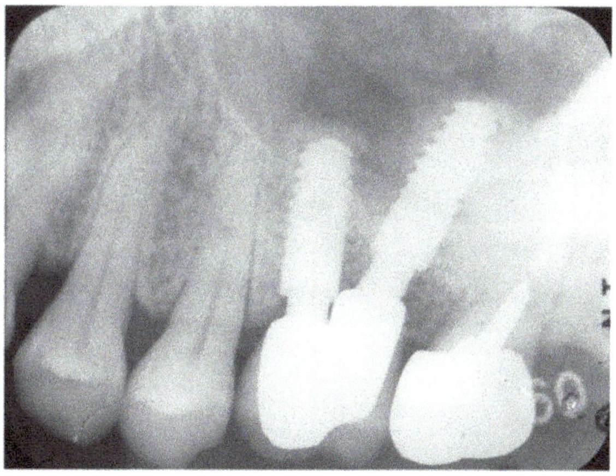

**Fig. 10** Case 1. Periapical X-ray film, April 2014. Seven years and 5 months after superstructure placement, showing no bone resorption around the double implant necks

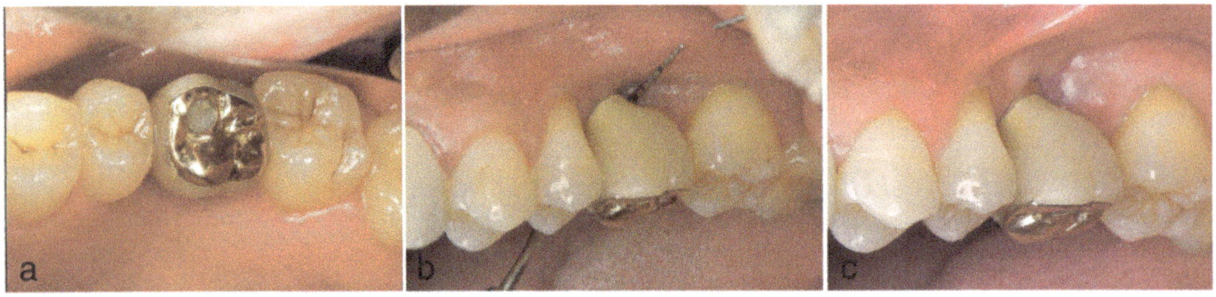


**Fig. 11** Case 2. **a** April 2013. Four years and 5 months after placement of the superstructure. Occlusal view. **b** Periodontal probe can easily pass through the interimplant space, allowing for easy cleaning and maintenance. **c** June 2015, 6 years and 7 months after placement of the superstructure

inter-implant distance was less than 3 mm, crestal bone resorption was prevented [30-34]. Previous studies thus support the advantages of platform-switched implants as compared with platform-matched implants when double implants are placed adjacently.

In patient 1, the platform-switched double-implant placement was performed very close to each other (Fig. 3). If platform-matched implants had been used, inter-implant bone loss might have occurred. Fortunately, there was no evidence of bone resorption on the periapical X-ray obtained 7 years and 5 months after superstructure placement (Fig. 10). In addition, there has been no problem with the emergence profile because platform-switched implants provide a larger volume of soft tissue around the connecting area between the implant and abutment.

In patient 2, severe bone resorption including the buccal cortical plate occurred after #26 extraction and was greater than we had anticipated. Therefore, only GBR was performed without implant insertion to repair the severe bone resorption (Fig. 6). CT was performed to evaluate the GBR site after 3 months. Then, a double-implant placement was performed diagonally with another session of GBR to increase bone volume (Fig. 7).

The use of platform-switched implants has been associated with coronal extension of the interimplant bone peak beyond an imaginary line connecting the two implant-abutment interfaces [22]. In patient 2, even

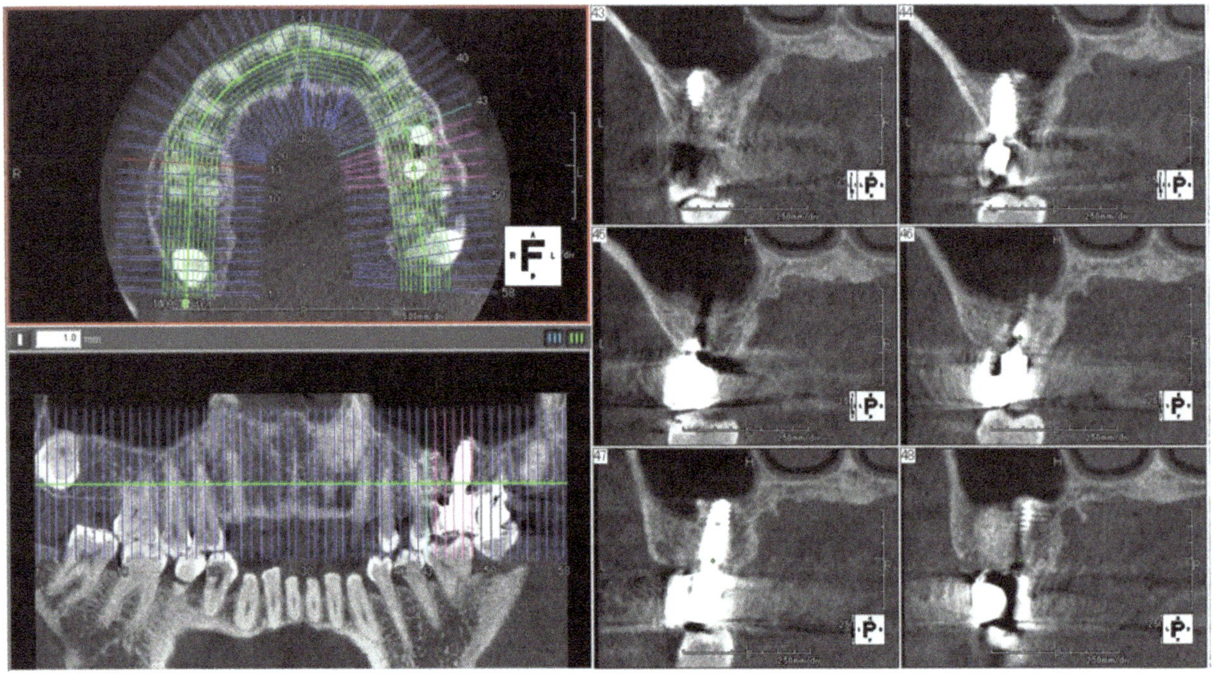

**Fig. 12** Case 1. April 2013. Cone-beam CT obtained 6 years and 5 months after superstructure placement. The double implants were surrounded by an adequate amount of hard tissue that acted as bone

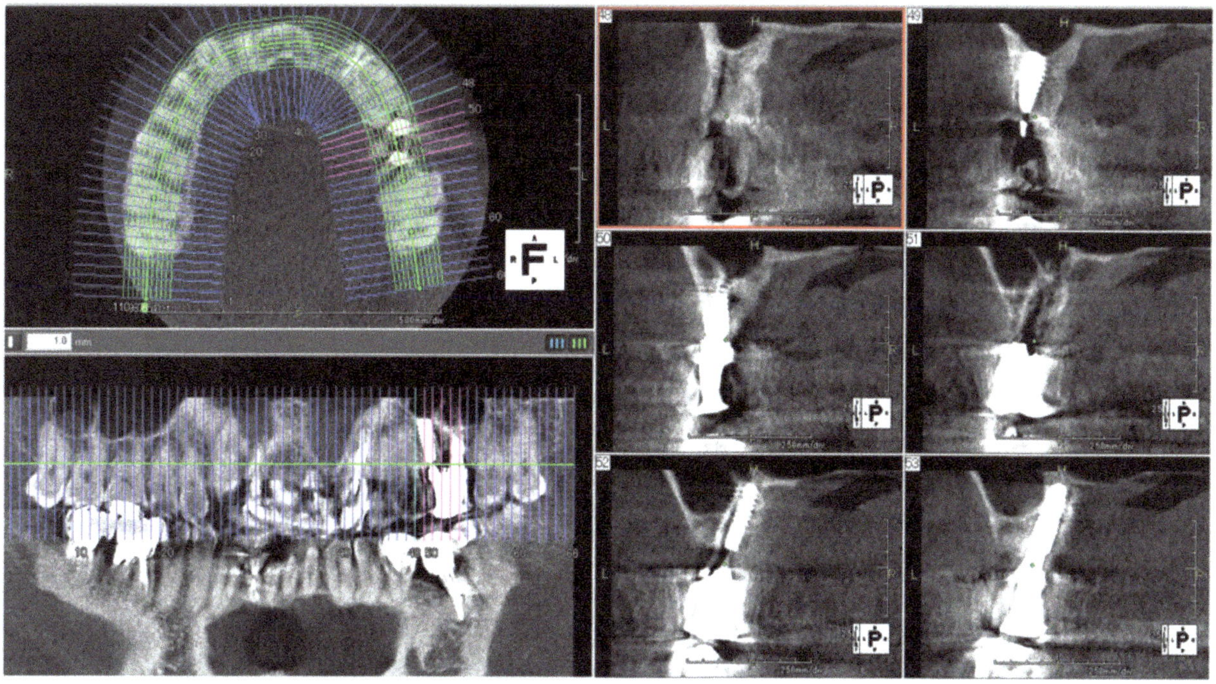

**Fig. 13** Case 2. Cone-beam CT scan obtained in February 2013 (4 years and 3 months after superstructure placement), showing that the double implants were surrounded by enough hard tissue to support the double implants

though the double-implant placement was performed adjacently, new bone formation over the implant shoulder was fortunately confirmed on a periapical X-ray (Fig. 14).

In diagonal double-implant placement, the mesial implant should be placed more buccally and the distal implant more palatally to improve esthetics [1]. In addition, oral hygiene is a very important factor related to inter-implant space. It might be easier for a patient to use an interdental brush from the palatal side rather than from the buccal side, especially in the maxillary molar region.

On the other hand, Bhat and Handelsman reported that there is a surgical risk due to the precision needed in a double-implant placement, because the mesiodistal space is often very limited. Therefore, any misplacement of double implants will ruin the mesial or the distal site, and misplacement also may damage the adjacent roots or compromise the embrasure space, so that only one implant can be placed [35]. This kind of careful attention should be paid when using a double-implant placement in single molar missing.

## Conclusions

We described two patients in whom diagonal platform-switched double-implant placement was performed for maxillary single-first-molar replacement. In such patients, diagonal double implants have some advantages over wide-diameter implants. There was no bone resorption around double implants' necks. We therefore

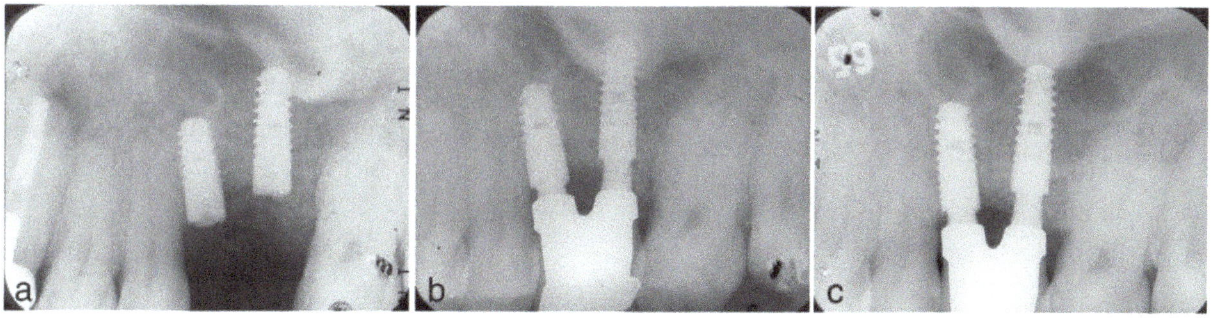


**Fig. 14** Case 2. Periapical X-ray films showing progression of intraimplant bone formation from implant date to 3 years and 8 months after procedure. **a** June 2008. **b** November 2008. **c** February 2012

consider this method as one option for maxillary single-first-molar replacement.

## Consent

Written informed consent was obtained from the patient for publication of this case report and any accompanying images. A copy of the written consent is available for review by the Editor-in-Chief of this journal.

### Competing interests

The authors declare that they have no competing interests.

### Authors' contributions

YH performed both of surgical and prosthodontic treatments. YH also drafted the manuscript. KI, SK, and TS participated in the diagnosis, the treatment plan, making of pictures, and collecting of references. All authors read and approved the final manuscript.

### Authors' information

YH is the director of Aichi Implant Center accredited by the Japanese Society of Oral Implantology (JSOI) and visiting professor of Asahi University, School of Dentistry, Japan. All of authors are implant specialists accredited by JSOI. YH, KI, and TS are fellow members of AAID (the American Academy of Implant Dentistry). SK is an associate fellow member of AAID.

### References


1. Misch CE. Posterior single-tooth replacement: surgical guidelines. In: Contemporary implant dentistry. Chapter 30. 3rd ed. St Louis: Mosby Year Book; 2008. p. 668–83.
2. Hotta Y. Recovery of alveolar bone by the guided bone regeneration technique. J Oral Implantol. 1996;22:138–46.
3. Hotta Y, Suzuki H. Clinical comparison between subperiosteal implant and sinus elevation in maxillary molar regions with minimal bone. J Jpn Soc Oral Implant. 1995;8:69–82.
4. Meijndert L, Raghoebar GM, Schupbach P, Meijer HJ, Vissink A. Bone quality at the implant site after reconstruction of a local defect of the maxillary anterior ridge with chin bone or deproteinised cancellous bovine bone. Int J Oral Maxillofac Surg. 2005;34:877–84.
5. Ersanli S, Olgac V, Leblebicioglu B. Histologic analysis of alveolar bone following guided bone regeneration. J Periodontol. 2004;75:750–6.
6. Papa F, Cortese A, Maltarello MC, Sagliocco R, Felice P, Claudio PP. Outcome of 50 consecutive sinus lift operations. Br J Oral Maxillofac Surg. 2005;43:309–13.
7. Barone A, Ricci M, Grassi RF, Nannmark U, Quaranta A, Covani U. A 6-month histological analysis on maxillary sinus augmentation with and without use of collagen membranes over the osteotomy window: randomized clinical trial. Clin Oral Implants Res. 2013;24:1–6.
8. Iezzi G, Degidi M, Piattelli A, Mangano C, Scarano A, Shibli JA, et al. Comparative histological results of different biomaterials used in sinus augmentation procedures: a human study at 6 months. Clin Oral Implants Res. 2012;23:1369–76.
9. Misch CE. Contemporary implant dentistry, Chapter 7. 3rd ed. St Louis: Mosby Year Book; 2008. p. 134–5.
10. Geramy A, Morgano SM. Finite element analysis of three designs of an implant-supported molar crown. J Prosthet Dent. 2004;92:434–40.
11. Balshi TJ, Wolfinger GJ. Two-implant-supported single molar replacement: interdental space requirements and comparison to alternative options. Int J Periodontics Restorative Dent. 1997;17:426–35.
12. Chou CT, Morris HF, Ochi S, Walker L, Des RD. AICRG, part II: crestal bone loss associated with the Ankylos implant: loading to 36 months. J Oral Implantol. 2004;30:134–43.
13. Bhutda G, Deo V. Five years clinical results following treatment of human intra-bony defects with an enamel matrix derivative: a randomized controlled trial. Acta Odontol Scand. 2013;71:764–70.
14. Mrozik KM, Gronthos S, Menicanin D, Marino V, Bartold PM. Effect of coating Straumann Bone Ceramic with Emdogain on mesenchymal stromal cell hard tissue formation. Clin Oral Investig. 2012;16:867–78.
15. Zhang FQ, Meng HX, Han J, Liu KN. Effects of emdogain on human periodontal ligament cells in vitro. Beijing Da Xue Xue Bao. 2012;18(44):6–10.
16. Levin L, Laviv A, Schwartz-Arad D. Long-term success of implants replacing a single molar. J Periodontol. 2006;77:1528–32.
17. Mazor Z, Lorean A, Mijiritsky E, Levin L. Replacement of a molar with 2 narrow diameter dental implants. Implant Dent. 2012;21:36–8.
18. Sullivan DY. Wide implants for wide teeth. Dent Econ. 1994;84:82–3.
19. Balshi TJ, Hernandez RE, Pryszlak MC, Rangert B. A comparative study of one implant versus two replacing a single molar. Int J Oral Maxillofac Implants. 1996;11:372–8.
20. Bakaeen LG, Winkler S, Neff PA. The effect of implant diameter, restoration design, and occlusal table variations on screw loosening of posterior single-tooth implant restorations. J Oral Implantol. 2001;27:63–72.
21. Desai SR, Karthikeyan I, Singh R. Evaluation of micromovements and stresses around single wide-diameter and double implants for replacing mandibular molar: a three-dimensional FEA. ISRN Dent. 2012;2012:680587.
22. Rodriguez-Ciurana X, Vela-Nebot X, Segala-Torres M, Calvo-Guirado JL, Cambra J, Mendez-Blanco V, et al. The effect of interimplant distance on the height of the interimplant bone crest when using platform-switched implants. Int J Periodontics Restorative Dent. 2009;29:141–51.
23. Vela X, Mendez V, Rodriguez X, Segala M, Tarnow DP. Crestal bone changes on platform-switched implants and adjacent teeth when the tooth-implant distance is less than 1.5 mm. Int J Periodontics Restorative Dent. 2012;32:149–55.
24. Matsumoto H, Funatsu T, Asakawa T, Harada R, Tanaka M. Changes of size in central incisors and first permanent molars of Japanese children—a comparison of the present status with that of 20 years ago. Jpn J Ped Dent. 2003;41:900–5.
25. Gurgel-Juarez NC, de Almeida EO, Rocha EP, Freitas AC, Anchieta RB, de Vargas LC, et al. Regular and platform switching: bone stress analysis varying implant type. J Prosthodont. 2012;21:160–6.
26. Atieh MA, Ibrahim HM, Atieh AH. Platform switching for marginal bone preservation around dental implants: a systematic review and meta-analysis. J Periodontol. 2010;81:1350–66.
27. Vela-Nebot X, Rodriguez-Ciurana X, Rodado-Alonso C, Segala-Torres M. Benefits of an implant platform modification technique to reduce crestal bone resorption. Implant Dent. 2006;15:313–20.
28. Lazzara RJ, Porter SS. Platform switching: a new concept in implant dentistry for controlling postrestorative crestal bone levels. Int J Periodontics Restorative Dent. 2006;26:9–17.
29. Cocchetto R, Traini T, Caddeo F, Celletti R. Evaluation of hard tissue response around wider platform-switched implants. Int J Periodontics Restorative Dent. 2010;30:163–71.
30. Nevins M, Nevins M, Gobbato L, Lee HJ, Wang CW, Kim DM. Maintaining interimplant crestal bone height via a combined platform-switched, Laser-Lok implant/abutment system: a proof-of-principle canine study. Int J Periodontics Restorative Dent. 2013;33:261–7.
31. de Oliveira RR, Novaes AB, Papalexiou V, Muglia VA, Taba M. Influence of interimplant distance on papilla formation and bone resorption: a clinical-radiographic study in dogs. J Oral Implantol. 2006;32:218–27.
32. Elian N, Bloom M, Dard M, Cho SC, Trushkowsky RD, Tarnow D. Effect of interimplant distance (2 and 3 mm) on the height of interimplant bone crest: a histomorphometric evaluation. J Periodontol. 2011;82:1749–56.
33. Barros RR, Novaes AB, Muglia VA, Iezzi G, Piattelli A. Influence of interimplant distances and placement depth on peri-implant bone remodeling of adjacent and immediately loaded Morse cone connection implants: a histomorphometric study in dogs. Clin Oral Implants Res. 2010;21:371–8.
34. Novaes AB, de Oliveira RR, Muglia VA, Papalexiou V, Taba M. The effects of interimplant distances on papilla formation and crestal resorption in implants with a morse cone connection and a platform switch: a histomorphometric study in dogs. J Periodontol. 2006;77:1839–49.
35. Bahat O, Handelsman M. Use of wide implants and double implants in the posterior jaw: a clinical report. Int J Oral Maxillofac Implants. 1996;11:379–86.

# Effect of implant design on primary stability using torque-time curves in artificial bone

Yoko Yamaguchi[1*], Makoto Shiota[2], Motohiro Munakata[3], Shohei Kasugai[2] and Masahiko Ozeki[1]


## Abstract

**Background:** Primary stability following implant placement is essential for osseointegration and is affected by both implant design and bone density. The aim of this study was to compare the relationships between torque-time curves and implant designs in a poor bone quality model.

**Methods:** Nine implant designs, with five implants in each category, were compared. A total of 90 implants (Straumann: Standard RN, Bone Level RC, Tapered Effect RN; Nobel Biocare: Brånemark MKIII, MKIV) were placed in type IV artificial bone. Torque-time curves of insertion and removal were recorded at the rate of 1000 samples/s by a torque analyzer.

**Results:** The torque-time curves were divided into initial, parallel, tapered, and platform areas. The mean torque rise rate of the parallel area was smallest at 0.36 N · cm/s, with a significant difference from those of the other areas ($p < 0.05$). Values of 2.14, 2.33, and 2.65 N · cm/s were obtained for the initial, tapered, and platform areas, respectively. The removal torque for six of the implant designs (Bone Level RC 8, 10, and 12 mm; Tapered Effect RN 10 mm; Brånemark MKIII 10 mm, MKIV 10 mm) was significantly smaller than the corresponding insertion torque ($p < 0.05$). However, the removal torque for ST6, 8, and 10 was almost the same as or slightly greater than the corresponding insertion torque.

**Conclusions:** The insertion torque-time curves and design features of the implants were accurately transferred. Increasing implant taper angle appeared to increase the torque rate. Torque was mainly generated from the superior surface to the valley of the thread and the inferior and axial surfaces of the platform, while the inferior and axial surfaces of the thread did not significantly affect torque generation.


**Keywords:** Primary stability; Implant design; Bone density; Torque-time curve; Insertion torque; Removal torque

## Background

Primary stability following implant placement is an essential condition for osseointegration. The primary stability is affected by the implant design, including surface-modifying or implant cavity-forming techniques, as well as by the bone quantity and bone density of the patient [1–3]. In recent years, the interest of implant manufacturers and clinicians has shifted to the acquisition of good fixation, especially for incurable cases in which the density of cancellous bone, such as the maxilla molar part, is low and the cortical bone is thin [4, 5], for which the effects of surface-modifying techniques are low and focus has been changing to the design of the entire implant [6]. Among implant designs, it has been described that good primary stability can be achieved for long and thick implants [7–10] with a small pitch [11] and a taper [6, 12–18], but the cited reports only evaluated primary stability for the entire implant. An implant has characteristic shapes such as parallel, tapered, and platform areas, and the overall design is constructed by placing these areas together. However, there have been no reports of studies that quantitatively measured and evaluated individual designs involved in primary stability. It has been reported that quantitative techniques are necessary to enable the criteria for successful endosseous implants to be more clearly defined [17]. Periotest [19, 20], resonant vibration frequency analysis [21], implant torque value [22], and removal torque value [23] are used as quantitative primary stability evaluations. However, in the

* Correspondence: blacklab87@gmail.com
[1]Department of Implant Dentistry, Showa University School of Dentistry, 2-1-1 Kitasenzoku Ota-ku, Tokyo 145-8515, Japan
Full list of author information is available at the end of the article

periotest and resonant vibration frequency analysis, only general numerical values can be obtained from an implant and it is impossible to perform analyses for individual designs. Furthermore, regarding the implant torque value and removal torque value, analyses for individual designs are impossible as long as only the maximum torque value is used in the conventional methods. Therefore, in this study, for the purpose of measuring the effects of individual implant designs quantitatively, simulation experiments with artificial bone were performed.

## Methods

### Implants

The type of implant used for the experiments and the characteristics of its design are shown in Table 1 and Fig. 1, respectively. Figure 1 shows that the implant is compressed longitudinally to one third. The outer surface of the implant is indicated with a solid line, and the inner surface of the implant is indicated with a dotted line.

### Preparation of an implant socket in artificial bone

For artificial bone, rigid polyurethane foam (Solid Rigid Polyurethane Foam 20 pcf; Sawbones; Pacific Research Laboratories Inc., USA) measuring 18 × 4 × 13 cm and approaching the maxilla molar part bone density (0.32 g/cc) and physical properties (compressive strength, 8.4 MPa; tensile strength, 5.6 MPa; shear strength, 4.3 MPa; coefficient of elasticity, 284 GPa) [24] was employed. An implant socket was formed by making an interval of more than 2 cm, while avoiding axis wobbling as much as possible, with a drill press (ASD-360; Ashina, Hiroshima, Japan) in the artificial bone.

### Measurement of torque-time curves

For measurement of torque-time curves, a torque measurement system capable of high-speed sampling at 1 sample/ms (PC torque analyzer TRQ-5DRU; Vectrix, Tokyo, Japan) was used. The rotational speed at the time of insertion was 15 rpm, the load was 500 g, and the maximum torque value indicated in the torque-time curve (and following implant torque curve) when inserting the implant (Osseoset 200; Nobel Biocare Japan, Tokyo, Japan) was assumed as the insertion torque value. In addition, the removal torque value (RT) was obtained from the removal torque curve when the implant was reversed immediately after insertion.

**Table 1** The type of the implant used for experiment

| System | Length (mm) | Pitch (mm) | Lead (mm) | Code | Manufacturer |
|---|---|---|---|---|---|
| Standard RN | 6, 8, 10 | 1.2 | 1.2 | ST | Straumann |
| Bone Level RC | 8, 10, 12 | 0.8 | 0.8 | BL | Straumann |
| Tapered Effect RN | 10 | 0.8 | 0.8 | TE | Straumann |
| Brånemark MKIII | 10 | 0.6 | 1.2 | MK3 | Nobel Biocare |
| Brånemark MKIV | 10 | 0.6 | 1.2 | MK4 | Nobel Biocare |

### Measurement of the rate of torque rise

The average torque rise rate (N · cm/s) in each region was obtained from the point that the origin and torque rose immediately after implantation, with both ends of the region indicating lines, both ends of the region indicating a quadratic function, and the torque values and implant time of both ends indicating a logarithmic function becoming gradual on the implant torque curve, and mean values and SD were calculated.

### Statistical analysis

It was confirmed that the measurement results for the insertion and removal torque values of each implant were normally distributed, and their significant differences were examined by Student's $t$ test and the Tukey–Kramer method (JMP software; SAS Institute Japan, Tokyo, Japan). The significance level was set at $p = 0.05$.

## Results

### Insertion torque

The insertion torque curve was divided into four regions. The first was the region where the torque rose suddenly immediately after insertion, which was seen in all implant bodies (shown as ① in the figure, and hereinafter called the initial area). The second was the region where the torque rose linearly with a moderate gradient, which was seen in all implant bodies except for Brånemark MKIV (MK4) (shown as ② in the figure, and hereinafter called the parallel area). The third was the region where torque rose suddenly, which was seen in Bone Level RC (BL), Tapered Effect RN (TE), and MK (shown as ③ in the figure, and hereinafter called the tapered area). The fourth was the region where the torque reached a critical point, rose suddenly, and then rose gently, which was seen in Brånemark MKIII (MK3) and MK4 (shown as ④ in the figure, and hereinafter called the tapered area).

Regarding the Standard RN (ST), the axial surface and lateral surface were parallel, while for ST6, 8, and 10, only the length was different. The insertion torque curve of the ST3 class shown in Fig. 2a resembled closely, and moderate gradient lines were presented after the initial area in which the torque rose immediately after implantation (parallel area). The length and insertion torque values of the parallel area varied as the length of the implant varied among 6, 8, and 10 mm.

The torque curve for BL3 in Fig. 3a presented a sudden rise in torque on a quadratic function in the initial area immediately after insertion and a subsequent parallel area (tapered area). As the length of the implant

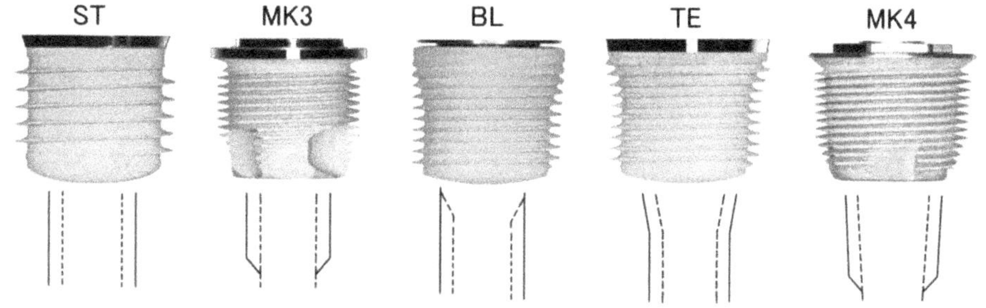


**Fig. 1** Compressed longitudinally to one third for characteristics of implant design. *ST* Straumann standard implant, *MK3* Nobel Biocare MKIII, *BL* Straumann bone level implant, *TE* Straumann tapered effect implant, *MK4* Nobel Biocare MKIV. Outer surface of implant (*solid line*). Inner surface of implant (*dotted line*)

varied among 8, 10, and 12 mm, only the length of the parallel area changed, and the initial area and tapered area had almost the same form. The lateral surface for BL was entirely parallel, while the axial surface had a taper only in the cervical region and the thread of the area was decreased in height. The torque curve for the BL3 class in Fig. 3a showed a rapid rise in torque in the form of a tapered area in the initial area immediately after implantation and in a subsequent parallel area. When the length of the implant varied among 8, 10, and 12 mm, only the length of the parallel area changed, and the initial area and tapered area had almost the same form. For the TE, the lower part of the implant was parallel and the lateral surface and axial surface had the same taper in the cervical region. TE10 in Fig. 4a showed a torque curve with a similar form to BL10 in Fig. 3 and had three kinds of areas. The torque curves for MK3 and MK4 in Fig. 4a had an area in which the torque finally rose suddenly after reaching its critical point and became moderate. This was distinguished from the tapered areas of BL and TE and assumed to be a platform area. MK4 had a gentle taper on the entire axial surface and platform. The platform area, shown in ④, was seen at the end of the torque curve in Fig. 5a, and its torque value was the maximum value among the nine kinds evaluated in this study. In past reports, MK3 was parallel, similar to ST, and had a platform, similar to MK4, and a platform area was seen in the last part of the torque curve. In MK3, the platform area followed the initial area and parallel area, although it presented a final torque value of 4.3 N · cm in the parallel area and then rose further to 10.7 N · cm in the platform area.

### Removal torque

In the removal torque curve, the characteristics of the implant design were not clearly recognized, compared with the implant torque curve. In all implants, the torque rose suddenly immediately after removal was started and reached a peak value. The changes in torque from the peak value were classified into two types. For ST shown in Fig. 2b, the torque fell gently from the peak value. For BL, TE, MK3, and MK4 in Figs. 3b, 4b, and 5b, a sudden fall in torque was seen immediately after the peak value, and it then fell gently. Table 2 shows the maximal values for insertion torque value (IT) and RT obtained from the torque curves and the $p$ values obtained by significance tests for RT and IT. The RT for six kinds of implants (BL8, 10, 12, TE10, MK3, MK4) was smaller than the corresponding IT, with statistical significance ($p < 0.05$), while the RT for ST6, 8, and 10 was almost the same as or slightly greater than the corresponding IT.

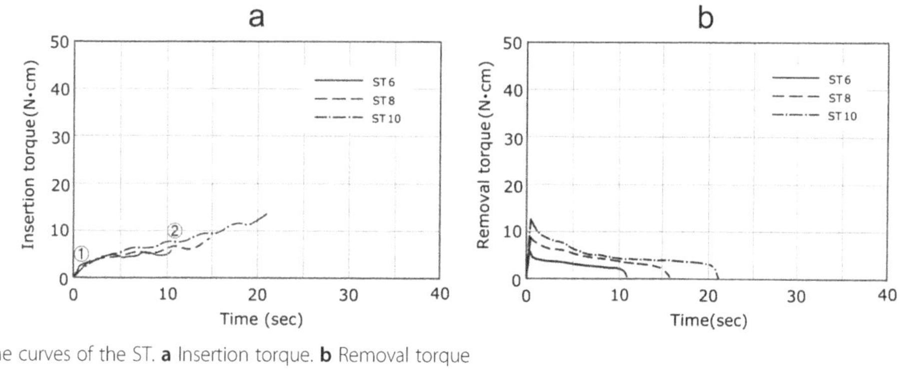


**Fig. 2** Torque-time curves of the ST. **a** Insertion torque. **b** Removal torque

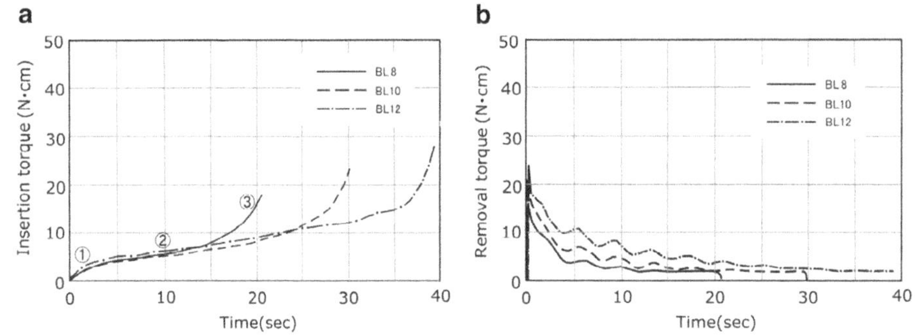


**Fig. 3** Torque-time curves of the BL. **a** Insertion torque. **b** Removal torque

### Torque rise rate

Table 3 shows the average torque rise obtained from the torque curve according to areas. The mean torque rise rate of the parallel area was the smallest at 0.36 N · cm/s and differed significantly from those of the other areas ($p < 0.05$). Specifically, the rates were 2.14, 2.33, and 2.65 N · cm/s for the initial area, tapered area, and platform area, respectively, and greater than those of the parallel area by 6–7 times, although significant differences were not recognized among the mean values of these three areas.

## Discussion

### Insertion torque curve

In 2000, O'Sullivan reported torque curves for a prosthetic implant for the first time, and evaluated the characteristics of the tapered type by torque curves obtained by inserting five kinds of implants into the maxillary bone of unembalmed human cadavers. In a subsequent review, Meredith [25] cited six kinds of torque curves when the final osteotomy diameter was changed and described that a torque curve rose more markedly with a thinner implant cavity. In 2011, Kim et al. [26] compared a case with a self-tapping blade and a case without a self-tapping blade using their torque curves with artificial bone. In 2012, Park et al. [27] obtained the maximum insertion torque, angular momentum, and total insertion energy by torque curves, although quantitative analyses on whether torque curves were correlated with implant designs were not conducted. Furthermore, most conventional studies on torque have focused on measurement [28–31] of the maximum torque value and/or RT at the time of IT or the relationship between the RFA value and IT and/or RT [6, 13, 16, 18, 32]. The present study was not limited to measurements of IT and RT, as the characteristics of the torque curves were divided into four areas designated as the initial, parallel, tapered, and platform areas, and quantitative analyses were performed for each area. For the initial area, a rapid rise in torque occurring immediately after insertion for 1–2 s was observed, and torque value rises of 1.43–2.26 N · cm were also recognized. This reflects torque generated by the implant placed at the predetermined position on the prepared hole rotating and rubbing with the artificial bone with the load of 500 g, and it is presumed that the rapid rise in the initial area was a phenomenon when the thread ridge was inserted into the artificial bone. This indicates that the friction at the time of rotating and pressing is greater than that at the time of rotating and cutting the bones with a tap and is a reasonable result. In the parallel area, the torque curve was a line with a moderate gradient, and the torque rise rate obtained from the gradient of the line was

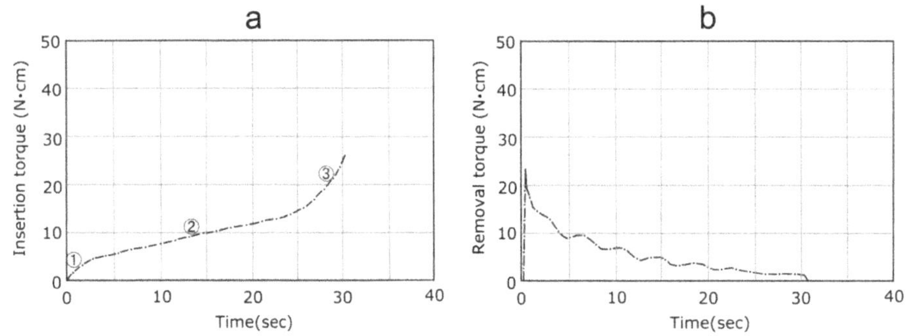


**Fig. 4** Torque-time curves of the TE. **a** Insertion torque. **b** Removal torque

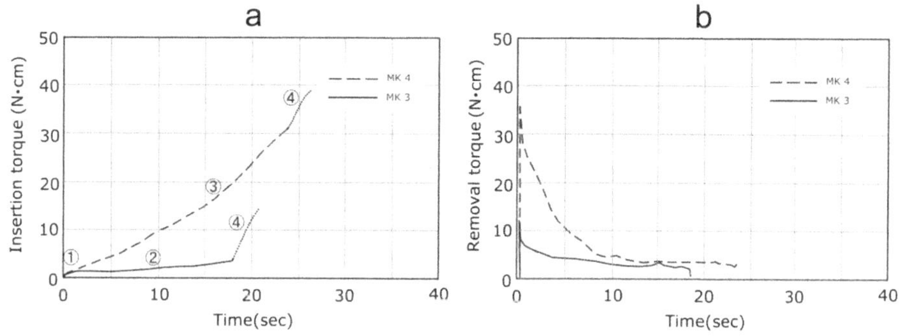


**Fig. 5** Torque-time curves of the MK3 and MK4. **a** Insertion torque. **b** Removal torque

0.36 N · cm/s. From this, it is estimated that the torque increase when one revolution is added to the parallel thread is about 1.44 N · cm. The preceding thread goes forward and spreads out the bones consistently, and the following thread of the same size does not cause new torque at the time of plastic deformation, and it is therefore presumed that the torque rise in the parallel area is moderate. In the tapered area, the torque curve presented a quadratic curve steadily, the torque rise rate was 2.33 N · cm/s, and the torque increase when one revolution was added was as great as 9.32 N · cm. From this, it is supposed that an increase in the tapered thread is an effective method to increase the torque efficiently. In the tapered area, the diameters of the following threads continued to increase consistently, plastic deformation was caused in all threads in the tapered area, and a torque curve in which the torque continued to increase was produced as a result. It is supposed that the first rapid rise in the platform area was observed when the platform bottom compressed the artificial bone and that stress relaxation of the artificial bone made it more moderate subsequently. The torque rise rate by the platform was 2.65 N · cm/s, which was greater than that of the tapered area.

#### Removal torque curve

There have been reports on the removal torque curve of a prosthetic implant. Although the removal torque curves measured in the present study had similar shapes to one another, they were divided into two groups upon detailed observation, comprising a group of ST with parallel only, and a group of BL, TE, MK3, and MK4 having tapers and platforms. Since the thread contacts the artificial bone sequentially at the time of insertion, the torque curves showed the characteristics of each area. At the time of removal, since all threads come in contact with the artificial bone at first, the torque curve did not present the characteristics of the design until it reached the peak value. However, it is estimated that when the thread begins to move subsequently, the difference in design of each area appeared in the torque curve. It seems that the change in torque after reaching the peak value at the time of removal is important information for predicting the influence of the change in primary stability occurring through instant load and the early load on secondary stability. The torque value that instantly decreased with a tapered implant was as small as 4–7 N · cm, and it is necessary to study this further in the future.

**Table 2** Insertion torque value and removal torque value

| Code | Insertion torque (N · cm) | Removal torque (N · cm) | Effective thread length (ETL) (×π mm) |
|---|---|---|---|
| ST6 | 6.19 ± 0.716 | 5.95 ± 0.718 | 11.53 |
| ST8 | 8.06 ± 1.038 | 9.09 ± 1.093 | 15.11 |
| ST10 | 13.13 ± 1.763 | 12.37 ± 1.746 | 21.48 |
| BL8 | 17.67 ± 1.290 | 16.67 ± 2.140 | 20.88 |
| BL10 | 23.56 ± 1.628 | 21.99 ± 1.530 | 31.00 |
| BL12 | 26.66 ± 3.897 | 24.40 ± 2.298 | 39.96 |
| TE10 | 25.17 ± 2.374 | 23.76 ± 2.027 | 31.11 |
| MK3 | 16.03 ± 0.516 | 10.30 ± 0.708 | 39.38 |
| MK4 | 39.35 ± 0.494 | 34.31 ± 0502 | 54.81 |
| | | | ±:SD |

**Table 3** Torque rise rate of the each area (N · cm/s)

| | Initial area | Parallel area | Tapered area | Platform area |
|---|---|---|---|---|
| ST6 | 1.42 ± 0.43 | 0.31 ± 0.14 | – | – |
| ST8 | 3.57 ± 1.62 | 0.35 ± 0.09 | – | – |
| ST10 | 2.49 ± 0.81 | 0.45 ± 0.05 | – | – |
| BL8 | 2.16 ± 0.21 | 0.50 ± 0.08 | 2.32 ± 0.52 | – |
| BL10 | 1.96 ± 0.49 | 0.35+0.04 | 2.45+0.23 | – |
| BL12 | 1.82 ± 0.27 | 0.33 ± 0.02 | 3.41 ± 0.64 | – |
| TE10 | 2.37 ± 0.42 | 0.44 ± 0.05 | 2.30 ± 0.29 | – |
| MK3 | 2.16 ± 0.28 | 0.15 ± 0.02 | – | 3.33 ± 0.85 |
| MK4 | 2.00 ± 0.00 | – | 1.30 ± 0.02 | 2.44 ± 0.09 |
| Average | 2.22 ± 0.60 | 0.36 ± 0.18 | 2.36 ± 0.75 | 2.89 ± 0.63 |
| | | | | ±:SD |

### Comparison between IT and RT

The purpose of measuring and evaluating RT in the present study was to clarify whether the implant stability evaluated by IT can be guaranteed even immediately after insertion. In this study, RT was smaller than IT in the implants having tapered and/or platform areas and a significant difference was recognized, while in the design with only a parallel area, no significant difference was seen between IT and RT or RT was slightly greater than IT. Previous studies that measured both IT and RT include those using artificial bone [19, 33], human bone [6, 16, 34], and animal bones [35, 36]. Among such studies, IT and RT were small in those using artificial bone, and RT was smaller than IT. Therefore, using IT to assess the primary stability of an implant revealed the need for certain adjustments.

### Influence of cortical bone

The reason why a simulation test for only cancellous bone without cortical bone was performed in the present study has already been described. It was reported that bone density and the ratio of cortical bone and cancellous bone have influence on the primary stability of an implant and that higher primary stability is achieved with thread, even at the slightest level, binding to cortical bone rather than being surrounded by only cancellous bones [32]. Therefore, it is expected that torque will rise at the end of the torque curve in the cortical bone region and that the torque will further grow by a synergistic effect with factors that increase the torque, such as a taper or platform of an implant. In the simulation experiments in this study, quantitative measurements were successfully performed by extracting only the effects of implant designs and by using a uniform pseudo bone without cortical bones. Sufficient torque is needed for primary stability of an implant, although the risk that excessive compressive force acts on the bone to cause bone resorption and further bone necrosis has been pointed out [37, 38]. To avoid such a situation, it is necessary to find a balance between local bone resorption and the torque, and Meredith [25] recommended insertion torque values of 25–30 N · cm. The torque value and torque rising rate according to the design of implant bodies obtained in the present study enabled estimation of the part of bones generating retention and identification of the part giving compressive force to bones. This will allow us to clarify the relationships among the design of an implant, the value of the torque generated by the implant, and the compressive force to the bones.

## Conclusions

In the torque-duration curve at the time of insertion, the characteristics of the implant design are well shown. It is presented as a straight line with a moderate gradient in the parallel thread area, a quadratic curve-like curve in the tapered area, and a hyperbola-like curve in the platform area. The torque rise rate was 2.14 N · cm/s for the initial area, 0.36 for the parallel area, 2.33 for the tapered area, and 2.65 for the platform area. The torque-duration curves at the time of removal were classified into tapered implants with the peak magnitude as the maximum torque value and straight implants with a maximum torque value greater than the peak magnitude. The RT of the implants having tapered or platform areas was significantly smaller than the corresponding IT, while the RT of the straight implants was the same as or slightly greater than the corresponding IT.

#### Abbreviations

BL: Bone Level RC; IT: insertion torque value; MK3: Brånemark MKIII; MK4: Brånemark MKIV; RT: removal torque value; ST: Standard RN; TE: Tapered Effect RN.

#### Competing interests

Dr. Yamaguchi reports grants from The Ministry of Education, Culture, Sports, Science and Technology, JSPS KAKENHI Grant Number 217919, non-financial support from Straumann LLC, during the conduct of the study. The other authors declare that they have no competing interests.

#### Authors' contributions

YY participated in the sequence alignment concept/design, data collection, and data analysis and drafted the manuscript. MS conceived of the study, participated in its design and coordination, and helped draft the manuscript. MM participated in the data collection and performed the statistical analysis. SK participated in the design of the study. MO participated in the critical revision of the article. All authors read and approved the final manuscript.

#### Acknowledgements

The authors thank the Vectrix Corporation for the technical knowledge of the torque analyzer and Straumann LLC for donating the implants used in this research. This study was supported by JSPS KAKENHI Grant Number 217919, The Ministry of Education, Culture, Sports, Science and Technology.

#### Author details

[1]Department of Implant Dentistry, Showa University School of Dentistry, 2-1-1 Kitasenzoku Ota-ku, Tokyo 145-8515, Japan. [2]Oral Implantology and Regenerative Dental Medicine, Department of Masticatory Function Rehabilitation, Division of Oral Health Sciences, Graduate School, Tokyo Medical and Dental University, 1-5-45 Yushima, Bunkyo-ku, Tokyo 113-8510, Japan. [3]Oral Implantology Department of Prosthodontic Dentistry for Function of TMJ and Occlusion, Kanagawa Dental University, 82, Inaokachou, Yokosuka-shi, Kanagawa 238-8580, Japan.

#### References

1. Friberg B, Sennerby L, Roos J, Johansson P, Strid CG, Lekholm U. Evaluation of bone density using cutting resistance measurements and microradiography. An *in vitro* study in pig ribs. Clin Oral Implants Res. 1995;6:164–71.
2. Chiapasco M, Gatti C, Rossi E, Haeflige W, Markwaldel TH. Implant-retained mandibular overdentures with immediate loading: a retrospective multicenter study on 226 consecutive cases. Clin Oral Implants Res. 1997;8:48–57.
3. Javed F, Romanos GE. The role of primary stability for successful immediate loading of dental implants. A literature review. J Dent. 2010;38:612–20.
4. Lekholm U, Zarb GA. Patient Selection and Preparation. In: Brånemark P-I, Zarb GA, Albrektsson T, editors. Tissue integrated prostheses: osseointegration in clinical dentistry. Chicago: Quintessence Publishing Co. Inc; 1985. p. 199–209.

5. Devlin H, Horner K, Ledgerton D. A comparison of maxillary and mandibular bone mineral densities. J Prosthet Dent. 1998;79:323–7.
6. O'Sullivan D, Sennerby L, Meredith N. Measurements comparing the initial stability of five designs of dental implants: a human cadaver study. Clin Implant Dent Relat Res. 2000;2:85–92.
7. Ochi S, Morris HF, Winkler S. The influence of implant type, material, coating, diameter, and length on periotest values at second-stage surgery: DICRG interim report no.4. Dental Implant Clinical Research Group. Implant Dent. 1994;3:159–62.
8. Winkler S, Morris HF, Ochi S. Implant survival to 36 months as related to length and diameter. Ann Periodontol. 2000;5:22–31.
9. Steigenga JT, Al-Shammari KF, Nociti FH, Misch CE, Wang HL. Dental implant design and its relationship to long-term implant success. Implant Dent. 2003;12:306–17.
10. Baggi L, Cappelloni I, Di Girolamo M, Maceri F, Vairo G. The influence of implant diameter and length on stress distribution of osseointegrated implants related to crestal bone geometry: a three-dimensional finite element analysis. J Prosthet Dent. 2008;6:422–31.
11. Orsini E, Giavaresi G, Trire A, Ottani V, Salgarello S. Dental implant thread pitch and its influence on the osseointegration process: an in vivo comparison study. Int J Maxillofac Implants. 2010;2:383–92.
12. Romanos GE, Ciornei G, Jucan A, Malmstrom H, Gupta B. In vitro assessment of primary stability of Straumann implant designs. Clin Implant Dent Relat Res. 2012;16:89–95.
13. Toyoshima T, Wagner W, Klein MO, Stender E, Wieland M, Al-Nawas B. Primary stability of a hybrid self-tapping implant compared to a cylindrical non-self-tapping implant with respect to drilling protocols in an ex vivo model. Clin Implant Dent Relat Res. 2011;13:71–8.
14. O'Sullivan D, Sennerby L, Jagger D, Meredith N. A comparison of two methods of enhancing implant primary stability. Clin Implant Dent Relat Res. 2004;6:48–57.
15. O'Sullivan D, Sennerby L, Meredith M. Influence of implant taper on the primary and secondary stability of osseointegrated titanium implants. Clin Oral Implants Res. 2004;15:474–80.
16. Akkocaoglu M, Uysal S, Tekdemir I, Akca K, Cehreli MC. Implant design and intraosseous stability of immediately placed implants: a human cadaver study. Clin Oral Impl Res. 2005;16:202–9.
17. Chong L, Khocht A, Suzuki JB, Gaughan J. Effect of implant design on initial stability of tapered implants. J Oral Implantol. 2009;3:130–5.
18. Meredith N. Assessment of implant stability as a prognostic determinant. Int J Prosthodont. 1998;11:491–501.
19. Olive J, Aparicio C. Periotest method as a measure of osseointegrated oral implant stability. Int J Oral Maxillofac Implants. 1990;5:390–400.
20. Teerlinck J, Quirynen M, Darius P, van Steenberghe D. Periotest: an objective clinical diagnosis of bone apposition toward implants. Int J Oral Maxillofac Implants. 1991;6:55–61.
21. Meredith N, Alleyne D, Cawley P. Quantitative determination of the stability of the implant-tissue interface using resonance frequency analysis. Clin Oral Implants Res. 1996;7:261–7.
22. Johansson P, Strid K. Assessment of bone quality from cutting resistance during implant surgery. J Prothodont. 1998;9:491–501.
23. Roberts WE, Smith RK, Zilberman Y, Mozsary PG, Smith RS. Osseous adaptation to continuous loading of rigid endosseous implants. Am J Orthod. 1984;86:95–111.
24. Doe J. Sawbone block 20 PCF. 2014. www.sawbones.com. Accessed 8 Dec 2014.
25. Meredith N. A review of implant design, geometry and placement. Appl Osseointegrantion Res. 2008;6:8–12.
26. Kim DR, Lim YJ, Kim MJ, Kwon HB, Kim SH. Self-cutting blades and their influence on primary stability of tapered dental implants in a simulated low-density bone model: a laboratory study. Oral Surg Oral Med Oral Pathol Oral Radiol Endo. 2011;112:573–80.
27. Park KJ, Kwon JY, Kim SK, Heo SJ, Koak JY, Lee JH, et al. The relationship between implant stability quotient values and implant insertion variables: a clinical study. J Oral Rehabil. 2012;39:151–9.
28. Ueda M, Matsuki M, Jacobsson M, Tjellstrom A. Relationship between insertion torque and removal torque analyzed in fresh temporal bone. Int J Oral Maxillofac Implants. 1991;6:442–7.
29. Niimi A, Ozeki K, Ueda M, Nakayama B. A comparative study of removal torque of endosseous implants in the fibula, iliac crest and scapula of cadavers: preliminary report. Clin Oral Implants Res. 1997;8:286–9.
30. Simon H, Caputo AA. Removal torque of immediately loaded transitional endosseous implants in human subjects. Int J Oral Maxillofac Implants. 2002;17:839–45.
31. Marin C, Granato R, Suzuki M, Gil JN, Piattelli A, Coelho G. Removal torque and histomorphometric evaluation of bioceramic grit-blasted/acid-etched and dual acid-etched implant surfaces: an experimental study in dogs. J Periodontol. 2008;79:1942–9.
32. Ahn SJ, Leesungbok R, Lee SW, Heo YK, Kang KL. Differences in implant stability associated with various methods of preparation of the implant bed: an in vitro study. J Prosthetic Dent. 2012;107:366–72.
33. Blickford JH. An introduction to the design and behavior of bolted joints. New York: Marcel Dekker Inc; 1995. p. 213.
34. Shalabi MM, Wolke JGC, Jansen JA. The effects of implant surface roughness and surgical technique on implant fixation in an in vitro model. Clin Oral Implants Res. 2006;17:172–8.
35. Sakoh J, Wahlmann U, Stender E, Nat R, Al-Nawas B, Wagner W. Primary stability of a conical implant and a hybrid, cylindric screw-type implant in vitro. Int J Oral Maxillofac Implants. 2006;21:560–6.
36. Tabassum A, Meijer GJ, Wolke JGC, Jansen JA. Influence of the surgical technique and surface roughness on the primary stability of an implant in artificial bone with a density equivalent to maxillary bone: a laboratory study. Clin Oral Implants Res. 2009;20:327–32.
37. Atsumi M, Park SH, Wang HL. Methods used to assess implant stability: current status. Int J Oral Maxillofac Implants. 2007;22:743–54.
38. Duyck J, Renold HJ, Van Oosterwyck H, Naert I, Vander Sloten J, Ellingsen JE. The influence of static and dynamic loading on marginal bone reactions around osseointegrated implants: an animal experimental study. Clin Oral Implants Res. 2001;12:207–18.

# The fracture strength by a torsion test at the implant-abutment interface

Fumihiko Watanabe[1*], Kazuhiko Hiroyasu[2] and Kazuhiko Ueda[2]


## Abstract

**Background:** Fractured connections between implants and implant abutments or abutment screws are frequently encountered in a clinical setting. The purpose of this study was to investigate fracture strength using a torsion test at the interface between the implant and the abutment.

**Methods:** Thirty screw-type implant with diameters of 3.3, 3.8, 4.3, 5.0, and 6.0 mm were submitted to a torsion test. Implants of each size were connected to abutments with abutment screws tightened to 20 N · cm. Mechanical stress was applied with a rotational speed of 3.6 °/min until fracture occurred, and maximum torque (fracture torque) and torsional yield strength were measured. The mean values were calculated and then compared using Tukey's test. The abutments were then removed, and the implant-abutment interfaces were examined using a scanning electron microscope (SEM).

**Result:** No significant differences in mean fracture torque were found among 3.3, 3.8, and 4.3 mm-diameter implants, but significant differences were found between these sizes and 5.0 and 6.0 mm-diameter implants ($p < 0.01$). Concerning mean torsional yield strength, significant differences were found between 3.3, 3.8, and 4.3 mm-diameter and 5.0 and 6.0 mm-diameter implants ($p < 0.01$). Observations under the SEM showed that all the projections of the abutment corresponding to the internal notches of the implant body had been destroyed.

**Conclusions:** Smaller diameter implants demonstrated lower fracture torque and torsional yield strength than implants with larger diameters. In internal tube-in-tube connections, three abutment projections corresponding to rotation-prevention notches were destroyed in each implant.


**Keywords:** Torsion test; Implant-abutment interface; Abutment connection deformation; Torque; Mechanical load

## Background

A single-tooth osseointegrated implant is composed of an implant body, an abutment, an abutment screw, and an artificial crown. The implant and abutment are typically connected by an abutment screw. The degree of mechanical integrity at the implant-abutment interface depends on screw preload, abutment connection design, the fitness of all components, and dynamic loading conditions. Fractures of the internal or external connection between implants and implant abutments or abutment screws are encountered in the clinical setting [1–3]. Fractures may occur as a result of excessive axial forces (bending moments), horizontal loading, or rotational torque during functional activities such as chewing or parafunctional activities such as grinding and clenching. Several studies [4, 5] have evaluated implant-abutment assemblies in dynamic cyclic fatigue testing according to ISO 14801 [6]. However, evaluation of the strength of the implant-abutment assembly has not been reported when subjected to torsion testing. Test methods and standard vales have not yet been established for such torsion testing of implant-abutment assemblies. Abutment connections are principally classified as either internal or external types and are available in a variety of designs, including hexagonal, octagonal, cone screw, cone hex, cylinder hex, spline, cam, cam tube, and pin/slot. Implants incorporate features for rotation-prevention at the implant-abutment interface. The advantages and disadvantages of various types of implant-abutment connections have been discussed in several studies [7–11]. Norton

* Correspondence: fumi@ngt.ndu.ac.jp
[1]Department of Crown and Bridge Prosthodontics, School of Life Dentistry at Niigata, The Nippon Dental University, 951-8580 1-8 Hamaura-cho, Chuo-ku, Niigata, Japan
Full list of author information is available at the end of the article

reported that internal implant-abutment interface connections have higher bending moment resistance than external connections [10]. Presently, although more than 200 kinds of implant systems are available on the market, most manufacturers do not provide specific data regarding system-specific implant-abutment connection design complications [12, 13]. In the oral cavity, implant restorations are exposed to vertical, horizontal, and rotational forces during chewing. The maximum torsional strength and proportional limited strength on crown and tooth restoration materials were measured, and the values were compared with a mechanical bending and pull test value [14].

The purpose of this in vitro study was to investigate fracture strength using a torsion test at the implant-abutment interface in order to assess the effect of torsion force on the connection.

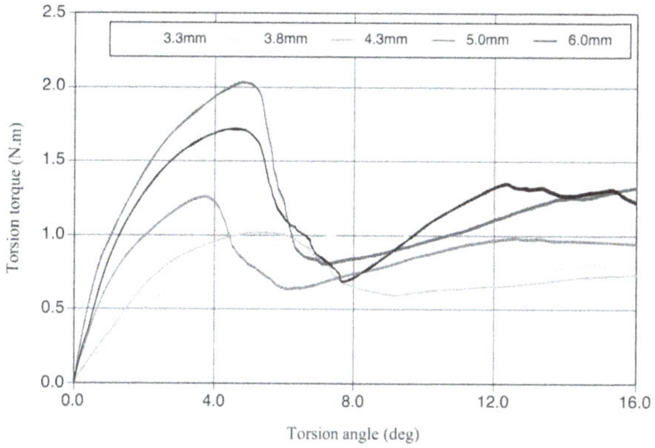


**Fig. 2** Torsional yield strength and maximum fracture torque strength of CAMLOG implant in each diameter

## Methods

Thirty titanium screw implants of five different diameters (3.3, 3.8, 4.3, 5.0, and 6.0 mm) with tube-in-tube implant-abutment connections (CAMLOG Biotechnologies, Wimsheim, Germany) were used as test specimens. Implants of each size were connected to abutments, and abutment screws were tightened to 20 N · cm using a digital torque meter (Hios HDM-5; Hios Inc, Chiba, Japan). A torsion testing device (AG-XR; Shimadzu, Kyoto, Japan) was used on all implant test specimens in this study (Fig. 1).

The specimens were mounted on the torsion testing device, and mechanical stress was applied with a rotational speed of 3.6 °/min until permanent deformation or fracture occurred. The maximum torque (fracture torque) and torsional yield strength were measured in each specimen. The mean values of measured data were calculated and compared using Tukey's test at 0.05 level of significance.

The specimens were then removed from the device and the abutments unscrewed, and the parts of the interface between the rotation-prevention structure of the implants and abutments were examined using a scanning electron microscope (SEM).

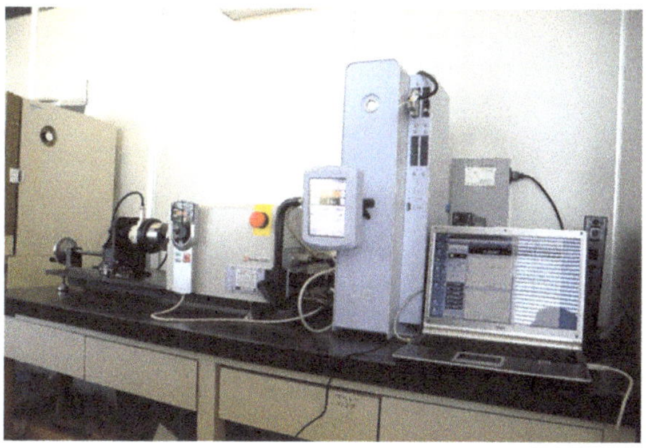

**Fig. 1** Torsion testing device

## Results

The relationship between torsional load and fracture occurrence followed a parabolic curve, and the maximum fracture torque and torsional yield strength of all sizes of implants were recorded (Fig. 2). The straight line of a primary curve in the initial phase represents the proportional limit. The transition point between the proportional straight line and the beginning of the curve is defined as the yield point and always occurs after plastic deformation. The mean values of these measured data are shown in Figs. 3 and 4. No significant differences in mean maximum fracture torque were found among 3.3, 3.8, and 4.3 mm-diameter implants, but significant differences were found between these sizes and 5.0 and 6.0 mm-diameter implants ($p < 0.01$). The mean torsional yield strengths demonstrated significant differences between 3.3, 3.8, and 4.3 mm-diameter and 5.0- and 6.0-mm-diameter implants ($p < 0.01$). The torsional fracture strength of the smaller diameter (3.3 and 3.8 mm) implants was markedly lower than that of the wider diameter implants. Observations under the SEM showed that all implan
t-abutment connections had been damaged. Specifically, the internal notches of the implant body remained intact, but all projections of abutment corresponding to internal notches had been destroyed (Fig. 5).

## Discussion

During the physiological function of chewing, or the non-physiological function of bruxism, compressive, bending, and torsional stresses are generated in teeth or prosthetics. These stress will cause the abutment screw loosening or fracture, fracture of the abutment, fracture of the implant, and the implant/abutment connection. The extent of the damage is influenced by the design of

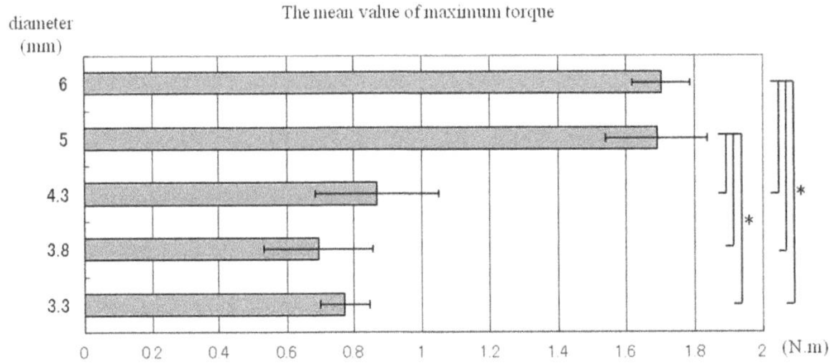


**Fig. 3** The mean value of maximum fracture torque strength

the prosthesis, the fit of the implant prosthesis, the implant inclination, and the loading force. In these circumstances, tolerable enough clinical implant/abutment joint strength is required and ISO 14801 is used as their fatigue strength test method. However, torsional stresses generated in the oral cavity should also be considered. For these reasons, this study was undertaken in order to compare the torsional strength required to deform the implant-abutment connection for various diameter implants. The mode of failure will be the future investigation to be resolved by observing the fractured surfaces. In all specimens tested in this study, the relationship between static torsional load and fracture occurrence followed a parabolic curve. The primary curve was determined to be the torsional torque under which plastic deformation occurred and subsequently proceeded, resulting in permanent deformation. The curves illustrated in Fig. 2 showed two patterns in all specimens. Smaller diameter (3.3 and 3.8 mm) implants fractured much easier and earlier at the implant-abutment interface. This load-displacement curve is similar to the result of statistic loading test that Huang HM et al. [5] reported.

Examining all SEM images of the implant-abutment connections, we found that although their anti-rotational notches had been destroyed, the corresponding internal grooves remained intact. When torsion was applied, the grooves, which are composed of grade 4 commercially pure titanium (CP-Ti), were compressed; however, the abutment interlocks, which are composed of a titanium alloy (Ti-6Al-4V), were completely sheared off. Although the tensile strength of the Ti-6Al-4V alloy is at least 2 % greater than that of CP-Ti, much more titanium is adjacent to the grooves, which are compressed and can therefore withstand the transmitted force. On the other hand, the interlocks contain less material and therefore shear off if the applied force is too high. Nagel et al. studied the implant-abutment connection of each of the Replace-Select and the CAMLOG implants using FEM and reported that each design was very similar [15]. When comparing each system, they reported that the Replace-Select implant may fail by fracture of the implant body at the thinnest part of the wall. This thin portion represents the internal design that prevents the implant-abutment from rotating.

For comparison between the mechanical strength of CP-Ti screw implants with internal tube-in-tube implant-abutment connections and that of external hexagonal-type connections, all abutments and CP-Ti implants with external hexagonal-type connections were heavily damaged or destroyed in all phases of loading. A typical fracture

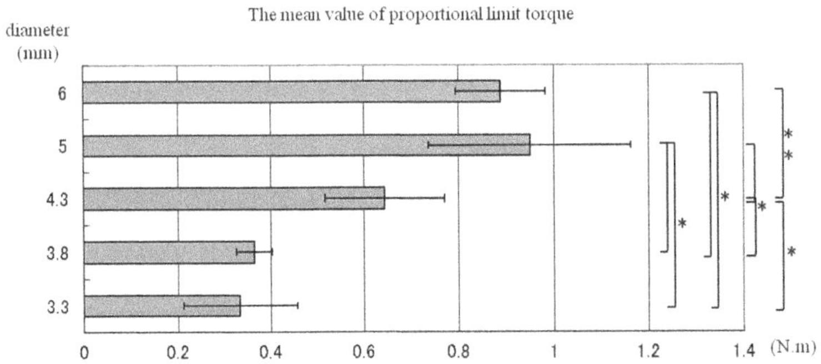


**Fig. 4** The mean value of torsional yield strength

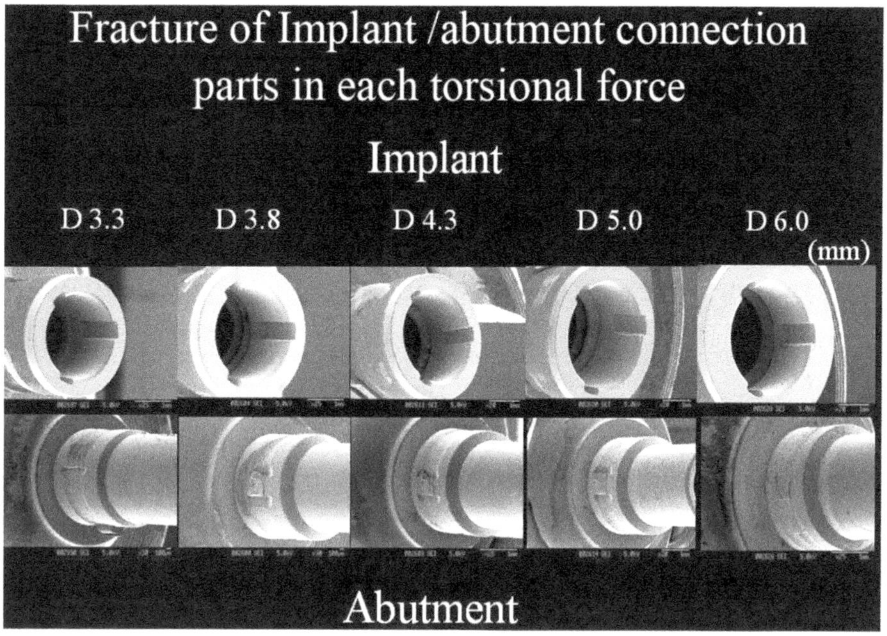


**Fig. 5** SEM picture of CAMLOG implant after torsion test

curve for CP-Ti implants with external connections is shown. The proportional limit and a parabola-like curve with eternal destruction were drawn. Torsion forces of 0.25, 0.50, 0.75, 1.00, 1.25, and 1.50 N · m were applied to the external CP-Ti implants. Deformation occurred in both the implant and the abutment at each torsion force (Fig. 6). This might have been the result of the abutment connection design or the physical properties of the implant materials. In addition, the deformation effect on the torsional yield strength of the implants and abutments is worth noting, as deformation occurred immediately before torsion fracture in all specimens.

Balfour and O'Brien tested the following three kinds of implants for maximum anti-rotational stability: external hexagon-type 0.7 mm-diameter CP-Ti implants, internal octagon-type 0.6 mm-diameter Ti-6Al-4V

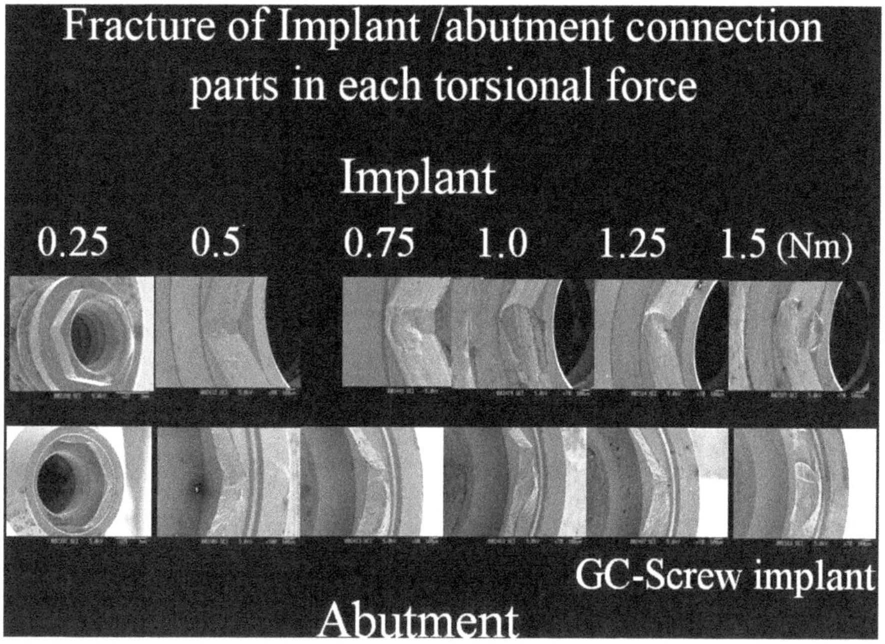


**Fig. 6** SEM picture of implant with external hexagonal connection

implants, and internal hexagon-type 1.7 mm-diameter Ti-6Al-4V implants and abutments [16]. Testing comprised rigidly fixing a calibrated torque gauge to the abutment sleeve and applying torque until failure of the components was apparent. The torques necessary to separate the single-tooth abutments from the implants were 8.7 in.-lb (98.3 N · cm) for the external hexagon-type, 3.3 in.-lb (37.3 N · cm) for the internal octagon-type, and 10.0 in.-lb (192.1 N · cm) for the internal hexagon-type. In the internal octagon and internal hexagon designs, failure was limited to the abutment connections. The Balfour and O'Brien result differed from those reported in this study (4.3 and 3.8 mm diameters, 87 and 70 N · cm, respectively). The results from this study confirmed that the torsional strengths were different depending on the connection dimensions as reported by Balfour and O'Brien. CAMLOG implants (5 and 6 mm diameter) achieved higher torsional strength than 4.3, 3.8, and 3.3 mm diameter. This resulted from a combination of increased implant diameter and thickness of the implant walls.

## Conclusions

The forces that led to permanent deformation of the abutment connections were dependent on the implant diameter. The differences between the implants used in this study were obvious, both macroscopically and microscopically. Significantly less force was needed to fracture smaller than larger diameter implants. Furthermore, in the CAMLOG implants only, abutment projections corresponding to anti-rotational notches were destroyed, which could have been due to differences in the strength and tensile properties of the materials.

#### Competing interests

Fumihiko Watanabe, Kazuhiko Hiroyasu, Kazuhiko Ueda declare that they have no competing interests.

#### Authors' contributions

FW contributed to conception, design, data acquisition, analysis, and interpretation, drafted the manuscript, and critically revised the manuscript; KH contributed to data analysis and interpretation and critically revised the manuscript; KU contributed to data acquisition and analysis and critically revised the manuscript. All authors gave final approval and agree to be accountable for all aspects of the work.

#### Acknowledgements

The authors are grateful to the CAMLOG foundation for providing dental implants for the experiments. The authors declare no potential conflicts of interest with respect to the authorship and/or publication of this article.

#### Author details

[1]Department of Crown and Bridge Prosthodontics, School of Life Dentistry at Niigata, The Nippon Dental University, 951-8580 1-8 Hamaura-cho, Chuo-ku, Niigata, Japan. [2]Oral Implant Care Unit Niigata Hospital, The Nippon Dental University, 1-8 Hamaura-cho, Chuo-ku, Niigata, Japan.

#### References

1. Goodacre CJ, Kan JK, Rungcharassaeng K. Clinical complications of osseointegrated implants. J Prosthet Dent. 1999;81(5):537–52.
2. Pjetursson BE, Tan K, Lang NP, Bragger U, Egger M, Zwahlen M. A systematic review of the survival and complication rates of fixed partial denture (FPDs) after an observation period of at least 5 years. Clin Oral Implants Res. 2004;15(6):625–42.
3. Schwarz MS. Mechanical complications of dental implants. Clin Oral Implants Res. 2000;11 Suppl 1:156–8.
4. Dittmer MP, Dittmer S, Borcher L, Kohorst P, Stiesch M. Influence of the interface design on the yield force of the implant-abutment complex before and after cyclic mechanical loading. J Prosthodont Res. 2012;56(1):19–24.
5. Huang HM, Tsai CM, Chang CC, Lin CT, Lee SY. Evaluation of loading conditions on fatigue-failed implants by fracture surface analysis. J Oral Maxillofac Implants. 2005;20(6):854–9.
6. ISO/DIS 14801 Dentistry-Implant-Dynamic fatigue test for endosseous dental implants.
7. Sailer I, Sailer T, Stawarczyk B, Jung RE, Hammerle CH. In vitro study of the influence of the type of connection on the fracture load of zirconia abutments with internal and external implant-abutment connections. Int J Oral Maxillofac Implants. 2009;24(5):850–8.
8. Coppedê AR, Bersani E, de Mattos Mda G, Rodrigues RS, Sartori IA, Ribeiro RF. Fracture resistance of the implant-abutment connection in implants with internal hex and internal conical connections under oblique compressive loading: an in vitro study. Int J Prosthodont. 2009;22(3):283–6.
9. Pedroza JE, Torrealba Y, Elias A, Psoter W. Comparison of the compressive strength of 3 different implant design systems. J Oral Implantol. 2007;33(1):1–7.
10. Norton MR. An in vitro evaluation of the strength of an internal conical interface compared to a butt joint interface in implant design. Clin Oral Implants Res. 1997;8(4):290–8.
11. Möllersten L, Lockowandt P, Linden LA. Comparison of strength and failure mode of seven implant systems: an in vitro test. J Prosthet Dent. 1997;78(6):582–91.
12. Eckert SE, Parein A, Myshin HL, Padilla JL. Validation of dental implant systems through a review of literature supplied by system manufacturers. J Prosthet Dent. 1997;77(3):271–9.
13. Eckert SE, Choi YG, Sanchez AR, Koka S. Comparison of dental implant systems: quality of clinical evidence and prediction of 5-year survival. Int J Oral Maxillofac Implants. 2005;20(3):406–15.
14. Seto M, Watanabe F. Torsion test of material for dental restoration. (in Japanese) J J Dent Mater. 2014;33(4):313–20.
15. Nagel RAK, Merkle H, Muller-Srorz H, Kirsch A, Sager D. Lateral load and torsion behavior of new internal abutment connections. Toronto: Presented at the 16th Annual Meeting of the Academy of Osseointegration; 2001.
16. Balfour A, O'Brien GR. Comparative study of antirotational single tooth abutments. J Prosthet Dent. 1995;73(1):36–43.

# Soft-tissue grafting for peri-implantitis—a treatment option in case of unsuitable skeletal basic morphology of the alveolar bone and lack of keratinized mucosa: a retrospective clinical cohort study

Michael Stiller[1,6], Rainer Mengel[2], Sebastian Becher[3], Bernhard Brinkmann[4], Barbara Peleska[2] and Esther Kluk[5,6*]

**Abstract**

**Background:** This retrospective study evaluated soft-tissue grafting as a surgical treatment option for peri-implantitis in case of unsuitable basic skeletal morphology of the alveolar bone and lack of keratinized mucosa.

**Methods:** Twenty-eight patients (21 females, 7 males, at a mean age 59.4 years) were included with a total of 54 implants. All implants showed peri-implantitis and attached keratinized buccal mucosa of ≤2 mm. A surgical procedure of soft-tissue grafting (STG) was made by inserting an inlay and inlay-onlay transplant. Clinical investigations were made prior to the STG (baseline) and after 9–180 months (Ø 43 months) including the following parameters: soft-tissue biotype, skeletal basic morphology of the alveolar bone, width of the peri-implant keratinized mucosa (KM), mobility of the KM, pocket probing depth (PPD), and bleeding on probing (BOP).

**Results:** Nearly all patients showed a thin soft-tissue biotype. The analysis of the skeletal basic morphology of the alveolar bone revealed a narrow apical base in 18 patients, middle base in 7 patients, and broad base in 3 patients. Width of the KM increased significantly ($p < 0.01$) from 0.4 ± 0,5 mm to 4.3 ± 1.5 mm after STG and PPD was significantly ($p < 0{,}01$) reduced from 6.3 ± 2,3 mm to 4.1 ± 1.9 mm. A significant reduction ($p < 0.01$) in BOP was recorded. All patients reported a clinical improvement of the inflammatory symptoms at follow-up.

**Conclusions:** The results of this study showed that the STG can be applied successfully as a surgical treatment of peri-implantitis. It remains unclear whether soft-tissue biotype or the skeletal basic morphology of the alveolar bone affects the outcome of this surgical treatment.

**Keywords:** Peri-implantitis treatment, Soft-tissue grafts, Apical skeletal basis, Keratinized mucosa

## Background

With an increasing number of patients with implant-supported dentures, dentists are increasingly confronted with diseases of the peri-implant hard and soft tissue [1].

Ten-year survival rates of about 95 % of dental implants were reported, but a high percentage of these implants showed peri-implantitis [2, 3]. In this case, the complications around the implant are so complex that the mechanic-physical, biological, chemical, and toxicological effects are often difficult to determine.

In addition to the etiologically relevant patient-related as well dentist-related factors of peri-implantitis, immunological foreign body response to the implant material was described [4].

The surgical and non-surgical treatment techniques are usually based on the peri-implant bone defect morphology [5, 6].

* Correspondence: kluk@implant-consult.de
[5]Department of Postgraduate Education - Master of Oral Implantology, Center for Oral and Maxillofacial Surgery, Johann Wolfgang Goethe University Frankfurt, Theodor-Stern-Kai 17, Frankfurt 60577, Germany
[6]Private Practice for Oral Surgery and Implantology, ECDI Center, Brahmsst. 11, 14193 Berlin, Germany
Full list of author information is available at the end of the article

Further, important anatomical factors such as the three-dimensional position of the implant and the resulting defect morphology in relation to the cephalometric basic pattern of the maxilla and the mandible remained unconsidered. The influence of the structural-biological factors with regard to the morphology of the peri-implant soft tissue remains also controversial [7].

Particularly, the quality and quantity of the peri-implant soft tissue affect significantly the dynamics of the marginal bone loss [8]. So that an adequate keratinized mucosa at the implant site leads to a reduced plaque accumulation, a reduced inflammatory mucosal infiltration, and a pro-inflammatory mediator release [9]. This was confirmed in an animal study of Benghazi et al., they showed in their study that in case of missed keratinized mucosa, bone resorption and prevalence of soft-tissue recession could be reduced through soft-tissue grafting [10].

The aim of this retrospective clinical cohort study is to evaluate the success of soft-tissue grafting (STG) as a surgical treatment of peri-implantitis in case of unsuitable skeletal basic morphology of the alveolar bone and the lack of keratinized mucosa. The null hypothesis of this study is that STG as an exclusive surgical treatment modality after initial treatment particularly in a case of thin skeletal basic morphology reduces clinical symptoms of peri-implantitis. In cases of an absence of the skeletal-related, three-dimensional defect, morphology in a relation to the implant position soft-tissue grafting seems to be the only reconstructive option. In such cases, STG allows recession of a peri-implant inflammatory process through stabilization of the peri-implant soft tissue.

## Methods

This study was conducted according to the guidelines of the ethics committee at the Johann Wolfgang Goethe University in Frankfurt/Main and strictly followed the ethical principles of the World Medical Association Declaration of Helsinki [11]. All patients were informed about the surgical procedure of this study and signed an informed consent.

### Patient population

The selection of the patients was made according to the data bank of the surgeon. All the patients were referred to a private clinic and to a department of oral surgery at the university. Patients who suffered from a peri-implantitis and were treated with STG were taken into consideration for this investigation. Patients were contacted by phone to ask for a participation in this study. From 62 patients, 28 agreed to participate in the study. The other 34 patients were either not available by phone or did not agree to participate in the study for personal reasons.

### Exclusion criteria

Patients with the following diseases were excluded from this study: untreated diabetes mellitus, pregnancy, bisphosphonate medication, current orthodontic treatment, tumors, and infectious diseases (HIV).

A total of 28 patients (21 females, 7 males, at a mean age 59.4 years) with a total of 54 implants were included. All patients were given a detailed description of the treatment procedures and were required to sign an informed consent form.

There was a total of 20 implants (13 in maxilla, 7 in mandible) in the anterior region (from canine to canine) and 34 implants (20 in maxilla, 14 in mandible) in the posterior region (up to the first premolar).

All implants suffered from peri-implantitis and showed attached keratinized buccal mucosa of ≤2 mm. The definition of peri-implantitis is according to established criteria defined when PPD (pocket probing depth) was >5 mm with or without BOP and with an annual bone loss of >0.2 mm [3]. The assessment of peri-implantitis was carried out 1 year after insertion of the superstructure in this study. The level of bone loss is according to the criteria of Albrektsson et al. [12] and the measurement of bleeding on probing according to the results of the study of Naert et al. [13].

To exclude falsification of a positive diagnosis of peri-implantitis in case of the absence of bleeding on probing in addition to excessive pocket probing depth patients' discomfort and pain were strict incoming criteria for STG.The following implant systems were used for a treatment before beginning of this retrospective study: 3 × Biomet 3i (Biomet 3i Deutschland GmbH, Munich, Germany), 31 × Ankylos (Dentsply IH GmbH, Mannheim, Germany), 1 × Astra Tech (Dentsply IH GmbH, Mannheim, Germany), 15 × Camlog (Camlog Vertriebs GmbH, Wimsheim, Germany), 3 × IMZ (Friadent, Mannheim, Germany), and 1 × Nobel Replace select (Nobel Biocare Holding AG, Zürich, Switzerland).

Three patients have bar overdentures (all in maxilla), three patients telescoping dentures (one in the maxilla and two in the mandible), and 22 patients fixed prosthesis; 8 of them have single crown restorations.

The average time from the placement of the implants to the soft-tissue grafting was 63.2 ± 44.4 months.

### Treatment procedures

#### *Non-surgical procedure*

A sub-mucosal ultrasonic curettage with ultrasonic system (Cavitron Ultrasonic scaler® with plastic Scalers, Dentsply, Mannheim, Germany) was made by all patients to reduce the inflammation signs as prerequisite before STG. Furthermore, an antibacterial treatment was made with a sub-mucosal irrigation using hydrogen peroxide 3 % and a local antibiotic application of doxycycline (Ligosan®, Heraeus Kulzer, Hanau, Germany).

If BOP was observed after this non-surgical therapy and during the following 6 months, a surgical treatment in terms of a soft-tissue grafting using onlay or inlay-onlay grafts with respect to the skeletal configuration was conducted. In case of persistent bleeding or other significant peri-implant inflammative symptoms, the protocol prevents, from the ethical point of view, further peri-implant bone loss, excessive antibiotic administration, and occurrence of systemic influence of the pathologic process. To increase comparability and measure reliability, all the baseline measurements used in the statistical analysis were strictly performed after initial phase. All surgical procedures were carried out by one surgeon from 1998–2012.

### Surgical procedure

The patient (Fig. 1) was anesthetized using (Ultracain® DS-forte, 1: 100,000, Sanofi-Aventis®, Frankfurt, Germany); then, a vestibular mucosal flap was raised with a preservation of a thin soft-tissue layer on the implant surface.

The thickness of the soft-tissue layer that remained on the implant surface was reduced as much as possible without perforating this layer or exposing the implant surface; for this procedure, microsurgical techniques were used in order to achieve immobility of the transplanted keratinized mucosa.

After decontamination of the exposed implant surfaces with 37 % phosphoric acid gel (Orbis Handels-GmbH, Münster, Germany), an onlay graft was inserted (Figs. 2 and 3). In cases with highly esthetic sensitive areas, an inlay-onlay graft was used, which had, in addition to the keratinized Onlay part, a sub-epithelial connective tissue part to about 50 % [14–16]. In contrast to inlay-onlay graft, an onlay graft consists only of keratinized mucosa with a thickness of approximately 1 mm harvested from palate as well.

The grafts were harvested from the palate in the region between the first premolars and second molars. The desire extension and shape of the graft was transferred with the help of a simple, tailored paper template before graft preparation from the palate, so that it fits exactly into the previously prepared peri-implant defect and thus accurately simulated the needed amount of keratinized mucosa. The appropriate connective tissue grafts were harvested by placing the template on the palate. The grafts' sizes were of 5–7 mm width and 7–20 mm length.

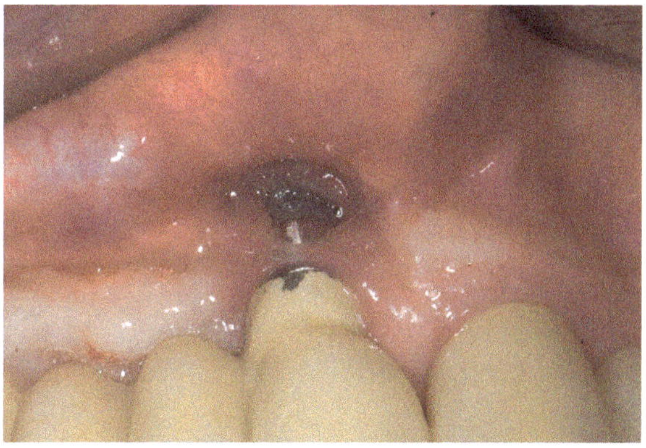

**Fig. 1** Patient 1: Buccal view of an implant regio 11. Implant (Camlog Vertriebs GmbH, Wimsheim, Germany, implant 10 years in situ) with buccal severe peri-implantitis. (8 mm PPD/pus+). Implant is partly exposed and its position is at the apical base. Reconstruction using bone grafting is therefore contraindicated. Patient (75 years old) refused explanation

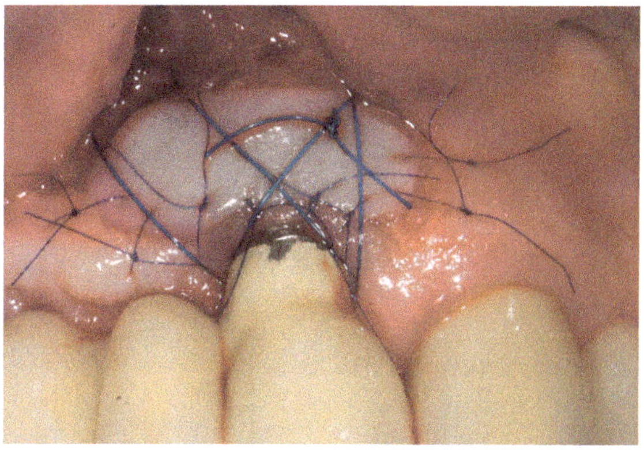

**Fig. 2** Intra-operative view after vestibulum-plasty and positioning of an onlay-transplant harvested from the palate. The coronal part of the graft was carefully fixed on the originally existing soft-tissue bridge, the apical part sits on the tissue that is denudated by vestibulum-plasty. Part of the exposed implant thread was covered directly by the graft. The graft was extended 5 mm mesially and 6 mm distally due to nutritive considerations, and it was fixed in the receptive site using suturing

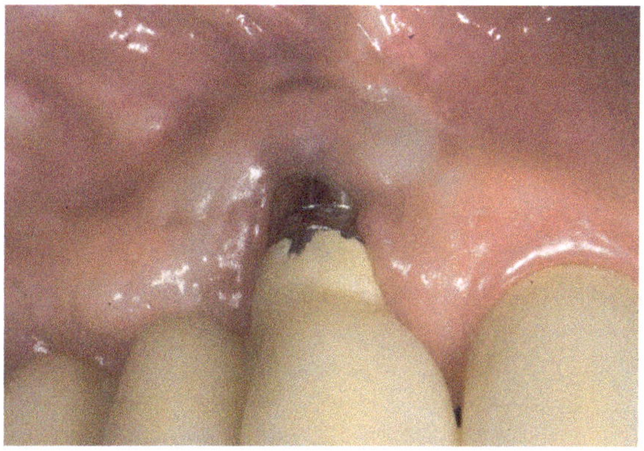

**Fig. 3** Implant 24 months after soft-tissue grafting. There is no sign of inflammation and a new mobile keratinized mucosa was built buccally, (4 mm PPD, Pu-/BOP-). Patient is symptom-free

The graft was degreased with a micro scissor, and then reduced with a scalpel to about 1 mm and after that fixed on the peri-implant lesion in a stable position using non-absorbable size 5–0 and 6–0 mono sutures.

In case of crater- shaped peri-implant defects, circular soft-tissue grafts were placed improving soft-tissue quality and quantity after severe peri-implant infections with BOP and massive suppuration. Because of diminished possibility of STG fixation especially in the lower jaw, onlay grafts were buried with help of deep bucco-lingual sutures and healing abutments in the immediate postoperative period until suture removal. (Figs. 4, 5, 6, 7, 8, 9, and 10)

The palatal donor site was covered with a preoperative custom-made (0.5 mm) plastic surgical bandage.

In all patients, a postoperatively systematic antibiotic medication 3000 mg per day (1000 mg Amoxicillin Ratiopharm, Ratiopharm GmbH, Ulm, Germany) was administrated for 7 days.

To reduce postoperative wound swelling and accompanying postoperative pain, a glucocorticoid was infiltrated sub-mucosal at the vestibular region (Dexabene® 4 mg/ml, Merckle Recordati-KGaA, Darmstadt, Germany).

As analgesic treatment, all patients were given ibuprofen (IBU-ratiopharm 400 acute, Ratiopharm GmbH, Ulm, Germany). The surgical bandage and the suturing were removed after 7 to 10 days.

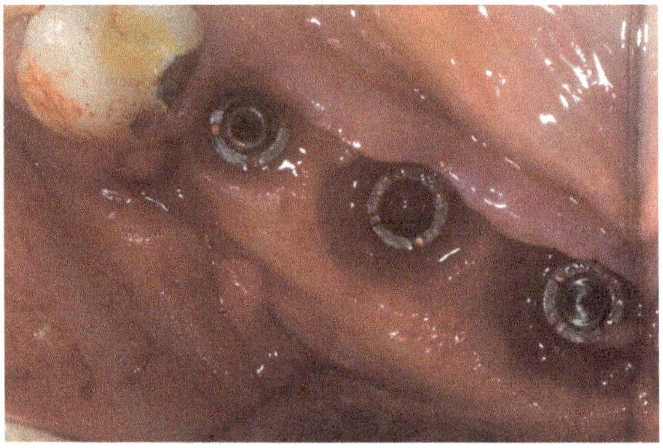

**Fig. 5** Crater-shaped peri-implant defects. Granulation tissue was removed followed by peri-implant osteotomie with the objective of optimizing subsequent soft-tissue transplantation

### Clinical parameters

The first clinical examination was carried out after initial anti-infective treatment before surgery (baseline), and the second one was made after a period of 9–180 months (Ø 43 months). In each clinical examination, the following parameters were assessed: the soft-tissue biotype, the skeletal biotype was classified, width and mobility of keratinized mucosa (KM), pocket probing depth (PPD), and bleeding on probing (BOP) as well.

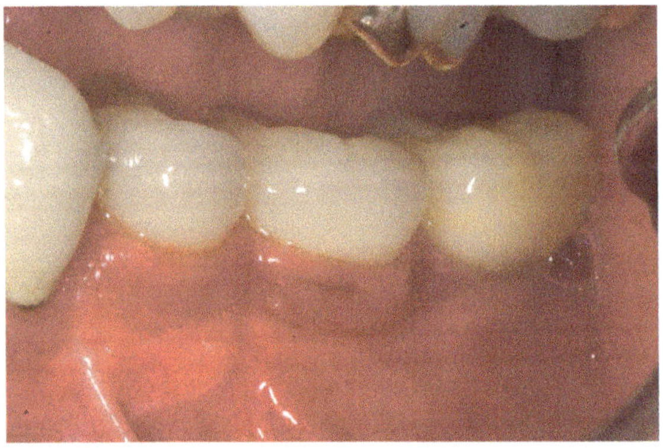

**Fig. 4** Female patient with severe peri-implantitis in regions 35, 36, 37. PPD ≥7 mm and BOP with suppuration and fistula 36, deficient keratinized mucosa due to hard tissue augmentation 5.5 years ago

The soft-tissue biotype was determined prior to the STG [17]. Differences were made between thick biotype and thin biotype. During this investigation, the transparency of the mucosa specified the suitable category when the periodontal probe was inserted into the sulcus. The probe was inserted vestibularly into the midpoint of the sulcus of an existing adjacent tooth (preferably at the maxillary central incisor), and by translucency, it was characterized as a thin biotype. A thick biotype was characterized if color impermeability through the mucosa was recognized.

Furthermore, the basic skeletal morphology of the alveolar bone was determined based on the classification of Cawood and Howell [18]. This was manually detected at the mandibular symphysis with a dental caliper (Caliper according to Beerendonk®, DCV instruments Seitingen-Oberflacht, Germany).

A classification as a broad apical base was made when the thickness of the jaw at the apical region in oral-vestibular direction was bigger than the thickness of the jaw at the marginal area of a natural tooth. A middle base was classified, when the thickness of the jaw had

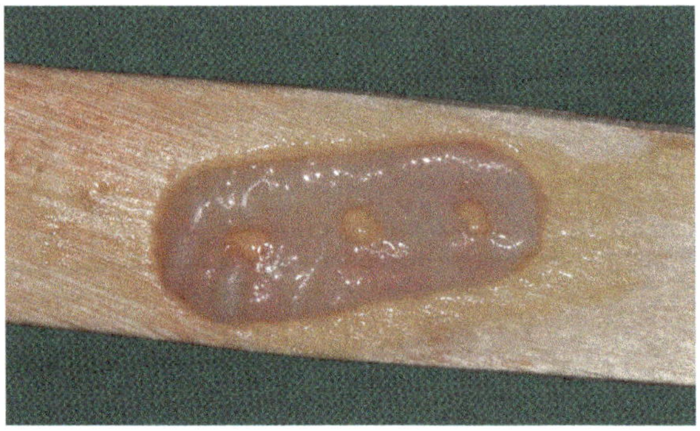

**Fig. 6** Free onlay graft harvested from the palate with perforations for sulcus formers

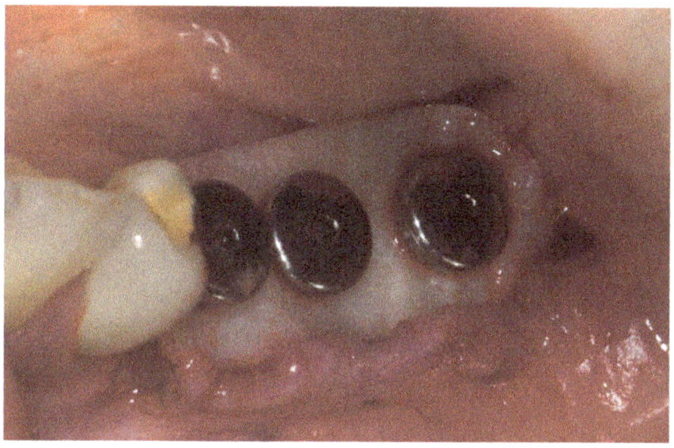

**Fig. 7** Free onlay graft try in fixed by sulcus formers after vestibular plasty at the lingual and buccal site

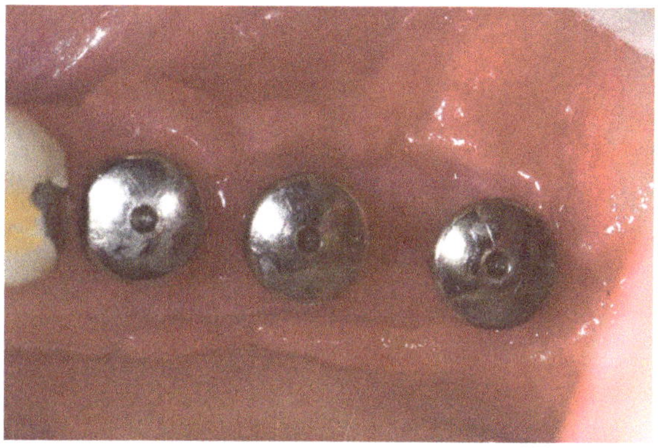

**Fig. 9** Postoperative examination after 2 weeks, perfect integration of free onlay graft with retracted wound margins at the lingual and buccal site

the same dimension at the two regions mentioned above and when the jaw at the apical region was thinner than it was at the marginal region of a natural tooth, then it was classified as narrow. If the mandibular symphysis was edentulous, the detection of skeletal biotype was performed at the maxillary anterior region. A schematic overview of various exemplary forms of the apical bases in the symphysis region is shown in Fig. 11.

After staining of the soft tissue using the Schiller iodine solution [19], the width of the KM at each implant was measured using a periodontal probe at midpoint of the vestibular surface.

The mobility of the KM was detected using the long side of the periodontal probe by vertical movement with slight pressure. According to the mobility of the mucosa, it was classified as "movable" or as "immovable". The worst value per implant and transplant was recorded, and in cases of more than one implant per patient, the worst value was recorded.

The PPD measurements were performed using a periodontal probe (PCP10, Hu-Friedy®, Rotterdam, Netherlands) with 25 N/mm force application on the four surfaces (mesial, distal, buccal/vestibular, and palatal/lingual). To ensure the evaluation in cases of unclear PPD values, the superstructures were removed, and PPD was measured. In patients with more than one implant, the worst PPD value was recorded.

The BOP measurements were made on four surfaces (mesial, distal, buccal/vestibular, and lingual/palatal) using the modified sulcus bleeding index by Lange et al. [20].

In addition, the suppuration was detected. The worst value per implant was recorded, and in cases of more than one implant per patient, the worst value was noted.

#### Follow-up

Nine to one-hundred eighty months after STG, the following clinical parameters were assessed again: width and mobility of keratinized mucosa (KM), pocket probing depth (PPD), bleeding on probing (BOP), and suppuration (pos./neg.). All the patients enrolled in a regular maintenance program during the follow-up period.

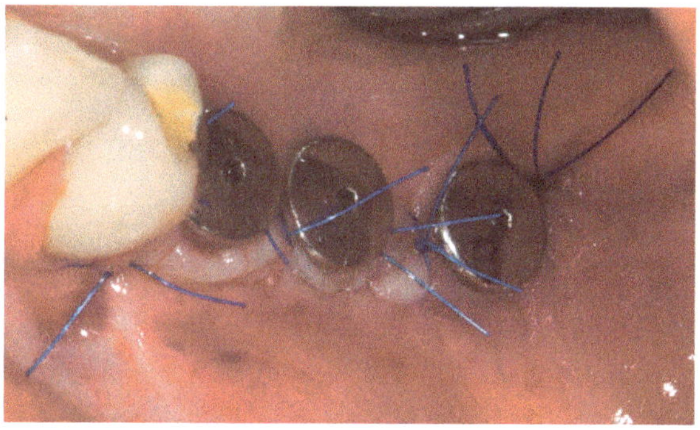

**Fig. 8** Free onlay graft buried by lingual and buccal split flap mucosa in the immediate postoperative time

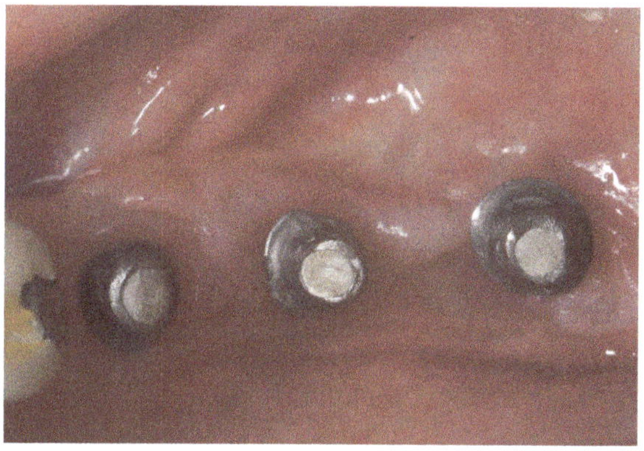

**Fig. 10** Clinical situation 2.5 years after soft-tissue transplantation without signs of inflammation

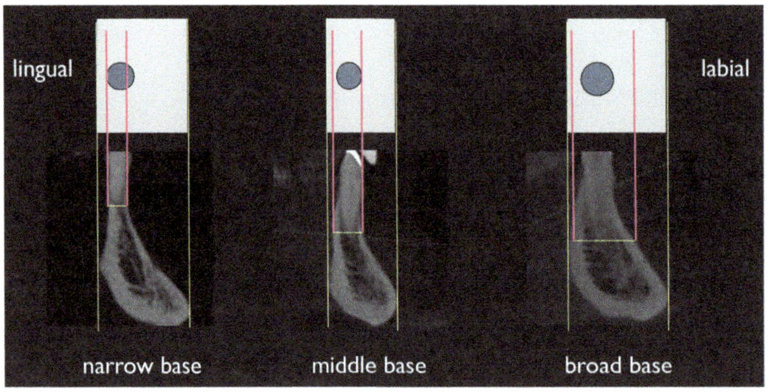


**Fig. 11** Schematic illustration of the apical base in the mandibular symphysis. A semi-quantitative measurement was made in this area. The *vertical red lines* represent the width of the alveolar bone in the apical region of the tooth/implant

### Statistical analysis

Collected data were documented anonymously using the Excel program (Microsoft©) and assessed using the statistical program SPSS 16.0 (SPSS Inc., Chicago, Illinois, USA).

For group comparisons and paired comparisons, paired *t* tests were applied with an error probability limit of 0.05. A linear regression analysis was performed as well.

## Results

All 28 patients were examined at baseline and after a period of time between 9 to 180 months. No implant was lost during this study. The soft-tissue biotype was thin in 26 of 28 patients and 2 patients as thick categorized. The analysis of the skeletal base morphology showed that 18 patients had a narrow base, 7 patients had a middle base, and 3 had a broad apical base.

The mean width of the KM was $0.4 \pm 0.5$ mm per implant before STG, and it was significantly ($p < 0.01$) improved to $4.3 \pm 1.5$ mm. Prior to the STG, 34 of 54 implants showed no keratinized mucosa, and 20 implants showed keratinized mucosa ≤1 mm. At the second measurement (follow-up), 16 implants showed KM of ≤3 mm and 38 implants showed 4–7 mm KM (Fig. 12).

High mobility of the keratinized mucosa was documented in all implants before STG. At the follow-up, 16

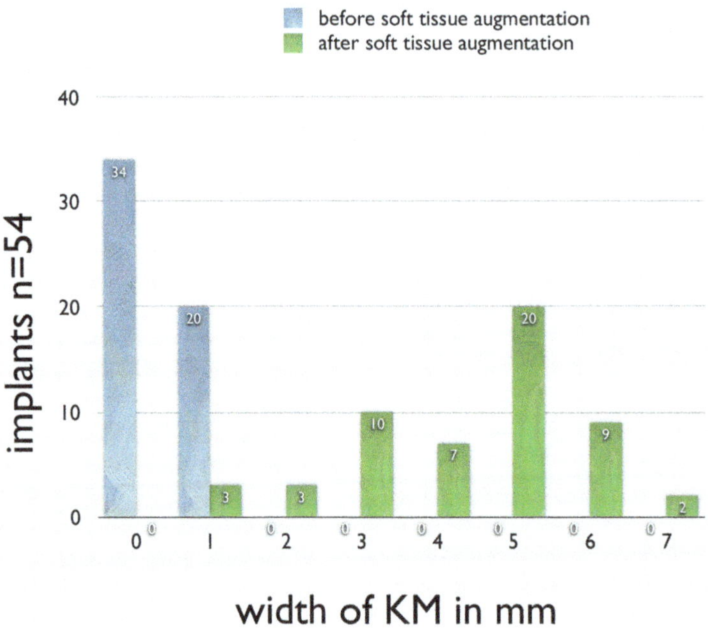


**Fig. 12** The width of the KM before and after STG. *t* test showed significant increase in KM width

implants had no mobility of the KM, and 12 implants showed slight mobility.

The mean PPD before soft-tissue augmentation was 6.3 ± 2.3 mm, and it was improved significantly ($p < 0.01$) to 4.1 ± 1.9 mm (Fig. 13). Prior to STG, 35 implants showed PPD of 4–6 mm, and 19 implants had PPD of ≥7 mm. To the time of the follow-up, the PPD was ≤3 mm at 19 implants, 4–6 mm at 30 implants, and ≥7 mm at 5 implants.

At baseline, suppuration could be detected in 11 patients but at follow-up only in 3 patients (Fig. 14).

The BOP was significantly ($p < 0.01$) reduced after grafting, it was observed in 23 implants at baseline but at the follow-up only in 8 implants (Fig. 14).

Due to the wide range of the follow-up period (Ø 43 months), we underwent a stratification of the patients cohort. They were subdivided into three time intervals. First group: 6–12 month follow-up ($n = 7$), second group 13–36 month follow-up ($n = 10$), and third group >36 month follow-up ($n = 11$).

The distribution of patients was as follows: in the first group, four patients = none BOP, one patient = moderate BOP, two patients = BOP with suppuration; in the second group, eight patients = none BOP, two patients = moderate BOP; in the third group, eight patients = none BOP, two patients = moderate BOP, one patient = BOP with suppuration.

At baseline, eight patients complained about significant discomfort and six patients about slight pressure pain or burning when the area of the lesion was touched.

At follow-up, all patients were pain-free and declared a subjective stable feeling at the implant region. The positive feeling after therapy was described as follows: "stable mucosa", "less sensitive to pain", "absence of the food niche", "cleaning is easier and", "no more taste of pus".

## Discussion

Until now, no methodology has been established as a gold standard approach for the treatment of peri-implantitis. The surgical phase comprises flap surgery or utilizing either resective or regenerative techniques. However, the selection criteria for the application of these different methods are not clearly defined.

The flap surgery with degranulation of the bony defect, decontamination of the implant surface, and postoperative antibiotic therapy could not achieve long-term stability [21]. In resective therapies, such as modeling osteoplasty, the success of the treatment depends on both the initial defect depth [22] and beginning of the disease [23]. Furthermore, the implantoplasty has been applied to smooth the supra-crestal implant surfaces [24].

The regenerative therapies aim to achieve re-osseointegration of implants, and it can be used with different materials. Long-term results are still unavailable for both of the resective and the regenerative methods, and therefore, it is still open as to which method is preferable. From a clinical point of view, these results are frustrating, and so they lead to the search for other surgical techniques, which can be used in combination with the above-mentioned methods in a certain decision-making process.

In the literature, there are no similar studies to compare with the present study. The results of the measured clinical parameters prove clearly that STGs can be

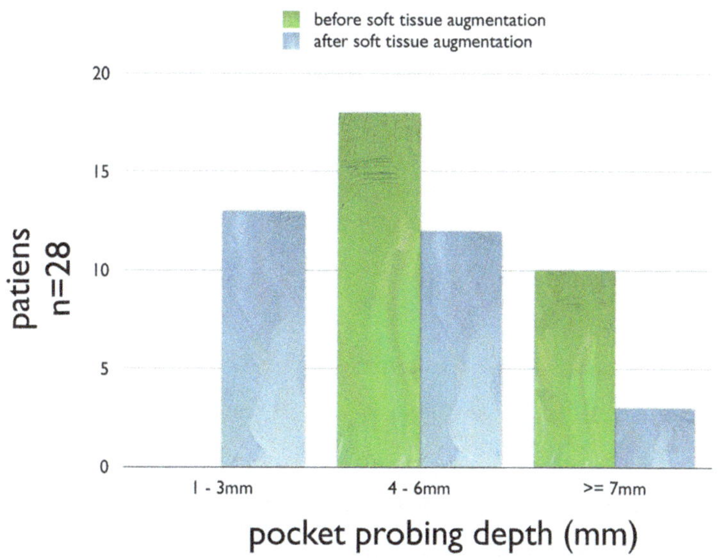


**Fig. 13** Results of the PPD before and after STG showing a significant reduction in PPD measurements ($p < 0.01$)

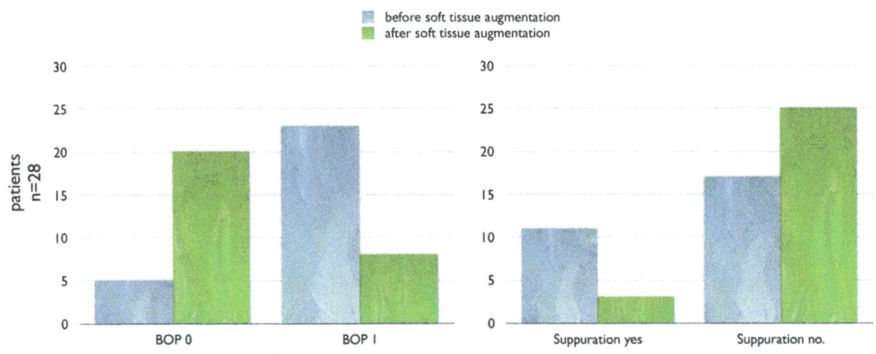


**Fig. 14** Results of BOP and suppuration before and after STG showing a significant reduction ($p < 0.01$)

applied for treatment of peri-implantitis particularly in cases of unfavorable bone defect morphology. This is the situation when the position of the planned implant is inaccurate in or outside the skeletal base of the alveolar bone. The soft-tissue grafting procedure seems to be reasonable from a palliative point of view because the peri-implant recurrent inflammatory symptoms lead to explantation with superstructure loss which affects the quality of life for patients.

Besides the soft-tissue biotype, the basic skeletal morphology of alveolar bone could be, therefore, a risk factor for the development of peri-implant disease and could also be a key factor for the successful treatment of peri-implantitis using soft-tissue grafting. The fact, that in the present cohort study approximately 65 % of patients have narrow apical base and only 10 % showed a broad base, lead to the suggestion that a narrow skeletal configuration of the upper and lower jaw as class IV according to Cawood and Howell [18] can be seen as an additional possible risk factor for the development of peri-implant inflammatory lesions. The reduced bone dimension above ossointegrated implants with respect to buccal and lingual site in case of narrowing with reduced bone vascularization especially in case of dense bone could be responsible for progressive bone loss and superinfection in such unfavorable skeletal configuration. In the literature, there are no references confirming that with certain skeletal conditions higher incidence rates can be expected. It is therefore advisable that future clinical trials consider this feature as a clinical evaluation criterion to validate this observation with clinical data. In recent years and especially in orthodontics, it is actively discussed that the development of the alveolar bone at different basic skeletal constitutions has a significant relation to the application of forces. It was found that fenestrations and dehiscences at orthodontically moved teeth will mainly be determined by the skeletal morphology, the corresponding growth pattern, and the bite situation [25, 26]. For example, patients with a horizontal skull structure and a broad apical alveolar bone base showed quantitatively less fenestrations and dehiscences of teeth than patients with a vertical skull structure and concomitant thin apical bone base. The importance of the position of the implant in relation to the skeletal basic morphology of the alveolar bone as a risk factor is still not clear. Further risk analysis using the predictive value of anatomical factors in relation to cephalometric basic pattern of the maxilla and mandible in the development of the peri-implantitis is advisable.

Similar to the fact that peri-implant lesions are quite different from periodontitis is the reaction behavior of the alveolar bone adjacent to the teeth completely different from its behavior at the implant sites. Although, it can be accepted that fenestrations and dehiscences occur at implants in the form of severe peri-implant inflammatory defects when the implants are set at or even outside the bone base. In this case, hardly reconstructable peri-implant defect morphology will result due to the 3D missed bone.

In spite of the fact that the quality and quantity of the peri-implant soft tissue has a very important effect on the marginal peri-implant bone loss [10, 27–30], there are no approaches in the literature for the soft-tissue grafting as a therapeutic method which can be used alone after initial treatment. The present study showed that in most cases and even by undesired peri-implant defect morphologies, stabilization of the soft tissue and reduction of the peri-implant inflammatory process could be achieved.

The reduced mobility of the soft tissue achieved in this study allows the conclusion that the presented methodology is strongly technical and surgeon sensitive. The degree of preoperative inflammatory activity did not correlate with the degree of immobilization of the KM gained, which means that the degree of postoperative gained immobility was not dependent on the severity of preoperative bleeding. The high proportion of patients with a thin mucosal biotype and the achieved changes in the local peri-implant biotypes emphasize this observation. In this context, the consequent anti-infective treatment performed before STG is of prime importance for patient outcome. Reduction of local bleeding and vulnerability allows proper transplant procedure and a reliable healing process.

It remains unsettled whether patients with a thick biotype will be less responsive to soft-tissue grafting than patients with a thin biotype. Therefore, it is recommended to conduct such investigation with a control group of patients with thick biotype in order to be able to answer this question. It is also recommended to investigate other approaches in larger cohort constitutional variations with different phenotypic forms of intra-oral soft and hard tissues of different ethnic groups similar to the study by Patil et al. [31].

According to the follow-up data that were stratified, it revealed that in the shorter period of follow-up, BOP could be rather present than in the longer healing period (>12 month, 2nd and 3rd group). The reason for that could be the slow-going scarification of the transplanted mucosa for many years. Depending on the increasing rigidity of the transplanted keratinized mucosa, the irritation of the mobile mucosa decreases and the signs of inflammation (BOP) is reduced. Besides the weak data, it seems that the new mucosa has to undergo a maturing process before a significant reduction of inflammatory symptoms occurs. Nevertheless, the study design cannot clearly answer this question; further controlled prospective trials have to be performed.

The reduction of PPD was possible through the stabilization and immobilization of the soft tissue accompanied by the establishment of an inflammation-free soft-tissue cuff, more than through the bone regeneration. The significant reduced values of BOP values are in accordance with the results of Boynueğri et al. [9] which confirmed that an adequate width of keratinized mucosa reduced plaque accumulation, inflammatory mucosal infiltration, and pro-inflammatory mediator release. Whether the STG at dental implants finally influences crestal bone changes remains unclear until now. Further controlled clinical trials with regular x-ray evaluation would be of tremendous interest.

## Conclusions

Considering the results of this retrospective study, it can be summarized that soft-tissue grafting as an additional surgical therapy option can be integrated in the treatment concept of peri-implantitis. The results showed as well that with certain clinical morphological conditions, the soft-tissue grafting can enhance a successful surgical treatment of peri-implantitis. It can be accepted as well that the implant system, and thus, the implant design has no direct influence on the indication of STG.

The soft-tissue grafting procedure seems to be reasonable from a palliative point of view because the peri-implant recurrent inflammatory symptoms lead to explantation with superstructure loss which affect the quality of life for patients.

### Abbreviations

BOP: bleeding on probing; KM: keratinized mucosa; PPD: pocket probing depth; STG: soft-tissue grafting.

### Competing interests

Michael Stiller, Rainer Mengel, Sebastian Becher, Bernhard Brinkmann, Barbara Peleska, Esther Kluk declare that they have no competing interests.

### Authors' contributions

MS and EK have made substantial contributions to conception and acquisition of data. MS and EK carried out the study and drafted the manuscript. RM, SB, BB, and BP participated in carrying out the study and drafting the manuscript. All authors read and approved the final manuscript.

### Acknowledgments

The authors gratefully acknowledge the assistance of Dr. Rim Hmaidouch, Department of Dental Prosthodontics, Faculty of Oral and Dental Medicine at Johann Wolfgang Goethe University, Frankfurt, Germany, in the translation and revision of this manuscript.
The authors thank Dr. Eva-Maria Stiller and Prof. Dr. Axel Bumann for the consultation in the orthodontic questions.

### Author details

[1]School of Dental Medicine, Section of Experimental Orofacial Medicine, Philipps University, Georg-Voigt-Str. 3, 35039 Marburg, Germany. [2]School of Dental Medicine, Department of Prosthodontics, Philipps University, Georg-Voigt-Str. 3, 35039 Marburg, Germany. [3]Practice of Oral and Maxillofacial Surgery, ECDI Center, Königsallee 68, 40212 Düsseldorf, Germany. [4]Clinic ABC Bogen, ECDI Center, ABC Strasse 19, 20354 Hamburg, Germany. [5]Department of Postgraduate Education - Master of Oral Implantology, Center for Oral and Maxillofacial Surgery, Johann Wolfgang Goethe University Frankfurt, Theodor-Stern-Kai 17, Frankfurt 60577, Germany. [6]Private Practice for Oral Surgery and Implantology, ECDI Center, Brahmsst. 11, 14193 Berlin, Germany.

### References

1. Atieh MA, Alsabeeha NH, Faggion Jr CM, Duncan WJ. The frequency of peri-implant diseases: a systematic review and meta-analysis. J Periodontol. 2013;84(11):1586–98.
2. Mombelli A, Müller N, Cionca N. The epidemiology of peri-implantitis. Clin Oral Implants Res. 2012;23(6):67–76.
3. Swierkot K, Lottholz P, Flores-de-Jacoby L, Mengel R. Mucositis, peri-implantitis, implant success, and survival of implants in patients with treated generalized aggressive periodontitis: 3- to 16-year results of a prospective long-term cohort study. J Periodontol. 2012;83:1213–25.
4. Albrektsson T, Buser D, Chen ST, Cochran D, DeBruyn H, Jemt T, et al. Statements from the Estepona Consensus Meeting on Peri-implantitis, 2012. Clin Implant Dent Relat Res. 2012;14:781–2.
5. Khoshkam V, Chan HL, Lin GH, MacEachern MP, Monje A, Suarez F, et al. Reconstructive procedures for treating peri-implantitis: a systematic review. J Dent Res. 2013;92(12):131–8.
6. Lang NP, Wilson TG, Corbet EF. Biological complications with dental implants: their prevention, diagnosis and treatment. Clin Oral Implants Res. 2000;11 Suppl 1:146–55.
7. Greenstein G, Cavallaro J. Failed dental implants: diagnosis, removal and survival of reimplantations. J Am Dent Assoc. 2011;145(8):835–42.
8. Lin GH, Chan HL, Wang HL. The significance of keratinized mucosa on implant health: a systematic review. J Periodontol. 2013;84(12):1755–67.

9. Boynueğri D, Nemli SK, Kasko YA. Significance of keratinized mucosa around dental implants: a prospective comparative study. Clin Oral Implants Res. 2013;24(8):928–33.
10. Bengazi F, Botticelli D, Favero V, Perini A, Urbizo Velez J, Lang NP. Influence of presence or absence of keratinized mucosa on the alveolar bony crest level as it relates to different buccal marginal bone thicknesses. An experimental study in dogs. Clin Oral Implants Res. 2014;25(9):1065–71.
11. World Medical Association. World Medical Association Declaration of Helsinki: ethical principles for medical research involving human subjects. JAMA. 2013;310(20):2191–4.
12. Albrektsson T, Zarb G, Worthington P, Eriksson AR. The long-term efficacy of currently used dental implants: a review and proposed criteria of success. Int J Oral Maxillofac Implants. 1986;1(1):11–25.
13. Naert I, Gizani S, Vuylsteke M, van Steenberghe D. A 5-year randomized clinical trial on the influence of splinted and unsplinted oral implants in the mandibular overdenture therapy. Part I: Peri-implant outcome. Clin Oral Implants Res. 1998;9(3):170–7.
14. Seibert JS, Louis JV. Soft tissue ridge augmentation utilizing a combination onlay-interpositional graft procedure: a case report. Int J Periodontics Restorative Dent. 1996;16(4):310–21.
15. Stiller M, Eisenmann E, Fritz H, Freesmeyer WB. Der lokale Alveolarkammaufbau bei Weichgewebsdefiziten. Z Zahnärztl Implantol. 1998;14:213–8.
16. Stiller M. Die Rekonstruktion des mukogingivalen Komplexes an Einzelzahnimplantaten zur Verbesserung von Funktion und Ästhetik mit Hilfe mikrochirurgischer Wundversorgungstechniken. ZWR - Das deutsche Zahnärzteblatt. 2001;110:578–84.
17. De Rouck T, Eghbali R, Collys K, De Bruyn H, Cosyn J. The gingival biotype revisited: transparency of the periodontal probe through the gingival margin as a method to discriminate thin from thick gingiva. J Clin Periodontol. 2009;36:428–33.
18. Cawood JI, Howell RA. A classification of the edentulous jaws. Int J Oral Maxillofac Surg. 1988;17(4):232–6.
19. Kern G, Stadler G, Hinderfeld E. Die Schillersche Jodprobe. Archiv für Gynäkologie. 1962;197(1):36–56.
20. Lange DE, Plagmann HC, Eenboom A, Promesberger A. Clinical methods for the objective evaluation of oral hygiene. Dtsch Zahnarztl T. 1977;32(1):44–7.
21. Heitz-Mayfield LJ, Lang NP. Comparative biology of chronic and aggressive periodontitis vs. peri-implantitis. Periodontol 2000. 2010;53:167–81.
22. Serino G, Turri A. Outcome of surgical treatment of peri-implantitis: results from a 2-year prospective clinical study in humans. Clin Oral Implants Res. 2011;22(11):1214–20.
23. Charalampakis G, Rabe P, Leonhardt A, Dahlén G. A follow-up study of peri-implantitis cases after treatment. J Clin Periodontol. 2011;38(9):864–71.
24. Schwarz F, John G, Mainusch S, Sahm N, Becker J. Combined surgical therapy of peri-implantitis evaluating two methods of surface debridement and decontamination. A two-year clinical follow up report. J Clin Periodontol. 2012;39(8):789–97.
25. Enhos S, Uysal T, Yagci A, Veli İ, Ucar FI, Ozer T. Dehiscence and fenestration in patients with different vertical growth patterns assessed with cone-beam computed tomography. Angle Orthod. 2012;82(5):868–74.
26. Evangelista K, Vasconcelos Kde F, Bumann A, Hirsch E, Nitka M, Silva MA. Dehiscence and fenestration in patients with Class I and Class II Division 1 malocclusion assessed with cone-beam computed tomography. Am J Orthod Dentofacial Orthop. 2010;138(2):133–7.
27. Gobbato L, Avila-Ortiz G, Sohrabi K, Wang CW, Karimbux N. The effect of keratinized mucosa width on peri-implant health: a systematic review. Int J Oral Maxillofac Implants. 2013;28(6):1536–45.
28. Linkevicius T, Apse P, Grybauskas S, Puisys A. The influence of soft tissue thickness on crestal bone changes around implants: a 1-year prospective controlled clinical trial. Int J Oral Maxillofac Implants. 2009;24(4):712–9.
29. Linkevicius T, Puisys A, Linkeviciene L, Peciuliene V, Schlee M. Crestal bone stability around implants with horizontally matching connection after soft tissue thickening: a prospective clinical trial. Clin Implant Dent Relat Res. 2013;17. doi:10.1111/cid.12155. [Epub ahead of print].
30. Brito C, Tenenbaum HC, Wong BK, Schmitt C, Nogueira-Filho G. Is keratinized mucosa indispensable to maintain peri-implant health? A systematic review of the literature. J Biomed Mater Res B Appl Biomater. 2014;102(3):643–50.
31. Patil R, van Brakel R, Mahesh K, de Putter C, Cune MS. An exploratory study on assessment of gingival biotype and crown dimensions as predictors for implant esthetics comparing caucasian and Indian subjects. J Oral Implantol. 2013;39(3):308–13.

# Focal osteoporotic bone marrow defect involving dental implant: a case report

Natália Galvão Garcia[1*], Francisco Barbara Abreu Barros[1], Márcia Maria Dalmolin Carvalho[2] and Denise Tostes Oliveira[1]

**Abstract**

In oral implantology, the most serious complications occur intraoperatively or within a short period. We describe an unusual case of focal osteoporotic bone marrow defect involving dental implant in the posterior mandibular region of the adult woman. Despite the fact that this condition requires no treatment, it could lead to the displacement of the dental implant. Additionally, this case report reinforces that histopathological analysis is mandatory for precise diagnosis of the radiolucency into posterior mandibular region of the adult woman associated or not with dental implant placement.

**Keywords:** Bone marrow; Defect; Dental implant

## Background

In oral implantology, the most serious complications and those most frequently described in the literature occur during surgery [1]. The well-known intraoperative complications and accidents related to surgery have included hemorrhage, nerve damage, mandibular fractures, damage to adjacent teeth, lack of primary stability, and displacement or migration of implants [2].

The displacement of an implant will occur intraoperatively or within a short period because of poor surgical technique or anatomic variances [2]. In addition, the presence of the medullar component in the jawbones causing the focal osteoporotic bone marrow defect can facilitate the displacement of dental implants during surgery [2, 3].

The focal osteoporotic bone marrow defect corresponds to the uncommon hematopoietic tissue found mainly in posterior mandibular region of the adult woman [2, 4, 5]. This condition is generally asymptomatic and discovered during radiographic exam of the jaws [2, 4]. Most of the focal osteoporotic bone marrow defects occur in edentulous areas region where tooth extraction was previously performed [5]. Recently, Sençimen et al. (2011) reported a case of the focal osteoporotic bone marrow occurring secondary to dental implant placement [6].

This paper describes an unusual case of focal osteoporotic bone marrow defect involving dental implant in posterior mandibular region of the adult woman.

## Case presentation

An 84-year-old white woman was referred to private dental clinic for an implant rehabilitation treatment. Intraoral examination revealed healthy mucosa and there was not any sign of infection. Her past medical history was unremarkable. The radiography of the molar region showed with a quite ill-defined radiolucent area presenting irregular borders associated to dental implant (Fig. 1). This condition was asymptomatic and no expansion of the mandibular cortical bone was detected. Under local anesthesia, a biopsy was performed and the tissue submitted to the Bauru School of Dentistry Oral Pathology Biopsy Service of the University of São Paulo. The histopathological examination revealed normal hematopoietic bone marrow characterized by erythroid, granulocytic, monocytic, and lymphocytic series (Fig. 2). In addition, megakaryocytes, fat cells, and bone trabeculae were also observed (Fig. 3). Abnormal morphology of the hematopoietic cells or malignant cells was not seen. The histopathological findings confirmed the diagnosis of focal osteoporotic bone marrow defect of the mandible.

## Discussion

Focal osteoporotic bone marrow defect is a condition that corresponds to the uncommon presence of hematopoietic

* Correspondence: natggalvao@hotmail.com
[1]Department of Stomatology, Area of Pathology, Bauru School of Dentistry, University of São Paulo, Bauru, São Paulo, Brazil
Full list of author information is available at the end of the article

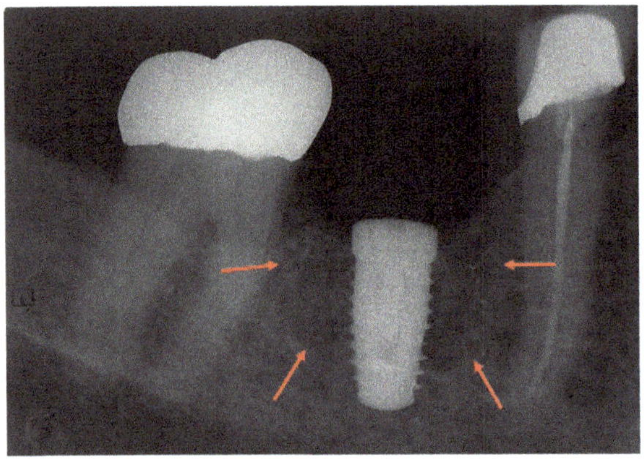

**Fig. 1** The periapical radiograph revealed the presence of an extensive and poorly circumscribed osteoporotic area around the proximal implant

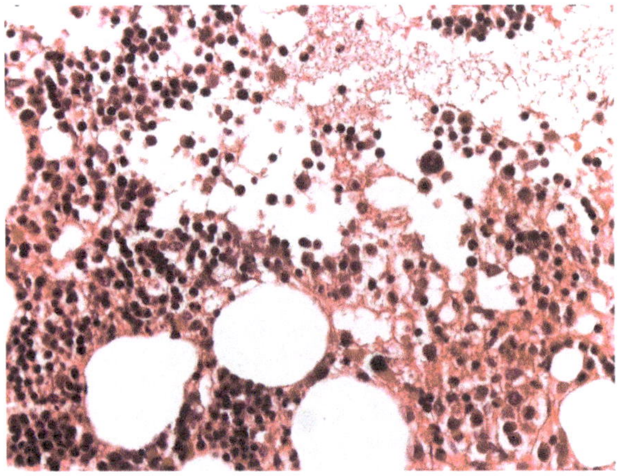

**Fig. 3** Erythroid, granulocytic, monocytic and lymphocytic series are illustrated, as well as megakaryocytes (hematoxylin and eosin, original magnification ×400)

tissue found in edentulous areas of the jaws in middle-age women [6].

Clinically, the focal osteoporotic bone marrow defect occurs as isolated or multifocal radiolucency with several millimeters to centimeters in diameter and ill-defined borders [4]. This condition is rarely mentioned in differential diagnosis of radiolucent lesions of the jaws, and the radiographic appearance may be confused with other intraosseous pathologic conditions such as osteomyelitis, traumatic bone cyst, and fibrous dysplasia [4, 6].

The exact cause of focal osteoporotic bone marrow defect is unknown but failure in bone repair in areas of trauma has been associated with its occurrence in edentulous region where tooth extraction [4, 5] or dental implant [3, 6] such as our case report, was previously performed. Sençimen et al. (2011) suggested that the proliferation of hematopoietic marrow elements around the dental implant may be a response of the healing spongious bone to surgically initiated trauma which may occur due to overheating of bone or peri-implant bone compression at the implant osteotomy site by drilling a narrower osteotomy [6].

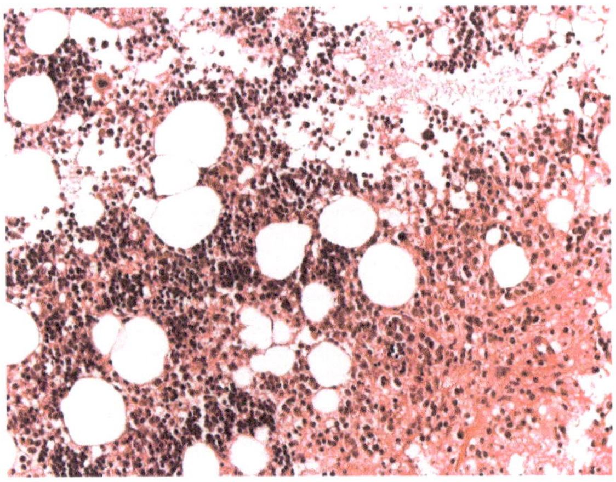

**Fig. 2** Normal hematopoietic cells, fat cells and bone trabeculae (hematoxylin and eosin, original magnification ×200)

Only few cases of the focal osteoporotic bone marrow defect associated with dental implants has been described in the English literature [3, 6]. Sençimen et al. (2011) reported a clinical case in which the focal osteoporotic bone marrow defect occurred 2 years postoperatively apical to a dental implant in posterior mandible region and the diagnosis was established based on the combination of clinical, radiographic, and microscopic features [6]. Posteriorly, Lee et al. (2013) reported three clinical cases of displacement of dental implants into the focal osteoporotic bone marrow defect, but the final diagnoses of this condition were based only on clinical and radiographic findings [3]. In this paper, we described a case of the focal osteoporotic bone marrow defect associated to dental implant which was diagnosed by histopathological analysis.

Microscopically, the presence of hematopoietic marrow composed of monocytic, erythroid, granulocytic, and lymphocytic series as well as megakaryocytes associated with fatty marrow is required for diagnosis of focal osteoporotic bone marrow defect [3, 4].

In the present case the final diagnosis was established based on the combination of radiographic and microscopic features. Some authors have based the focal osteoporotic bone marrow defect diagnosis on age, site, and clinical and radiographic findings [3], but it is important to reinforce that the final diagnosis of this condition should be established on microscopic features rather than clinical and radiographic parameters [4].

## Conclusions
This is the second well-documented case report including clinical, radiographic, and microscopic analysis of focal osteoporotic bone marrow defect involving dental implant. Despite the fact that this condition requires no treatment, it could lead to the displacement of the dental implant. In addition, we would like to alert that histopathological analysis is mandatory for precise diagnosis of the radiolucency into posterior mandibular region of the adult woman associated or no with dental implant placement.

## Consent
Written informed consent was obtained from the patient for publication of this case report and any accompanying images. A copy of the written consent is available for review by the Editor-in-Chief of this journal.

### Competing interests
Author Garcia NG, Barros FBA, Carvalho MMD, and Oliveira DT states that there are no conflicts of interest.

### Author's contributions
G NG and B FBA have made substantial contributions to analysis and interpretation of data and in drafting the manuscript. C MMD has made substantial contribution to conception and acquisition of data. O DT has been involved in drafting the manuscript and revising it critically for important intellectual content and also has given final approval of the version to be published. All authors read and approved the final manuscript.

### Authors' information
Garcia NG is a PhD student in Department of Stomatology, Area of Pathology, Bauru School of Dentistry, University of São Paulo, Bauru, São Paulo, Brazil. Barros FBA is a MSc student in Department of Stomatology, Area of Pathology, Bauru School of Dentistry, University of São Paulo, Bauru, São Paulo, Brazil. Carvalho MMD is a DDs in Private Practice, Campinas, São Paulo, Brazil. Oliveira DT is an associate professor in Department of Stomatology, Area of Pathology, Bauru School of Dentistry, University of São Paulo, Bauru, São Paulo, Brazil.

### Acknowledgements
We would like to thank the "National Counsel of Technological and Scientific Development" (CNPq) (141641/2013-4).

### Author details
[1]Department of Stomatology, Area of Pathology, Bauru School of Dentistry, University of São Paulo, Bauru, São Paulo, Brazil. [2]Dentist, Private Practice, Campinas, São Paulo, Brazil.

### References
1. Lamas Pelayo J, Peñarrocha Diago M, Martí Bowen E, Peñarrocha DM. Intraoperative complications during oral implantology. Med Oral Patol Oral Cir Bucal. 2008;13:E239–43.
2. Bayram B, Alaaddinoglu E. Implant-box mandible: dislocation of an implant into the mandible. J Oral Maxillofac Surg. 2011;69:498–501.
3. Lee SC, Jeong CH, Im HY, Kim SY, Ryu JY, Hy Y, et al. Displacement of dental implants into the focal osteoporotic bone marrow defect: a report of three cases. J Korean Assoc Oral Maxillofac Surg. 2013;39:94–9.
4. Bravo-Calderón DM, Oliveira DT, Santos WHM. Bilateral osteoporotic bone marrow defects of the mandible: a case report. Head Face Med. 2012;8:22.
5. Makek M, Lello GE. Focal osteoporotic bone marrow defects of the jaws. J Oral Maxillofac Surg. 1986;44:268–73.
6. Sençimen M, Delilbasi C, Gülses A, Okçu KM, Gunhan O, Varol A. Focal osteoporotic hematopoietic bone marrow defect formation around a dental implant: a case report. Int J Oral Maxillofac Implants. 2011;26:e1–4.

# 23

# In vitro immunological and biological evaluations of the angiogenic potential of platelet-rich fibrin preparations: a standardized comparison with PRP preparations

Mito Kobayashi[1,2], Tomoyuki Kawase[1,3*], Kazuhiro Okuda[2], Larry F. Wolff[4] and Hiromasa Yoshie[2]

**Abstract**

**Background:** Platelet-rich fibrin (PRF), a platelet-rich plasma (PRP) derivative mainly composed of fibrin networks, has been increasingly demonstrated to be effective in wound healing in clinical and pre-clinical animal studies. However, there has still been a concern that major growth factors may significantly be loss from PRF during its preparation through the slow clotting process. To address this concern, we compared the angiogenic potential of PRF and PRP by standardization of procedures based on volume ratios.

**Methods:** PRP, PRF, and platelet-poor plasma (PPP) were prepared from the peripheral blood of healthy donors. PRF preparations were squeezed or homogenized to produce exudate (PRF*exu*) or extract (PRF*ext*), respectively. Concentrations of the angiogenic factors and their bioactivities were determined using ELISA kits, a scratch assay using endothelial cells and a chicken chorioallantoic membrane (CAM) assay.

**Results:** In PRP and PRF preparations, both VEGF and PDGF-BB were significantly more concentrated than PPP. In the scratch assay, PRF*exu* and PRF*ext* were the most effective for wound closure. In the CAM assay, PRF membranes were the most effective for neovascularization.

**Conclusions:** It is suggested that PRF preparations efficiently preserve the angiogenic factors and function not only as a scaffolding material but as a reservoir of angiogenic factors in wound healing.

**Keywords:** Platelets, Fibrin, Plasma, Angiogenesis, Endothelial cells

## Background

Since Marx's publications [1, 2], platelet-rich plasma (PRP) has been widely applied in regenerative therapy. However, because the preparation protocol is relatively complex and not standardized between laboratories, its clinical outcomes have often varied significantly among individual clinical research groups [3]. To overcome this disadvantage, Choukroun and his co-workers developed platelet-rich fibrin (PRF) by modifying the process of PRP preparation [3–5]. PRF can be prepared solely through the activation of an endogenous coagulation process without the aid of animal-derived coagulants such as bovine thrombin. Its advantages include operator-friendly preparation procedures and doctor-friendly handling when used in a clinical setting. However, the primary and more important advantage of PRF should be attributed to its clinical effectiveness rather than efficiency in preparation and handling.

Because PRF is mainly composed of fibrin fibers, it has been generally thought that PRF preparations must be distinguished from PRP, a "cocktail" of growth factors. Furthermore, there has been a concern that most growth factors may diffuse and be loss during the PRF preparation process. To address this concern, clinical and pre-

* Correspondence: kawase@dent.niigata-u.ac.jp
[1]Division of Oral Bioengineering, Institute of Medicine and Dentistry, Niigata University, Niigata, Japan
[3]Advanced Research Center, The Nippon Dental University School of Life Dentistry at Niigata, Niigata, Japan
Full list of author information is available at the end of the article

clinical animal studies have increasingly been performed over the past 2 years [6–16]. The majority of published articles to date have concluded that PRF preparations were more effective or equally effective to PRP preparations in wound healing and tissue regeneration. These findings are not surprising because fibrin fibers would be expected to function as an efficient carrier to form a delivery system of growth factors [17]; however, the methods for PRF preparation and application are often not fully disclosed or vary across individual studies. Therefore, for a more precise comparison, it is necessary to standardize the procedures for preparation of PRF and to normalize their effectiveness by utilizing known volumes of blood samples.

For example, to standardize the handling of PRF exudate (PRF*exu*), in a previous study [18], we developed a compression device and proposed the use of this device to create a PRF membrane with uniform thickness and to minimize loss of PRF*exu* assuming that PRF*exu* contains significant amounts of important growth factors for wound healing. As a result of this comparative study using an ex vivo chick embryo chorioallantoic membrane (CAM) assay, it turned out that growth factors were distributed both in the exudate portion and in the fibrin network. Therefore, to more precisely compare the PRF with PRP preparations at the cellular and molecular levels, it is necessary to standardize the preparation procedures and to evaluate their potency by the volume ratios of the originally collected peripheral blood samples with the resulting preparation samples.

In this study, because the primary site of PRP action in wound healing and tissue regeneration is the formation of blood vessels [17, 19], we focused on vascular endothelial growth factor (VEGF) and its target action of angiogenesis and compared the concentrations of PRP and PRF preparations as to their biological effectiveness using ELISA and bioassay systems after performing the appropriate normalization.

## Methods

### Preparation and clotting of PRP

As previously described [20, 21], blood was collected from three healthy and non-smoking volunteers aged 28, 30, and 54 years (two females; one male), and PRP was prepared along with platelet-poor plasma (PPP) using the two-step centrifugation protocol. The number of platelets in the freshly prepared PRP and PPP samples was determined using an automated hematology analyzer (pocH 100iV diff: Sysmex, Kobe, Japan). Then, PRP and PPP preparations were frozen and stored at −20 °C until further used (usually within 2 weeks).

Preparation of PPP and PRP samples is shown in Fig. 1a. For clotting, bovine thrombin (180 U) (Haematologic Technologies, Inc., Essex Junction, VT, USA) and 10 % $CaCl_2$ (30 μL) were added to the indicated volumes of PRP or PPP preparations to form 5 × 5 × 1 mm (width × length × thickness) membranes. The relative volumes of individual preparations against the original blood samples were calculated and are summarized in Table 1.

The study design and consent forms for all procedures performed with the study subjects were approved by the ethical committee for human subject use at Niigata University Medical and Dental Hospital in accordance with the Helsinki Declaration of 1975 and as revised in 2008.

### Preparation, compression, and homogenization of PRF

As described previously [18], blood was collected from the same donors and immediately centrifuged by a Medifuge centrifugation system (Silfradent S. r. l., Santa Sofia, Italy). Preparation of PRF samples, PRF*exu* and PRF*ext* are shown in Fig. 1b. After eliminating the red thrombus, the

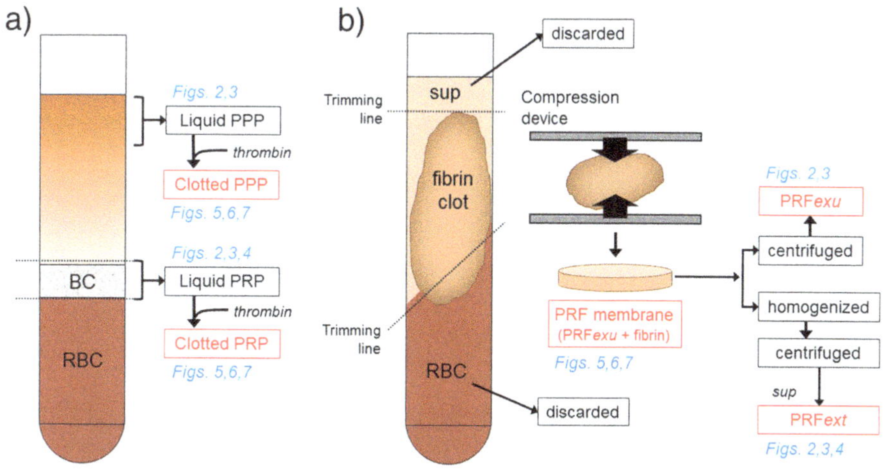


**Fig. 1** **a** Preparation of PPP and PRP samples. **b** Preparations of PRF samples (PRF*exu* and PRF*ext*)

**Table 1** Comparison of sample volumes and preparation volumes

| | Platelet-poor plasma (PPP) | PPP clot | Platelet-rich plasma (PRP) | PRP clot | Platelet-rich fibrin exudate (PRF*exu*) | Platelet-rich fibrin extract (PRF*ext*) | Platelet-rich fibrin (PRF) membrane |
|---|---|---|---|---|---|---|---|
| Starting blood sample volume (mL) | 10[a] | 10[a] | 10[a] | 10[a] | 10 | 10 | 10 |
| Resulting sample volume (mL) (vs. starting volume) | 2.5 (1:4) | | 1 (1:10) | | 1 (1:10) | 1 (1:10) | 1[b] (1:10) |
| Relative condensation (fold) | 1 | | 2.5 | | 2.5 | 2.5 | |
| Volume needed to mold a clot (mL) (vs. resulting sample volume) | | 0.25 (1:10) | | 0.2 (1:5) | | | |
| Number of 5 × 5 × 1-mm membrane | | 10[c] | | 5[c] | | | 5–7[d] |
| Relative condensation (fold) | | 1 | | 2 | | | 1.4–2.0 |

[a]This sample volume does not include the volume of acid citrate dextrose solution (ACD; 1.5 mL)
[b](Acquired sample volume) = (blood sample volume) – (RBC fraction) – (serum volume)
[c]Estimated number of membranes
[d]Acquired number of membranes

resulting PRF preparations were compressed by the PRF compression device [18]. As described earlier, the stainless steel PRF compression device developed for PRF membrane preparation was composed of two spoon shaped parts. The clearance between the spoon parts when compressed was adjusted to be 1 mm. Thus, when the PRF clots were compressed with this device, a standard 1-mm thick PRF membrane was consistently prepared.

After compression, PRF membranes were centrifuged to squeeze out the PRF*exu*. Alternatively, PRF membranes were minced and homogenized on ice for 1 min with a micro-Multimixer (Ieda Trading, Corp., Tokyo, Japan) and centrifuged to obtain supernatants (PRF*ext*) (Fig. 1b). The resulting PRF*exu* and PRF*ext* were directly used along with PRP and PPP preparations for ELISA and the bioassays. Comparison of sample and preparation volumes is shown in Table 1. PPP, PRP, and PRF membrane preparations were standardized by preparing them from the same volume (10 mL) of blood samples.

#### Determination of growth factor levels by ELISA

The concentrations of VEGF, PDGF-BB, and soluble DLL1 in frozen PPP, PRP, and PRF samples were determined using human VEGF, PDGF-BB, and DLL1 Quantikine ELISA Kits (R&D Systems, Inc., Minneapolis, MN, USA).

#### Cell culture and scratch assay

Human umbilical vein endothelial cells (HUVECs) were obtained from Cell Applications, Inc., (San Diego, CA, USA) and cultured with HuMedia-EB2 supplemented with growth factors (Kurabo, Tokyo, Japan). For the scratch assay, the cells were seeded into 6-well plates at a density of $1 \times 10^5$ cells/well and cultured in a $CO_2$ incubator until they reached early confluence. The medium was then replaced with HuMedia-EB2 supplemented with reduced amounts of growth factors (1:5 in dilution). The monolayer was scratched using a scraper with a 1-mm blade and incubated for an additional 24 h with 2 % (*v*/*v*) PRF*exu*, PRF*ext*, PRP, or PPP. The wound areas were photographed at specific time points, and the width of the scratched gap was determined using ImageJ (National Institutes of Health, Bethesda, MD, USA).

#### Western blotting analysis

HUVECs were seeded onto 6-well plates at a density of $1 \times 10^4$ cells/well and pre-cultured for 2 days to form subconfluent cultures. After washing, the cells were treated with PPP, PRP, or PRF*ext* in a $CO_2$ incubator (5 % $CO_2$) for 10 min in serum-free Hank's balanced saline solution (HBSS). After washing twice with ice cold PBS, the cells were lysed with Laemmli sample buffer as previously described [22]. Protein samples were fractionated using 10 % SDS-PAGE (ATTO, Tokyo, Japan) and electro-blotted onto PVDF membranes using the Trans-Blot® Turbo™ Transfer System (Bio-Rad Laboratories, Hercules, CA, USA).

After blocking with diluted Block A (1:2) (DS Pharma, Osaka, Japan) or 5 % BSA (Fraction V) (Sigma, St. Louis, MO, USA) in 0.1 % Tween 20-containing TBS (T-TBS) for 4–5 h at 4 °C, the membranes were probed overnight at 4 °C with the following primary antibodies: rabbit polyclonal anti-phospho-VEGFR2 (Y996) (1:2000 in dilution) (Cell Signaling Technology, Danvers, MA, USA), rabbit polyclonal anti-VEGFR2 (D5B1) (1:2,000) (Cell Signaling Technology), or goat polyclonal anti-actin antibody (1:1,000) (Santa Cruz Biotechnology, Inc., Santa Cruz, CA, USA). After washing three times with T-TBS, the membranes were probed with horseradish peroxidase-conjugated goat polyclonal anti-rabbit IgG H&L (1:5,000) (Abcam, Cambridge, MA, USA) or horseradish peroxidase-conjugated donkey anti-goat IgG (Santa Cruz Biotechnology) for 45 min at 4 °C. After washing, images were visualized using Clarity™ Western ECL Substrate (Bio-Rad) and imaged using a cooled CCD camera system (Image Capture; ATTO, Tokyo, Japan).

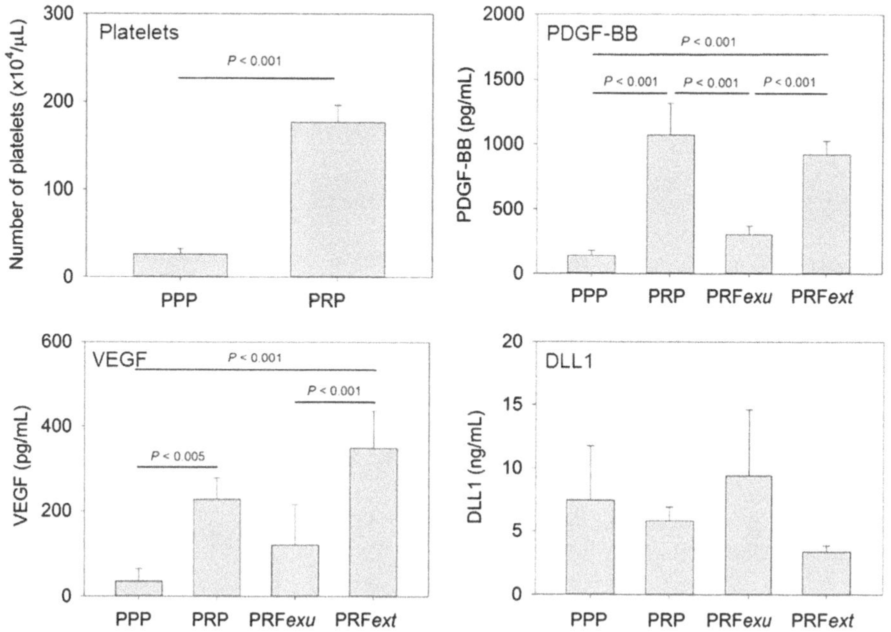


**Fig. 2** The concentration of platelets, VEGF, PDGF-BB, and DLL1 in PPP, PRP, PRF*exu*, and PRF*ext* preparations. $n = 5$

## The ex vivo chorioallantoic membrane model

As described previously [18], fertilized chicken eggs were incubated in a hatching incubator equipped with an automatic rotator (KingSURO20; Belbird, Siki, Japan) at 37 °C with a relative air humidity of 65 %. On embryo developmental day 11, a hole approximately 16 mm in diameter was opened in the eggshell, and clots of PPP and PRP and PRF membranes (5 × 5 mm) were placed on the central area of the CAMs. After the holes were sealed, the eggs were incubated for an additional 3 days. The CAM vasculature was macroscopically photographed at the initial time point (day 0) and the end point (day 3).

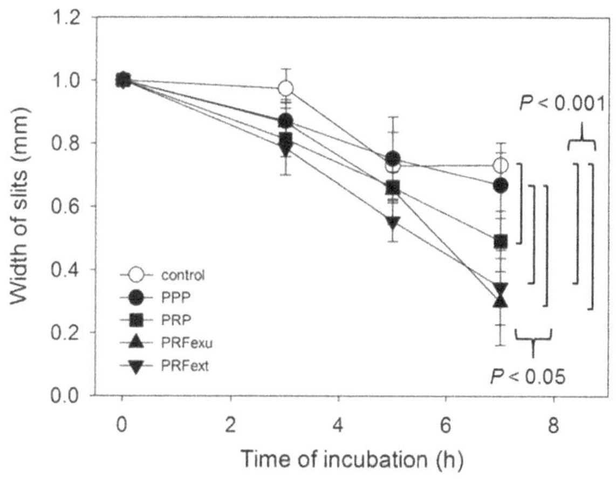


**Fig. 3** The time-course effects of PPP, PRP, PRF*exu*, or PRF*ext* preparations on the wound prepared in HUVEC cultures. The controls included no plasma-derived supplements. $n = 5$

The number of vessels in the center circle (1 $cm^2$) was determined using image analysis software (WinROOF, Mitani Corp., Fukui, Japan). In brief, RGB (red-green-blue) channel layers were separated, and the blue channel layer was manually adjusted to its threshold. After the images were binarized to clearly show blood vessels [23], the number of vessels was counted manually per $cm^2$.

## Histological and immunohistochemical examination of CAM

After counting the number of blood vessels, CAMs were harvested, fixed, and embedded in paraffin for histological examination. As described previously [24], deparaffinized sections were subjected to hematoxylin-eosin (HE) staining and Masson's trichrome staining.

Alternatively, the sections were antigen-retrieved and blocked with 2.5 % normal horse serum (Vector Labs, Burlingame, CA) and subsequently probed with a mouse monoclonal anti-α-smooth muscle actin (α-SMA) antibody (1:100) (Abcam, Cambridge, MA, USA) overnight at 4 °C, followed by incubation in the ImmPRESS® anti-mouse IgG (Vector). Immunoreactive proteins were visualized by a DAB substrate solution (Kirkegaard & Perry Laboratories, Inc., Gaithersburg, MD).

The number of α-$SMA^+$ vessel-like structure (shown by arrows) inside the CAM was determined using image analysis software (WinROOF, Mitani Corp., Fukui, Japan). In brief, after the contrast of the images was enhanced manually, the number of vessels was counted. The area of the CAM in the cross-sections was also evaluated. Then, the number of vessels was normalized

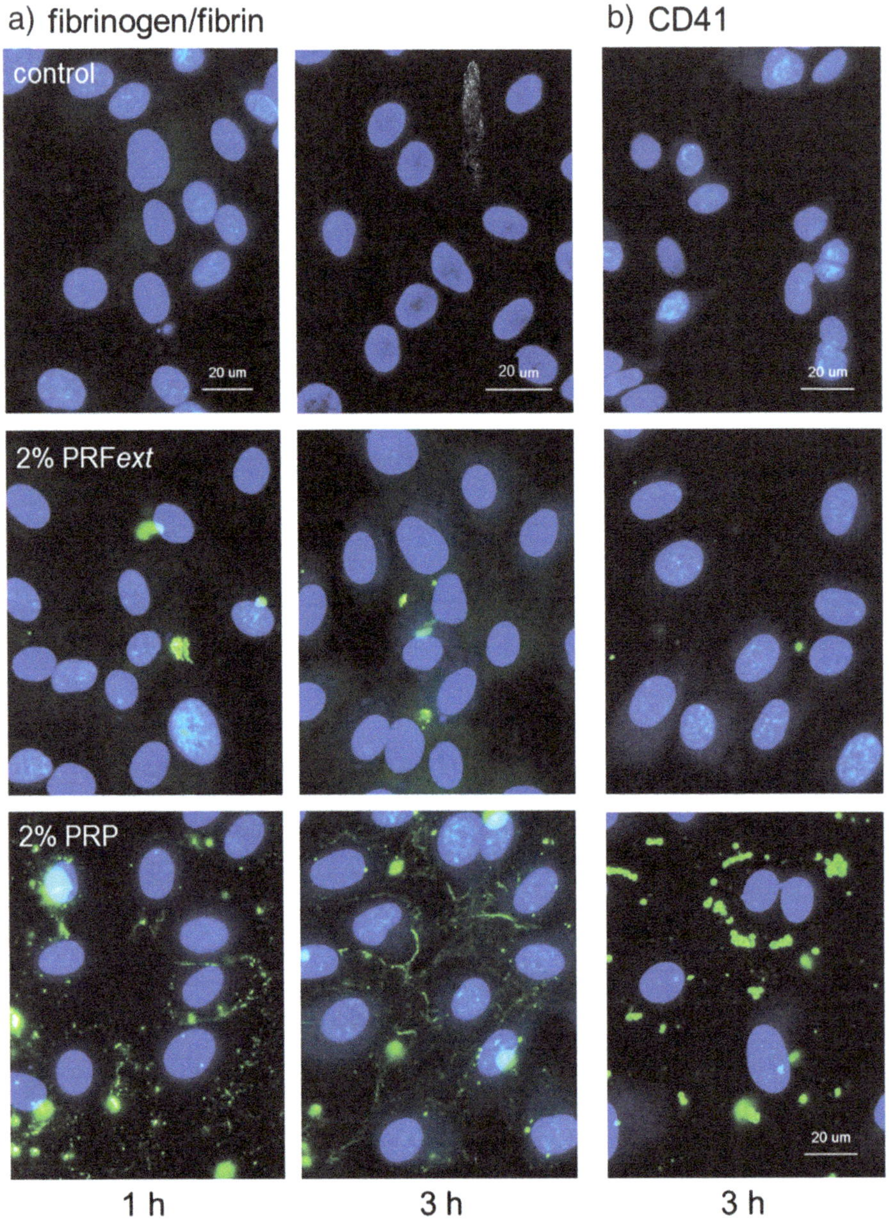


**Fig. 4** Immunofluorescence examination of fibrin fiber formation (**a**) and CD41$^+$ platelet distribution (**b**) in PRP-treated HUVEC cultures. HUVECs were treated with 2 % PRFext- or 2 % PRP-containing media for up to 3 h. The cells were fixed and subjected to immunofluorescence examination. Similar data were obtained from two additional independent experiments ($n = 3$). Bar = 20 μm

by utilizing the ratio of the area to the number of vessels per unit square ($mm^2$).

### Immunofluorescence examination

HUVECs were seeded onto glass coverslips and pre-cultured for 24 h to form subconfluent cultures. The cells were treated with 2 % PRP or PRF*ext* for up to 3 h. The cells were then fixed and treated with FITC-conjugated mouse monoclonal anti-CD41 (1:5) (Beckman Coulter, Inc., Brea, CA, USA) or FITC-conjugated rabbit polyclonal anti-human fibrinogen (1:20) (Medical & Biological Laboratories Co., Ltd, Nagoya, Japan) for 1 h at 4 °C, as described previously [25]. After three washes with T-PBS, the cells were mounted with VECTASHIELD Mounting Medium with DAPI (Vector Laboratories, Burlingame, CA, USA) and examined using a fluorescence microscope (Nikon, Tokyo, Japan).

### Statistical analysis

The data were reported as the mean value ± standard deviation (S.D.). For multi-group comparisons, statistical analyses were performed to compare the mean values

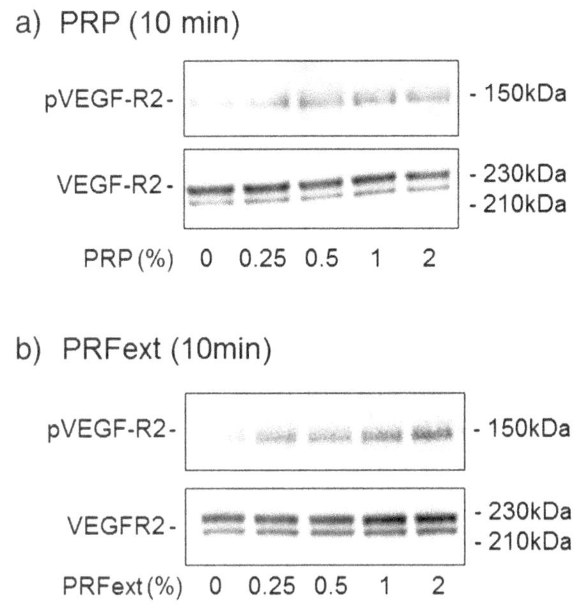

**Fig. 5** The dose-dependent effects of PRP (**a**) and PRF*ext* preparations (**b**) on phosphorylation of VEGFR2 in HUVEC at 10 min. Similar data were obtained from three additional independent experiments ($n = 4$)

using one-way analysis of variance (ANOVA) followed by Tukey's multiple comparison test (SigmaPlot 12.5; Systat Software, Inc., San Jose, CA, USA). $P$ values <0.05 were considered significant.

## Results

The concentration of platelets and growth factors in PPP, PRP, and PRF preparations are shown in Fig. 2. In PRP preparations, platelets were concentrated approximately 6.8-fold over PPP preparations. Although it is challenging to accurately count platelets in PRF preparations, we previously observed by SEM examination that platelets aggregated and attached to the surface of the PRF membrane, suggesting that platelets were concentrated on PRF membrane surfaces [18]. In support of this finding, PDGF-BB, a platelet-specific growth factor, was concentrated 7.6 and 6.5-fold in PRP and PRF*ext* preparations, respectively, when compared with PPP preparations. The potent angiogenic factors, VEGF and soluble DLL1, demonstrated contrasting results. VEGF was concentrated in PRP and PRF*ext* preparations 6.5 and 10.0-fold, respectively, when compared with PPP preparations, whereas soluble DLL1 was not concentrated in either PRP or PRF*ext* when compared with PPP. In addition, the concentration of another angiogenic factor, bFGF, was too low to reproducibly be detected in any of the preparations tested in this study (data not shown).

The time-course effects of PPP, PRP, and PRF preparations on simulated wounds prepared in HUVEC confluent cultures are shown in Fig. 3. The wound closure was facilitated by PRP (2 %) and PRF preparations (2 %), but not PPP preparations (2 %). The order of potency was PRF*exu* ≥ PRF*ext* > PRP > > PPP at 7 h of incubation. The statistical significances are $P < 0.05$ (PPP vs. PRF*exu; PPP vs. PRFext; control vs. PPP*) and $P < 0.001$ (control vs. PRF*ext*; control vs. PRF*exu*). The controls included no plasma-derived supplements.

The time-course effects of PRF*ext* and PRP on the formation of fibrin fibers in HUVEC cultures are shown in Fig. 4a. Typical fibrin fibers were formed time dependently only in PRP-added cultures, but not in controls without plasma-derived supplements or in PRF-added cultures. The distributions of CD41$^+$ platelets in PRP-treated HUVEC cultures are shown in Fig. 4b. Significant numbers of CD41$^+$ particles were found in PRP-added cultures, but not in the control cultures without plasma-derived supplements. A low number of CD41$^+$ particles were found in PRF-added cultures.

The dose-dependent effects of PRP and PRF*ext* preparations on the phosphorylation of VEGFR2 are shown in Fig. 5. PRP and PRF preparations (0.25–2 %) dose-dependently phosphorylated VEGFR2 when compared with pan VEGFR2, and the potency of PRF*ext* preparations were similar to that of PRP preparations.

The effects of clotted PPP, clotted PRP, and PRF membrane preparations on new blood capillary formation in the CAM assay are shown in Fig. 6. New capillary formation at 3 days after application was macroscopically examined. The image analysis for quantitation demonstrated that both PRP and PRF preparations significantly increased the number of blood capillaries. The order of potency was PRF ≥ PRP ≥ PPP and the statistical significances are $P < 0.05$ (control vs. PPP), $P < 0.01$ (PPP vs. PRF), and $P < 0.001$ (control vs. PRP; control vs. PRF). The controls included no plasma-derived supplements.

These effects were further confirmed by determining the number of mature blood vessels based on the concept that α-SMA is a marker of vascular smooth muscle cells. Alpha-SMA was immunohistochemically evaluated to determine the number of blood vessels. Immunohistochemical examination of the effects of clotted PPP, clotted PRP, and PRF membrane preparations on formation of α-SMA$^+$ mature blood vessels in the CAM. As earlier demonstrated in the macroscopic examination of new capillary formation (Fig. 6), both PRP and PRF preparations significantly increased the number of mature blood vessels (Fig. 7). Here again, a similar trend of α-SMA-staining potency for estimating the number of mature blood vessels was PRF ≥ PRP > PPP. The statistical significances were $P < 0.05$ (control vs. PRP) and $P < 0.01$

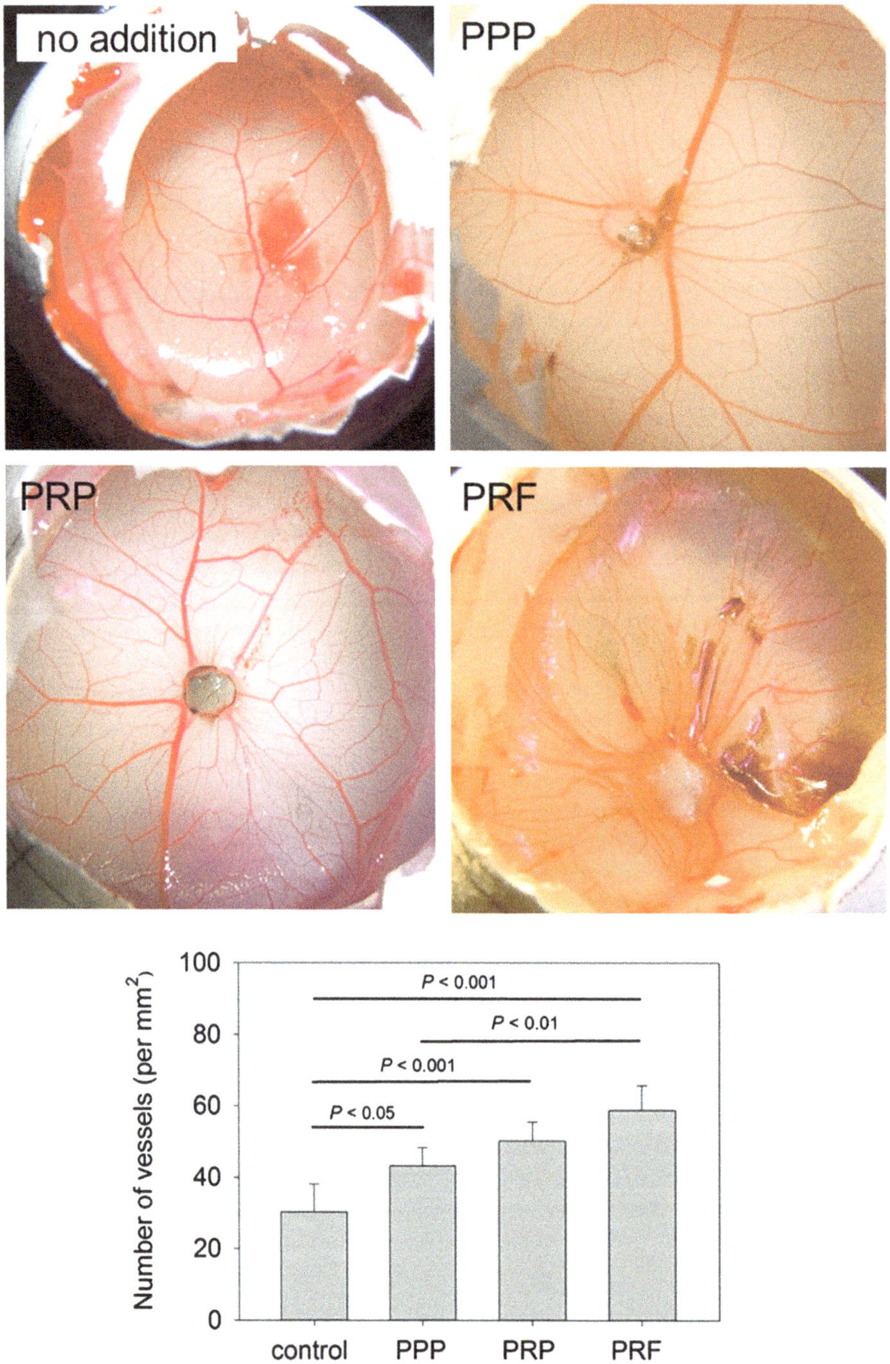


**Fig. 6** The effects of clotted PPP, clotted PRP, and PRF membrane preparations on new blood vessel formation in the CAM assay. The controls included no plasma-derived supplements. $n = 5$

(control vs. PRF; PPP vs. PRF). The controls included no plasma-derived supplements.

Further histological examination with Masson's trichrome staining was performed to examine the changes taking place in the CAM assay. The effects of clotted PPP, clotted PRP, and PRF membrane preparations on the thickness and the structure of the CAM are shown in Fig. 8. These preparations all significantly thickened the CAM by stimulating fibroblast proliferation and extracellular matrix (ECM) deposition. However, both PRP and PRF preparations were more potent at stimulating fibroblast proliferation and collagen deposition

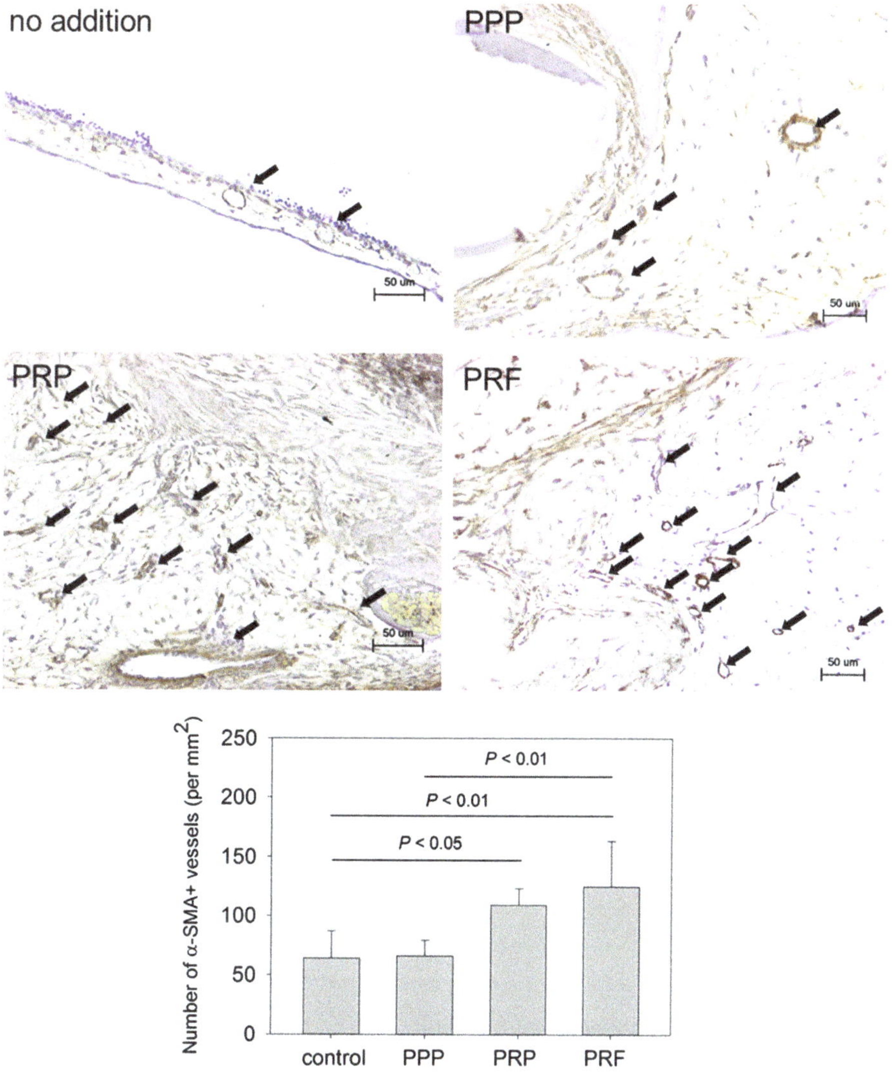


**Fig. 7** Immunohistochemical examination of the effects of clotted PPP, clotted PRP, and PRF membrane preparations on formation of α-SMA$^+$ matured blood vessels in the CAM. Representative photomicrographs of α-SMA$^+$ matured blood vessels (indicated by *arrows*). The controls included no plasma-derived supplements. $n = 5$

than PPP preparations. The controls included no plasma-derived supplements.

## Discussion

The PRF preparation procedure presented here is simple and less technique-sensitive than previously reported; however, it cannot be ruled out that, because of slow clotting, the centrifugation process possibly activates platelets to release growth factors more than what was predicted. It has widely been thought; however, without clear evidence, that even though they function as a scaffolding material, PRF preparations may not provide growth factors to the level that will synergistically facilitate wound healing and tissue regeneration. Dohan Ehrenfest and co-workers first reported that PRF preparations contain significant amounts of growth factors [5], and we independently demonstrated that the growth factors are distributed not only in PRF*exu* but also on and among fibrin fibers [18] (Kawase et al., unpublished observations). Therefore, evidence supports the notion that PRF preparations contain and deliver growth factors to the site of wound-healing.

Furthermore, it has recently been demonstrated in clinical and pre-clinical animal studies that PRF preparations have the potential of tissue regeneration at levels almost identical to or even greater than PRP preparations [6–16]. However, the majority of these results were obtained from macroscopic and/or histological examinations and therefore, these studies were phenomenological and did not investigate the mechanism or the mode of PRF

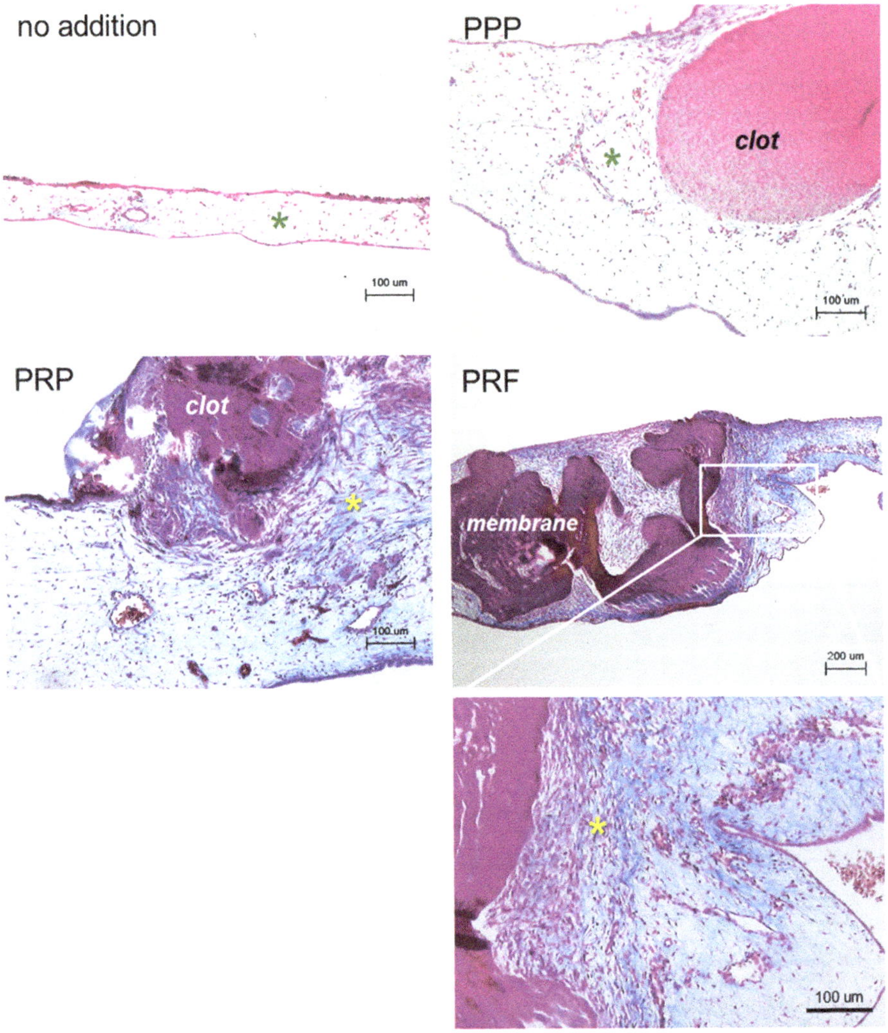


**Fig. 8** Histological examination of the effects of clotted PPP, clotted PRP, and PRF membrane preparations on the thickness and the structure of the CAM. Representative photomicrographs of Masson's trichrome staining ($n = 5$). Cell nuclei and collagen are stained red and blue, respectively. *Asterisks* represent the regions for evaluation of cell density and collagen deposition. The controls included no plasma-derived supplements

action. To our knowledge, the potency and efficacy of PRP and PRF preparations have not precisely been compared with each other at the cellular and molecular levels. One of the possible reasons is that clinicians require evidence to support their clinical use of PRF. From a more experimental point of view, the lack of appropriate standardization or normalization methods between laboratories has hindered the comparison of PRP with PRF in wound-healing investigations. In this study, individual samples were normalized based on the volume ratio of the original whole blood samples to the resulting products (Table 1). It may not be the most suitable for quantitative comparison; however, we believe that the data we obtained will support or explain the previously published data [26–28].

In our study, the ELISA results of the PDGF-BB and VEGF, representative growth factors stored in platelets, demonstrated that platelets were highly concentrated in PRF preparations as well as in PRP preparations. In bioassays, PRF preparations exerted significant effects on wound closure and neovascularization at levels somewhat greater than PRP preparations. We speculate that a factor(s) existing in PRP, but not in PRF preparations, may attenuate the effect of PRP. The most plausible candidate is fibrinogen/fibrin because insoluble fibrin functions not only as a scaffolding material for many cell types but also as a carrier of growth factors [18, 29]. In previous studies [30] (Kawase et al., unpublished observations), we observed that fibrin fibers were formed by the addition of PRP preparations within 30 min and grown thereafter in human periodontal ligament cell cultures and osteoblastic MG63 cell cultures. In this study, an immunofluorescence examination demonstrated that fibrin fibers were similarly formed in HUVEC cultures within 60 min of PRP application, but not PRF*ext* application, and grown over time. Therefore, it is plausible that many growth factors can be trapped by the newly formed fibrin fibers.

Furthermore, it was demonstrated that many CD41$^+$ particles, i.e., platelets and/or their membrane debris, were present in HUVEC cultures treated with PRP preparations, but not PRF*ext* preparations. It is known that endothelial cells bind to platelets through integrin $\alpha_v\beta_3$ and CD40 [31]. Activation of integrin $\alpha_v\beta_3$ facilitates cell migration [32], whereas activation of CD40 inhibits cell migration [33]. In our case, activation of CD40 was probably more dominant than the integrin to reduce HUVEC migration.

When the two PRF preparation forms, i.e., PRF*exu* and PRF*ext*, were compared by ELISA, both PDGF-BB and VEGF were contained at significantly higher levels in PRF*ext* than in PRF*exu*. However, the bioassay using the HUVEC scratch assay demonstrated that the potencies of the PRF*ext* and PRF*exu* were almost identical. At present, we do not have strong evidence to explain the discrepancy between the concentrations evaluated by ELISA and the order of potency obtained in the scratch assay for PRF*ext* and PRF*exu*. In conjunction with the well-known fact that PRP preparations contain a variety of growth factors [17], it seems likely that PDGF and VEGF, even at lower concentrations in PRF*exu* may act synergistically with other growth factors, such as TGFβ, bFGF, EGF, and IGF-I, to exert the maximum effects on cell migration.

In a previous study [25], we demonstrated using Western blotting analysis that PRP stimulates VEGF receptor type 2 (VEGFR2) to accelerate endothelial cell motility and wound closure. In this study, we demonstrated that PRF*ext* acted on HUVEC and phosphorylated VEGFR2 in a dose-dependent manner that was almost identical to that of PRP. This finding is essentially consistent with the data obtained from the immunological determinations. In this study, we did not demonstrate the direct activation of PDGF receptors by PRF and PRP preparations. However, judging from the literature previously published [34], it is anticipated that PDGF and VEGF synergistically function to facilitate neovascularization during the wound healing process.

The CAM assay provided additional interesting as well as informative data. The CAM was thickened by all preparations, and both PRP and PRF preparations were more potent than PPP preparations. This phenomenon could be explained by the direct action of TGF-β and PDGF, in addition to the probable indirect action of VEGF, all of which are concentrated in both PRP and PRF preparations [17, 20, 35, 36] and capable of stimulating the proliferation of fibroblasts. Among them, TGF-β is stored in a latent form in the extracellular matrix [37] and functions as the most potent known growth factor involved in collagen production [38, 39]. According to a recent review article [38], it was suggested that VEGF, TGF-β, and PDGF provided by PRP or PRF preparations in high concentrations cooperatively induced dynamic reciprocal interactions between the cells and ECM to thicken the CAM. In addition, it turns out that this simple ex vivo experimental system can be applied in examining possible dynamic interactions between ECM and CAM.

## Conclusions

These findings suggest that the major angiogenic growth factors, such as PDGF and VEGF, are not significantly diffused away from platelets activated by endogenous thrombin during centrifugation but efficiently preserved in PRF preparations and that the angiogenic potential of PRF preparations is compatible with that of PRP preparations. In conjunction with the user-friendly preparation procedure and high-handling efficiency, we would recommend the clinical use of PRF preparations as a higher-quality, clinically effective substitute for PRP preparations in wound healing therapy.

#### Abbreviations

ACD: acid citrate dextrose solution; ANOVA: one-way analysis of variance; CAM: chick embryo chorioallantoic membrane; DLL1: delta-like protein 1; ECM: extracellular matrix; EGF: epidermal growth factor; ELISA: enzyme-linked immunosorbent assay; HE: hematoxylin-eosin; HUVEC: human umbilical vein endothelial cells; IGF-I: insulin-like growth factor-I; PDGF: platelet-derived growth factor; PPP: platelet-poor plasma; PRF: platelet-rich fibrin; PRF*ext*: platelet-rich fibrin extract; PRF*exu*: platelet-rich fibrin exudate; PRP: platelet-rich plasma; RGB: red-green-blue; TGFβ: transforming growth factor-β; T-TBS: 0.1 % tween 20-containing Tris-based saline; VEGF: vascular endothelial growth factor; VEGFR2: VEGF receptor type 2; α-SMA: α-smooth muscle actin.

#### Competing interests

Author MK, TK, KO, HY, and LFW state that there are no conflicts of interest.

#### Authors' contributions

MK and TK conceived and designed the study, performed the experiments, and wrote the manuscript. KO performed the experiments and data analysis. HY and LFW participated in manuscript preparation. All authors read and approved the final version of the manuscript.

#### Acknowledgements

This project was funded through support by JSPS KAKENHI (Grant #23592881, #24390443, and #24390465).

#### Author details

[1]Division of Oral Bioengineering, Institute of Medicine and Dentistry, Niigata University, Niigata, Japan. [2]Division of Periodontology, Institute of Medicine and Dentistry, Niigata University, Niigata, Japan. [3]Advanced Research Center, The Nippon Dental University School of Life Dentistry at Niigata, Niigata, Japan. [4]Division of Periodontology, Department of Developmental and Surgical Sciences, University of Minnesota School of Dentistry, Minneapolis, MN, USA.

## References


1. Marx RE, Carlson ER, Eichstaedt RM, Schimmele SR, Strauss JE, Georgeff KR. Platelet-rich plasma: growth factor enhancement for bone grafts. Oral Surg Oral Med Oral Pathol Oral Radiol Endod. 1998;85:638–46.
2. Marx RE. Platelet-rich plasma: evidence to support its use. J Oral Maxillofac Surg. 2004;62:489–96.
3. Choukroun J, Diss A, Simonpieri A, Girard MO, Schoeffler C, Dohan SL, et al. Platelet-rich fibrin (PRF): a second-generation platelet concentrate. Part V: histologic evaluations of PRF effects on bone allograft maturation in sinus lift. Oral Surg Oral Med Oral Pathol Oral Radiol Endod. 2006;101:299–303.
4. Dohan DM, Choukroun J, Diss A, Dohan SL, Dohan AJ, Mouhyi J, et al. Platelet-rich fibrin (PRF): a second-generation platelet concentrate. Part I: technological concepts and evolution. Oral Surg Oral Med Oral Pathol Oral Radiol Endod. 2006;101:e37–44.
5. Dohan DM, Choukroun J, Diss A, Dohan SL, Dohan AJ, Mouhyi J, et al. Platelet-rich fibrin (PRF): a second-generation platelet concentrate. Part II: platelet-related biologic features. Oral Surg Oral Med Oral Pathol Oral Radiol Endod. 2006;101:e45–50.
6. Gassling VL, Acil Y, Springer IN, Hubert N, Wiltfang J. Platelet-rich plasma and platelet-rich fibrin in human cell culture. Oral Surg Oral Med Oral Pathol Oral Radiol Endod. 2009;108:48–55.
7. Giannini S, Cielo A, Bonanome L, Rastelli C, Derla C, Corpaci F, et al. Comparison between PRP, PRGF and PRF: lights and shadows in three similar but different protocols. Eur Rev Med Pharmacol Sci. 2015;19:927–30.
8. Jeong KI, Kim SG, Oh JS, Lee SY, Cho YS, Yang SS, et al. Effect of platelet-rich plasma and platelet-rich fibrin on peri-implant bone defects in dogs. J Biomed Nanotechnol. 2013;9:535–7.
9. Kim TH, Kim SH, Sandor GK, Kim YD. Comparison of platelet-rich plasma (PRP), platelet-rich fibrin (PRF), and concentrated growth factor (CGF) in rabbit-skull defect healing. Arch Oral Biol. 2014;59:550–8.
10. Lichtenfels M, Colome L, Sebben AD, Braga-Silva J. Effect of platelet rich plasma and platelet rich fibrin on sciatic nerve regeneration in a rat model. Microsurgery. 2013;33:383–90.
11. Narang I, Mittal N, Mishra N. A comparative evaluation of the blood clot, platelet-rich plasma, and platelet-rich fibrin in regeneration of necrotic immature permanent teeth: a clinical study. Contemp Clin Dent. 2015;6:63–8.
12. Passaretti F, Tia M, D'Esposito V, De Pascale M, Del Corso M, Sepulveres R, et al. Growth-promoting action and growth factor release by different platelet derivatives. Platelets. 2014;25:252–6.
13. Hatakeyama I, Marukawa E, Takahashi Y, Omura K. Effects of platelet-poor plasma, platelet-rich plasma, and platelet-rich fibrin on healing of extraction sockets with buccal dehiscence in dogs. Tissue Eng Part A. 2014;20:874–82.
14. He L, Lin Y, Hu X, Zhang Y, Wu H. A comparative study of platelet-rich fibrin (PRF) and platelet-rich plasma (PRP) on the effect of proliferation and differentiation of rat osteoblasts in vitro. Oral Surg Oral Med Oral Pathol Oral Radiol Endod. 2009;108:707–13.
15. Pradeep AR, Rao NS, Agarwal E, Bajaj P, Kumari M, Naik SB. Comparative evaluation of autologous platelet-rich fibrin and platelet-rich plasma in the treatment of 3-wall intrabony defects in chronic periodontitis: a randomized controlled clinical trial. J Periodontol. 2012;83:1499–507.
16. Bajaj P, Pradeep AR, Agarwal E, Rao NS, Naik SB, Priyanka N, et al. Comparative evaluation of autologous platelet-rich fibrin and platelet-rich plasma in the treatment of mandibular degree II furcation defects: a randomized controlled clinical trial. J Periodontal Res. 2013;48:573–81.
17. Kawase T. Platelet-rich plasma and its derivatives as promising bioactive materials for regenerative medicine: basic principles and concepts underlying recent advances. Odontology. 2015;103:126–35.
18. Kobayashi M, Kawase T, Horimizu M, Okuda K, Wolff LF, Yoshie H. A proposed protocol for the standardized preparation of PRF membranes for clinical use. Biologicals. 2012;40:323–9.
19. Bir SC, Esaki J, Marui A, Yamahara K, Tsubota H, Ikeda T, et al. Angiogenic properties of sustained release platelet-rich plasma: characterization in-vitro and in the ischemic hind limb of the mouse. J Vasc Surg. 2009;50:870–9. e2.
20. Okuda K, Kawase T, Momose M, Murata M, Saito Y, Suzuki H, et al. Platelet-rich plasma contains high levels of platelet-derived growth factor and transforming growth factor-beta and modulates the proliferation of periodontally related cells in vitro. J Periodontol. 2003;74:849–57.
21. Nakajima Y, Kawase T, Kobayashi M, Okuda K, Wolff LF, Yoshie H. Bioactivity of freeze-dried platelet-rich plasma in an adsorbed form on a biodegradable polymer material. Platelets. 2012;23:594–603.
22. Uematsu K, Kawase T, Nagata M, Suzuki K, Okuda K, Yoshie H, et al. Tissue culture of human alveolar periosteal sheets using a stem-cell culture medium (MesenPRO-RS): in vitro expansion of CD146-positive cells and concomitant upregulation of osteogenic potential in vivo. Stem Cell Res. 2013;10:1–19.
23. Nagata M, Hoshina H, Li M, Arasawa M, Uematsu K, Ogawa S, et al. A clinical study of alveolar bone tissue engineering with cultured autogenous periosteal cells: coordinated activation of bone formation and resorption. Bone. 2012;50:1123–9.
24. Kawase T, Okuda K, Kogami H, Nakayama H, Nagata M, Nakata K, et al. Characterization of human cultured periosteal sheets expressing bone-forming potential: in vitro and in vivo animal studies. J Tissue Eng Regen Med. 2009;3:218–29.
25. Kawase T, Tanaka T, Okuda K, Tsuchimochi M, Oda M, Hara T. Quantitative single-cell motility analysis of platelet-rich plasma-treated endothelial cells in vitro. Cytoskeleton (Hoboken). 2015;72:246–55.
26. Sahni A, Francis CW. Vascular endothelial growth factor binds to fibrinogen and fibrin and stimulates endothelial cell proliferation. Blood. 2000;96:3772–8.
27. Wong C, Inman E, Spaethe R, Helgerson S. Fibrin-based biomaterials to deliver human growth factors. Thromb Haemost. 2003;89:573–82.
28. Kumar RV, Shubhashini N. Platelet rich fibrin: a new paradigm in periodontal regeneration. Cell Tissue Bank. 2013;14:453–63.
29. Janmey PA, Winer JP, Weisel JW. Fibrin gels and their clinical and bioengineering applications. J R Soc Interface. 2009;6:1–10.
30. Kawase T, Okuda K, Wolff LF, Yoshie H. Platelet-rich plasma-derived fibrin clot formation stimulates collagen synthesis in periodontal ligament and osteoblastic cells in vitro. J Periodontol. 2003;74:858–64.
31. Kaplan ZS, Jackson SP. The role of platelets in atherothrombosis. Hematology Am Soc Hematol Educ Program. 2011;2011:51–61.
32. Gao B, Saba TM, Tsan MF. Role of alpha(v)beta(3)-integrin in TNF-alpha-induced endothelial cell migration. Am J Physiol Cell Physiol. 2002;283: C1196–205.
33. Urbich C, Dernbach E, Aicher A, Zeiher AM, Dimmeler S. CD40 ligand inhibits endothelial cell migration by increasing production of endothelial reactive oxygen species. Circulation. 2002;106:981–6.
34. Richardson TP, Peters MC, Ennett AB, Mooney DJ. Polymeric system for dual growth factor delivery. Nat Biotechnol. 2001;19:1029–34.
35. De Pascale MR, Sommese L, Casamassimi A, Napoli C. Platelet derivatives in regenerative medicine: an update. Transfus Med Rev. 2015;29:52–61.
36. Amable P, Carias RB, Teixeira MV, da Cruz PI, Correa do Amaral RJ, Granjeiro J, et al. Platelet-rich plasma preparation for regenerative medicine: optimization and quantification of cytokines and growth factors. Stem Cell Research Therapy. 2013;4:67.
37. Robertson IB, Horiguchi M, Zilberberg L, Dabovic B, Hadjiolova K, Rifkin DB. Latent TGF-beta-binding proteins. Matrix Biol. 2015; DOI: 10.1016/j.matbio.2015.05.005.
38. Schultz GS, Wysocki A. Interactions between extracellular matrix and growth factors in wound healing. Wound Repair Regen. 2009;17:153–62.
39. Barrientos S, Stojadinovic O, Golinko MS, Brem H, Tomic-Canic M. Growth factors and cytokines in wound healing. Wound Repair Regen. 2008;16:585–601.

# 24

# Modality and risk management for orthodontic extrusion procedures in interdisciplinary treatment for generating proper bone and tissue contours for the planned implant: a case report

Sachiko Maeda[1*] and Takeshi Sasaki[2]

**Abstract**

In adult interdisciplinary treatments with using dental implants, limited orthodontic treatment, especially orthodontic extrusion (OE), offers many benefits by both correcting teeth alignment and by contributing to the regeneration of periodontal tissues. However, orthodontic procedures carry some risks and unpredictabilities that might compromise tooth and/or periodontal tissue health. Especially in complex cases, it is difficult to decide which orthodontic treatment modalities should be combined, in what sequences they should be applied, and what their force systems and treatment times are.

To achieve optimum results, some cases require two or more OEs to the same site being carried out at different times while taking the treatment effects into consideration. Such staged OE offers minimum intervention and maximum efficiency. In this case report, OE was first applied for orthodontic extraction. After bone regeneration followed by an implant placement and another surgical operation, a second OE was applied to align the inclination of an adjacent tooth. As a result, a predictable prognosis of implants as well as greatly improved esthetics and periodontal tissue health were achieved.

**Keywords:** Interdisciplinary treatment; Implant; Orthodontic extrusion (OE); Combination of orthodontic modalities; Risk management; Orthodontic extraction; Esthetics; Periodontal tissue health; Minimum intervention

## Background

Adjunctive orthodontic treatment for adults is tooth movement that is carried out to facilitate other dental procedures necessary to control disease, restore function, and/or enhance appearance [1]. Orthodontic extrusion is an adjunctive orthodontic treatment with the potential to improve bone anatomy in consideration of implant placement [2].

Several studies have reported that orthodontic extrusion (OE) has many benefits in adult interdisciplinary treatment [3–6].

Because OE is regarded as being simpler and easier than comprehensive orthodontic treatment, this treatment can be mistakenly considered simple and completed without careful planning, which can lead to an unsatisfactory clinical outcome. Orthodontic treatments involve some risks for tooth and/or periodontal tissue that may lead to unpredictable and unsatisfactory results regardless of the complexity of treatments [7–9].

To achieve optimum results, it is important to decide which orthodontic treatment modalities should be combined. In addition, the sequence in which they are applied, the force system, and their treatment time must be considered [10].

In this case report, two LOTs were applied to the same site at different times, along with tooth extraction and guided bone regeneration followed by implant

* Correspondence: maedas@cwa.bai.ne.jp
[1]Private practice limited to orthodontics, 8F Hankyu-Terminal-Bldg. 1-1-4 Shibata, Kitaku, Osaka 530-0012, Japan
Full list of author information is available at the end of the article

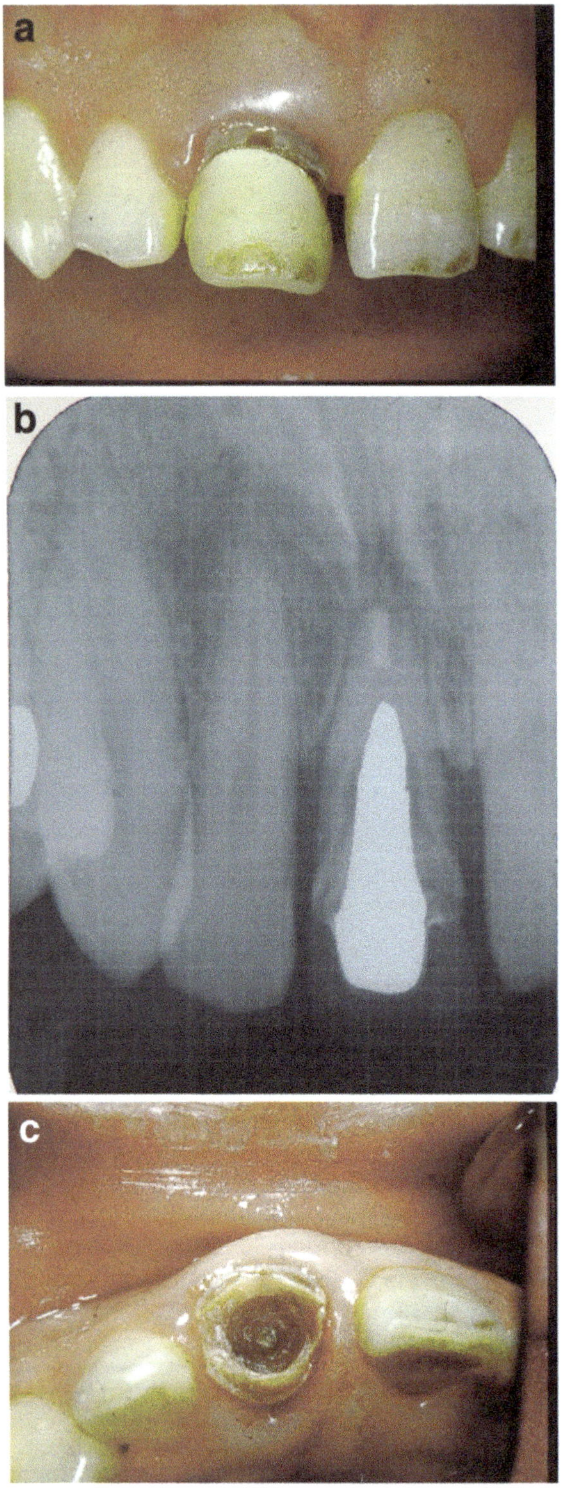

**Fig. 1** Initial clinical situation. **a** Flaring of the right maxillary incisors. **b** Initial dental radiograph showing short root, bone defect of the right maxillary incisor, and a fracture in the middle of the root. **c** After removal of the facial crown and metal post, the right maxillary incisor is seen to have large subgingival caries

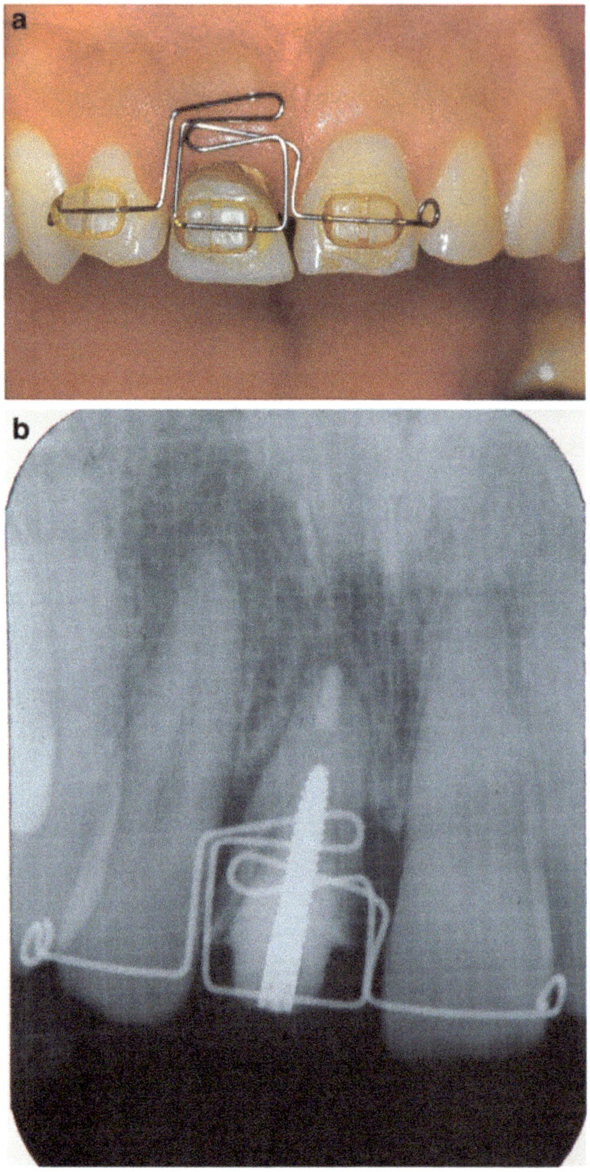

**Fig. 2** Initial orthodontic extrusion. **a** After the initial OE with the 016 NITI sectional arch wire, a 016 stainless steel wire with horizontal loops was placed to advance the extrusion. **b** Radiograph after OE

placement. For this patient, limited orthodontic treatment provided twice during the sequence of overall treatment resulting in improved esthetics and soft tissue health.

## Case presentation

A 28-year-old male visited our clinic with a chief complaint of poor esthetics in the maxillary anterior region. The patient was in good general health, and his medical

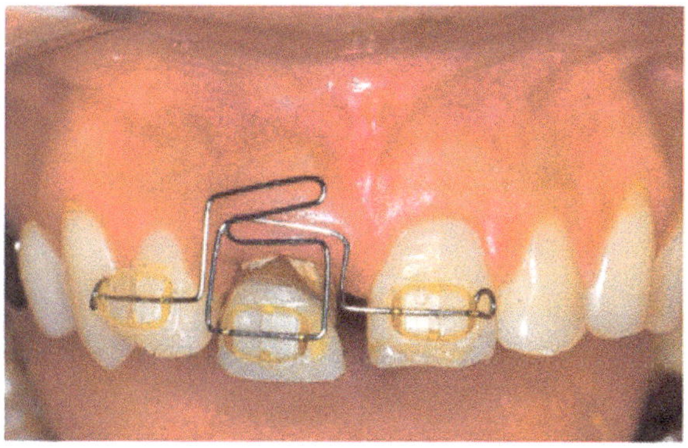

**Fig. 3** One month after the initiation of OE

and dental history indicated no contraindications to dental treatment.

The right maxillary central incisor had previously been restored with a porcelain veneer, while the right lateral incisor was inclined labially and distally. This resulted in spaces of 1.5 and 1.0 mm on the mesial and distal proximal area of the central incisor, respectively. Intraoral examination indicated that the right central incisor was elongated along with gingival recession. Radiographic examination revealed a large diameter metal post, bone resorption of up to one half of the resorbed short root, and a fracture in the middle of the root. Moderate bone resorption was also observed on the mesial aspect of the right lateral and left central maxillary teeth. Deep caries was found under the veneer and along the post space on the right central incisor (Fig. 1a–c).

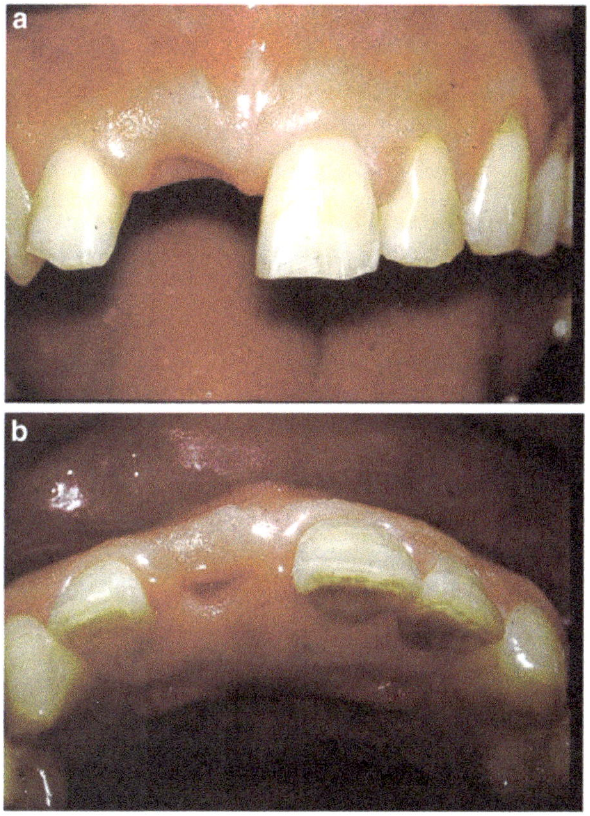

**Fig. 4** After the extraction of the maxillary central incisor (**a** frontal view, **b** occlusal view)

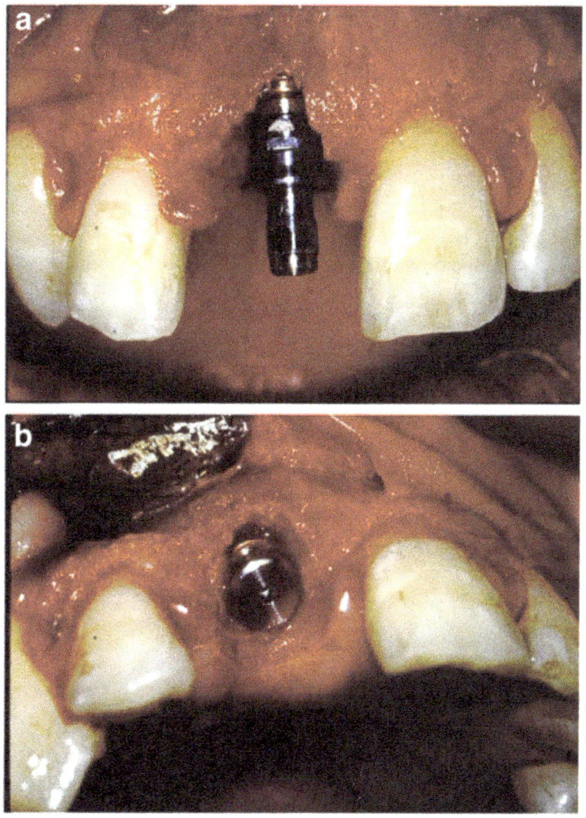

**Fig. 5** Placement of an implant and GBR (**a** frontal view, **b** occlusal view)

The treatment plan consisted of the following items:

- Initial preparation with scaling and root planing
- Orthodontic extrusion and extraction of the right maxillary central incisor
- Implant placement with a bone grafting procedure
- A second implant operation for an abutment connection
- Orthodontic treatment for the right lateral incisor
- Final restoration and retention

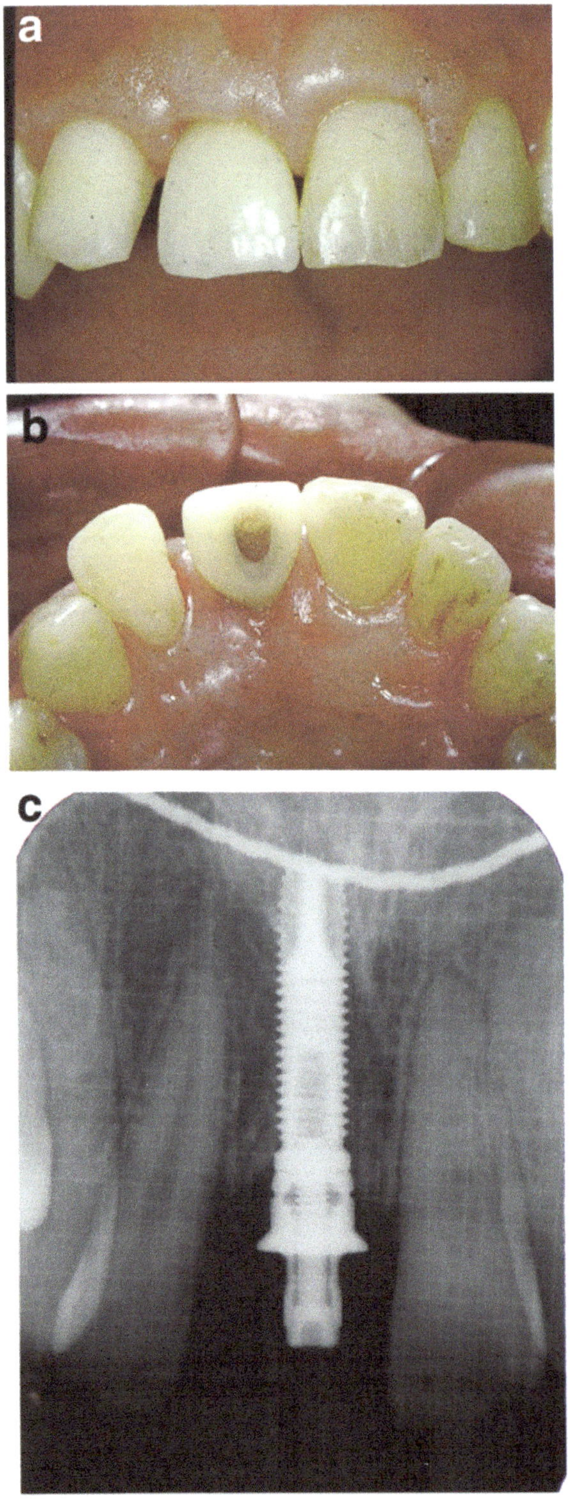

**Fig. 6** Provisional restoration on the implant (**a** frontal view, **b** occlusal view, **c** radiograph after placement of the provisional crown)

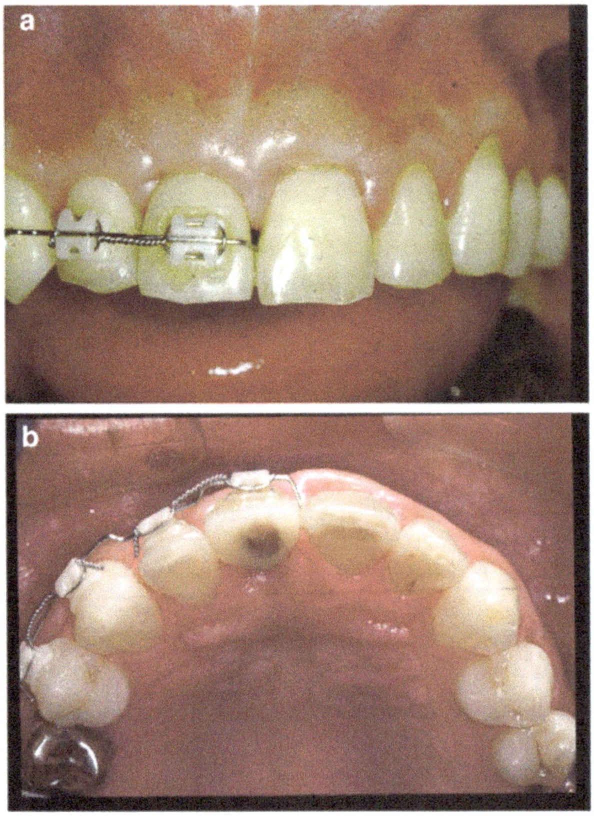

**Fig. 7** After the second orthodontic treatment to move the right maxillary lateral incisor in the mesio-lingual direction (**a** frontal view, **b** occlusal view)

After removal of the existing restoration and the provisionalization of the right maxillary central incisor, scaling and root planing and open flap curettage were carried out. Brackets were then placed onto maxillary right lateral incisor, central incisor, and left central incisor (12, 11, 21 according to FDI system) and extrusion of 11 was completed by using a sectional arch wire with anchorage on #12, #21 with light force(30~50 g) in an incisal direction. Initially, a 016(0.016 mm diameter) nickel and titanium sectional wire and then a 016 stainless steel sectional wire with horizontal loop were used (Fig. 2a, b). Occlusal adjustments were made by grinding off the incisor area of the tooth. After 3 months, approximately 4 mm of tooth extrusion was achieved. (Fig. 3). The tooth was extracted 1 month after completing the extrusion (Fig. 4a, b). Six weeks after the extraction, a root form type implant (Osseotite Implant415, 3i )(4 × 15 mm) was placed into the site with tissue regeneration therapy using deproteinized cancellous bovine xenograft particles (Bio-Oss, Osteohealth) and enamel matrix derivative (Emdogain, Biora) and subepithelial connective tissue graft with dissolvable collagen membrane (Os-sx, Colbar) (10 × 10 mm) (Fig. 5a, b). Five months after the initial implant surgery, a second surgery for flap reflection was performed and provisional restoration was done with a temporary cylinder fixed on to the implant (Fig. 6a–c). A second orthodontic treatment to move the right maxillary lateral incisor in the mesio-palatal direction was initiated at this time by applying brackets on the right maxillary canine and provisional crown of the implant (Fig. 7a, b). Active tooth movement took 2.5 months, and 9 months retention was done with a wire-retainer cemented on the palatal side of the anterior teeth until a final implant crown was cemented on the abutment (Fig. 8a–c).

An esthetic implant-supported crown with symmetric soft tissue contours was achieved with the combined orthodontic extrusion, orthodontic alignment, and grafting procedures. The maintenance phase has been uneventful.

Orthodontic treatment plays a major role in adult interdisciplinary dentistry. In this case, orthodontic treatments were applied in two stages. In the first stage, OE of the right maxillary central incisor was carried out. In the second stage, the flaring adjacent lateral incisor on the same side was corrected. The first orthodontic treatment made optimal implant placement possible because of regenerated hard and soft tissue after the extraction. In addition, the first stage facilitated esthetic restoration with regenerated alveolar bone and soft tissue [11–13].

The second orthodontic treatment was employed to correct the position and angulation of the lateral incisor using an osseointegrated implant as the orthodontic anchor.

It was important that these orthodontic treatments were not applied simultaneously or with the same force system (orthodontic term: combination of all the forces and moments acting on these teeth).

There were two reasons for selecting a staged approach instead of a simultaneous one. First, if these tooth movements were attempted simultaneously, not only would the extrusion of the central incisor not be effectively achieved, but also the mesio-palatal movement of the right lateral incisor could not be sufficiently controlled. Since a lateral incisor will move to an unhealthy bone-defected area close to a central incisor, there could be the risk of an attachment loss of the lateral incisor [14–16]. In contrast, a staged approach would not incur the risk of attachment loss of the lateral incisor because regenerative therapy was applied first [17–19].

Second, with an edgewise appliance, tooth movement can be controlled most efficiently when both adjacent teeth work as anchors [20] (Fig. 9a–c), and a symmetric counteractive orthodontic force can be applied between

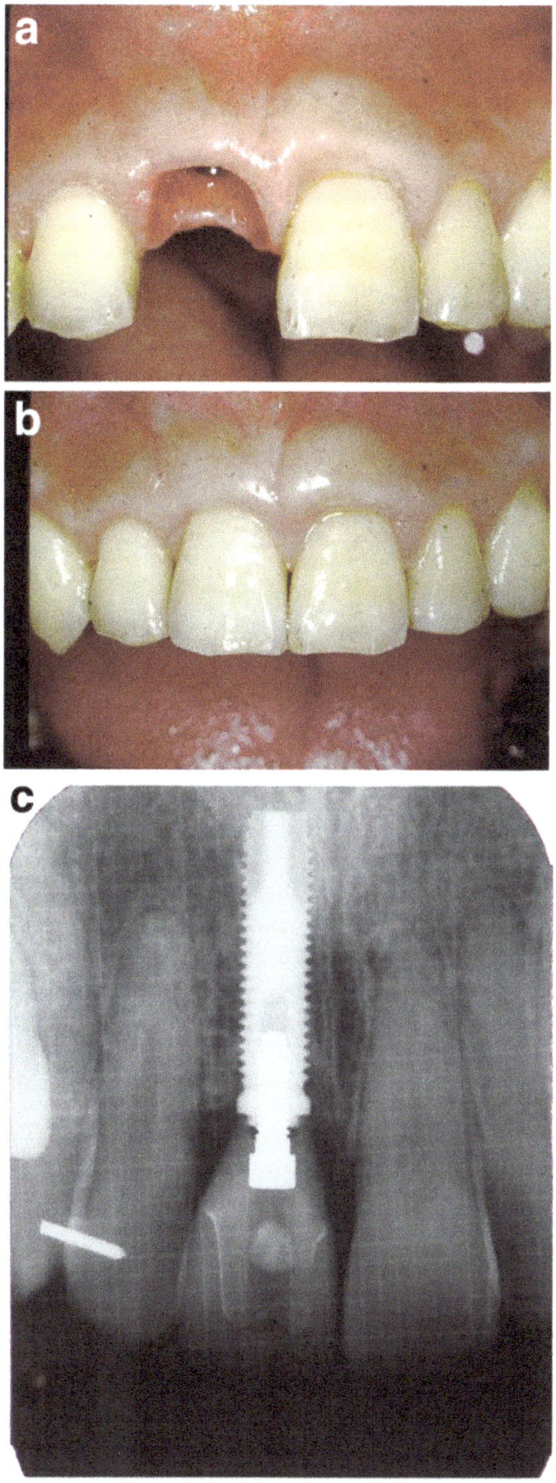

**Fig. 8** Definitive restoration. **a** Before definitive restoration on the implant cemented on the abutment. **b** Definitive restoration on the implant cemented on the abutment. **c** Radiograph of the definitive restoration

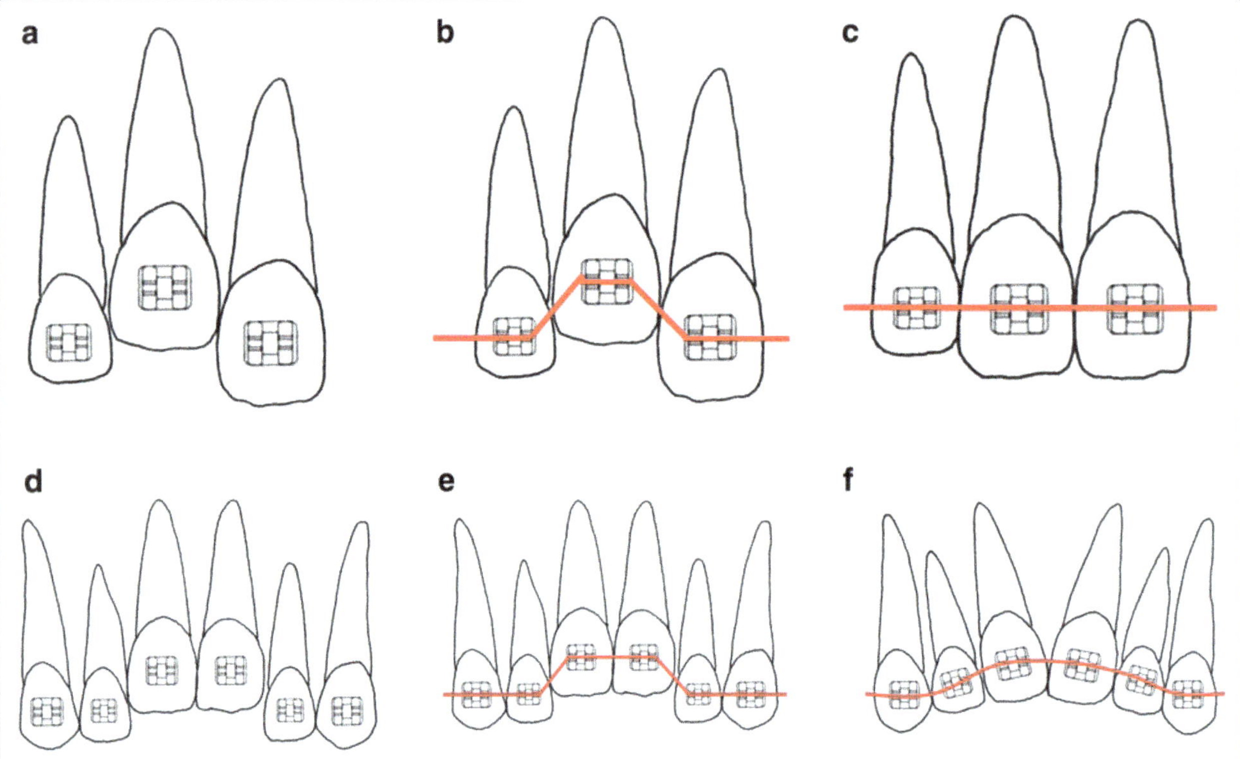


**Fig. 9** For extrusion of the right maxillary central incisor (**a**), the force system (**b**) would provide the desired result (**c**).For extrusion of the two maxillary central incisors (**d**), the force system (**e**) would provide inadequate results (**f**)

adjacent teeth (Fig. 9d–f). It is impossible to simultaneously perform a 4-mm extrusion of a central incisor (4 mm vertical movement) and a 1.5-mm mesio-palatal movement of a lateral incisor (1.5 mm lateral movement) (Fig. 10). Both an extrusion and a mesial movement of about 1 mm can be treated at the same time with one continuous arch wire using a leveling sequence [21]. However, it is not possible to move two teeth adjacent to each other in different directions and by different amounts using the same force system efficiently.

Orthodontic treatments in adults carry higher risks, such as gingival recession, alveolar bone resorption, and root resorption, compared with those in children [22, 23]. When a continuous arch wire is placed on many teeth to provide anchorage, balancing forces can result in unintended outcomes. In this case, the movement of the lateral

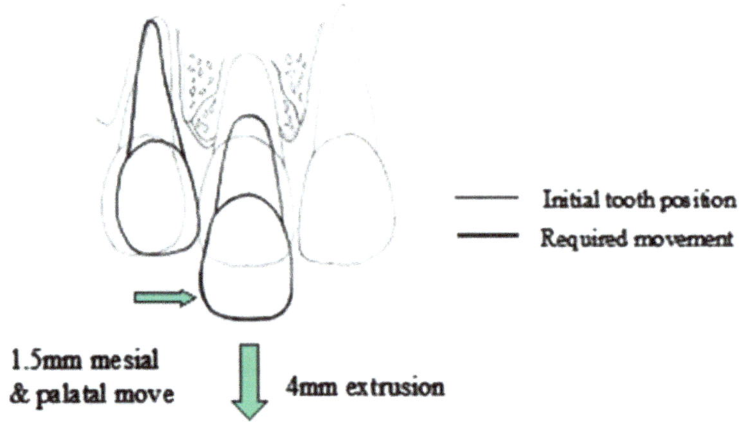


**Fig. 10** Required teeth movement (4 mm extrusion of the upper right central incisor and 1.5 mm mesial and palatal movement of the upper right lateral incisor). No force system with just one arch wire can facilitate this movement

incisor was achieved in a short period of time by using only one adjacent tooth as anchor because the anchorage for the implant was already in place. Adverse effects of orthodontic force could be minimized because the orthodontic treatment was performed in the shortest period of time possible and in a limited treatment area. The staged approach of orthodontic treatment in this study was carried out with minimum intervention and maximum efficiency.

## Conclusions

To prepare optimum implant placement site with improved esthetics and healthy periimplant tissue, orthodontic extrusion is one of the most effective and minimum invasive modalities, however, some cases require staged process with different type of orthodontic approach at different times.

## Consent

Written informed consent was obtained from the patient for the publication of this report and any accompanying images.

### Competing interests

The authors declare that they have no competing interests.

### Authors' contributions

Dr. SM carried out the clinical procedure and study, participated in the sequence alignment, and drafted the manuscript. Dr. TS also carried out the clinical procedure and study with SM. Both authors read and approved the final manuscript.

### Author details

[1]Private practice limited to orthodontics, 8F Hankyu-Terminal-Bldg. 1-1-4 Shibata, Kitaku, Osaka 530-0012, Japan. [2]Private practice in general practice, 9F Nissei-Shinosaka-Bldg. 3-4-30 Miyahara, Yodogawa-ku, Osaka 532-0003, Japan.

### References

1. Proffit WR, Fields HW, Sarver DM. Contemporary orthodontics. Fourth edition. In: Proffit WR, editors. St. Louis: Mosby; 2007. p. 377–394,644–647.
2. Daskalogiannakis J. Glossary of orthodontic terms. Chicago: Quintessence; 2000. p. 158.
3. Maeda S, Maeda Y, Ono Y, Nakamura K, Matsui T. Interdisciplinary approach and orthodontic options for treatment of advanced periodontal disease and malocclusion: a case report. Quintessence Int. 2007;38:653–62.
4. Maeda S, Ono Y, Nakamura K, Kuwahara T. Molar uprighting with extrusion for implant site bone regeneration and improvement of the periodontal environment. Int J Period Res Dent. 2008;28:374–81.
5. Mantzikos T & Shamus I. Case report: Forced eruption and implant site development. Angle Orthod 1998; 68: 179-186.
6. Cardaropoli D, Re S, Corrente G, Abundo R. Reconstruction of the maxillary midline papilla following a combined orthodontic-periodontic treatment in adult periodontal patients. J Clin Periodontol. 2004;31:79–84.
7. Hollender L, Rönnerman A, Thilander B. Root resorption, marginal bone support and clinical crown length in orthodontically treated patients. Eur J Orthod. 1980;2:197–205.
8. Zachrisson BU, Alnaes L. Periodontal condition in orthodontically treated and untreated individuals. I. Loss of attachment, gingival pocket depth and clinical crown height. Angle Orthod. 1973;43:402–11.
9. Zachrisson BU. Cause and prevention of injuries to teeth and supporting structures during orthodontic treatment. Am J Orthod. 1976;69:285–300.
10. Salzmann JA. Problems of the adult as an orthodontic patient. Am J Orthod. 1970;57:84–5.
11. López SG, Gaya MVO, Capilla MV. Esthetic restoration with orthodontic traction and single-tooth implant: case report. Int J Periodont Rest Dent. 2005;25:239–45.
12. Mantzikos T, Shamus I. Forced eruption and implant site development: soft tissue response. Am J Orthod Dentfac Orthop. 1997;112:596–606.
13. Mantzikos T, Shamus I. Case report: forced eruption and implant site development. Angle Orthod. 1998;68:179–86.
14. Ericsson I, Thilander B, Lindhe J, Okamoto H. The effect of orthodontic tilting movements on the periodontal tissues of infected and non-infected dentitions in dogs. J Clin Periodontol. 1977;4:278–93.
15. Lindskog-Stokland B, Wennström JL, Nyman S, Thilander B. Orthodontic tooth movement into edentulous areas with reduced bone height. An experimental study in the dog. European J Orthod. 1993;15:89–96.
16. Polson AM, Caton J, Polson A, Nyman S, Novak J, Reed B. Periodontal response after tooth movement into intrabony defects. J Periodontol. 1984;55:197–202.
17. Araújo MG, Carmagnola D, Berglundh T, Thilander B, Lindhe J. Orthodontic movement in bone defects augmented with Bio-Oss. An experimental study in dogs. J Clin Periodontol. 2001;28:73–80.
18. Diedrich P, Fritz U, Kinzinger G, Angelakis J. Movement of periodontally affected teeth after guided tissue regeneration (GTR)-an experimental piOE study in animals. J Orofac Orthop. 2003;64:214–27.
19. Re S, Corrente G, Abundo R, Cardaropoli D. Orthodontic movement into bone defects augmented with bovine bone mineral and fibrin sealer: a reentry case report. Int J Periodont Rest Dent. 2002;22:138–45.
20. Daskalogiannakis J. Glossary of orthodontic terms. Chicago: Quintessence; 2000. p. 118–9.
21. Daskalogiannakis J. Glossary of orthodontic terms. Chicago: Quintessence; 2000. p. 157.
22. Harris EF, Baker WC. Loss of root length and crestal bone height before and during treatment in adolescent and adult orthodontic patients. Am J Orthod Dentofac Orthop. 1990;98:463–9.
23. Lupi JE, Handelman CS, Sadowsky C. Prevalence and severity of apical root resorption and alveolar bone loss in orthodontically treated adults. Am J Orthod Dentofac Orthop. 1996;109:28–37.

# Use of a trephine bur and curette for minimally invasive harvesting of particulate cancellous bone and marrow from the iliac crest: a case of alveolar ridge reconstruction

Yukimori Isoda[1], Eisaku Imamura[2*], Daisuke Ueno[3], Tsubasa Akaike[2] and Yoshiki Hamada[4]

**Abstract**

Iliac particulate cancellous bone and marrow (PCBM) is still the most predictable autogenous graft material for vertical ridge reconstruction because of its high cell content as well as osteoinductive and osteoconductive properties. However, postoperative meralgia paresthetica, gait disturbance, pain, and bleeding have been reported following conventional harvesting from the anterior iliac crest. We present a case of minimally invasive harvesting of iliac PCBM. A short incision was made, and the iliac crest was exposed after elevation of the periosteal membrane. Only the iliac cortical bone was removed using a trephine bur to avoid perforation. PCBM was harvested with hand curettes and grafted into the vertical ridge defect. Because of the small surgical field, gait disturbance was resolved within 1 day without other postoperative complications. This technique is potentially useful for harvesting a small amount of iliac PCBM.

**Keywords:** Bone graft, Particulate cancellous bone and marrow, Trephine bur, Minimally invasive surgery

## Background

Recently, bone substitute materials have been used in prosthetic treatment with dental implants to reduce surgical invasion, cost, and potential resorption. These products have shown predictable results for localized defects and sinus floor augmentation [1, 2]. However, autogenous particulate cancellous bone and marrow (PCBM) is still the gold standard for extensive bone reconstructions because of the high level of osteocompetent cells for new bone formation. The ilium is the best donor site in terms of cellular quality, and the posterior ilium contains the largest amount of PCBM [3]. The disadvantage of conventional harvesting methods from the iliac crest is the increased risk of postoperative meralgia paresthetica, gait disturbance, pain, and bleeding [4–6]. To prevent these complications, less invasive procedures are required. This case report describes an alveolar ridge reconstruction with harvested PCBM from the iliac crest using a new minimally invasive technique.

## Case presentation

### Case report

This clinical report was approved by the Ethics Committee of Yokohama General Hospital, Yokohama, Japan (No. 27–002). A 42-year-old man visited the Department of Oral and Maxillofacial Surgery, Yokohama General Hospital in June 2006 with the chief complaint of pain arising from the maxillary right lateral incisor (tooth #7) and impacted canine (tooth #6). A fistula and slight swelling were observed on the alveololabial gingiva of tooth #7. No pus discharge from the fistula was found. Radiographic examination revealed apical periodontitis with root resorption of tooth #6. Furthermore, the radiolucent area extended to the labial alveolar bone of tooth #7. Because the infection had spread around the impacted tooth #6, teeth #6 and

* Correspondence: eitaro@wa2.so-net.ne.jp
[2]Department of Oral and Maxillofacial Surgery, Yokohama General Hospital, 2201-5 Kurogane-cho, Aoba-ku, Yokohama-shi, Kanagawa 225-0025, Japan
Full list of author information is available at the end of the article

#7 were extracted under local anesthesia in August 2006. A prophylactic antibiotic[1] was prescribed at 1 day prior to extraction.

At 4 months after the extraction, the patient requested implant treatment in the missing teeth region. However, severe alveolar bone resorption was observed on radiographic images (Fig. 1). We decided to perform alveolar ridge reconstruction prior to the placement of dental implants. Under general anesthesia, we made a 15-mm skin incision and exposed the iliac crest covered with the periosteum (Fig. 2). The periosteum on the medial aspect was elevated, and a window in the cortical bone was created with a motor-driven trephine bur (8-mm diameter). About 2 g of PCBM was harvested with bone curettes (Fig. 3), before the removed cortical bone was replaced in its original position. The wound was completely closed. A pressure dressing was used for 48 h postoperatively [7].

Following the above procedure, the recipient site was exposed after elevation of a full-thickness flap (Fig. 4a). Multiple small cortical penetrations were made, and the PCBM was closely placed on the recipient site followed by the setting of a shape-adapted titanium micromesh sheet[2] (Fig. 4b). A periosteum-releasing incision of the flap was made, and the grafted site was completely closed by the flap using 4-0 nylon sutures. At the postoperative 2-week follow-up, a 3-mm-diameter wound dehiscence was found at the grafted site. An antibiotic[3] was prescribed (200 mg twice-daily for 7 days). No infections were observed up to the 9-month follow-up, and CT images revealed an adequate reconstructed alveolar ridge for placement of dental implants (Fig. 5). Therefore, the titanium micromesh sheet was removed, and two dental implants[4] of 3.5-mm diameter (lengths, 13 and 11 mm) were placed on the reconstructed alveolar ridge (Fig. 6). The implant stability quotient (ISQ) values were 77 in site #6 and 76 in site #7, as measured by an Osstell™ Mentor,[5] indicating excellent stability at the time of implant placement [8].

Alveolar ridge reconstruction using iliac PCBM achieved sufficient vertical bone regeneration for implant placement. At the 3-year follow-up, radiographs showed excellent results (Fig. 7).

## Discussion

The present case demonstrated a minimally invasive approach for extraoral harvesting compared with conventional methods [6]. The iliac crest is one of the most popular donor sites for major maxillofacial reconstruction, because it contains the greatest volume of PCBM and includes a rich supply of osteocompetent cells [3]. However, meralgia paresthetica and gait disturbance have been reported as major postoperative complications [4–6]. A literature review reported 0–20 % temporary and 0–5 % permanent sensory disturbances of the lateral femoral cutaneous nerve (LFCN) [9]. When the LFCN is located in the vicinity of the anterior superior iliac spine (ASIS), flap retraction causes damage, leading to dysesthesia [9]. Harvesting from the anterior iliac crest carries a risk of LFCN injury because the course of the LFCN is rarely superolateral to the ASIS. In such cases, a layer-by-layer dissection of the soft tissues can reduce the risk of nerve injury. The LFCN should be considered the most susceptible to iatrogenic injury [9]. Majkrzak et al. [10] reported that the LFCN was observed to cross the inguinal ligament at 1.4 ± 0.4 cm medial to the ASIS and traverse the inguinal ligament at 1.0 ± 0.1 cm deep to the ligament. For the best approach to the anterior ilium, a skin incision should be made parallel to and

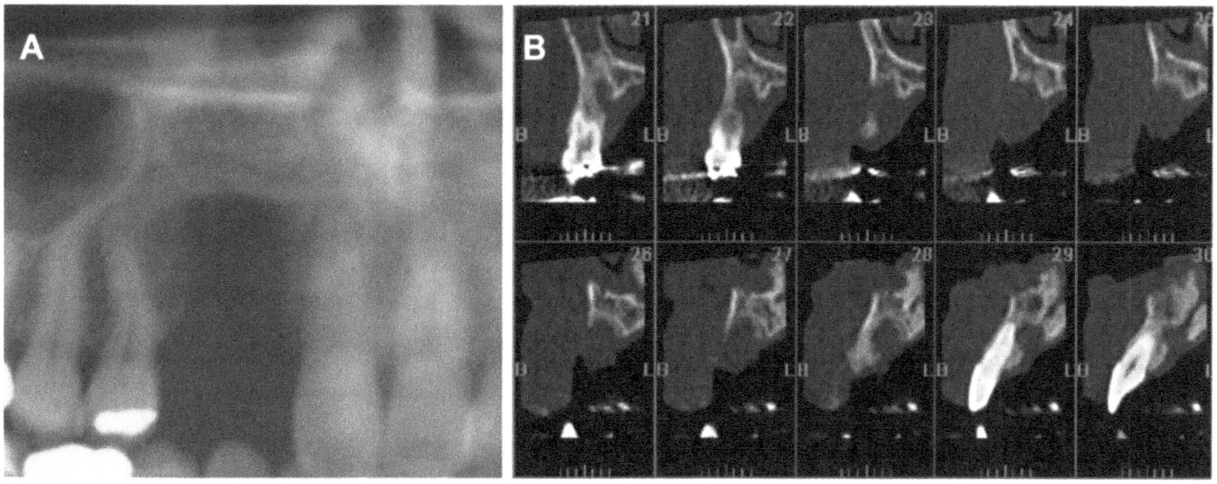


**Fig. 1** Preoperative radiographic images. **a**, **b** Panoramic radiograph (**a**) and cross-sectional CT images (**b**) show vertical bone resorption in the missing teeth region of #6 and #7

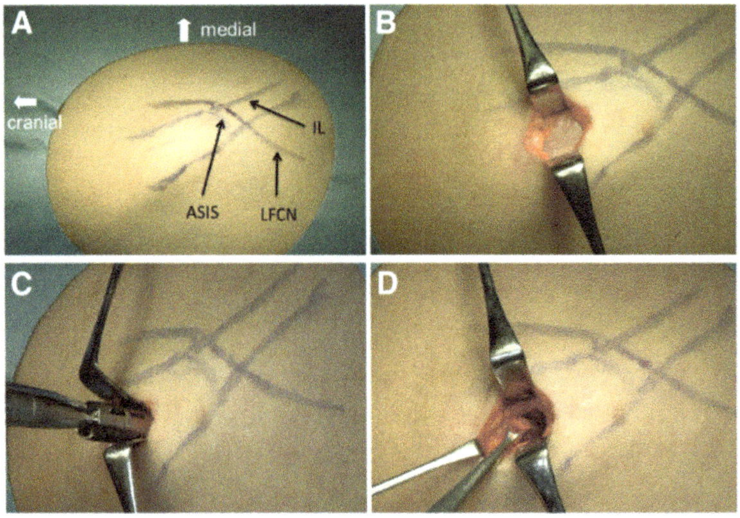


**Fig. 2** Surgical procedures for harvesting of PCBM from the iliac crest. **a** Planning of the anatomic landmarks before the incision. The inguinal ligament (*IL*), anterior superior iliac spine (*ASIS*), and lateral femoral cutaneous nerve (*LFCN*) are indicated by pyoktanin blue. **b** Preparation of the full-thickness flaps following a short incision. **c** Cutting of the cortical bone using a trephine bur. **d** Harvesting of PCBM with a surgical curette through the window in the cortical bone

below the iliac crest by beginning at least 2 cm superior and lateral to the ASIS [9].

A recent clinical report evaluated morbidity associated with iliac crest harvesting [11]. At 1 week after harvesting, 28 and 72 % of the subjects felt severe pain and moderate pain, respectively. At 1 month after harvesting, 22 and 67 % of the subjects felt moderate pain and mild pain, respectively. The scars after harvesting were also evaluated, based on the patient satisfaction score, revealing that 22 % of the subjects felt bad about their condition [11]. Furthermore, Joshi et al. [12] reported that approximately 56 % of patients who underwent conventional iliac crest harvesting had postoperative gait disturbance for more than 2 weeks. Because gait disturbance is associated with the degree of invasiveness, a short incision can minimize the risk of complications [6]. To our knowledge, few articles have reported harvesting techniques using a trephine bur [4, 6, 13]. Burstein et al. [6] reported that the trephine bur technique can reduce incision length compared with conventional methods (2 vs. 5 cm). As a result, the use of the trephine bur technique permitted earlier ambulation and discharge from hospital [4, 6, 13]. Missiuna et al. [14] reported the morbidity associated with iliac crest harvesting using a trephine bur. They found that 69 and 100 % of the subjects were completely without pain at 1 and 8 weeks, respectively,

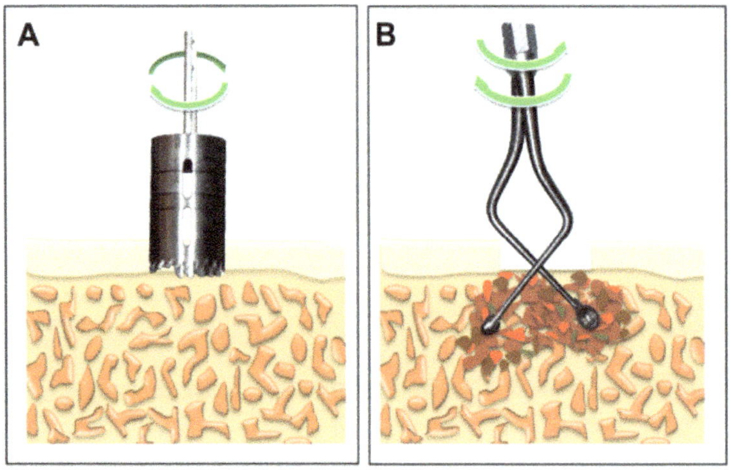


**Fig. 3** **a** Cortical bone was hollowed out using a trephine bur. **b** PCBM was gently harvested from the hollowed region using a curette

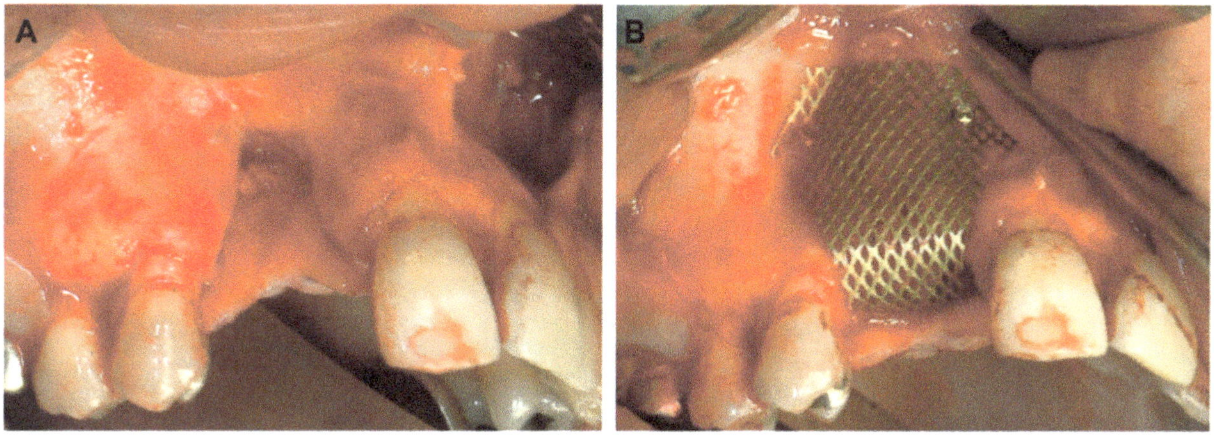


**Fig. 4 a** Intraoral view immediately after flap elevation. A vertical bone defect without the buccal and palatal walls is seen. **b** Intraoral view immediately after PCBM grafting covered by a trimmed titanium micromesh sheet

after harvesting. Furthermore, none of the subjects reported any unpleasant signs and symptoms related to the residual scar. In another study, the use of a trephine to procure corticocancellous bone cores from the anterior iliac crest was found to carry a high risk of peritoneal perforation [15]. In our case, the trephine bur was used only for cutting of the cortical bone, and the cancellous bone was gently harvested with hand curettes. Consequently, there were no surgical complications.

Although the present technique can reduce surgical invasion, harvesting volume is limited compared with the conventional methods. When a defect is not too large, but requires graft material with high osteogenic ability, this technique is suitable for harvesting a small amount of cancellous bone. When a large amount of grafting volume is required, the conventional techniques should be selected. Currently, the most common extraoral donor sites other than the anterior iliac crest are the proximal tibia and posterior iliac crest, because both of these sites can yield a significantly greater mean volume of compressed cancellous bone than the anterior iliac crest [16]. Since hormonal as well as constitutional factors seem to be more relevant to the iliac crest than to the tibia, significantly higher bone density and volume with better osteogenic potential were observed compared with the tibia in elderly patients [17]. A disadvantage of tibial bone harvesting may be that the postoperative scar often causes cosmetic disturbance when patients wear short trousers or skirts. In contrast, the postoperative scar from harvesting of iliac bone is inconspicuous because of its location. Therefore, the

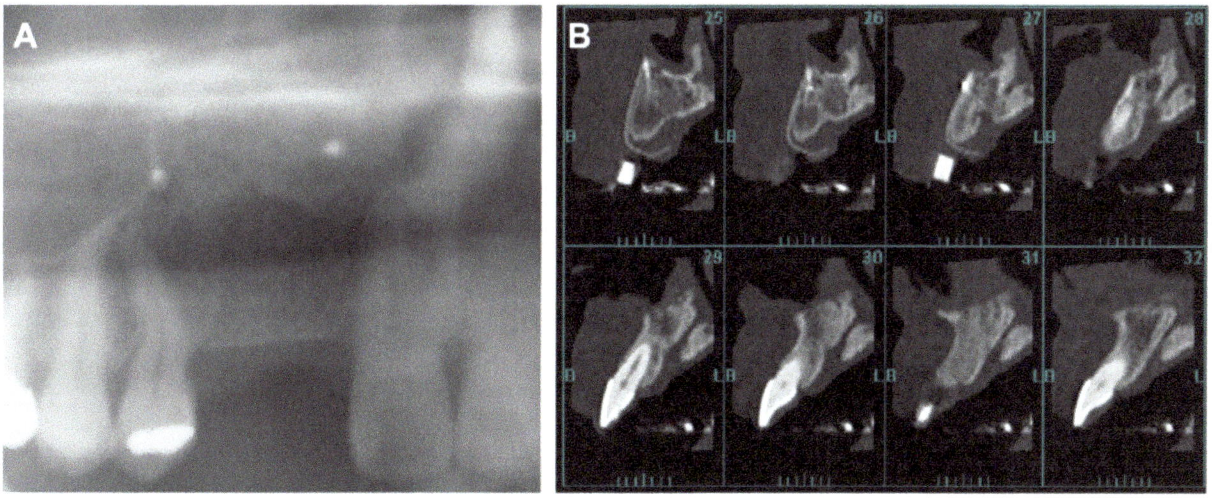


**Fig. 5** Preoperative radiographic images at 9 months after bone grafting. **a**, **b** Panoramic radiograph (**a**) and cross-sectional CT images (**b**) show significant bone regeneration in the missing teeth region of #6 and #7

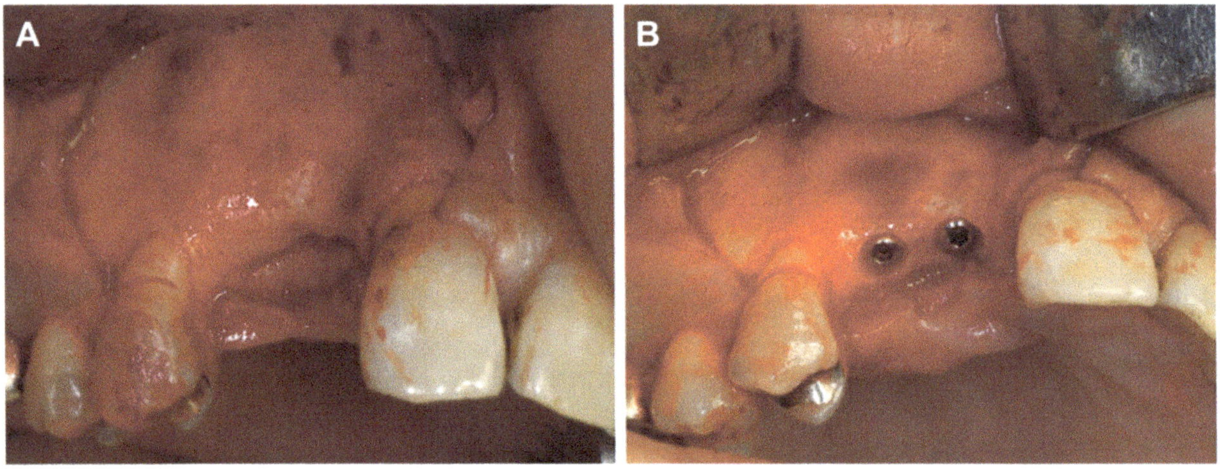


**Fig. 6 a** Intraoral view immediately after flap elevation at 9 months after bone grafting. Significant vertical bone regeneration is observed. **b** Two dental implants were placed in the optimal sites

properties of each harvesting methodology should be considered when extraoral harvesting is required.

The present case demonstrated significant bone regeneration in a two-wall bone defect. Because PCBM underwent remodeling and became mature bone at 9 months after grafting [18], two implants were able to be placed in the optimal site with excellent primal stability (ISQ values 77 in site #6 and 76 in site #7). It is generally accepted that implant stability can be reliably confirmed for implants with an ISQ of more than 47 [19]. The present results indicate that bone grafting using PCBM can lead to the acquisition of excellent bone quality in the grafted site even though the bone grafting was performed in a setting of advanced bone resorption.

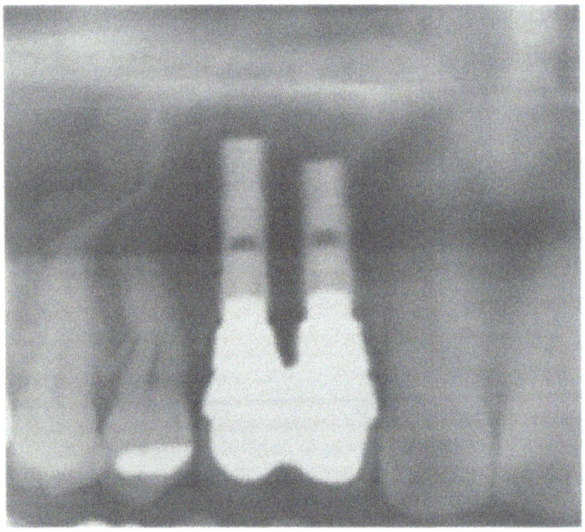

**Fig. 7** Vertical bone height is maintained at 3 years after fixation of the prosthesis

## Conclusions

The present case report demonstrates a minimally invasive harvesting technique of PCBM from the iliac crest. The following important points need to be considered: (1) to avoid LFCN injury, a skin incision should be made parallel to and below the iliac crest by beginning at least 2 cm superior and lateral to the ASIS and (2) to minimize the risk of postoperative complications, the trephine bur should only be used for cutting of the cortical bone, and cancellous bone should be softly harvested with hand curettes after a short incision.

## Consent

Written informed consent was obtained from the patient for publication of this case report and any accompanying images.

## Endnotes

[1]Cefdinir; Sawai Pharmaceutical Co. Ltd., Osaka, Japan.

[2]Titanium micromesh sheet 0.1-mm thickness; M-TAM; Stryker Leibinger GmbH & Co., MI, USA.

[3]Clarithromycin; Taisho Pharmaceutical Co. Ltd., Tokyo, Japan.

[4]MicroThread™; AstraTech, Mölndal, Sweden.

[5]Osstell™ Mentor; Integration Diagnostics Ltd., Göteborg, Sweden.

### Competing interests

Yukimori Isoda, Eisaku Imamura, Daisuke Ueno, Tsubasa Akaike, and Yoshiki Hamada declare that they have no competing interests.

### Author's information

YI is a Visiting Assistant Professor in the Unit of Oral and Maxillofacial Implantology, Tsurumi University Dental Hospital, Yokohama, Japan.
EI is the Chief in the Department of Oral and Maxillofacial Surgery, Yokohama General Hospital, Yokohama, Japan.

DU is a Senior Assistant Professor in the Department of Implantology and Periodontology, Kanagawa Dental University, Graduate School of Dentistry, Yokohama, Japan.
TA is a Part-time Resident in the Department of Oral and Maxillofacial Surgery, Yokohama General Hospital, Yokohama, Japan.
YH is the Professor and Chairman in the Department of Oral and Maxillofacial Surgery, Tsurumi University School of Dental Medicine, Yokohama, Japan.

**Authors' contributions**

EI and YI designed and performed the surgery and wrote the paper; TA wrote the paper; DU and YH compiled the paper. All authors read and approved the final manuscript.

**Author details**

[1]Unit of Oral and Maxillofacial Implantology, Tsurumi University Dental Hospital, Yokohama, Japan. [2]Department of Oral and Maxillofacial Surgery, Yokohama General Hospital, 2201-5 Kurogane-cho, Aoba-ku, Yokohama-shi, Kanagawa 225-0025, Japan. [3]Department of Implantology and Periodontology, Graduate School of Dentistry, Kanagawa Dental University, Yokohama, Japan. [4]Department of Oral and Maxillofacial Surgery, Tsurumi University School of Dental Medicine, Yokohama, Japan.

**References**

1. Klein MO, Al-Nawas B. For which clinical indications in dental implantology is the use of bone substitute materials scientifically substantiated? Eur J Oral Implantol. 2011;4:11–29.
2. Tonetti MS, Hämmerle CH, European Workshop on Periodontology Group C. Advances in bone augmentation to enable dental implant placement: Consensus Report of the Sixth European Workshop on Periodontology. J Clin Periodontol. 2008;35:168–72.
3. Marx RE. Mandibular reconstruction. J Oral Maxillofac Surg. 1993;51:466–79.
4. Sharma S, Schneider LF, Barr J, Chibbaro P, Grayson B, Cutting CB. Comparison of minimally invasive versus conventional open harvesting techniques for iliac bone graft in secondary alveolar cleft patients. Plast Reconstr Surg. 2011;128:485–91.
5. Sàndor GK, Nish IA, Carmichael RP. Comparison of conventional surgery with motorized trephine in bone harvest from the anterior iliac crest. Oral Surg Oral Med Oral Pathol Oral Radiol Endod. 2003;95:150–5.
6. Burstein FD, Simms C, Cohen SR, et al. Iliac crest bone graft harvesting techniques: a comparison. Plast Reconstr Surg. 2000;105:34–9.
7. Freilich MM, Sándor GK. Ambulatory in-office anterior iliac crest bone harvesting. Oral Surg Oral Med Oral Pathol Oral Radiol Endod. 2006; 101:291–8.
8. Al-Khaldi N, Sleeman D, Allen F. Stability of dental implants in grafted bone in the anterior maxilla: longitudinal study. Br J Oral Maxillofac Surg. 2011;49: 319–23.
9. Mischkowski RA, Selbach I, Neugebauer J, Koebke J, Zöller JE. Lateral femoral cutaneous nerve and iliac crest bone grafts—anatomical and clinical considerations. Int J Oral Maxillofac Surg. 2006;35:366–72.
10. Majkrzak A, Johnston J, Kacey D, Zeller J. Variability of the lateral femoral cutaneous nerve: an anatomic basis for planning safe surgical approaches. Clin Anat. 2010;23:304–11.
11. Matsa S, Murugan S, Kannadasan K. Evaluation of morbidity associated with iliac crest harvest for alveolar cleft bone grafting. J Maxillofac Oral Surg. 2012;11:91–5.
12. Joshi A, Kostakis GC. An investigation of post-operative morbidity following iliac crest graft harvesting. Br Dent J. 2004;196:167–71.
13. Sàndor GK, Rittenberg BN, Clokie CM, Caminiti MF. Clinical success in harvesting autogenous bone using a minimally invasive trephine. J Oral Maxillofac Surg. 2003;61:164–8.
14. Missiuna PC, Gandhi HS, Farrokhyar F, Harnett BE, Dore EMG, Roberts B. Anatomically safe and minimally invasive transcrestal technique for procurement of autogenous cancellous bone graft from the mid-iliac crest. Can J Surg. 2011;54:327–32.
15. Caminiti MF, Sándor GK, Carmichael RP. Quantification of bone harvested from the iliac crest using a power-driven trephine. J Oral Maxillofac Surg. 1999;57:801–5.
16. Engelstad ME, Morse T. Anterior iliac crest, posterior iliac crest, and proximal tibia donor sites: a comparison of cancellous bone volumes in fresh cadavers. J Oral Maxillofac Surg. 2010;68:3015–21.
17. Gerressen M, Prescher A, Riediger D, van der Ven D, Ghassemi A. Tibial versus iliac bone grafts: a comparative examination in 15 freshly preserved adult cadavers. Clin Oral Implants Res. 2008;19:1270–5.
18. Iino M, Ishii H, Sato J, Seto K. Histological evaluation of autogenous iliac particulate cancellous bone and marrow grafted to alveolar clefts—a preliminary report of five young adult cases. Cleft Palate Craniofac J. 2000; 37:55–60.
19. Nedir R, Bischof M, Szmukler-Moncler S, Bernard JP, Samson J. Predicting osseointegration by means of implant primary stability. Clin Oral Implants Res. 2004;15:520–8

# 26

# Occlusal rehabilitation in patients with congenitally missing teeth—dental implants, conventional prosthetics, tooth autotransplants, and preservation of deciduous teeth—a systematic review

Hendrik Terheyden[1*] and Falk Wüsthoff[2]

**Abstract**

**Background:** Implant patients with congenitally missing teeth share some common charateristics and deserve special attention.

**Methods:** The PICO question was "In patients with congenitally missing teeth, does an early occlusal rehabilitation with dental implants in comparison to tooth autotransplants, conventional prosthetics on teeth or preservation of deciduous teeth have better general outcomes in terms of survival, success and better patient centered outcomes in terms of quality of life, self-esteem, satisfaction, chewing function?"
After electronic database search, a total of 63 relevant studies were eligible, of which 42 qualified for numerical data synthesis, 26 being retrospective studies. A data synthesis was performed by weighted means for survival/success/annual failure rates.

**Results:** The mean survival of implants was 95.3 % (prosthesis survival 97.8 %), autotransplants 94.4 %, deciduous teeth 89.6 %, and conventional prostheses 60.2 %. The implant survival in children, adolescents, and adults was 72.4, 93.0, and 97.4 %. Annual failure rates of implants 3.317 %, autotransplants 1.061 %, deciduous teeth 0.908 %, and conventional prostheses 5.144 % indicated better results for natural teeth and more maintenance needs for the both prosthetic treatments. The mean OHIP score was 27.8 at baseline and a mean improvement of 14.9 score points was reported after implant prosthetics. The mean satisfaction rates were 93.4 (implants), 76.6 (conventional prostheses), 72.0 (autotransplants), and 65.5 % (orthodontic space closure).

**Conclusions:** In synopsis of general and patient-centered outcomes, implants yielded the best results, however, not in children <13 years. Autotransplants and deciduous teeth had low annual failure rates and are appropriate treatments in children and adolescents at low costs. Conventional prosthetics had lower survival/success rates than the other options. Due to heterogeneity and low number of studies, patient-reported outcomes in this review have to be interpreted with caution.

**Keywords:** Hypodontia; Oligodontia; Anodontia; Tooth aplasia; Tooth agenesis; Congenitally missing teeth; Tooth autotransplantation; Deciduous tooth; Dental implants; Ectodermal dysplasia

* Correspondence: Terheyden@rkh-kassel.de
[1]Department of Oral and Maxillofacial Surgery, Red Cross Hospital, Hansteinstr. 29, D-34121 Kassel, Germany
Full list of author information is available at the end of the article

## Background

Congenitally missing teeth, also called hypodontia, is the most frequent human malformation. The prevalence of hypodontia in white populations is estimated to be 5.5 %, with a higher incidence in women than in men. Hypodontia varies in severity, from a single missing tooth to the absence of all permanent teeth called anodontia. Oligodontia is usually defined as the absence of 6 or more permanent teeth, the third molars excluded, and its prevalence is estimated at 0.14 % in the white population [1]. Hypodontia can occur in isolation (non-syndromal) or as a part of numerous inherited syndromes of which the different forms of ectodermal dysplasia are the predominant entity [2]. Patients with congenitally missing teeth comprise a special group of patients deserving special attention, especially when dental implants are needed.

In cases with congenitally missing teeth, the defect in the dentition occurs very early in life, in contrast to many other implant patients who lost their teeth due to caries or periodontitis at later stages. The early time point has an advantage that the young patients are usually well adapted to the defects. However, prosthetic treatments are often necessary already in childhood. In childhood and adolescence, prosthetic treatments can be complicated, because teeth should not be ground as abutments for crowns due to the large pulp cavity, and dentures may not be splinted if the jaws still grow. It is also questionable whether dental implants can be placed before termination of growth due to the well-known problems of secondary infraocclusion due to the ankylotic healing of osseointegrated implants and due to other biological reasons [3]. Furthermore, children and their young parents and families often have a cost problem, since unlike other implant patient groups, the tooth defects appear in early phases of life when the income is low or needed elsewhere. In some public health systems, occlusal rehabilitation in childhood and adolescence is covered by public insurances and has to be finished before the 18th year of life.

The local implant site can be special, too. A site with aplasia of the primary or secondary tooth usually is different from implant sites in conventional implant patients. Usually, there is a severe lack of alveolar bone width and often height and bone has never been there, since alveolar bone is unlike the basal jaw bone, a development of the erupting tooth. In addition, bone quality can be more cortical and brittle than in conventional implant sites, which can influence implant placement as well as orthodontic tooth movement. The same applies to the fixed masticatory gingiva in a site with tooth aplasia, which can be narrow or missing at all. Due to these common general properties of an implant site with tooth agenesis irrespective of the number of missing teeth, this systematic review includes articles with single or few missing teeth (mild hypodontia), multiple (>6) missing teeth (oligodontia), and also total absence of teeth (anodontia).

There may be mainly four or five treatment options for occlusal rehabilitation in cases with congenitally missing teeth, including dental implant-borne prosthetics. First option is the preservation of a primary deciduous tooth. Such decision has to be made first, if a primary tooth is still present in the site due to missing eruption of a permanent successor. A second option may be the autotransplantation of other teeth, if such transplants are available. This is a well-accepted method in childhood, since tooth autotransplants can heal with a functional periodontium which enables orthodontic movement and enables the tooth to participate in growth of the alveolar crest. Furthermore, tooth transplants in childhood have a better prognosis, when root development is still incomplete and the apical foramen is still open, compared to mature teeth in adults with closed foramen. A third option is conventional prosthetics on teeth, which in childhood will typically include unsplinted overdentures, which should not interfere with jaw growth or resin-bonded bridges, since juvenile teeth should not be ground for crowns. The fourth option is dental implants. Each of the four options has its advantages and limitations and a differential indication has to be made in every single case of congenitally missing teeth. The fifth option may be orthodontic space closure as a single treatment. Of course, adjunctive orthodontic treatment is a very important part of occlusal rehabilitation in patients with congenitally missing teeth. However, this is not in the focus of this systematic review, because this therapy is not generally applicable to cases with multiple missing teeth.

To the knowledge of the authors, narrative literature reviews [4–7] and consensus meetings [8–10] have been published on the topic in the literature. There is only one systematic review without numerical meta-analysis [11]. In the latter, Yap and Klineberg addressed studies on dental implants in patients with ectodermal dysplasia (ED) and tooth agenesis but not on the alternative treatments. They found documented implant survival rates of 88.5–97.6 % in ED cases and 90–100 % in tooth agenesis. The authors concluded that implants placed in adolescent patients with ED do not have a significant negative influence on facial growth and that implants in ED patients younger than 18 years have a high risk of failure.

The aim of this study is a systematic review of the literature of treatment of patients with congenitally missing teeth and a meta-analysis in from of weighted means of survival and success data. The aim is to elucidate the role of dental implants in the group of patients with congenitally missing teeth in comparison with the other treatment options. In addition to the general treatment outcome parameters, the aim was also to include patient-centered and patient-reported outcome parameters. This paper was prepared as the basis of a consensus meeting of the German Implant Association to be held on 9th–10th of September 2015 in Aerzen, Germany.

## Methods

This systematic review was structured and performed according to the preferred reporting items of the PRISMA statement [12].

### Focused question

The focused question serving for literature search was structured according to the PICO format (Table 1) "In patients with congenitally missing teeth, does an early occlusal rehabilitation with dental implants in comparison to tooth autotransplants, conventional prosthetics on teeth or preservation of deciduous teeth have better general outcomes in terms of survival, success and better patient centered outcomes in terms of quality of life, self-esteem, satisfaction, chewing function?".

### Search strategy

PubMed of the US National Library of Medicine and EMBASE were used as electronic databases to perform a systematic search for relevant articles published in the dental literature between 1980 up to 31 May 2015.

A first probatory screening using only the MeSH terms "anodontia" and "dental implants" yielded too few results. It became clear that there are numerous synonyms of anodontia, which had to be included in the search (Table 1). A search strategy based on the elements of the PICO question was constructed: (tooth OR teeth OR dental) AND ((anodontia OR aplas* OR agenesis OR oligodontia OR hypodontia OR developmentally absent OR congenitally missing OR noncarious OR birth defect OR ectodermal dysplasia) AND ((rehabilitation OR dental implant* OR bone augment* OR alveolar bone grafting)

**Table 1** Logical deduction of the literature search phrase from the PICO questionable

| Patients | Intervention | Control | Outcomes |
|---|---|---|---|
| Patients with congenitally missing teeth | Rehabilitation | Tooth autotransplants | General: |
| | Dental implants | Preservation of deciduous teeth | Implant/tooth survival/success |
| | Bone augmentation | Conventional prosthodontic treatment | Prosthesis survival/success |
| | | Orthodontic treatment | Craniofacial growth |
| | | | Patient reported: |
| | | | Quality of life |
| | | | Self-esteem |
| | | | Satisfaction |
| | | | Chewing function |
| Synonyms, search terms, search phrase | | | |
| • Anodontia (MeSH) | • Rehabilitation | • Autotransplan* | • Survival |
| • Hypodontia | • Dental implan* (MeSH) | • Crown (MeSH) | • Success |
| • Oligodontia | • Alveolar bone grafting (MeSH) | • Dentur* (MeSH) | • Growth |
| • Tooth aplasia | • Bone augmentation | • Dental Prosthe* (MeSH) | • Quality of life (MeSH) |
| • Tooth agenesis | | • Orthodonti* (MeSH) | • Satisfaction |
| • Congenitally missing teeth | | • Tooth deciduous (MeSH) | • Self-esteem |
| • Developmentally absent teeth | | | • Chewing |
| • Birth defects | | | • Masticat* (MeSH) |
| • Noncarious defects | | | • Masticat* (MeSH) |
| • Ectodermal dysplasia | | | |
| AND (tooth OR teeth OR dental) | | | |

Boolean operators: (Within column OR, columns AND except intervention and control OR) AND (tooth OR teeth OR dental)
NOT cancer, ophthalm*, brain, cataract
Filter: humans
Search phrase
(tooth OR teeth OR dental) AND ((anodontia OR aplas* OR agenesis OR oligodontia OR hypodontia OR developmentally absent OR congenitally missing OR noncarious OR birth defect OR ectodermal dysplasia) AND ((rehabilitation OR dental implant* OR bone augment* OR alveolar bone grafting) OR (autotransplan* OR crown OR denture* OR dental prosth* OR orthodont* OR deciduous )) AND (survival OR success OR growth OR quality of life OR satisfaction OR self-esteem OR chewing OR masticat*) NOT cancer NOT ophthalm* NOT brain NOT cataract))

OR (autotransplan* OR crown OR denture* OR dental prosth* OR orthodont* OR deciduous )) AND (survival OR success OR growth OR quality of life OR satisfaction OR self-esteem OR chewing OR masticat*) NOT cancer NOT ophthalm* NOT brain NOT cataract)).

Screening was performed independently by the two authors. Disagreement regarding inclusion during the first and second stage of study selection was resolved by discussion.

Electronic search was complemented by an iterative hand-search in the reference lists of the already identified articles. If required, the corresponding authors were contacted and requested to provide missing data or information by email.

### Study inclusion and exclusion criteria

During the first stage of study selection, the titles and abstracts were screened and evaluated according to the following inclusion criteria:

(1) English language.
(2) Retrospective and prospective clinical trials, observational studies, cross sectional studies, cohort studies, case series.

During this procedure, the pre-selected publications were evaluated according to the following exclusion criteria:

(1) Inclusion of minimum 5 patients (exclusion of case reports).
(2) Inadequate case definition or missing follow-up times.
(3) Double publication of the same sample
(4) Lack of clinical data
(5) Studies in cleft lip and palate patients

### Quality and risk of bias assessment of selected studies

A quality assessment of all selected full-text articles was performed. It made no sense to use the Cochrane collaborations' tool for assessing risk of bias for randomized controlled studies since the majority of the included studies were retrospective case series. Instead, a system modified from the US Agency for Healthcare Research and Quality Methods Guide for Comparative Effectiveness Reviews was used, which asked for the sources of possible bias [13]. The criteria were each judged with low, medium, and high risk of bias: case selection bias and confounding, attrition bias (loss of participants), detection bias (reliable measures?), reporting bias (selective or incomplete reporting), followed by a summary of the risk. Exclusion and quality assessment was performed independently by both authors. Disagreements were resolved by discussion.

### Data extraction

A data extraction template was generated and based on the treatment types for the general outcome parameters and for the patient-centered outcome parameters. Due to incomplete reporting, old studies, and changing definitions in some papers, the required data on survival and success were often not found directly listed in the publications. In this case, they had to be retrieved from side informations or recalculated from tables. The following rules were applied: survival meant that the unit (implant, tooth, prosthesis) was reported to be present in the oral cavity. Success definition of an implant followed the criteria of Buser and coworkers [14] which are the following: absence of persistent subjective complaints such as pain, foreign body sensation and/or dysesthesia, absence of a peri-implant infection with suppuration, absence of mobility, absence of a continuous radiolucency (severe bone resorption) around the implant. A prosthesis either conventional or implant borne was counted as a success, if there were no complications reported like fracture, soft tissue recessions, or documented treatment needs. A deciduous tooth was counted as a success, if there was no ankylosis and infraocclusion reported. A tooth autotransplant was regarded as a success if there were no reports of ankylosis or severe root resorption, infection, or mobility.

### Statistics and data synthesis

For data synthesis, the survival and success data of the individual studies were pooled by the weighted mean method and 95 % confidence intervals were calculated as estimations of variance. A meta-analysis was not possible due to the structure of the underlying survival success data as simple percentages without a measure of variance and without control groups in most studies. The survival/success data were weighted both based on patients and units (either implants/teeth/prostheses). Because the studies showed large differences in follow-up times, these were standardized by calculating annual failure rates by dividing the success and survival data through the follow-up time in years. All spreadsheet calculations and statistics were made with the Microsoft Excel program.

## Results

### Study selection

A total of 1508 potentially relevant titles and abstracts were found by the electronic search. Twelve titles found additionally by evaluation of reference lists of included articles were added. During first screening, 1020 publications were excluded based on database information. One hundred twenty-eight full-text articles were thoroughly evaluated. A total of 65 papers had to be excluded at this stage because they did not fulfill the inclusion criteria of the present systematic review. Sixty-three articles went into qualitative assessment (Fig. 1). One article had to be excluded or pooled with another because of possible double publication of the same cohort (Grecchi (b) [15]), one article because of missing follow-up times (Hvaring [16]), one because of missing clinical data (Kjaer [17]), and two articles because of missing numerical data (Dellavia [18, 19]). The study of Bergendal [20] could be kept in the analysis after contacting the author for clarification (no follow-up time reported). The implants in that study were observed only over the healing period (estimated 6 months in average). Because of too few studies and incompletely reported data studies on orthodontic gap closure, facial growth and masticatory performance were not included into the quantitative data synthesis. Forty-two studies were included in the assessment of general outcome parameter survival and success. For 16 studies on patient-centered variables, also weighted means were calculated.

#### Evaluation of study quality and risk of bias

The majority ($n = 25$) of the 42 studies were retrospective, 14 were prospective including one RCT 2 were cross sectional studies, and 1 remained unclear. Despite a low evidence level in terms of study design, there were no major concerns about risk of bias. The 30/42 studies were rated with a low risk of bias, and 12/42 had a medium risk. No study had a high risk of bias and consequently no further study was excluded at this stage because of bias (Table 2).

#### Studies on general outcome parameters

##### *Studies on dental implants and implant-supported prosthetics*

A total of 19 studies with a mean follow-up time of 4.6 years (maximum 15.1 years) was included (Table 3). Most studies were of retrospective character. The heterogeneity of the studies concerning survival and success data was low and acceptable for the numerical data synthesis. The studies showed some heterogeneity in patient inclusion, because in some studies, missing single teeth and treatments with single crowns on implants were mixed with severe oligodontia and varying prosthetic treatment including overdentures on implants. Also, management of bone defects and necessity of bone grafting were heterogenous between the studies. This heterogeneity did not lead to exclusion from the present numerical evaluation. The study of Bergendal and coworkers [20] was considered important, because a high ratio of implant failures was reported in childhood. It was one of the very few studies in the literature on implantation in childhood. However, no follow-up time was reported because it was a cross-sectional survey. The author was contacted via email

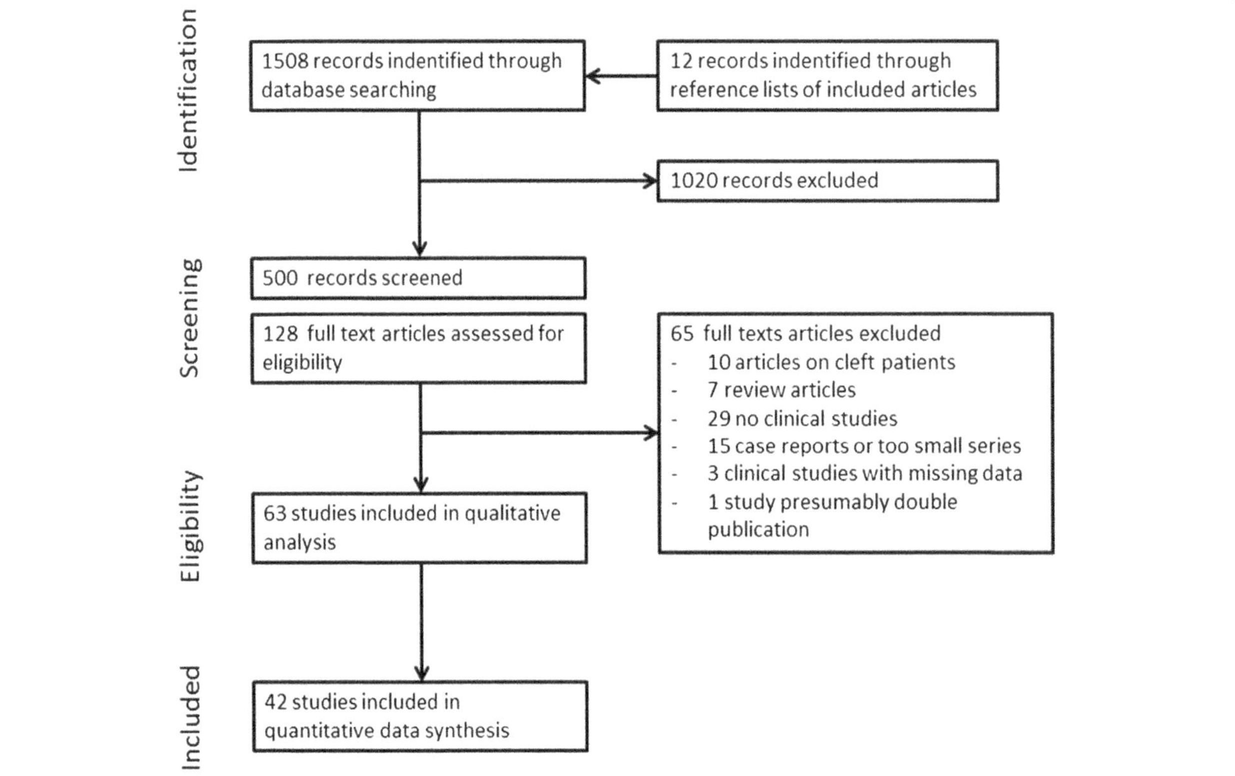


**Fig. 1** Flow diagram of literature search and inclusion

**Table 2** Summary of the selected studies and quality assessement

| Author | Year | Study type | Case selection bias (homogeneity and confounders) | Performance bias (fidelity to protocol) | Attrition bias (loss of participants) | Detection bias (reliable measures) | Reporting bias (selective reporting or conflicting interests) | Summary assessments Risk of bias |
|---|---|---|---|---|---|---|---|---|
| Implant studies | | | | | | | | |
| Ledermann [40] | 1993 | Retrospect | M | M | L | M | H | M |
| Kearns [41] | 1999 | ProspObs | L | L | L | L | M | L |
| Thilander [3] | 2001 | ProspObs | L | L | L | L | L | L |
| Guckes [42] | 2002 | ProspObs | M | L | L | L | M | L |
| Sweeney [43] | 2005 | Retrospect | L | L | L | L | M | L |
| Finnema [27] | 2005 | Retrospect | L | L | M | L | M | L |
| Poggio [44] | 2005 | Retrospect | M | M | M | M | M | M |
| Zarone [45] | 2006 | ProspObs | L | L | L | L | L | L |
| Becelli [46] | 2007 | Retrospect | L | L | L | L | M | L |
| Bergendal [20] | 2008 | Survey | M | L | H | M | M | M |
| Dueled [26] | 2008 | Retrospect | M | L | M | L | L | L |
| Krieger [25] | 2009 | Retrospect | M | L | L | M | M | L |
| Degidi [47] | 2009 | RCT | L | L | L | L | L | L |
| Creton [1] | 2010 | Retrospect | L | L | M | L | M | L |
| Grecchi [15](a), [22](b) | 2010 | Retrospect | H | M | M | L | L | M |
| Nissan [48] | 2011 | Unclear | H | L | M | M | M | M |
| Heuberer [38] | 2012 | Retrospect | L | L | L | L | M | L |
| Hosseini [49] | 2013 | ProspObs | L | L | L | L | L | L |
| Zou [50] | 2014 | Retrospect | M | L | L | L | L | L |
| Autotransplants | | | | | | | | 14/19 L 5/19 M |
| Kristersson [51] | 1991 | Retrospect | M | L | L | L | L | L |
| Kugelberg [52] | 1994 | ProspObs | M | L | L | L | L | L |
| Marcusson [53] | 1996 | ProspObs | M | L | L | L | L | L |
| Josefsson [54] | 1999 | Retrospect | M | L | M | L | L | L |
| Czochrowska [55] | 2002 | Retrospect | H | L | M | L | L | M |
| Bauss [23] | 2004 | prospCT | M | L | M | M | M | M |
| Jonsson [56] | 2004 | ProspObs | M | L | L | L | M | L |
| Tanaka [57] | 2007 | Retrospect | M | L | M | L | M | M |
| Mensink [58] | 2010 | Retrospect | M | L | L | L | M | L |
| Kvint [59] | 2010 | Retrospect | M | L | L | L | L | L |
| Bokelund [24] | 2013 | Retrospect | L | L | L | L | L | L |
| Deciduous teeth | | | | | | | | 8/11 L 3/11 M |
| Bjerklin [60] | 2000 | ProspObs | M | L | M | L | L | L |
| Ith-Hansen [61] | 2000 | ProspObs | L | L | L | L | L | L |
| Sletten [62] | 2003 | Retrospect | L | L | M | L | M | L |
| Bjerklin [63] | 2008 | ProspObs | M | L | M | L | L | L |
| Kjaer [17] | 2008 | Retrospect | L | L | M | L | L | L |
| Hvaring [16] | 2013 | Cross section | L | L | L | L | L | L |

**Table 2** Summary of the selected studies and quality assessement *(Continued)*

| | | | | | | | | |
|---|---|---|---|---|---|---|---|---|
| Convent. Prosth. | | | | | | | | 2/6 L 4/6 M |
| Hobkirk [64] | 1989 | Retrospect | H | M | M | L | M | M |
| Pröbster [65] | 1997 | Retrospect | M | L | M | L | M | M |
| Garnett [66] | 2005 | Retrospect | M | L | M | L | M | M |
| Dueled [26] | 2008 | Retrospect | M | L | M | L | L | L |
| Krieger [25] | 2009 | Retrospect | M | L | L | M | M | M |
| Spinas [67] | 2013 | ProspObs | L | L | L | L | M | L |
| | | | | | | | | 2/6 L 4/6 M |
| Total | $n = 42$ | 25 retrosp 14 prosp | | | | | | 30/42 L12/42 M |

and confirmed that all implant losses had occurred during healing time before prosthetic restoration. Since healing time was has usually a maximum of 6 months, the follow-up time was set on arbitrary 0.6 year. The study of Durstberger et al. [21] had to be excluded because of vague follow-up data and no information of implant losses during follow-up and most of the mentioned patients were only planned for implant placement but had no implants placed. The studies of Grecchi (a) [22] were pooled with Grecchi (b) [15] for numerical analysis, because of assumed double publication of the same samples. In most of the studies, implants had been placed in conjunction with bone grafting, but only Grecchi (a) [22] had presented outcome data on this aspect. There were no prominent differences for implants placed in grafted bone compared with non-grafted sites. Secondary infraocclusion of approximately 1 mm was a problem of implant placements in the maxillary incisor region in childhood [3]. Marginal bone resorption at implants was not a prominent finding and ranged from 0.2 to 1.2 mm in the studies which reported this aspect. The success/survival data and further subgroup analysis for implant survival data is presented below.

***Studies on tooth autotransplantation***

A total of 11 studies with a mean follow-up time of 7.6 years (maximum 26.4 years) were included, all of which qualified also for the numerical analysis (Table 4). The study heterogeneity concerning survival and success data was low and acceptable for numerical data analysis. The studies showed some heterogeneity in patient inclusion, because in most studies a tooth agenesis sample was mixed also with missing teeth due to trauma and other reasons, which did not lead to exclusion from the present evaluation. According to the table, three studies found a better survival between 10 and 46 % of immature teeth compared to mature teeth. The Bauss study [23] demonstrated better pulpal and periodontal conditions if a transplantated tooth was not moved orthodontically, in comparison of the different orthodontic treatments derotation was more harmful than extrusion. According to the Bokelund study [24], premolar transplants performed better than molars. A preceding primary tooth at the receptor site of a tooth autotransplant was connected with a lower transplant success than a normal primary tooth. The numerical success/survival data are presented below.

***Studies on preservation of deciduous teeth***

A total of 6 studies with a mean follow-up time of 12.5 years (maximum 16.5 years) was included, of which only 4 qualified for the numerical analysis (Table 5). The studies were homogenous in terms of outcome parameters and inclusion of only tooth agenesis patients. Two studies (Kjaer [17], Hvaring [16] ) contained no data on follow-up times. The Kjaer study made an important statement that in patients in whom the dentitions shows morphological signs of ectodermal dysplasia (screw driver shaper incisors, taurodontism, invaginations of incisors or slim incisors, typical ED sites of aplasia), the risk of root resorption fatal prognosis of a deciduous tooth was elevated by the factor 1.46 compared to patients with normal tooth appearance. In general, root resorption, ankylosis, and consecutive infraocclusion were a problem of preservation of deciduous second molars at the site of a secondary premolar aplasia. The absence of root resorption was interpreted as success criterion in most studies, therefore, in contrast to high survival figures, the success of deciduous teeth was lower. The numerical success/survival data are presented below.

***Studies on conventional prosthetics on teeth***

A total of 6 studies with a mean follow-up time of 7.2 years (maximum 15.1 years) was included, all of which qualified for the numerical analysis (Table 6). This relatively small group of studies showed a high level of heterogeneity in patient inclusion, because this group comprised various indications from single missing incisors up to severe hypodontia treated with

**Table 3** Synopsis of included studies on dental implants and prosthetics on dental implants in order of publication year

| Author | Year | Study type | Population | Treatment | Comparison | Patients | Implants | Implant survival [%] | Implant success [%] | Prosthes. survival [%] | Marginal resorpt. [mm] | Infra occlusion [mm] | Follow-up [y] | Risk of bias |
|---|---|---|---|---|---|---|---|---|---|---|---|---|---|---|
| Ledermann [40] | 1993 | Retrospect | Agenesis, trauma | FPD | 9–18 years | 34 | 42 | 90 | 90 | 100 | | | 3 | M |
| Kearns [41] | 1999 | ProspObs | ED 5–17 years | Full denture | All | 6 | 41 | 97.6 | | | | | 7.8 | L |
| | | | | | <6 years | 2 | 9 | 100 | 44.4 | 0 | | | 7.8 | |
| | | | | | >12 years | 4 | 32 | 96.9 | 96.9 | 100 | | | 7.8 | |
| Thilander [3] | 2001 | ProspObs | Agen,<18 years trauma | SC, FPD | All | 18 | 47 | 100 | 100 | 93.9 | | | 10 | L |
| | | | | | Incisors | 12 | 26 | 100 | 100 | 88.2 | 0.75 | 0.98 | 10 | |
| | | | | | Canines | 4 | 8 | 100 | 100 | 100 | 0.6 | 0 | 10 | |
| | | | | | Premolars | 5 | 13 | 100 | 100 | 100 | 0.5 | 0.1–0.6 | 10 | |
| Guckes [42] | 2002 | ProspObs | ED 5–18 years | Full denture | All | 51 | 264 | 90 | | | | | 2 | L |
| | | | | | Maxilla | | 21 | 71 | | | | | 2 | |
| | | | | | Mandible | | 243 | 91 | | | | | 2 | |
| | | | | | <11 years | | 46 | 85 | | | | | 2 | |
| | | | | | 11–18 years | | 122 | 87 | | | | | 2 | |
| | | | | | >18 years | | 96 | 95 | | | | | 2 | |
| Sweeney [43] | 2005 | Retrospect | ED adolesc. | FPD, full denture | All | 14 | 61 | 88.5 | | 94 | | | 3.33 | L |
| | | | | | Maxilla | 4 | 15 | 80 | | | | | 3.33 | |
| | | | | | Mandible | 14 | 46 | 91.3 | | | | | 3.33 | |
| Finnema [27] | 2005 | Retrospect | Oligodont. adults | FPD | All | 13 | 87 | 89.7 | | | | | 3 | L |
| | | | | | Maxilla | | | 86 | | | | | 3 | |
| | | | | | Mandible | | | 96 | | | | | 3 | |
| Poggio [44] | 2005 | Retrospect | Oligodont. adults | SC | No | 24 | 46 | 100 | | 82.6 | | | 5.25 | M |
| Zarone [45] | 2006 | ProspObs | Ag incisors adults | SC | No | 30 | 34 | 97.1 | 94.1 | | 1.2 | | 3.75 | L |
| Becelli [46] | 2007 | Retrospect | Oligodont. adults | SC, FPD | No | 8 | 60 | 96.6 | | | | | 8.5 | L |
| Bergendal [20] | 2008 | Survey | ED, adoles children | n.s. | All | 26 | 47 | 76.6 | | | | | 0.6 | M |
| | | | | | 14–15 years | 21 | 33 | 93.9 | | | | | 0.6 | |
| | | | | | <13 years | 5 | 14 | 35.7 | | | | | 0.6 | |
| Dueled [26] | 2008 | Retrospect | Oligodont | SC, FPD | Implant supported | 110 | 179 | 100 | 87.3 | 99 | | | 3.8 | L |

**Table 3** Synopsis of included studies on dental implants and prosthetics on dental implants in order of publication year *(Continued)*

| | | | | | | | | | | | | |
|---|---|---|---|---|---|---|---|---|---|---|---|---|
| Krieger [25] | 2009 | Retrospect | Oligodont. adults | SC, FPD | All impl | 17 | 40 | 92.5 | | 87.9 | | 15.1 | L |
| | | | | | SCImpl | 12 | 24 | 87.5 | 62 | 83.3 | | 15.1 | |
| | | | | | FDP Impl | 6 | 16 | 100 | 100 | 100 | | 15.1 | |
| Degidi [47] | 2009 | RCT | Ag Incisors adults | SC | All | 60 | 60 | 100 | 98.3 | 100 | | 3 | L |
| | | | | | Imm. load | 30 | 30 | 100 | 100 | 100 | 0.85 | 3 | |
| | | | | | Conv. load | 30 | 30 | 100 | 96.6 | 93.3 | 0.75 | 3 | |
| Creton [1] | 2010 | Retrospect | Oligodont. adults | FPD | No | 44 | 214 | 89.8 | | | | 2.9 | L |
| Grecchi (a) [15] | 2010 | Retrospect | ED adults | FPD | All | 4 | 44 | 100 | 90.9 | | 0.4 | 1.8 | M |
| | | | | | Grafted | 3 | | 100 | | | 0.3 | | |
| | | | | | Non-graft | 1 | | 100 | | | 1.2 | | |
| | | | | | Maxilla | | 20 | 100 | | | 0.2 | | |
| | | | | | Mandible | | 24 | 100 | | | 0.7 | | |
| Grecchi (b) [22] | 2010 | Retrospect | ED adults | FPD | No | 8 | 78 | 98.7 | | | 0.5–0.6 | 1.8 | Pooled |
| Nissan [48] | 2011 | Unclear | Agenesis | SC | No | 12 | 21 | 95.2 | 95.2 | | | 2.5 | M |
| Heuberer [38] | 2012 | Retrospect | Mixed ED < 12 years | Full denture | All | 6 | 16 | 93.8 | | 100 | | 4 | L |
| | | | | | Maxilla, onplants | 4 | 8 | 87.5 | | 100 | | 5 | |
| | | | | | Mandible | 3 | 8 | 100 | | 100 | | 3 | |
| Hosseini [49] | 2013 | ProspObs | Hypodontia | SC | No | 59 | 98 | 100 | 99 | 97.2 | | 3 | L |
| Zou [50] | 2014 | Retrospect | ED Adults | FPD | No | 25 | 169 | 98.3 | 97.2 | 100 | 1.4 | 5 | L |

**Table 4** Synopsis of included studies on tooth autotransplantation in order of publication year

| Author | Year | Study type | Population | Comparison | Patients | Transplants | Transplant survival [%] | Transplant success [%] | Pulp vitality [%] | Intact periodont. [%] | Follow-up [y] | Risk of bias |
|---|---|---|---|---|---|---|---|---|---|---|---|---|
| Kristersson [51] | 1991 | Retrosp. | Agen, incis, trauma | All | 50 | 50 | 98 | 82 | | | 7.5 | L |
| | | | | Immature | | 41 | | 90 | | | 7.5 | |
| | | | | Mature | | 9 | | 44 | | | 7.5 | |
| Kugelberg [52] | 1994 | Prosp.Ob | Ag, Tr | All | 40 | 45 | 96 | 89 | | | 4 | L |
| | | | | Immature | | 23 | | 96 | 100 | 96 | 4 | |
| | | | | Mature | | 22 | | 82 | 0 | 82 | 4 | |
| Marcusson [53] | 1996 | Prosp.Ob | Ag, missing | No | 29 | 31 | 87 | | | | 8 | L |
| Josefsson [54] | 1999 | Retrosp. | Oligodontia | All | 80 | 110 | 91 | | | | 4 | L |
| | | | | Immature | | 11 | | 92 | | | 4 | |
| | | | | Mature | | 99 | | 82 | | | 4 | |
| Czochrowska [55] | 2002 | Retrosp. | Agenesis | No | 28 | 33 | 90 | 79 | | | 26.4 | M |
| Bauss [23] | 2004 | Retrosp. | Ag, missing | All | 88 | 91 | 100 | 84.6 | | | 4 | M |
| | | | | OrthDerot | 27 | 28 | 100 | | 71.4 | 67.8 | 4 | |
| | | | | OrthExtru | 20 | 21 | 100 | | 90.5 | 85.7 | 4 | |
| | | | | NoOrthod | 41 | 42 | 100 | | 97.6 | 95.2 | 4 | |
| Jonsson [56] | 2004 | Prosp.Ob | Ag, missing | No | 32 | 40 | 92.5 | | 76 | 100 | 10 | L |
| Tanaka [57] | 2007 | Retrosp. | Ag, missing | No | 24 | 28 | 100 | | 60.7 | | 4 | M |
| Mensink [58] | 2010 | Retrosp. | Ag, missing | No | 44 | 63 | 100 | | 89 | | 1 | L |
| Kvint [59] | 2010 | Retrosp. | Ag, missing | No | 215 | 215 | 88.4 | 81 | | | 4.8 | L |
| Bokelund [24] | 2013 | Retrosp. | Agenesis | All | 157 | 211 | 100 | | | | 10 | L |
| | | | | Premolar | | 162 | | 93 | | 93 | 10 | |
| | | | | Molars | | 49 | | 60 | | 60 | 10 | |
| | | | | NormalPrim | | 71 | | 95 | | 95 | 10 | |
| | | | | InfraoccPrim | | 140 | | 87 | | 87 | 10 | |

**Table 5** Synopsis of included studies on preservation of deciduous teeth in order of publication year

| Author | Year | Study type | Population | Comparison | Patients | Deciduous teeth | Deciduous tooth survival [%] | No Infra-occlusion (success) [%] | No root resorption [%] | Odds ratio | Follow-up [y] | Risk of bias |
|---|---|---|---|---|---|---|---|---|---|---|---|---|
| Bjerklin [60] | 2000 | ProspObs | Agenes | no | 41 | 59 | 88 | 45 | 40 | | 9 | L |
| Ith-Hansen [61] | 2000 | ProspObs | Agenes | no | 18 | 26 | 89.6 | 88.4 | 88.4 | | 16.5 | L |
| Sletten [62] | 2003 | Retrospect | Agenes | No | 20 | 28 | 86 | | | | 12.4 | L |
| Bjerklin [63] | 2008 | ProspObs | Agenes | No | 99 | 149 | 91 | 48 | 16.7 | | 12.2 | L |
| Kjaer [17] | 2008 | Retrospect | Agenes | ED shaped versus normal | 105 | n.s. | | | | 1.46 | No | L |
| Hvaring [16] | 2013 | Cross section | Agenes | No | 111 | 188 | | 57.4 | 66.6 | | No | L |

overdentures on teeth. Nevertheless, it was decided to keep these results in the numerical analysis, because of relatively consistent success and survival data across the different prosthetic therapies. The numerical success/survival data are presented below.

### Data synthesis

#### *Comparison of the four treatments*

The results of the weighted mean method and annual failure rates are presented in Table 7. In addition, the results are visualized in Figs. 2, 3, 4, 5, 6, 7, 8, and 9.

There is a marked difference in survival data if implants, autotransplants, and preservation of deciduous teeth are compared with conventional prosthetics on teeth, which has only a prosthesis survival of 60.2 % (CI 9.4) at a mean follow-up of 8.4 years. If not the patient but implants/teeth or prosthetic units are used to weigh the means, the results do not change markedly (Fig. 2).

Looking upon the success data, both deciduous teeth and autotransplants have markedly lower success than survival, which is mainly due to the high rate of ankyloses and root resorption in both treatment options using the natural teeth (Fig. 2).

Implants have higher annual failure rates than the natural tooth alternatives. This is also an effect of the shorter follow-up times in implants (4.6 years) compared to autotransplants (7.6 years) and deciduous teeth (12.5 years) (Fig. 3).

A direct comparison of implant and conventional prosthetics was made in two retrospective studies of Krieger and coworkers [25] and Dueled and coworkers [26]. In both studies, prostheses on implants had better

**Table 6** Synopsis of included studies on conventional prosthetics on teeth in order of publication year

| Author | Year | Study type | Population | Treatment | Comparison | Patients | Teeth | Prostheses | Prosthesis survival [%] | Prosthesis success [%] | Follow-up [y] | Risk of bias |
|---|---|---|---|---|---|---|---|---|---|---|---|---|
| Hobkirk [64] | 1989 | Retrospect | Hypodontia | Overdenture | All | 138 | | 138 | 51.5 | | 6 | M |
| | | | | | Mandible | 48 | | 48 | 33 | | 6 | |
| | | | | | Maxilla | 90 | | 90 | 61 | | 6 | |
| Pröbster [65] | 1997 | Retrospect | HypodTrauma | Single crown | No | 264 | 392 | 325 | 60 | | 10 | M |
| Garnett [66] | 2005 | Retrospect | Hypodontia | Single incis crown | | 45 | 73 | 73 | 59 | | 6 | M |
| Dueled [26] | 2008 | Retrospect | Oligodont adults | SC, FPD | On teeth | 19 | | 30 | 89.5 | 80 | 3.8 | L |
| | | | | SC, FPD | On implants | 110 | | 179 | 99 | 91 | 3.8 | |
| Krieger [25] | 2009 | Retrospect | Hypodontia | All | On teeth | 5 | | 25 | 85.7 | 42 | 15.1 | M |
| | | | | Single Cr. | On teeth | 5 | | 5 | 80 | 80 | 15.1 | |
| | | | | FDP | On teeth | 10 | | 20 | 84.1 | 72.8 | 15.1 | |
| | | | | All | On implants | 17 | | 33 | 87.9 | 53 | 15.1 | |
| | | | | SC | On implants | 12 | | 24 | 83.3 | 62.5 | 15.1 | |
| | | | | FDP | On implants | 6 | | 9 | 100 | 66.7 | 15.1 | |
| Spinas [67] | 2013 | Prosp.Obs. | Hypodontia | Resin bridge single Incis | | 30 | 32 | 32 | 93.8 | | 5 | L |

**Table 7** Numerical results of general outcome parameters (weighted mean values)

| [%] | Survival patient weighted | 95 % confid. interval | Success patient weighted | 95 % confid. interval | Survival impl/tooth/ unit weighted | 95 % confid. interval | Success impl/tooth/ unit weighted | 95 % confid. interval | Annual failure rate survival patient weighted | 95 % confid. interval | Annual failure rate success patient weighted | 95 % confid. interval | annual failure rate survival impl/tooth/ unit weighted | 95 % confid. interval | Annual failure rate success impl/tooth/ unit weighted | 95 % confid. interval |
|---|---|---|---|---|---|---|---|---|---|---|---|---|---|---|---|---|
| Treatment comparisons | | | | | | | | | | | | | | | | |
| Implants | 95.3 | 1.9 | 92.7 | 4.6 | 94.1 | 1.8 | 95.6 | 4.1 | 3.317 | 0.196 | 0.815 | 0.055 | 3.280 | 0.150 | 1.987 | 0.159 |
| AutoTX | 94.4 | 4.1 | 82.5 | 11.7 | 94.8 | 4.0 | 85.0 | 4.0 | 1.061 | 0.112 | 1.832 | 0.638 | 1.167 | 0.100 | 2.334 | 0.184 |
| Deciduous | 89.6 | 19.1 | 51.8 | 12.6 | 89.7 | 19.8 | 51.7 | 13.1 | 0.908 | 0.157 | 2.928 | 1.472 | 0.903 | 0.161 | 4.333 | 1.494 |
| ConvProsth | 60.2 | 9.4 | 59.4 | 44.3 | 62.6 | 7.6 | 59.4 | 44.3 | 5.144 | 0.851 | 5.368 | 4.947 | 11.098 | 1.477 | 9.863 | 6.895 |
| Implant subgroup analysis | | | | | | | | | | | | | | | | |
| Children | 72.4 | 18.8 | 44.4 | n.a. | 80.1 | 17.6 | 44.4 | n.a. | 50.177 | 32.083 | 7.128 | n.a. | 25.532 | 9.836 | 7.128 | n.a. |
| Adolescents | 93.0 | 9.5 | 93.7 | 27.0 | 82.0 | 8.3 | 95.7 | 7.5 | 4.610 | 1.029 | 2.052 | 1.313 | 4.626 | 0.712 | 1.262 | 0.724 |
| Adults | 97.4 | 4.0 | 92.2 | 7.5 | 95.6 | 3.3 | 91.4 | 6.8 | 0.670 | 0.001 | 1.850 | 0.272 | 1.280 | 0.122 | 2.188 | 0.276 |
| Ectod.Dyspl. | 89.6 | 8.4 | 93.4 | 30.3 | | | | | 11.665 | 2.520 | 1.431 | 0.219 | | | | |
| Hypo/oligodo | 97.2 | 3.9 | 92.4 | 5.4 | | | | | 0.864 | 0.067 | 1.899 | 0.199 | | | | |
| Prosthesis on implants | 97.8 | 2.3 | 94.5 | 2.4 | | | | | 0.864 | 0.032 | 0.884 | 0.029 | | | | |
| Prosthesis on teeth | 61.4 | 7.9 | 77.9 | 19.2 | 62.1 | 7.7 | 77.4 | 20.6 | 5.060 | 0.726 | 3.666 | 1.695 | 12.111 | 1.496 | 3.046 | 1.650 |
| Sing. crowns | 98.5 | 24.5 | | | | | | | | | | | | | | |
| FPD | 96.3 | 7.7 | | | | | | | | | | | | | | |
| Full dentures | 90.6 | 9.0 | | | | | | | | | | | | | | |
| Maxilla | | | | | 84.2 | 8.3 | | | | | | | | | | |
| Mandible | | | | | 91.9 | 30.3 | | | | | | | | | | |
| Single aplas | 99.1 | 14.5 | | | | | | | | | | | | | | |
| Mild hypodo | 94.6 | 5.3 | | | | | | | | | | | | | | |
| Severe Oligo | 93.1 | 11.0 | | | | | | | | | | | | | | |

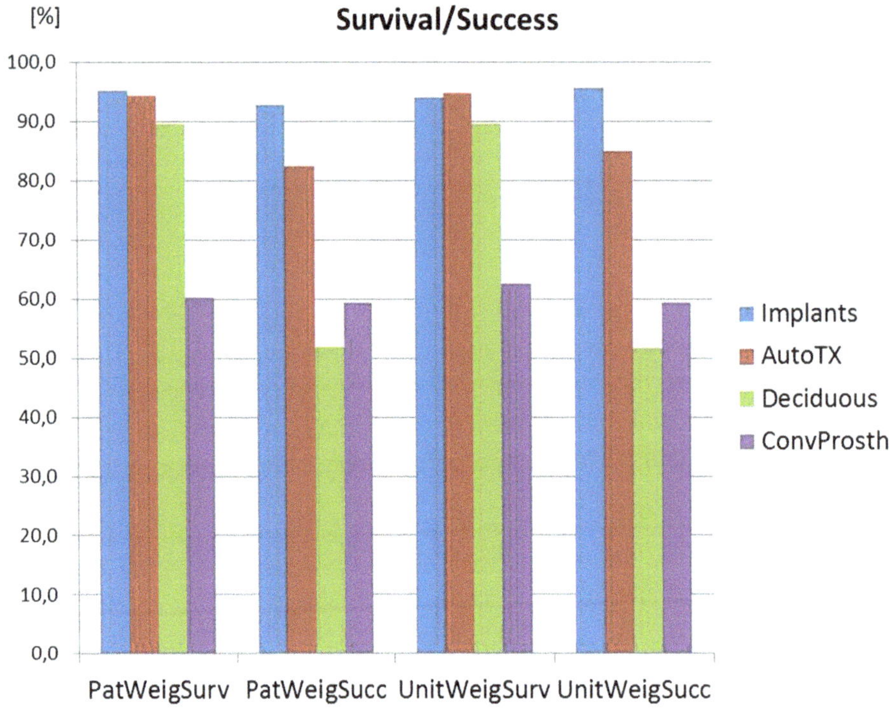


**Fig. 2** The diagram shows survival and success data of implants, tooth autotransplants, preserved deciduous teeth, and conventional prostheses on teeth. The means of the underlying studies are displayed either weighed on patients' base (=PatWeigSurv, PatWeigSucc) or on units' base (implant, tooth, or prosthesis) (=UnitWeigSurv, UnitWeigSucc)

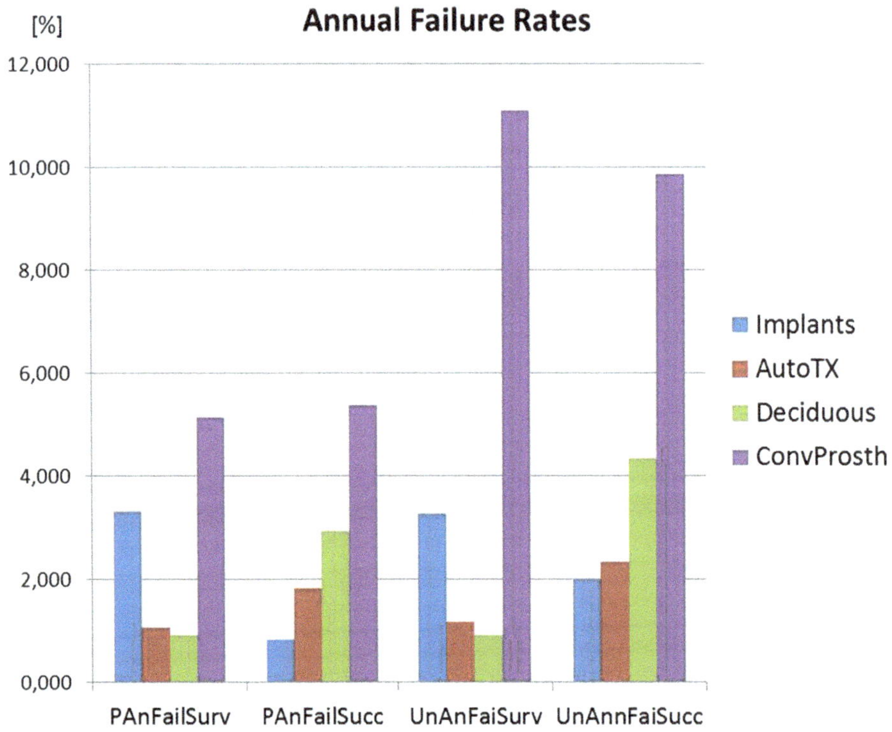


**Fig. 3** The diagram shows annual failure rates of the four treatments (implants, tooth autotransplants, preserved deciduous teeth, and conventional prostheses on teeth). The data are differentiated as in Fig. 2, either weighed on patients' base (=PAnFailSurv, PAnFailSucc) or on units' base (implant, tooth, or prosthesis) (=UnAnFaiSurv, UnAnnFaiSucc)

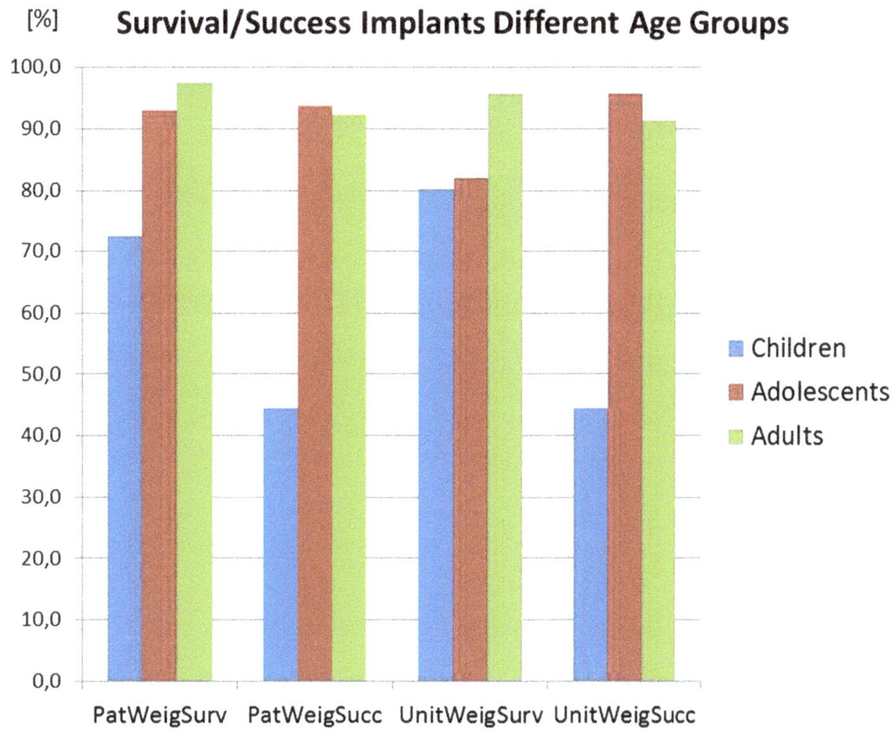


**Fig. 4** The diagram shows the same data types as Fig. 2, however here differentiated according to three age groups, children <13 years, adolescents <18 years, and adults >18 years

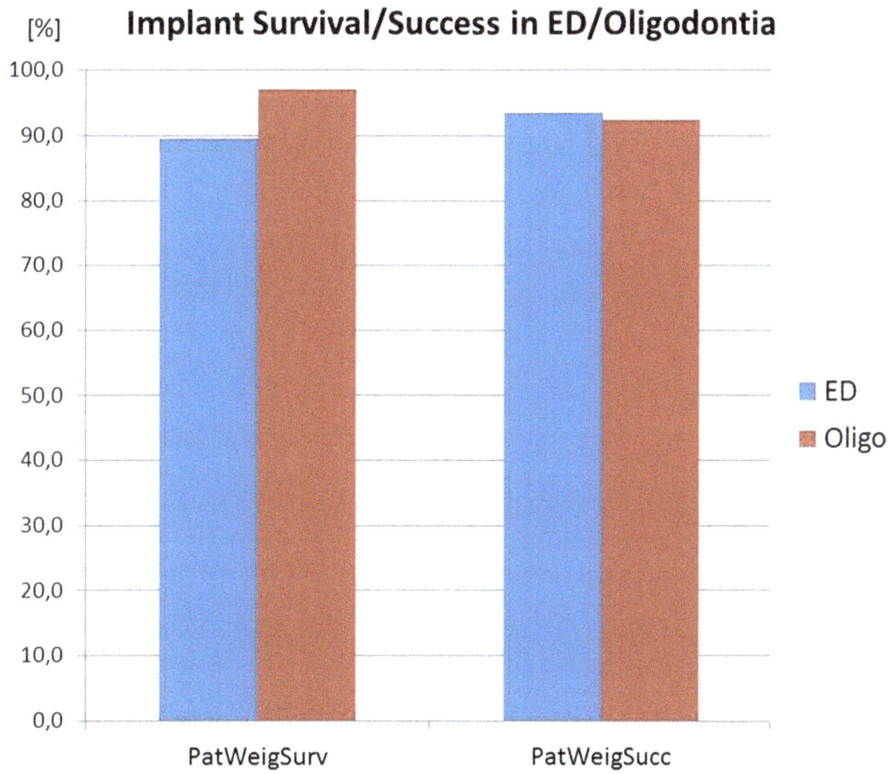


**Fig. 5** Only slight differences in implant prognosis were observed between studies with syndromic (ED) and non-syndromic cases

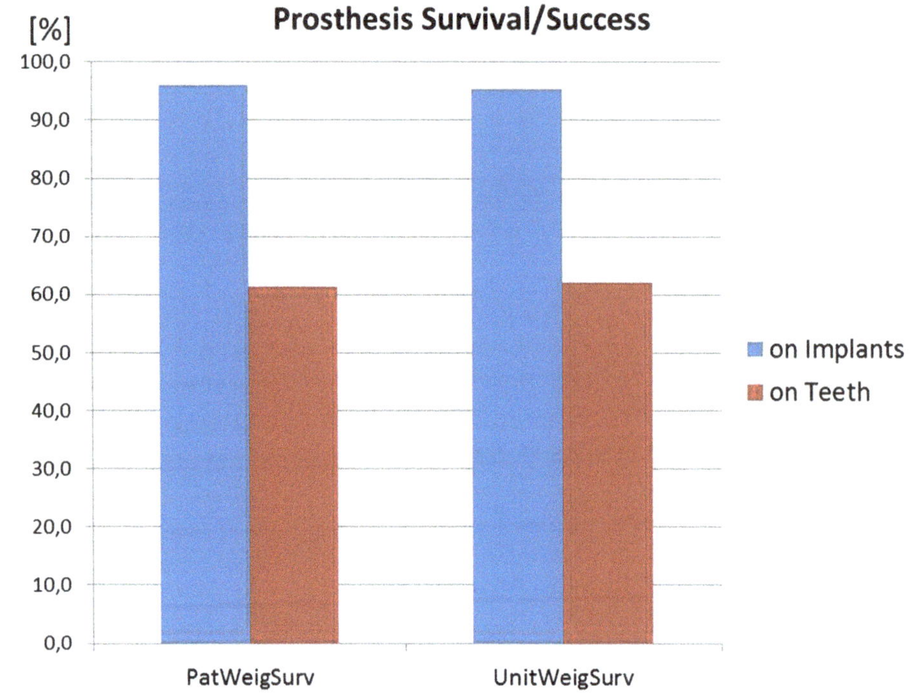


**Fig. 6** Prostheses on implants had a better prognosis than prostheses on teeth

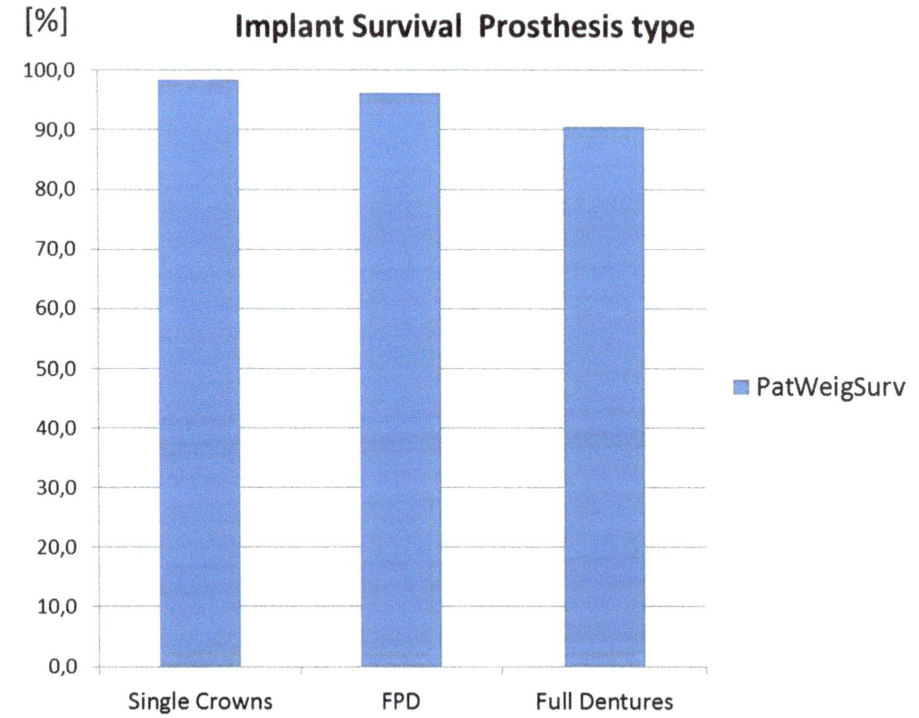


**Fig. 7** Compared to the difference between prostheses on implants and teeth (Fig. 6), the type of prosthesis plays a minor role on implant survival

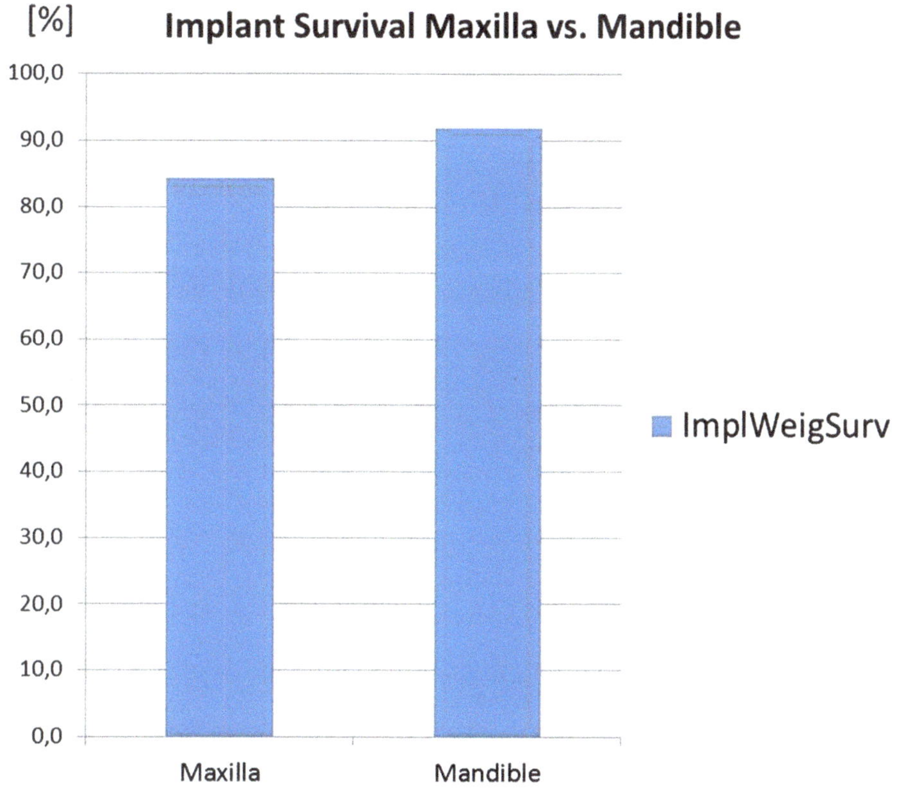


**Fig. 8** Implants in the maxilla had a lower prognosis than implants placed in the mandible

survival than on teeth. In the Dueled study, the difference of the prosthesis survival rates between implants and teeth was 9.5 % and the success rates differed by 11 % in favor of implants. The respective differences in the Krieger study were a survival difference of 2.2 % and a prosthesis success difference of 11 %. Krieger and coworkers observed also marked differences of >40 % between prosthesis success and survival, as an indicator for prosthetic maintenance and repair needs over a very long follow-up time of 15.1 years.

**Subgroup analysis of dental implant treatment**

***Children versus adolescents versus adults***

There is a clearly lower implant survival with 72.4 % (CI 18.8) when dental implants are used in childhood below the age of 13 (Fig. 4). In most included studies, implant losses in children occurred early during the healing phase. Also in adolescents below the age of 18 years with a success of 93.0 % (CI 9.5) dental implants performed slightly lower than in adults with a success of 97.4 % (CI 4.0) (Fig. 3). The annual implant failure rates in children were 50.177 % (CI 32.083), in adolescents 4.610 % (CI 1.029) and in adults 0.670 % (CI 0.001) (Table 7). The mean observation time of the here included studies in children was 4.1 year, in adolescents 4.9 years, and in adults with congenitally missing teeth 6.4 years.

***ED versus non-syndromic congenitally missing teeth (oligodontia)***

The implant success/survival data of ED patients are slightly lower than of non-syndromic patients (Fig. 5). The difference is more marked looking upon annual failure rates (Table 7), indicating that these losses occurred after short observation times. These losses were observed mainly during healing time in children suffering from ED.

***Prosthesis survival on teeth versus implants***

The prosthesis survival on teeth is 61.4 % (CI 7.9) after a mean observation time of 7.2 years. On implants, this figure is markedly higher with 97.8 % (CI 2.3) prosthesis survival after a mean observation of 4.6 years (Fig. 6).

***Prosthesis type***

The survival data of implants restored with single crowns are slightly higher than restored with fixed partial dentures than restore with full dentures (Fig. 7).

***Maxilla versus mandible***

The mandible shows with 91.9 % (CI 30.3) a better implant prognosis in patients with congenitally missing teeth than the maxilla with 84.2 % (CI 8.3) (Fig. 8).

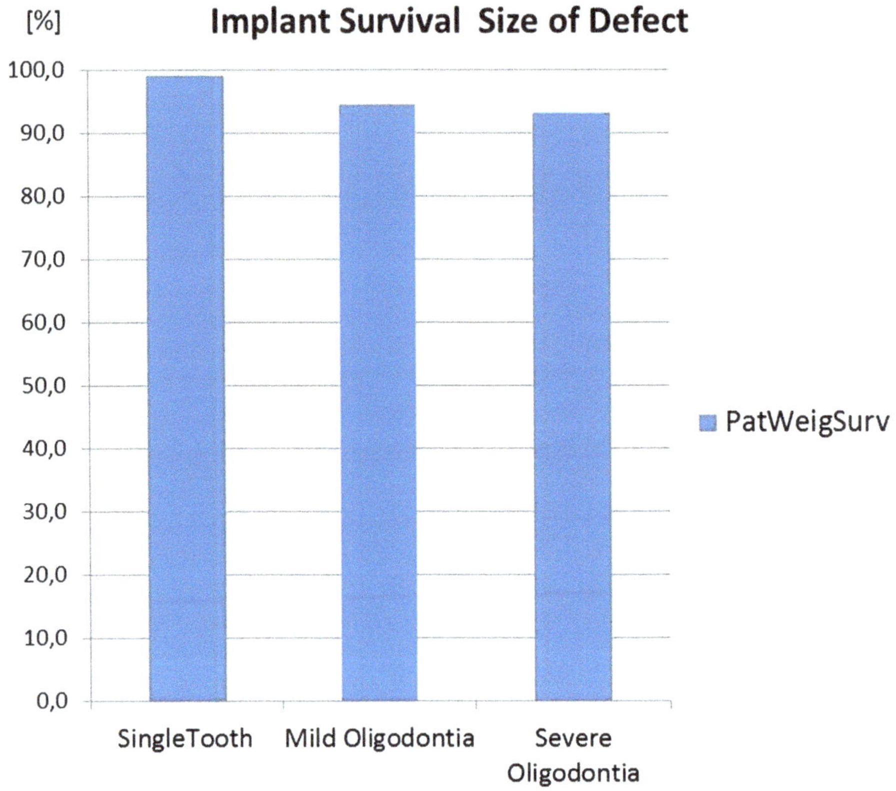


**Fig. 9** Compared to the difference between prostheses on implants and teeth (Fig. 6), the size of the defect either single missing teeth or mild or severe hypodontia plays a minor role for implant survival

***Size of defect***

Patients with single tooth aplasias (99.1 % (CI 14.5)) had better implant survivals than patients with mild hypodontias (94.6 (CI 5.3) and patients with severe hypodontias (93.1 (CI 11.0)) (Fig. 9).

**Studies on patient-centered outcome parameters**

***Studies on quality of life, self-esteem, and patient satisfaction***

A total of 16 retrieved studies included numerical assessment data of patient-centered parameters (Table 8). Many studies were cross-sectional studies with description of a baseline situation in hypodontia patiendraw 1ts. The patient inclusion was relatively homogenous between the studies. However, the studies were relatively heterogenous in the outcome parameters and study treatments because implant, conventional prosthetism, autotransplants, and orthodontic gap closure were included in this table. The number of studies in each treatment was in some cases $n = 1$ making numerical comparisons difficult.

Nevertheless, a numerical evaluation using the weighted mean method of the parameters OHIP49 (Oral Health Impact Profile), CPQ11-14 (Child Perceptions Questionnaire), and patient satisfaction was performed. The results are displayed in Table 9. The mean baseline score of the Oral Health Impact Profile 49 in prosthetically not treated adults was 27.8 (CI 0.9) points of a possible maximum of 196 points (14.1 % of maximum) indicating that the patients were not strongly limited by the disease. The baseline scores of the Children Perceptions Questionnaire 11–14 in untreated children with oligodontia was 26.2 (CI 2.2) of 148 maximum score points (17.7 % of maximum). A mean improvement of 14.9 OHIP points after prosthetic treatment and occlusal rehabilitation was calculated from three reporting studies. The reported improvement with conventional prosthetics was 19.5 points (only one study), with implant prosthetics 12.5 score points (only two studies). Patient satisfaction rates after treatment was 66.5 % (one study) with orthodontic space closure 75 % in autotransplants (one study), 76.6 % with conventional prosthetics (two studies), and 93.4 % with implant prosthetics (3 studies) in hypodontia patients (Table 9).

Two assessments of self-esteem were available. Hashem found self-esteem not significantly affected in hypodontia patients compared to normal control patients. Finnema observed an improvement of patients'

**Table 8** Synopsis of included studies on patient centered outcome parameters in order of publication year

| Autor | Year | Study type | Population | Treatment | Comparison | Patients | Implants/ missing tooth units | Baseline OHIP [scores] | OHIP improvement [scores] | OHIP esthetic [scores] | Rosenberg self-esteem [scores] | Self-esteem improvement [%] | CPQ [scores] | Satisfact [% sample or vas [%] | Risk of bias |
|---|---|---|---|---|---|---|---|---|---|---|---|---|---|---|---|
| Marcusson [53] | 1996 | Retrospective | Agenesis missing | AutoTX | no | 29 | 31 | | | | | | | 75 | M |
| Robertsson [29] | 2000 | Cross section | Agen lat inc | Orthod versus bridge | Orthod clos | 30 | 30 | | | | | | | 66.5 | L |
| | | | | | Orthod open | 20 | 20 | | | | | | | 69.5 | |
| Finnema [27] | 2005 | Retrospective | Oligodontia | FPD implants | Posttreatment | 13 | 87 | | | | | 61 | | 80 | M |
| Wong [68] | 2006 | Cross section | Oligodontia | n.r. | No | 25 | 93 | | | | | | 29 | | M |
| Stanford [69] | 2008 | Cross section | ED | FPD implants | Posttreatment | 109 | 624 | | | | | | | 91 | M |
| Dueled [26] | 2008 | Retrospective | Oligodont | SC, FPD | All | 129 | 215 | 13.4 | | | | | | | M |
| | | | | | Control | | | 8.2 | | 14 | | | | 96 | |
| | | | | | Implants | 110 | | | | 41 | | | | 98 | |
| | | | | | Convent. | 19 | | | | 47 | | | | 84 | |
| Locker [70] | 2010 | Cross section | Oligodontia | n.r. | No | 36 | 245 | | | | | | 22.3 | | |
| Laing [71] | 2010 | Cross section | Oligodontia | n.r. | Oligodontia all | 62 | | | | | | | 26.8 | | L |
| | | | | | Normal control | 61 | | | | | | | 28.5 | | |
| Goshima [28] | 2010 | ProspObs | Hypodontia | Implant SC | No | 18 | 37 | 35.2 | −26.3 | | | | | | L |
| Kohli [72] | 2011 | Cross section | ED | n.r. | 11–14 years | 35 | n.g. | | | | | | 25.1 | | L |
| | | | | | 15–19 years | 14 | | | | | | | 35.9 | | |
| | | | | | Self perceived | | | | | | | | 31.6 | | |
| | | | | | By caregivers | | | | | | | | 35.0 | | |
| Meaney [73] | 2012 | Cross section | ED | n.g. | no | 10 | n.g. | 61 | | | | | | | L |
| Hosseini [49] | 2013 | ProspObs | Hypodontia | Implant SC | No | 59 | 98 | 16.2 | −8.3 | | | | | | L |
| Hashem [37] | 2013 | Cross section | Oligodontia | n.g. | ED | 41 | n.g. | 62 | | | 22 | | | | M |
| | | | | | Normal control | 41 | n.g. | 31 | | | 22.3 | | | | |

**Table 8** Synopsis of included studies on patient centered outcome parameters in order of publication year *(Continued)*

| | | | | | | | | | | | |
|---|---|---|---|---|---|---|---|---|---|---|---|
| Anweigi (a) [74] | 2013 | Long Prosp Obs | Hypodontia | Bridges orthod. | FPD completed | 40 | n.g. | 35 | −19.5 | | L |
| | | | | | Orthodontic phase | 37 | n.g. | 32 | 22 | | |
| Anweigi (b) [75] | 2013 | Cross section | NonsyndrOligodonti | n.g. | 16–18 years | 40 | n.g. | 28 | | | L |
| | | | | | 19–34 years | 42 | n.g. | 33.5 | | | |
| Zou [50] | 2014 | Retrospective | ED | Implants | No | 25 | 169 | | | 91 | M |

**Table 9** Numerical results of patient-centered outcome parameters (weighted mean values)

| OHIP | Baseline OHIP | 95 % confid. interval | OHIP improvement general | 95 % confid. interval | OHIP improvement implants | 95 % confid. interval | OHIP improvement conventional | 95 % confid. interval |
|---|---|---|---|---|---|---|---|---|
| [Score units] | 27.8 | 0.9 | 14.9 | 1.7 | 12.5 | 0.2 | 19.5 | n.a. |
| CPQ | Baseline CPQ | | | | | | | |
| [Score units] | 26.6 | 2.2 | | | | | | |
| Patient satisfaction | Satisfaction orthod. clos | | Satisfaction AutoTX | | Satisfaction conventional | | Satisfaction implants | |
| [%] | 66.5 | n.a. | 75.0 | n.a. | 76.6 | 5.2 | 93.4 | 19.3 |

self-esteem in 61 % of cases after treatment with dental implants (Table 9).

#### Studies on chewing efficacy

Two studies were retrieved on chewing efficacy data after prosthetic treatment of hypodontia with implants. Both studies used different methods of assessment. In the study of Finnema and coworkers [27], the mandibular function impairment questionnaire (MFIQ) dropped from 2.23 (44.6 % of maximum scoring range of 5) at baseline to 0.31 after occlusal rehabilitation. The study of Goshima and coworkers [28] reported a marked improvement of bite force, masticatory index and functional impairment index, reduced chewing time, and increased occlusal contact area after prosthetic treatment with dental implants (Table 10).

### Further studies

#### Studies on orthodontic treatments in patients with congenitally missing teeth

The literature search according to the applied criteria revealed four relevant studies on orthodontic therapy. Since orthodontic therapy is in most cases a supportive therapy and no competing therapy orthodontics were not included into the numerical evaluation. Robertsson and Mohlin [29] compared directly in a cross-sectional study of 50 patients with missing lateral incisors, orthodontic space closure with orthodontic gap opening, and a bridge. The patients were slightly more satisfied with the esthetics of the space closure. There were slight differences in general patient satisfaction (see there) in favor of the bridge and no differences in any functional parameters. A remarkable finding in two studies of Uribe and coworkers [30] was that after orthodontic opening of a gap of an agenesis of a lateral incisor, the alveolar ridge lost 1.6 mm ridge width and 0.6 mm ridge height, measured retrospectively in stone models of 31 patients. In their second study [31], the same problem was measured with cone beam CT and a shrinkage of the width of the alveolar of 0.9 mm and no height reduction was measured in 11 patients. Dueled [26] observed in severe hypodontia the patients' root resorption in 36 % of oligodontia cases, who received adjunctive orthodontic therapy, which was not found in patients without orthodontic therapy. According to the authors, possible explanations for this finding may have been narrower and more cortical alveolar ridges in edentulous sites of tooth agenesis patients and different tooth root morphology (taurodontism).

#### Studies on craniofacial growth

In this group, 3 studies were retrieved according to the search criteria. The two studies of Dellavia and coworkers [18, 19] contained drawings (polar diagrams) but not the underlying numerical data. Their evaluation of facial photographies demonstrated that patients with ectodermal dysplasia had a slightly reduced global facial growth in comparison with normal reference peers, with a delay of about 2 years in mandibular and maxillary peak developments. The cross-sectional study of Johnson and coworkers [32] analyzed lateral cephalograms of 50 ED patients without treatment with dental implants and compared them with 45 ED patients, who had received dental implants. Craniofacial morphology did not differ significantly between implant-treated and non-treated ED patients.

## Discussion

This systematic review of the literature made a few noticeable findings. Dental implants and implant-borne prostheses demonstrated high survival and success data with approximately 30 % higher survival/success figures than conventional prostheses on teeth. However, in children implant and prosthesis, success was 20 % lower and success 40 % lower than in adults and adolescents. The factor severity of hypodontia, syndromal versus non-syndromal tooth defects, size and type of the prosthesis, maxilla versus mandible, were in comparison to the age group of minor significance for the implant prognosis. The two other non-prosthetic treatment options using natural teeth, tooth autotransplants, and preservation of the

**Table 10** Synopsis of studies of chewing performance before and after treatment with dental implants

| Autor | Year | Study type | Population | Treatment | Comparison | Patients | Replaced teeth | Bite force [N] | Color change chew.gum [a*] | Chewing time [s] | Occlusal contact area [mm$^2$] | Masticatory index 0–3 | MFIQ | Study quality |
|---|---|---|---|---|---|---|---|---|---|---|---|---|---|---|
| Finnema [27] | 2005 | Retrospect. | Oligodontia | Implant FPD | Before treatment | 13 | 156 | | | | | | 2.23 | M |
| | | | | | After treatment | | | | | | | | 0.31 | |
| Goshima [28] | 2009 | ProspObs | Oligodontia | Implant sing. crown | Before treatment | 18 | 37 | 1087.3 | 18.8 | 21.1 | 34.3 | 0.3 | | L |
| | | | | | After treatment | | | 1383 | 23.2 | 17.9 | 44.9 | 0 | | |

deciduous teeth had survival rates in the range of dental implants but lower success rates due to a considerable incidence of ankylosis, root resorption, and infraocclusion. Also, patient satisfaction rates were higher for dental implants compared to the other treatment options.

According to the present data, dental implants in patients with congenitally missing teeth have an excellent documented prognosis with survival rates of 95.3 % after a mean follow-up of 4.6 years. The prognosis even rises to 97.4 %, if only adults are considered taking into account the higher failure rates in children as discussed below. These figures are well lined with currently published data on implant prognosis in conventional dental implant patients. For example, a 95.5–96.3 % 5-year survival rate has been published in a recent meta-analysis [33].

The pictures changes slightly in favor of autotransplants and preservation of deciduous teeth when annual failure rates are calculated by dividing the survival/success data through the years of observation. Still, conventional prosthetics have the highest annual failure rates with approximately 5 %, 5 times higher than the annual failure rates after tooth autotransplantation and preservation of natural teeth with approximately 1 %. The annual failure rate is first of all the mathematical result of the 2–3 times longer observation time in the included studies on the treatment options using natural teeth. On the other hand, this finding confirms the clinical experience that a once healed autotransplant or a once preserved deciduous tooth has in contrast to prosthetic components causes hardly any maintenance and repair expenditures. The latter problem is even more evident, if in the present data, the annual survival-based failure rate of 5 % for conventional prosthetics is compared with the annual success-based failure rate of conventional prosthetics of 11 %. Survival means that the prosthetic component is still in the oral cavity whereas success can be much lower due to prosthetic complications and treatment needs. Here, the presented 3 % annual failure rate for dental implants ranges in the middle between conventional prosthetics and treatments with natural teeth. Again, this figure is pretty much in line with recent findings on annual failure rates in implants in conventional dental implant patients. A recently published meta-analysis on implants in conjunction with sinus floor augmentations reported an annual failure rate of 3.5 % [34].

The low prognosis of dental implants in children (72.4 %) compared to adolescents (93.0 %) and adults (97.4 %) was not surprising. Also, the systematic review of Yap and Klineberg [11] came to this conclusion. But the large difference of 25 % was remarkable and is clinically relevant. The high annual failure rates of implants in children according to the included studies of 50.2 % compared to 4.6 % in adolescents and 0.7 % in adults with congenitally missing teeth can be alarming. This is in part again an effect of the lower observation times in the included studies (factor 1.5). At this point, also the inclusion of the observation of Bergendal and coworkers [20] has to be discussed, who observed in a survey in Swedish specialist dental clinics an implant loss rate of 6.1 in adolescents and 64.3 % in children under the age of 13. She reported only healing failures of the implants and no long-term problems in children. The data have been included in this systematic review of the literature here, although it is not a true clinical study and the observation time of 6 months is arbitrary and short. The relevance of the observation of Bergendal has already been discussed elsewhere in the literature [35]. The study was also included because the finding fits to other studies in this review. A biological explanation of healing problems of dental implants in young children may be the brittle cortical bone structure and a more active immune system in children compared to adults and adolescents. An international Delphi consensus group, too, did not reach consensus on the use of dental implants in growing children affected by hypodontia [9, 10]. Decision making for dental implants in children and adolescents cannot only be based on survival data. It includes also secondary infraocclusion of restorations on implants which can account for the upper incisor region up to 2.2mm [3]. Less infraocclusion had been observed for teeth in the lower jaw and upper canines [3].

According to the setting of the second consensus conference of the German Implant Association, in this systematic review, special emphasis had to be laid on patient-reported and patient-centered outcomes. In summary, the retrieved studies showed that patients with hypodontia are less disabled than expected, as demonstrated by the moderate OHIP and CPQ scores. For example, according to a study in edentulous wearers of full dentures before implant stabilization, the baseline OHIP score was much higher (54.2) [36], compared to a mean baseline score in the studies included here of 27.8. This observation may be explained by the adaptation of the juvenile hypodontia patients to the situation from early childhood. Patients do not know it differently. This has also an impact on measurements of self-esteem, which according to Hashem and coworkers was not significantly different between hypodontia patients and control patients [37]. Nevertheless, an effect of occlusal rehabilitation was measurable with quality of life data in three available studies on that topic in the present data. Obviously, there is a lack of clinical studies using quality of life data in the field of congenitally missing teeth. Due to heterogeneity and low number of studies, data with patient-reported outcomes in this review have to be interpreted with caution. The same restrictions apply to interpretations of the presented data on the effect of occlusal rehabilitation on masticatory performance in hypodontia patients.

The PICO question asked whether an early occlusal rehabilitation with dental implants in comparison to tooth autotransplants, conventional prosthetics on teeth, or preservation of deciduous teeth has a better outcome. Based on the presented data here, the question can be answered with yes.

However, each treatment has its time. Preservation of deciduous teeth and autotransplantation is an ideal option in children and adolescents, when dental implants have reduced success rates. The latter option can also be used as a temporary solution until completion of growth. As shown here by the OHIP and self-esteem data and facial growth data, patients with severe oligodontia benefit from early occlusal rehabilitation. A practicable way to safe application of implants in children affected by severe oligodontia may be the proposal by Heuberer and coworkers [38], who used with good success onplants in the maxilla placed in the palate behind the teeth to fix an overdenture prosthesis. In this region, less infraocclusion and less interference with transversal palatal growth are expected. Accordingly for the same reasons, implants can be placed in the mandibular canine region. Also, costs play a role in clinical decision-making with tooth autotransplantation being the most cost-effective option [39] along with preservation of primary teeth, which virtually causes no costs. If the costs are manageable, in clinical decision-making, conventional tooth-borne prosthetic solutions should be thoroughly weighted against implants.

## Conclusion

In synopsis of general and patient-centered outcomes, implants yielded the best results, however, not in children younger than 13 years. Autotransplants and deciduous teeth had low annual failure rates and are appropriate treatments in children and adolescents at low costs. Conventional prosthetics had lower survival/success rates than the other options. Due to heterogeneity and low number of studies, patientreported outcomes in this review have to be interpreted with caution.

#### Competing interests

HT received lecture fees and/or unrestricted research grants from Geistlich Biomaterials, Wolhusen, Switzerland; Osteology Foundation, Lucerne, Switzerland; Straumann, Freiburg, Germany; Dentsply Implants, Mannheim, Germany; and Camlog Biotechnologies, Wimsheim, Germany. The authors declare that they have no competing interests related to this systematic review.

#### Authors' contributions

HT has written the manuscript and calculated the statistics. FW has managed the literature search and collected the original literature. Both have made substantial contributions to study conception, interpretation of data as well as manuscript preparation. Both authors read and approved the final manuscript.

#### Acknowledgements

The authors appreciate the additional information provided during the process from Dr. Birgitta Bergendal, Övertandläkare, Odontologiska Institutionen, Jönköping, Sweden.

#### Funding information

This study is funded by the German Association of Dental Implantology (Deutsche Gesellschaft für Implantologie im Zahn-, Mund- und Kieferbereich e.V.).

#### Author details

[1]Department of Oral and Maxillofacial Surgery, Red Cross Hospital, Hansteinstr. 29, D-34121 Kassel, Germany. [2]Department of Oral and Maxillofacial Surgery, Schleswig-Holstein University Hospital, Arnold-Heller-Straße 3, Haus 26, 2D-4105 Kiel, Germany.

#### References

1. Créton M, Cune M, Verhoeven W, Muradin M, Wismeijer D, Meijer G. Implant treatment in patients with severe hypodontia: a retrospective evaluation. J Oral Maxillofac Surg. 2010;68:530–8.
2. Bergendal B. Oligodontia ectodermal dysplasia—on signs, symptoms, genetics, and outcomes of dental treatment. Swed Dent J Suppl. 2010;205:13–78. 7–8.
3. Thilander B, Odman J, Lekholm U. Orthodontic aspects of the use of oral implants in adolescents: a 10-year follow-up study. Eur J Orthod. 2001;23:715–31.
4. Pigno MA, Blackman RB, Cronin Jr RJ, Cavazos E. Prosthodontic management of ectodermal dysplasia: a review of the literature. J Prosthet Dent. 1996;76:541–5.
5. Bergendal B. When should we extract deciduous teeth and place implants in young individuals with tooth agenesis? J Oral Rehabil. 2008;35 Suppl 1:55–63.
6. Kramer FJ, Baethge C, Tschernitschek H. Implants in children with ectodermal dysplasia: a case report and literature review. Clin Oral Implants Res. 2007;18:140–6.
7. Aydinbelge M, Gumus HO, Sekerci AE, Demetoğlu U, Etoz OA. Implants in children with hypohidrotic ectodermal dysplasia: an alternative approach to esthetic management: case report and review of the literature. Pediatr Dent. 2013;35:441–6.
8. Hobkirk JA, Nohl F, Bergendal B, Storhaug K, Richter MK. The management of ectodermal dysplasia and severe hypodontia. International conference statements. J Oral Rehabil. 2006;33:634–7.
9. Klineberg I, Cameron A, Hobkirk J, Bergendal B, Maniere MC, King N, et al. Rehabilitation of children with ectodermal dysplasia. Part 2: an international consensus meeting. Int J Oral Maxillofac Implants. 2013;28:1101–9.
10. Klineberg I, Cameron A, Whittle T, Hobkirk J, Bergendal B, Maniere MC, et al. Rehabilitation of children with ectodermal dysplasia. Part 1: an international Delphi study. Int J Oral Maxillofac Implants. 2013;28:1090–100.
11. Yap AK, Klineberg I. Dental implants in patients with ectodermal dysplasia and tooth agenesis: a critical review of the literature. Int J Prosthodont. 2009;22:268–76.
12. Moher D, Liberati A, Tetzlaff J, Altman DG, The PRISMA Group. Preferred Reporting Items for Systematic Reviews and Meta-Analyses: the PRISMA Statement. PLoS Med. 2009;6:e1000097. doi:10.1371/journal.pmed1000097.
13. Viswanathan M, Ansari MT, Berkman ND, Chang S, Hartling L, McPheeters LM, et al. Assessing the Risk of Bias of Individual Studies in Systematic Reviews of Health Care Interventions. Agency for Healthcare Research and Quality Methods Guide for Comparative Effectiveness Reviews. March 2012. AHRQ Publication No. 12-EHC047-EF. Available at: http://www.effectivehealthcare.ahrq.gov/ehc/products/322/998/MethodsGuideforCERs_Viswanathan_IndividualStudies.pdf.
14. Buser D, Janner SF, Wittneben JG, Brägger U, Ramseier CA, Salvi GE. 10-year survival and success rates of 511 titanium implants with a sandblasted and acid-etched surface: a retrospective study in 303 partially edentulous patients. Clin Implant Dent Relat Res. 2012;14:839–51.
15. Grecchi F, Zingari F, Bianco R, Zollino I, Casadio C, Carinci F. Implant rehabilitation in grafted and native bone in patients affected by ectodermal dysplasia: evaluation of 78 implants inserted in 8 patients. Implant Dent. 2010;19:400–8.
16. Hvaring CL, Øgaard B, Stenvik A, Birkeland K. The prognosis of retained primary molars without successors: infraocclusion, root resorption and restorations in 111 patients. Eur J Orthod. 2014;36:26–30.
17. Kjaer I, Nielsen MH, Skovgaard LT. Can persistence of primary molars be predicted in subjects with multiple tooth agenesis? Eur J Orthod. 2008;30:249–53.

18. Dellavia C, Catti F, Sforza C, Tommasi DG, Ferrario VF. Craniofacial growth in ectodermal dysplasia. Angle Orthod. 2010;80:733–9.
19. Dellavia C, Catti F, Sforza C, Grandi G, Ferrario VF. Non-invasive longitudinal assessment of facial growth in children and adolescents with hypohidrotic ectodermal dysplasia. Eur J Oral Sci. 2008;116:305–11.
20. Bergendal B, Ekman A, Nilsson P. Implant failure in young children with ectodermal dysplasia: a retrospective evaluation of use and outcome of dental implant treatment in children in Sweden. Int J Oral Maxillofac Implants. 2008;23:520–4.
21. Durstberger G, Celar A, Watzek G. Implant-surgical and prosthetic rehabilitation of patients with multiple dental aplasia: a clinical report. Int J Oral Maxillofac Implants. 1999;14:417–23.
22. Grecchi F, Pagliani L, Mancini GE, Zollino I, Carinci F. Implant treatment in grafted and native bone in patients affected by ectodermal dysplasia. J Craniofac Surg. 2010;21(6):1776–80.
23. Bauss O, Engelke W, Fenske C, Schilke R, Schwestka-Polly R. Autotransplantation of immature third molars into edentulous and atrophied jaw sections. Int J Oral Maxillofac Surg. 2004;33:488–96.
24. Bokelund M, Andreasen JO, Christensen SS, Kjaer I. Autotransplantation of maxillary second premolars to mandibular recipient sites where the primary second molars were impacted, predisposes for complications. Acta Odontol Scand. 2013;71:1464–8.
25. Krieger O, Matuliene G, Hüsler J, Salvi GE, Pjetursson B, Brägger U. Failures and complications in patients with birth defects restored with fixed dental prostheses and single crowns on teeth and/or implants. Clin Oral Implants Res. 2009;20:809–16.
26. Dueled E, Gotfredsen K, Trab Damsgaard M, Hede B. Professional and patient-based evaluation of oral rehabilitation in patients with tooth agenesis. Clin Oral Implants Res. 2009;20:729–36.
27. Finnema KJ, Raghoebar GM, Meijer HJ, Vissink A. Oral rehabilitation with dental implants in oligodontia patients. Int J Prosthodont. 2005;18:203–9.
28. Goshima K, Lexner MO, Thomsen CE, Miura H, Gotfredsen K, Bakke M. Functional aspects of treatment with implant-supported single crowns: a quality control study in subjects with tooth agenesis. Clin Oral Implants Res. 2010;21:108–14.
29. Robertsson S, Mohlin B. The congenitally missing upper lateral incisor. A retrospective study of orthodontic space closure versus restorative treatment. Eur J Orthod. 2000;22:697–710.
30. Uribe F, Chau V, Padala S, Neace WP, Cutrera A, Nanda R. Alveolar ridge width and height changes after orthodontic space opening in patients congenitally missing maxillary lateral incisors. Eur J Orthod. 2013;35:87–92.
31. Uribe F, Padala S, Allareddy V, Nanda R. Cone-beam computed tomography evaluation of alveolar ridge width and height changes after orthodontic space opening in patients with congenitally missing maxillary lateral incisors. Am J Orthod Dentofacial Orthop. 2013;144:848–59.
32. Johnson EL, Roberts MW, Guckes AD, Bailey LJ, Phillips CL, Wright JT. Analysis of craniofacial development in children with hypohidrotic ectodermal dysplasia. Am J Med Genet. 2002;112:327–34.
33. Wittneben JG, Millen C, Brägger U. Clinical performance of screw- versus cement-retained fixed implant-supported reconstructions—a systematic review. Int J Oral Maxillofac Implants. 2014;29(Suppl):84–98.
34. Pjetursson BE, Tan WC, Zwahlen M, Lang NP. A systematic review of the success of sinus floor elevation and survival of implants inserted in combination with sinus floor elevation. J Clin Periodontol. 2008;35(Suppl):216–40.
35. Bergendal B. Interpretive and report bias in publications on implants in patients with ectodermal dysplasia. Int J Prosthodont. 2011;24:505–6.
36. Jabbour Z, Emami E, de Grandmont P, Rompré PH, Feine JS. Is oral health-related quality of life stable following rehabilitation with mandibular two-implant overdentures? Clin Oral Implants Res. 2012;23:1205–9.
37. Hashem A, Kelly A, O'Connell B, O'Sullivan M. Impact of moderate and severe hypodontia and amelogenesis imperfecta on quality of life and self-esteem of adult patients. J Dent. 2013;41:689–94.
38. Heuberer S, Dvorak G, Zauza K, Watzek G. The use of onplants and implants in children with severe oligodontia: a retrospective evaluation. Clin Oral Implants Res. 2012;23:827–31.
39. Antonarakis GS, Prevezanos P, Gavric J, Christou P. Agenesis of maxillary lateral incisor and tooth replacement: cost-effectiveness of different treatment alternatives. Int J Prosthodont. 2014;27:257–63.
40. Ledermann PD, Hassell TM, Hefti AF. Osseointegrated dental implants as alternative therapy to bridge construction or orthodontics in young patients: seven years of clinical experience. Pediatr Dent. 1993;15:327–33.
41. Kearns G, Sharma A, Perrott D, Schmidt B, Kaban L, Vargervik K. Placement of endosseous implants in children and adolescents with hereditary ectodermal dysplasia. Oral Surg Oral Med Oral Pathol Oral Radiol Endod. 1999;88:5–10.
42. Guckes AD, Scurria MS, King TS, McCarthy GR, Brahim JS. Prospective clinical trial of dental implants in persons with ectodermal dysplasia. J Prosthet Dent. 2002;88:21–5.
43. Sweeney IP, Ferguson JW, Heggie AA, Lucas JO. Treatment outcomes for adolescent ectodermal dysplasia patients treated with dental implants. Int J Paediatr Dent. 2005;15:241–8.
44. Poggio CE, Salvato M, Salvato A. Multidisciplinary treatment of agenesis in the anterior and posterior areas: a long term retrospective analysis. Prog Orthod. 2005;6:262–9.
45. Zarone F, Sorrentino R, Vaccaro F, Russo S. Prosthetic treatment of maxillary lateral incisor agenesis with osseointegrated implants: a 24-39-month prospective clinical study. Clin Oral Implants Res. 2006;17:94–101.
46. Becelli R, Morello R, Renzi G, Dominici C. Treatment of oligodontia with endo-osseous fixtures: experience in eight consecutive patients at the end of dental growth. J Craniofac Surg. 2007;18:1327–30.
47. Degidi M, Nardi D, Piattelli A. Immediate versus one-stage restoration of small-diameter implants for a single missing maxillary lateral incisor: a 3-year randomized clinical trial. J Periodontol. 2009;80:1393–8.
48. Nissan J, Mardinger O, Strauss M, Peleg M, Sacco R, Chaushu G. Implant-supported restoration of congenitally missing teeth using cancellous bone block-allografts. Oral Surg Oral Med Oral Pathol Oral Radiol Endod. 2011;111:286–91.
49. Hosseini M, Worsaae N, Schiødt M, Gotfredsen K. A 3-year prospective study of implant-supported, single-tooth restorations of all-ceramic and metal-ceramic materials in patients with tooth agenesis. Clin Oral Implants Res. 2013;24:1078–87.
50. Zou D, Wu Y, Wang XD, Huang W, Zhang Z, Zhang Z. A retrospective 3- to 5-year study of the reconstruction of oral function using implant-supported prostheses in patients with hypohidrotic ectodermal dysplasia. J Oral Implantol. 2014;40:571–80.
51. Kristerson L, Lagerström L. Autotransplantation of teeth in cases with agenesis or traumatic loss of maxillary incisors. Eur J Orthod. 1991;13:486–92.
52. Kugelberg R, Tegsjö U, Malmgren O. Autotransplantation of 45 teeth to the upper incisor region in adolescents. Swed Dent J. 1994;18:165–72.
53. Marcusson KAM, Lilja-Karlander EK. Autotransplantation of premolars and molars in patients with tooth aplasia. J Dent. 1996;24:355–8.
54. Josefsson E, Brattström V, Tegsjö U, Valerius-Olsson H. Treatment of lower second premolar agenesis by autotransplantation: four-year evaluation of eighty patients. Acta Odontol Scand. 1999;57:111–5.
55. Czochrowska EM, Stenvik A, Bjercke B, Zachrisson BU. Outcome of tooth transplantation: survival and success rates 17–41 years posttreatment. Am J Orthod Dentofacial Orthop. 2002;121:110–9.
56. Jonsson T, Sigurdsson TJ. Autotransplantation of premolars to premolar sites. A long-term follow-up study of 40 consecutive patients. Am J Orthod Dentofacial Orthop. 2004;125:668–75.
57. Tanaka T, Deguchi T, Kageyama T, Kanomi R, Inoue M, Foong KW. Autotransplantation of 28 premolar donor teeth in 24 orthodontic patients. Angle Orthod. 2008;78:12–9.
58. Mensink G, Merkesteyn R. Autotransplantation of premolars. Brit Dent J. 2010;208:109–11.
59. Kvint S, Lindsten R, Magnusson A, Nilsson P, Bjerklin K. Autotransplantation of teeth in 215 patients. A follow-up study. Angle Orthod. 2010;80:446–51.
60. Bjerklin K, Bennett J. The long-term survival of lower second primary molars in subjects with agenesis of the premolars. Eur J Orthod. 2000;22:245–55.
61. Ith-Hansen K, Kjaer I. Persistence of deciduous molars in subjects with agenesis of the second premolars. Eur J Orthod. 2000;22:239–43.
62. Sletten DW, Smith BM, Southard KA, Casko JS, Southard TE. Retained deciduous mandibular molars in adults: a radiographic study of long-term changes. Am J Orthod Dentofacial Orthop. 2003;124:625–30.

63. Bjerklin K, Al-Najjar M, Kårestedt H, Andrén A. Agenesis of mandibular second premolars with retained primary molars: a longitudinal radiographic study of 99 subjects from 12 years of age to adulthood. Eur J Orthod. 2008;30:254–61.
64. Hobkirk JA, Goodman JR, Reynolds IR. Component failure in removable partial dentures for patients with severe hypodontia. Int J Prosthodont. 1989;2:327–30.
65. Pröbster B, Henrich GM. 11-year follow-up study of resin-bonded fixed partial dentures. Int J Prosthodont. 1997;10:259–68.
66. Garnett MJ, Wassell RW, Jepson NJ, Nohl FS. Survival of resin-bonded bridgework provided for post-orthodontic hypodontia patients with missing maxillary lateral incisors. Br Dent J. 2006;21(201):527–34.
67. Spinas E, Aresu M, Canargiu F. Prosthetic rehabilitation interventions in adolescents with fixed bridges: a 5-year observational study. Eur J Paediatr Dent. 2013;14:59–62.
68. Wong AT, McMillan AS, McGrath C. Oral health-related quality of life and severe hypodontia. J Oral Rehabil. 2006;33:869–73.
69. Stanford CM, Guckes A, Fete M, Srun S, Richter MK. Perceptions of outcomes of implant therapy in patients with ectodermal dysplasia syndromes. Int J Prosthodont. 2008;21:195–200.
70. Locker D, Jokovic A, Prakash P, Tompson B. Oral health-related quality of life of children with oligodontia. Int J Paediatr Dent. 2010;20:8–14.
71. Laing E, Cunningham SJ, Jones S, Moles D, Gill D. Psychosocial impact of hypodontia in children. Am J Orthod Dentofacial Orthop. 2010;137:35–41.
72. Kohli R, Levy S, Kummet CM, Dawson DV, Stanford CM. Comparison of perceptions of oral health-related quality of life in adolescents affected with ectodermal dysplasia relative to caregivers. Spec Care Dentist. 2011;31:88–94.
73. Meaney S, Anweigi L, Ziada H, Allen F. The impact of hypodontia: a qualitative study on the experiences of patients. Eur J Orthod. 2012;34:547–52.
74. Anweigi L, Finbarr Allen P, Ziada H. Impact of resin bonded bridgework on quality of life of patients with hypodontia. J Dent. 2013;41:683–8.
75. Anweigi L, Allen PF, Ziada H. The use of the Oral Health Impact Profile to measure the impact of mild, moderate and severe hypodontia on oral health-related quality of life in young adults. J Oral Rehabil. 2013;40:603–8.

# Palatal window osteotomy technique improves maxillary sinus augmentation in previously insufficient augmentation case

Daisuke Ueno[1*], Takashi Kurokawa[2], Katsuichiro Maruo[3], Tsuneaki Watanabe[2] and Jayanetti Asiri Jayawardena[4]

**Abstract**

**Introduction:** Perforation of the Schneiderian membrane is the most common complication in sinus floor augmentation (SFA). When volume of grafting is qualified to prevent enlargement of the membrane perforation, lack of bone volume may occur in optimal site.

**Case presentation:** SFA was performed in sites #24 to 26 in a 63-year-old male. However, a 10-mm size perforation of the Schneiderian membrane occurred in site #26. Although the sinus cavity was grafted with deproteinized bovine bone mineral (DBBM) after repair of membrane perforation, insufficient bone formation was observed on palatal and distal aspects of site #26 at 5 months after SFA. Although additional SFA was required for implant placement, it seemed to be difficult to elevate the membrane by a conventional lateral approach in the palatal aspect of the sinus floor (site #26). Considering the configuration of new bone formation, it was decided to perform the palatal antrostomy approach. The Schneiderian membrane was elevated without perforation, and the sinus cavity was grafted with DBBM mixed with venous blood. Two 12-mm long, 4.1-mm diameter implants were placed in sites #14 and 16. Four months after implant placement, abutment-connection surgery was successfully performed. The radiographic image indicated improved radiopacity, without obvious bone resorption in site #26.

**Conclusion:** The palatal window osteotomy technique could be considered as an alternative method for augmentation of maxillary sinus in cases where difficulty is encountered to elevate a membrane by a conventional approach (e.g., in cases in which buccal bone height is long).

**Keywords:** Sinus floor augmentation; Dental implants; Surgical technique; Palatal osteotomy

## Introduction

Sinus floor augmentation (SFA) is the most common technique to obtain bone height for implant placement in posterior maxilla. The most common method is the classical lateral antrostomy approach; After raising a full-thickness flap on the buccal side of the alveolar ridge, a trap door is created by a round bur [1]. The sinus membrane is dissected, and the trap door is rotated medially to push the Schneiderian membrane apically. Then the graft material is placed on the sinus floor. Although a conventional lateral window technique is known to be very predictable with good long-term success, only few reports have been introduced to evaluate the palatal antrostomy approach [2, 3]. The authors reported slight usability such as postoperative comfort compared to conventional buccal antrostomy approach [3]. This case demonstrates significant bone augmentation using a palatal antrostomy technique in the palatal aspect of the sinus floor which makes it difficult to elevate the Schneiderian membrane by a conventional approach.

## Clinical report

A 63-year-old male patient was introduced to the Unit of Oral and Maxillofacial Implantology, Tsurumi University Dental Hospital for implant treatment in April 2013 (Fig. 1). Since vertical bone heights in sites # 24 (4 mm) and 26 (less than 1 mm) were not enough for implant placement, SFA was performed prior to implant placement.

* Correspondence: ueno@kdu.ac.jp
[1]Department of Implantology and Periodontology, Kanagawa Dental University, Graduate School of Dentistry, 3-31-6 Tsuruya-cho, Kanagawa-ku, Yokohama, Japan
Full list of author information is available at the end of the article

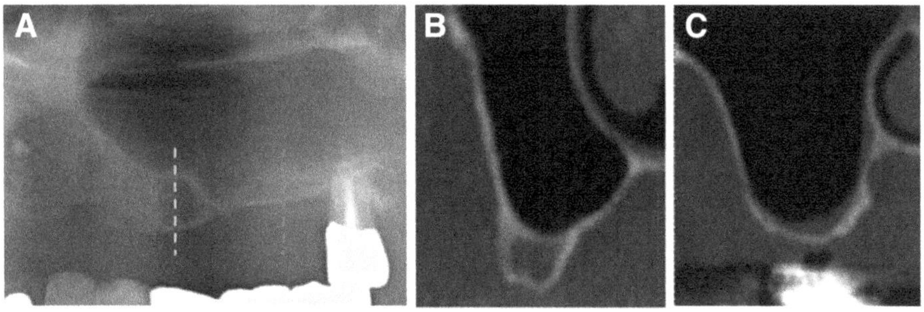


**Fig. 1** Preoperative radiographic images. **a** Orthopantomography shows that inadequate bone height was observed in sites #24 (*blue line*) and #26 (*red line*). **b** Coronal CT image of the *blue line*; vertical bone height is 4 mm. **c** Coronal CT image of the *red line*; vertical bone height is only 1 mm

However, a 10-mm size perforation of the Schneiderian membrane occurred in site #26 during sinus floor elevation. The membrane perforation was covered with a sheet-like collagen sponge[1]. Then, the sinus cavity was grafted with deproteinized bovine bone mineral (DBBM)[2] mixed with venous blood [4]. Use of DBBM was approved by the ethical committee of Tsurumi University. Nevertheless, volume of grafting in the posterior area was qualified to prevent enlargement of the membrane perforation. Site #24 was augmented with guided bone regeneration to increase bone width for implant placement.

No complications, such as postoperative nose bleeding, occurred during the healing period. Five months after sinus floor augmentation, a cone beam computed tomography (CBCT) image showed that an adequate volume of bone augmentation was achieved in site #24 (Fig. 2). In contrast, lack of bone formation was observed in palatal and distal aspects of site #26. Therefore, additional bone augmentation was planned in order to place implants with optimal position and direction.

A pala-crestal incision performed from site #21 to the interproximal aspects of the #27. The incision was extended intrasulcaly, and vertical release incisions were made at the mesiobuccal angle of the maxillary pad (Fig. 3). Full-thickness flaps were elevated buccal and palatal aspects. The palatal wall of the maxillary sinus was exposed after the elevation of a mucoperiosteal flap. A piezoelectric device[3] and diamond-coated round bur was used with copious saline irrigation to create the palatal window of the maxillary sinus. Then, the Schneiderian membrane was elevated by sinus lift elevator without perforation (Fig. 3). Since the palatal vault is steep, and palatal bone is thick, Tinti sinus lift elevator[4] which can be bent hard was used to separate the palatal Schneiderian membrane. Then, Memmingen sinus lift elevator[5] was used to elevate the membrane apically. After the sinus cavity was grafted with DBBM[2] mixed with venous blood, two 12-mm long, 4.1-mm diameter implants[6,7] were placed in sites #24 and 26 (Fig. 3). Then, further bone augmentation was performed on the buccal implant from the palatal bony window. The insertion torques of implants #24 and 26 were 35 and 25 Ncm, respectively. The graft sites were covered with a sheet-like collagen sponge to improve graft stability[1]. After periosteal-releasing incisions, flaps were sutured without flap tension. The post-surgical course was uneventful.

Four months after implant placement, abutment-connection surgery was performed. The radiographic

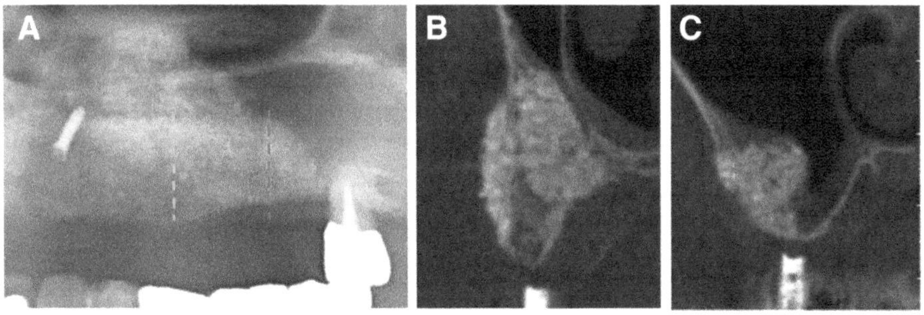


**Fig. 2** Radiographic image, 5 months after sinus bone augmentation. **a** Orthopantomography shows inadequate bone height observed in sites #26 (*red line*). **b** Coronal CT image of the *blue line*; vertical bone height is 15 mm. Horizontal augmentation is also achieved. **c** Coronal CT image of the *red line*; no bone augmentation was achieved in the palatal aspect of sinus cavity

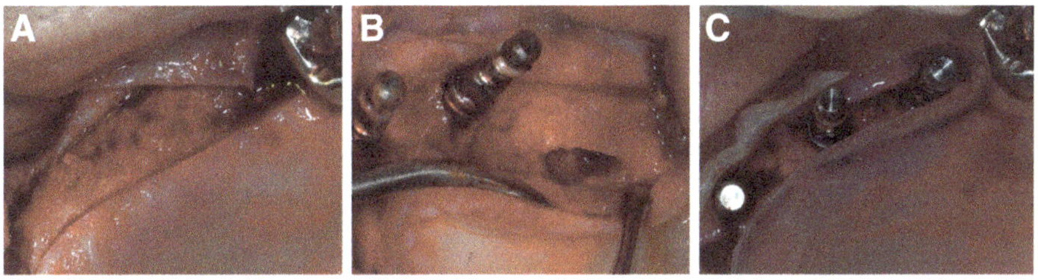


**Fig. 3** Sinus bone augmentation with implant placement after palatal window osteotomy. After pala-crestal incision (**a**) and raising full-thickness flaps on the buccal and palatal sides of the alveolar ridge, palatal antrostomy is performed by a round bur (**b**). An implant was placed in optimal position after bone grafting in the palatal aspect of sinus cavity (**c**)

image improved radiopacity without obvious bone resorption in the optimal site (Fig. 4). The values of the implant stability quotient (ISQ) of the implants in #24 and 26 were 78 and 71, respectively. All implants were functioning well 6 months after occlusal loading.

## Discussion

The palatal window osteotomy technique is previously described as beneficial because it has a higher postoperative comfort, especially for edentulous patients, because full dentures could be incorporated directly after surgery with an almost perfect fit [3, 5]. As another advantage, this case demonstrated significant bone augmentation in the palatal aspect of the sinus floor which makes it difficult to elevate membrane by conventional approach.

Perforation of the sinus membrane is the most common intra-operative complication in maxillary sinus floor augmentation. According to a systematic review, mean prevalence of membrane perforation was 19.5 % [6]. Membrane perforation was usually closed by fibrin glue, suturing or, covering them with a collagen membrane. Depending on the size and location of the perforation, a sufficient quantity of bone augmentation is not possible in the optimal site. In cases of larger perforations, discontinuation of SFA, and reoperation after healing of the sinus membrane may be a more reliable method. However, the staged recovery approach requires an additional treatment period. In the present case, bone volume required for implant placement was supplemented by the first SFA. Additional SFA with the palatal window osteotomy technique was able to graft in palatal sinus cavity which is the insufficient bone volume area. A particular advantage of the palatal window osteotomy is that it can easily approach the cavity compared to buccal window osteotomy, when buccal bone in maxillary sinus is thick and long. From these findings, it may be suggested that maxillary sinus augmentation with the palatal window osteotomy approach is useful in compensation of the palatal sinus cavity. Caution should be exercised during elevation of the palatal flap and osteotomy preparation in the palatal wall to avoid damage to the greater palatine neurovascular bundle (GPB) which contains greater palatine artery, vein, and nerve. Since GPB exits through the greater palatine foramen and runs anteriorly in the bone groove of the palate, three-dimensional analysis using CBCT or CT would reduce surgical complications [7]. Further studies are needed to confirm the efficiency of the palatal window osteotomy technique.

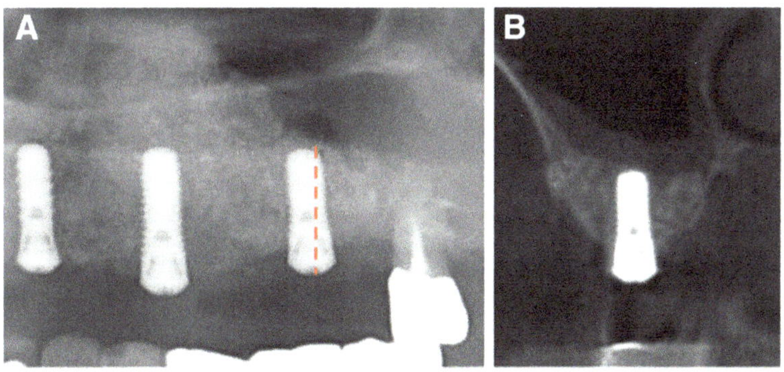


**Fig. 4** Radiographic image. Four months following 2nd sinus floor augmentation with implant placements. **a** Significant bone augmentation is achieved in site #26. **b** Coronal CT image of the *red line* shows that sufficient bone support with improved radiopacity was achieved in the palatal aspect of sinus cavity

## Consent

Written informed consent was obtained from the patient for publication of this report and any accompanying images.

## Endnotes

[1]TERUDERMIS, Orinpus-Termo Biomaterials, Tokyo, Japan.
[2]Bio-Oss®, Geistlich, Biomaterials, Wolhuser, Switzerland.
[3]Sonic Surgeon 300, Morita Corporation, Tokyo, Japan.
[4]Stoma Tinti Sinus Lift Elevator, Stoma, Germany.
[5]Stoma Memmingen Sinus Lift Elevator, Stoma, Germany.
[6]Straumann® Bone Level Implant, Basel, Switzerland.
[7]Straumann® Tapered Effect Implant, Basel, Switzerland.

### Competing interests

Daisuke Ueno, Takashi Kurokawa, Katsuichiro Maruo, Tsuneaki Watanabe and Jayanetti Asiri Jayawardena declare that they have no competing interests.

### Authors' contributions

DU designed and performed surgery, and wrote the paper; JAJ wrote and compiled the paper; TK and TW assisted in the surgery; and KM compiled the paper. All authors read and approved the final manuscript.

### Authors' information

DU is a senior assistant professor of the Department of Implantology and Periodontology, Kanagawa Dental University, Graduate School of Dentistry, Yokohama, Japan.
TK and TW are clinical research associates of the Unit of Oral and Maxillofacial Implantology, Tsurumi University Dental Hospital, Yokohama, Japan.
K.M. is an assistant professor of the Department of Removable Prosthodontics, Kanagawa Dental University, Graduate School of Dentistry, Yokosuka, Japan.
JAJ is an assistant professor of the Department of General Education, Tsurumi University, School of Dental Medicine.

### Author details

[1]Department of Implantology and Periodontology, Kanagawa Dental University, Graduate School of Dentistry, 3-31-6 Tsuruya-cho, Kanagawa-ku, Yokohama, Japan. [2]Unit of Oral and Maxillofacial Implantology, Tsurumi University Dental Hospital, Yokohama, Japan. [3]Department of Removal Prosthodontics, Kanagawa Dental University, Graduate School of Dentistry, Yokosuka, Japan. [4]Department of General Education, Tsurumi University, School of Dental Medicine, Yokohama, Japan.

### References

1. Tatum Jr H. Maxillary and sinus implant reconstructions. Dent Clin North Am. 1986;30:207–29.
2. Cabezas-Mojón J, Barona-Dorado C, Gómez-Moreno G, Fernández-Cáliz F, Martínez-González JM. Meta-analytic study of implant survival following sinus augmentation. Med Oral Patol Oral Cir Bucal. 2012;17:e135–9.
3. Stübinger S, Saldamli B, Landes CA, Sader R. Palatal piezosurgical window osteotomy for maxillary sinus augmentation. Int J Oral Maxillofac Surg. 2010;39:606–9.
4. Kasabah S, Simůnek A, Krug J, Lecaro MC. Maxillary sinus augmentation with deproteinized bovine bone (Bio-Oss) and Impladent dental implant system. Part II. Evaluation of deprotienized bovine bone (Bio-Oss) and implant surface. Acta Medica (Hradec Kralove). 2002;45:167-71.
5. Stübinger S, Saldamli B, Seitz O, Sader R, Landes CA. Palatal versus vestibular piezoelectric window osteotomy for maxillary sinus elevation: a comparative clinical study of two surgical techniques. Oral Surg Oral Med Oral Pathol Oral Radiol Endod. 2009;107:648–55.
6. Pjetursson BE, Tan WC, Zwahlen M, Lang NP. A systematic review of the success of sinus floor elevation and survival of implants inserted in combination with sinus floor elevation. J Clin Periodontol. 2008;35:216–40.
7. Ueno D, Sekiguchi R, Morita M, Jayawardena A, Shinpo S, Sato J, et al. Palatal mucosal measurements in a Japanese population using cone-beam computed tomography. J Esthet Restor Dent. 2014;26:48–58.

# A prospective cross-over study to evaluate the effect of two different occlusal concepts on the masseter muscle activity in implant-retained mandibular overdentures

Ahmed M. Abdelhamid[1], Kenda I. Hanno[2*] and Mohamed H. Imam[3]

**Abstract**

**Background:** The purpose of this prospective cross-over study is to evaluate the effect of bilateral balanced occlusion and canine guidance occlusion on the masseter muscle activity using implant-retained mandibular overdentures.

**Methods:** After evaluation of 12 completely edentulous patients using cone beam computed tomography (CBCT), mucoperiosteal flaps were reflected exposing the mandibular interforaminal region. Two implants were placed in the interforaminal region for each of the 12 patients. After a healing period of 3 months, acrylic maxillary complete dentures and mandibular overdentures were fabricated with bilateral balanced occlusion for 6 patients and canine guidance occlusion for the other 6 patients. Electromyographic evaluation of the masseter muscles, during clenching on a silicon index and chewing peanuts and cake, was conducted on the patients after using their dentures for 4 weeks. Each occlusion concept was then converted into the other concept using the same dentures, and the procedure of evaluation was repeated after 4 weeks. The recordings were analyzed statistically using Wilcoxon signed ranks test. $p < 0.05$ was considered statistically significant.

**Results:** The highest electromyographic activity of the masseter muscles was recorded during clenching on a preformed silicon index followed by chewing peanut then cake for both occlusal concepts. The recordings of the masseter muscle associated with canine guidance occlusion were higher than bilateral balanced occlusion but with no statistically significant difference except between the right masseter muscles during clenching ($p = 0.042$*).

**Conclusions:** Both bilateral balanced occlusion and canine guidance occlusion can be used successfully in implant-retained mandibular overdentures without affecting masseter muscle activity.

**Keywords:** Balanced occlusion, Canine guidance, Electromyography, Implant-retained overdentures, Muscle activity

## Background

Treatment of edentulous patients using a conventional complete removable denture is a common clinical undertaking. However, those patients may experience problems which include pain during mastication, reduced masticatory ability, as well as insufficient stability and retention of the mandibular denture [1].

The introduction of dental implants and, subsequently, the implant-supported mandibular overdenture has improved the quality of life for edentulous patients [2]. The biomechanical aspects of occlusal design, configuration, and anatomy significantly influence the ultimate success of implant. The development of occlusal concepts that is in harmony with the rest of the stomatognathic system is a major contributing factor in the long-term success rate of the implant-supported prosthesis [3].

Many authors [4] emphasized the role of occlusion as a key factor in implant success. James [5] stated that "nearly all problems of the implants that develop between the first and sixth week post-insertion are directly related to the occlusion." Lindquist et al., [6] and Miyata et al., [7]

* Correspondence: kendahanno@gmail.com
[2]Prosthodontics, Faculty of Dentistry, Alexandria University, Alexandria, Egypt
Full list of author information is available at the end of the article

studied the longitudinal effects of occlusal forces on osseointegrated implants and found that overloading was the main cause for bone loss around fixtures and/or loss of osseointegration of successfully integrated implants. The prosthesis must therefore be fabricated as accurately as possible in order to achieve long-term success, and occlusion should be a key factor of the overall success rate.

Currently, the occlusal philosophies that are proposed for implant overdentures are based on those for conventional complete dentures [8]. These philosophies include bilateral balanced occlusion and lingualized occlusion.

Balanced occlusion concept has been recommended in removable implant overdentures especially for patients with complete maxillary denture and mandibular implant-retained overdentures to distribute the loads and to provide better stability [9]. The chewing forces are applied to the working and balancing sides simultaneously and over all of the surfaces of the edentulous ridge, resulting in the decrease in pressure on the edentulous jaw and preventing residual ridge reduction [10].

For more than a hundred years, textbooks and undergraduate teaching have stated that canine guided dentures should be avoided, since they would result in denture instability and impaired muscle function; however, recent research has shown that conventional complete dentures can function successfully without balanced occlusion [11].

Canine guidance disengages the posterior teeth during excursive mandibular movements by vertically and horizontally overlapping the canines [12]. Grubwieser et al., [13] stated that canine guidance occlusion (CGO) can be used successfully in complete dentures as it improves mandibular denture retention, esthetic appearance, and masticatory ability. They also observed that CGO reduced muscle activity during lateral movement and protrusion when compared with BBO.

Canine guidance is easier and faster to be provided. It seems to be rational to recommend this occlusal concept for the excursive movements of the mandible in complete dentures wearers until future research can solve this question [14].

The various methods for assessment of masticatory function include food particle size estimation [15], sieving method [16], colorimetric determination [17], optical scanning method [18], biting force [15], and weight loss of viscoelastic food [19].

Occlusion may alter muscle activity and related jaw movements in mastication. Muscle activity, which is a reflection of masticatory function of the patient, can be objectively evaluated using surface electromyography (EMG) [20]. EMG is a valuable parameter to assess muscular dysfunction. Surface EMG measures muscle activity noninvasively using surface electrodes placed on the skin overlying the muscle to determine the timing of the muscle contraction and to investigate the behavior of the muscle during functions of the stomatognathic system [21].

Aziz et al., (2008) compared the effect of two different occlusal schemes on the muscle activity in implant-supported mandibular overdentures using electromyography. The results revealed slight increase in the muscle activity in patients rehabilitated with dentures constructed following the lingualized concept of occlusion compared to dentures constructed following the monoplane concept of occlusion [22].

The choice of an occlusal design or configuration for implant-retained prosthesis is broad and often controversial. To date, there is no evidence to recommend a specific occlusal design for implant-retained overdentures. No sufficient scientific evidence was found on applying canine guidance in implant-retained overdentures. Therefore, this study was conducted to investigate the effects of balanced occlusion and canine guidance on masseter muscle activity in implant-retained overdentures.

## Methods

The study design is a prospective cross-over study.

Twelve completely edentulous patients aged 45–65 years, having acceptable maxillomandibular relationship, sufficient inter-ridge space, and with no previous denture experience, were selected for this study. Complete maxillary and mandibular dentures were fabricated for each patient.

Since the type of opposing occlusion is a critical factor that influences the magnitude of forces transmitted to the implant bone interface, the opposing occlusion was selected to be mucosa-supported complete denture. This was done to standardize and control the amount of occlusal forces applied to the abutments. Complete dentures were proved to exert less amount of force compared to the natural teeth [23].

The selection of the interforaminal area of the mandible, where two implants were placed, was based on the recommendation by Lekholm and Zarb [24] and Hong et al., [25] as the bone in this area is of good quality. Implants are demonstrated to have fewer micro-movements, increased initial stability, and reduced stress concentration in high-quality bone [26]. Furthermore, it has been established that the survival of the root form titanium implants is very high in the anterior mandible and that the incidence of surgical complications is very low [27, 28].

A clear acrylic radiographic/surgical mandibular template including gutta-percha radiopaque indicators allowed implant alignment along planned prosthetic axes during implant surgery and ensured good visual access [29].

The previously fabricated denture was duplicated in clear acrylic resin and used as a radiographic surgical guide using gutta-percha as radiopaque markers. Each

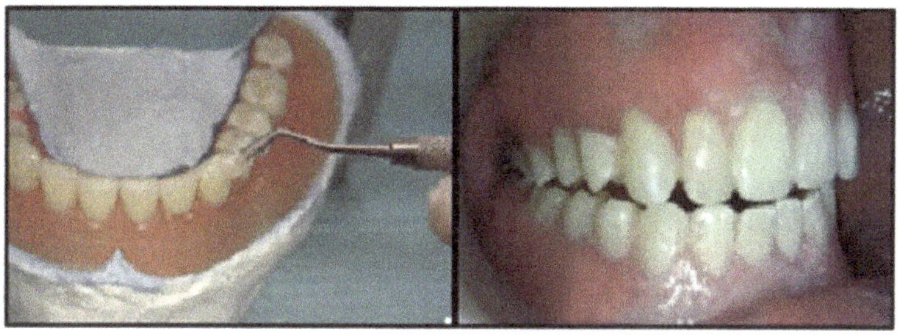

**Fig. 1** Application of light-cure composite resin on the mandibular canines and a view of canine guidance occlusion intraorally

patient was evaluated radiographically using cone beam computed tomography (CBCT) before surgical implant placement. A mucoperiosteal flap was reflected exposing the mandibular interforaminal region for optimal implant placement. Two implants (Dentium Superline, Dentium Co. Ltd., Korea) were screwed in position. The length of the implants was 10 mm and the diameter is 3.6 mm.

After a healing period of 3 months, acrylic maxillary and mandibular overdentures were fabricated with bilateral balanced occlusion for all patients. Positioner attachments were used and incorporated into the dentures using direct pickup method. Six patients used their dentures with bilateral balanced occlusion for 4 weeks then were evaluated by EMG. Following evaluation, it was converted into canine guidance occlusion using the same denture. This was achieved clinically by remounting using the semi-adjustable articulator.

Light-cured composite resin was then added in the mandibular canines to provide an interarch disocclusion space of 2 mm during eccentric movements.

For the other six patients, canine guidance occlusion was applied first in the try-in stage through application of light-cure composite resin on the mandibular canines (Fig. 1).

The patients used their dentures for 4 weeks then were evaluated using EMG. After evaluation, canine guidance occlusion was converted into bilateral balanced occlusion by removal of the composite resin from the mandibular canines (Fig. 2). The positioner attachments (positioner abutment and socket set, Dentium Co.Ltd, Korea) were placed on the implants and attached to the dentures by direct pickup method (Fig. 3).

### Recording the electromyographic activity

EMG has also been used to assess the masticatory function of mandibular implant-retained overdentures. The electrical output of a muscle, measured by electromyography, is proportional to the energy consumed to produce contractions. The masseter and anterior temporalis muscles on both sides were evaluated because they are the largest and strongest of the masticatory muscles, the most superficial and are accessible to surface EMG examination. The surface EMG recordings provided a safe, easy, and noninvasive method that allowed objective quantification of the energy of the muscle [30].

Standard amounts and sizes of cake and peanuts were used to reduce patient variability. These test foods were an example of soft and hard food, respectively, and they gave an idea about the effect of different types of food on muscle activity during function. Preformed silicon index was used to measure the muscle activity during clenching [31].

Evaluation of muscle activity was performed by measuring activity of the masseter muscles on both sides for both occlusal concepts at the end of 2 weeks using electromyography (Nicolet VikingQuest version 11, USA) with three types of test foods.

During all recordings, the patients were seated with their head unsupported and were asked to maintain a naturally erect position. The masseteric myoelectric activity of both sides (right and left) were recorded by means of disposable bipolar electrodes positioned on the bellies of the muscles parallel to the fiber orientation (Fig. 4).

Electroconductive gel was applied on the electrodes before they contacted the skin. The recording electrodes

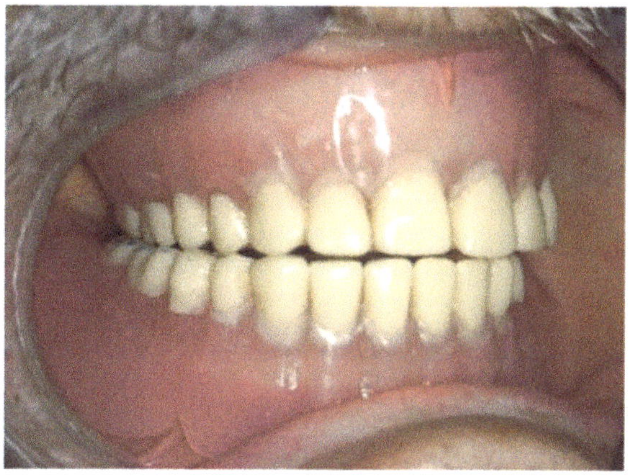

**Fig. 2** Bilateral balanced occlusion intraorally

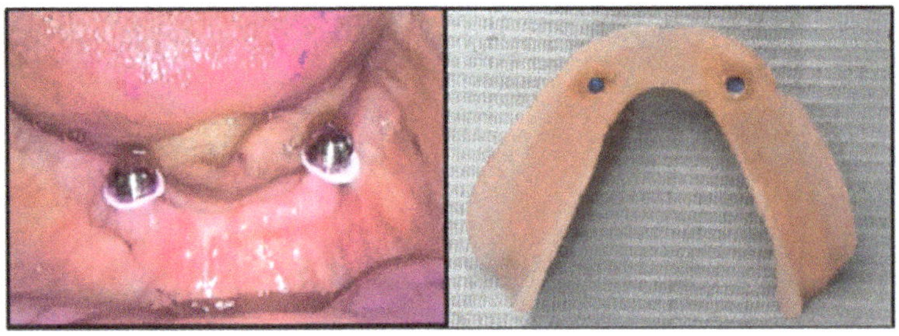

**Fig. 3** The white blockout spacers in place with the locator caps on top and the positioner socket with blue nylon cap

were positioned approximately 20 mm apart. The patient was grounded by using a grounding electrode. The third electrode was fixed on the palm of the patient's hand.

Each patient was instructed to clench with a preformed silicon index made by using vinyl polysiloxane material (putty) of standardized size positioned at the premolar region for 30 s to measure the muscle activity during clenching. Then the patients were instructed to chew on one peanut of similar size and diameter, and the EMG was recorded. Then the patients were instructed to chew on a piece of cake of standardized size (2 cm × 2 cm), and the EMG was recorded. The patients chewed the test samples on the right and left sides at 10-s intervals using their arbitrary chewing frequency until they are ready to swallow before the EMG was recorded.

At the end of the record and before removing the surface electrodes, the positions of the electrodes were marked to be used as a guide for accurate reproducibility. The previous tasks were separated by a recovery rest period of 2 min. The computerized data showed the root mean square (RMS) of the EMG signals (Fig. 5).

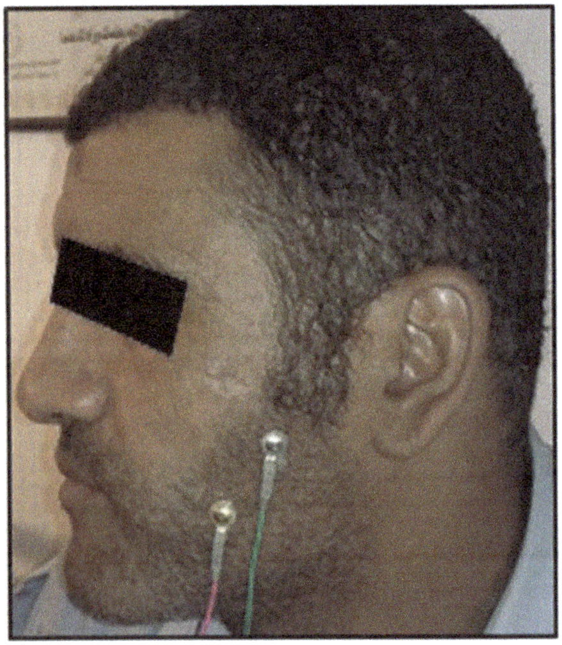

**Fig. 4** Bipolar electrodes positioned at the masseter muscle belly

### Statistical analysis

Data were fed to the computer. Quantitative data were described using range (minimum and maximum), mean, standard deviation, and median. Wilcoxon signed ranks test was applied. Significance of the obtained results was judged at the 5 % level. A $p$ value less than 0.05 was considered statistically significant.

### Ethical approval

This study protocol was approved by the research ethics committee of the Faculty of Dentistry, Alexandria University, Egypt.

### Ethics, consent, and permissions

All the patients signed an informed consent form before participation in this study.

### Consent to publish

All the patients who participated in the study provided consent to publish the data obtained from them during the study.

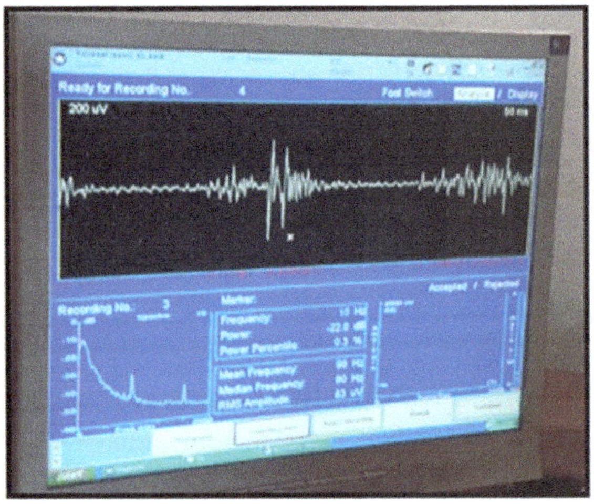

**Fig. 5** EMG signal on the monitor of the computer

## Results

In the right masseter muscle, bilateral balanced occlusion has shown lower RMS values on clenching with the silicon index, chewing peanut, and chewing cake compared to the RMS values of canine guidance occlusion (Table 1).

However, the table shows no statistically significant difference between the two occlusal concepts for the right masseter muscle. The difference was statistically significant only during clenching on a silicon index ($p = 0.042^*$).

In the left masseter muscle, bilateral balanced occlusion has shown lower RMS values on clenching with the silicon index, chewing peanut, and chewing cake compared to the RMS values of canine guidance occlusion. The table shows no statistically significant difference between the two occlusal concepts for the left masseter muscle (Table 1).

In the right masseter muscle, clenching on silicon index showed the highest RMS values followed by chewing peanut, and the least RMS value was for chewing cake. The results showed a statistical significant difference between them ($p = 0.006$).

In the left masseter muscle, clenching on silicon index showed the highest RMS values followed by chewing peanut and the least RMS value was for chewing cake. The results showed no statistical significant difference between them ($p = 0.082$). There was a statistical significant difference between clenching on silicon index and chewing cake ($p_1 = 0.037^*$) (Table 2).

In the right masseter muscle, clenching on silicon index showed the highest RMS values followed by chewing peanut and the least RMS value was for chewing cake. The results showed no statistical significant difference between them ($p = 0.778$).

In the left masseter muscle, clenching on silicon index showed the highest RMS values followed by chewing peanut, and the least RMS value was for chewing cake

**Table 1** Comparison between bilateral balanced occlusion and canine guidance occlusion according to EMG signals (RMS values) of the masseter muscle

| Food type | Bilateral Balanced Occlusion (n = 12) | | Canine Guidance Occlusion (n = 12) | |
|---|---|---|---|---|
| | Right | Left | Right | Left |
| **Silicon index** | | | | |
| Min. – Max. | 26.0 – 66.0 | 33.0 – 78.0 | 29.0 – 289.0 | 11.0 – 150.0 |
| Mean ± SD. | 55.75 ± 13.05 | 62.17 ± 15.86 | 61.67 ± 72.14 | 68.75 ± 42.86 |
| Median | 60.0 | 64.50 | 43.0 | 69.0 |
| **Z (p)** | → | 2.032*(0.042*) | ← | |
| | | → | 0.347 (0.728) | ← |
| **Peanut** | | | | |
| Min. – Max. | 28.0 – 63.0 | 21.0 – 108.0 | 34.0 – 185.0 | 24.0 – 126.0 |
| Mean ± SD. | 45.67 ± 12.34 | 57.33 ± 28.65 | 55.08 ± 41.27 | 61.50 ± 26.21 |
| Median | 43.50 | 50.50 | 44.0 | 62.0 |
| **Z (p)** | → | 0.116 (0.908) | ← | |
| | | → | 0.753 (0.452) | ← |
| **Cake** | | | | |
| Min. – Max. | 28.0 – 54.0 | 23.0 – 85.0 | 21.0 – 87.0 | 29.0 – 143.0 |
| Mean ± SD. | 38.33 ± 8.24 | 42.50 ± 21.66 | 46.83 ± 20.70 | 54.75 ± 31.19 |
| Median | 37.50 | 40.50 | 39.0 | 51.50 |
| **Z (p)** | → | 0.696 (0.487) | ← | |
| | | → | 1.159 (0.246) | ← |

*Z* Mann-Whitney test
*Statistically significant at $p \le 0.05$

**Table 2** Comparison between the different test foods according to RMS values of the EMG signals of right and left masseter muscles in bilateral balanced occlusion

| | Silicon index ($n = 12$) | Peanut ($n = 12$) | Cake ($n = 12$) | $^{KW}\chi^2$ | $p$ |
|---|---|---|---|---|---|
| Right | | | | | |
| Min.–Max. | 26.0–66.0 | 28.0–63.0 | 28.0–54.0 | | |
| Mean ± SD | 55.75 ± 13.05 | 45.67 ± 12.34 | 38.33 ± 8.24 | 10.180* | 0.006* |
| Median | 60.0 | 43.50 | 37.50 | | |
| | $p_1 = 0.005^*$, $p_2 = 0.037^*$, $p_3 = 0.063$ | | | | |
| Left | | | | | |
| Min.–Max. | 33.0–78.0 | 21.0–108.0 | 23.0–85.0 | | |
| Mean ± SD | 62.17 ± 15.86 | 57.33 ± 28.65 | 42.50 ± 21.66 | 5.013 | 0.082 |
| Median | 64.50 | 50.50 | 40.50 | | |
| | $p_1 = 0.037^*$, $p_2 = 0.354$, $p_3 = 0.131$ | | | | |

$^{KW}\chi^2$ chi square for Kruskal-Wallis test, $p_1$ $p$ value for Mann-Whitney test for comparing between Silicon index and Cake, $p_2$ $p$ value for Mann-Whitney test for comparing between silicon index and peanut, $p_3$ $p$ value for Mann-Whitney test for comparing between cake and peanut
*Statistically significant at $p \leq 0.05$

(54.75 ± 31.19). The results should no statistical significant difference between them ($p = 0.344$). (Table 3)

## Discussion

Many authors stated that bilateral balanced occlusion promotes better masticatory efficiency by bringing a larger amount of grinding surfaces into contact at each movement [32, 33]. The results of the current study did not show a significant difference for muscle function by EMG between the studied occlusal concepts. This finding coincides with El-Okel who compared masticatory efficiency through evaluation of electromyographic activity between bilateral balanced occlusion, canine guidance occlusion, lingualized, and monoplane occlusion schemes and found no significant difference [34]. The results also coincide with Grunert et al., [20] who found no difference in muscle activity between bilateral balanced occlusion and canine guidance occlusion in complete dentures. These results were also similar to Neto AF et al., who stated that bilateral balanced occlusion did not improve masticatory efficiency when compared with canine guidance [11]. Abd Elmonem evaluated masticatory efficiency in complete denture wearers with bilateral balanced occlusion and canine guidance using the colorimetric method and also found no statistical significant difference between them [35].

Despite the insignificant difference between EMG activity of the masseter muscles in bilateral balanced occlusion and canine guidance occlusion, the mean EMG activity was higher in canine guidance compared to bilateral balanced occlusion. This could be due to larger amount of grinding surfaces brought into contact at each movement in balanced occlusion resulting in less effort needed by the muscles during chewing. This could

**Table 3** Comparison between the different test foods according to RMS values of the EMG signals of right and left masseter muscles in canine guidance occlusion

| | Silicon index ($n = 12$) | Peanut ($n = 12$) | Cake ($n = 12$) | $^{KW}\chi^2$ | $p$ |
|---|---|---|---|---|---|
| Right | | | | | |
| Min.–Max. | 29.0–289.0 | 34.0–185.0 | 21.0–87.0 | | |
| Mean ± SD | 61.67 ± 72.14 | 55.08 ± 41.27 | 46.83 ± 20.70 | 0.501 | 0.778 |
| Median | 43.0 | 44.0 | 39.0 | | |
| | $p_1 = 1.000$, $p_2 = 0.488$, $p_3 = 0.602$ | | | | |
| Left | | | | | |
| Min.–Max. | 11.0–150.0 | 24.0–126.0 | 29.0–143.0 | | |
| Mean ± SD | 68.75 ± 42.86 | 61.50 ± 26.21 | 54.75 ± 31.19 | 2.134 | 0.344 |
| Median | 69.0 | 62.0 | 51.50 | | |
| | $p_1 = 0.225$, $p_2 = 0.728$, $p_3 = 0.202$ | | | | |

$^{KW}\chi^2$ chi square for Kruskal-Wallis test, $p_1$ $p$ value for Mann-Whitney test for comparing between silicon index and cake, $p_2$ $p$ value for Mann-Whitney test for comparing between silicon index and peanut, $p_3$ $p$ value for Mann-Whitney test for comparing between cake and peanut
*Statistically significant at $p \leq 0.05$

also be due to bilateral balanced occlusion facilitating adaptation to the new denture as stated by Rehmann et al. [36]. These results are in contrast with Grubweiser et al., [13] and Miralles et al., [37] who found that canine guidance occlusion reduced masseter muscle activity in complete denture wearers. They stated that neuromuscular function in edentulous subjects is similar to that found in dentate people and that canine guided dentures prevent parafunctional habits.

The results of this study showed that the EMG activity of the masseter muscles during clenching on a preformed silicon index was significantly higher than during chewing peanut and chewing cake. This finding is in line with Miralles et al., [37] who pointed out that the increased EMG activity may be due to increased vertical dimension leading to increased muscle activity during maximum voluntary clenching. This finding is also in line with Darwish et al., [38]. The results also show higher mean EMG activity when chewing peanut than when chewing cake in this study. This coincides with van der Bilt et al., [39] who stated that harder food consistency required higher muscle activity levels due to higher muscle force needed to comminute hard food. The results are also in agreement with Karkazis [40] who found that harder foods required higher chewing rates, higher electrical activity of the masseter muscle, and higher relative contraction periods, accompanied by shorter cycle durations.

### Limitations of the study

These include short follow-up periods, no subjective assessment of the dentures with different occlusion concepts using questionnaires and depending entirely on electromyography for the assessment of masticatory function.

## Conclusions

Within the limitations of this study of short follow-up periods of mandibular implant-retained overdenture and maxillary complete denture, the results lead to that both bilateral balanced occlusion and canine guidance occlusion can be used successfully in implant-retained overdentures without affecting masticatory function. However, the procedures involved in construction of dentures with bilateral balanced occlusion are more complex and time consuming. Greater muscle activity of both muscles is shown when chewing hard food due to higher muscle force needed to comminute hard food compared to soft food.

### Recommendations

The present study recommends the following:

- Further investigations for a longer follow-up period and for a larger sample to confirm widespread use of canine guidance occlusal concept and involving subjective assessment using questionnaires for the patients' satisfaction
- Evaluation of the effect of different attachment types on masticatory function using the canine guidance concept in implant-retained overdentures
- Evaluation of canine guidance occlusal concept using a different method of evaluation of masticatory function other than electromyography

### Abbreviations

BBO: Bilateral Balanced Occlusion; CBCT: Cone Beam Computed Tomography; CGO: Canine Guidance Occlusion; EMG: Electromyography; ME: Masticatory Efficiency.

### Competing interests

The authors Prof. Dr. Ahmed Mohamed Abdelhamid, Kenda Ibrahim Hisham Hanno, and Prof. Dr. Mohamed Hassan Imam state that they have no competing interests.

### Authors' contributions

KIH performed all the clinical procedures of the research and writing of the research article. The clinical procedures involve selection of the patients, surgical placement of the dental implants, construction of the maxillary and mandibular complete dentures and overdentures, conversion of the occlusal concepts, and electromyographic evaluation twice for each patient using the three test samples. AMA supervised the clinical work and revised the intellectual content of the research article. MHI supplied the electromyography machine in his clinic to measure the activity of the masseter muscles and provided the sheets containing the EMG signals for each test sample for each patient. All authors read and approved the final manuscript.

### Acknowledgements

I would like to express my sincere gratitude to my father, Dr. Ibrahim Hisham Hanno (pedodontist), who supplied all the materials used for the research and funded the research.
I would also like to express my deepest gratitude to my mother, Dr. Mervat M. Ghoneim (prosthodontist), for her continuous support and revision of both the prosthodontic clinical steps and intellectual content of the article.

### Author details

[1]Prosthodontics Department, Faculty of Dentistry, Alexandria University, Alexandria, Egypt. [2]Prosthodontics, Faculty of Dentistry, Alexandria University, Alexandria, Egypt. [3]Physical Medicine, Rheumatology and Rehabilitation, Faculty of Medicine, Alexandria University, Alexandria, Egypt.

### References

1. Al-Ghafli SA, Michalakis KX, Hirayama H, Kang K. The in vitro effect of different implant angulations and cyclic dislodgement on the retentive properties of an over denture attachment system. J Prosthet Dent. 2009;102:140–7.
2. Burns DR. Mandibular implant overdenture controversy-consensus and controversy. J Prosthod. 2000;90:45–58.
3. Skalak R. Biomechanical considerations in osseointegrated prostheses. J Prosthet Dent. 1983;49:843–8.
4. Branemark PI. Osseointegration and its experimental background. J Prosthet Dent. 1983;50:399–410.
5. James RA. Periodontal considerations in implant dentistry. J Prosthet Dent. 1973;30:202–9.
6. Lindquist LW, Rockler B, Carlson GE. Bone resorption and fixtures on edentulous patients treated with mandibular fixed tissue integrated prothesis. J Prosthet Dent. 1988;59:59–63.
7. Miyata T, Kobayashi Y, Araki H, Ohto T, Shin K. The influence of controlled occlusal overload on peri-implant tissue. Part 3: a histologic study in monkeys. Int J Oral Maxillofac Implants. 2000;15:425–31.
8. Kim Y, Oh TJ, Misch CE, Wang HL. Occlusal considerations in implant therapy: clinical guidelines with biomechanical rationale. Clin Oral Impl Res. 2005;16:26–35.

9. Misch CE. Contemporary implant dentistry, 3rd ed. Mosby Inc, St. Louis. 2008. pp: 38–67, 645–67.
10. Pera P, Bassi F, Schierano G, Appendino P, Preti G. Implant anchored complete mandibular denture: evaluation of masticatory efficiency, oral function and degree of satisfaction. J Oral Rehabil. 1998;25:462–7.
11. Farias Neto A, Mestriner Junior W, Carreiro AF. Masticatory efficiency in denture wearers with bilateral balanced occlusion and canine guidance. Braz Dent J. 2010;21:165–9.
12. Peroz I, Leuenberg A, Haustein I, Lange KP. Comparison between balanced occlusion and canine guidance in complete denture wearers—a clinical, randomized trial. Quintessence Int. 2003;34:607–12.
13. Grubwieser G, Flatz A, Grunert I, Kofler M, Ulmer H, Gausch K, et al. Quantitative analysis of masseter and temporalis EMGs: a comparison of anterior guided versus balanced occlusal concepts in patients wearing complete dentures. J Oral Rehabil. 1999;26:731–6.
14. Farias-Neto A, Carreiro AF. Complete denture occlusion: an evidence-based approach. J Prosthodont. 2013;22:94–7.
15. Fontijn-Tekamp FA, Slagter AP, Van Der Bilt A, Hof MA V 'T, Witter DJ, Kalk W, et al. Biting and chewing in overdentures, full dentures, and natural dentitions. J Dent Res. 2000;79:1519–24.
16. Mowlana F, Heath MR, Van der Bilt A, Van der Glas HW. Assessment of chewing efficiency: a comparison of particle size distribution determined using optical scanning and sieving of almonds. J Oral Rehabil. 1994;21:545–51.
17. Santos CE, De Freitas O, Cesar A, Spadaro C, Mestriner-Junior W. Development of a colorimetric system for evaluation of masticatory efficiency. Braz Dent J. 2006;17:95–9.
18. Mowlana F, Heath R. Assessment of masticatory efficiency: new methods appropriate for clinical research in dental practice. Eur J Prosthodont Restor Dent. 1993;1:121–5.
19. Poyiadjis YM, Likeman PR. Some clinical investigations of the masticatory performance of complete denture wearers. J Dent. 1984;12:334–41.
20. Grunert I, Kofler M, Gausch K, Kronenberg M. Masseter and temporalis surface electromyography in patients wearing complete dentures comparing anterior and posterior occlusal concepts—a pilot study. J Oral Rehabil. 1994;21:337–47.
21. Miles TS, Nauntofte B, Svensson P. Clinical Oral Physiology. Copenhagen: Quintessence Publishing Co. Ltd; 2004. p. 214–5.
22. Aziz H, El Afandy M, Elsayed M. The effect of occlusal design on muscle activity in implant supported mandibular overdentures. CDJ. 2008;2:335–50.
23. Reitz PV, Weiner MG, Levin B. An overdenture survey. J Prosthet Dent. 1980;43:457.
24. Lekholm U, Zarb G. Patient selection and preparation. In: Branemark PI, Zarb GA, Albrektsson T, editors. Tissue integrated prosthesis: osseointegration in clinical dentistry. Chicago: Quintessence; 1985. p. 199–209.
25. Hong HR, Pae A, Kim Y, Paek J, Kim HS, Kwon KR. Effect of implant position, angulation, and attachment height on peri-implant bone stress associated with mandibular two-implant overdentures: a finite element analysis. Int J Oral Maxillofac Implants. 2012;27:e69–76.
26. Kitagawa T, Tanimoto Y, Nemoto K, Aida M. Influence of cortical bone quality on stress distribution in bone around dental implant. Dent Mater J. 2005;24:219–24.
27. Karabuda C, Yaltirik M, Bayrakatar M. A clinical comparison of prosthetic complications of implant-supported over dentures with different attachment systems. Implant Dent. 2008;17:74–81.
28. Roe P, Kan JY, Rungcharassaeng K, Lozada JL. Immediate loading of unsplinted implants in the anterior mandible for overdentures: 3-year results. Int J Oral Maxillofac Implants. 2011;26:1296–302.
29. Wulfman C, Hadida A, Rignon-Bret C. Radiographic and surgical guide fabrication for implant-retained mandibular overdenture. J Prosthet Dent. 2010;103:53–7.
30. Castroflorio T, Bracco P, Farina D. Surface electromyography in the assessment of jaw elevator muscles. J Oral Rehabil. 2008;35:638–45.
31. Uçankale M, Akoğlu B, Ozkan Y, Ozkan YK. The effect of different attachment systems with implant retained overdentures on maximum bite force and EMG. Gerodontology. 2012;29:24–9.
32. Zarb GA, Bolender CL, Eckert SE, Fenton AH, Jacob RF, Mericske-Stern R. Prosthodontic treatment for edentulous patients: complete dentures and implant-supported prostheses. 12th ed. St. Louis: Mosby; 2004. p. 294.
33. Ohguri T, Kawano F, Ichikawa T, Matsumoto N. Influence of occlusal scheme on the pressure distribution under a complete denture. Int J Prosthodont. 1999;12:353–8.
34. El-Okel AB. The effect of different occlusal schemes on the electromyographic activity and masticatory efficiency in complete denture wearers. Ph.D. Thesis. Department of Removable Prosthodontics, Faculty of Dentistry, Al-Azhar University. Egypt. 2006.
35. Abd Elmonem E. Colorimetric comparative analysis of masticatory efficiency in complete denture wearers with two different occlusal concepts. M.Sc. Thesis. Removable Prosthodontics Department, Faculty of Dentistry, Alexandria University. Egypt. 2014.
36. Rehmann P, Balkenhol M, Ferger P, Wostmann B. Influence of the occlusal concept of complete dentures on patient satisfaction in the initial phase after fitting: bilateral balanced occlusion versus canine guidance. Int J Prosthodont. 2008;21:60–1.
37. Miralles R, Bull R, Manns A, Roman E. Influence of balanced occlusion and canine guidance on electromyographic activity of elevator muscles in complete denture wearers. J Prosthet Dent. 1989;61:494–8.
38. Darwish AA, Segaan LG, El Shorbagy ZA, Abd El Hamid AM. Electromyographic activity of masseter muscle of patients wearing complete dentures with different occlusal concepts. Alex Dent J. 1989;14:3.
39. van der Bilt A, van Kampen FMC, Cune MS. Masticatory function with mandibular implant-supported overdentures fitted with different attachment types. Eur J Oral Sci. 2006;114:191–6.
40. Karkazis HC. EMG activity of the masseter muscle in implant supported overdenture wearers during chewing of hard and soft food. J Oral Rehabil. 2002;29:986–91.

# Arterial blood supply variation in the anterior midline mandible: Significance to dental implantology

Joseph Gakonyo[1*], Fawzia Butt[2], Philip Mwachaka[2] and Evelyn Wagaiyu[3]

## Abstract

**Background:** Inter-foraminal implant placement poses a risk to the sublingual artery as it enters the mandibular midline lingual foramen. Lack of consensus on the source of this artery poses a dilemma to surgeons during management of haemorrhagic episodes. Determination of the exact source of this artery is therefore pivotal.

**Methods:** This was a cross-sectional descriptive study involving 34 adult human cadavers. The facial and lingual arteries were followed from the external carotid artery to determine whether they terminated as the sublingual artery. Statistical significance tests were done using the Mann-Whitney *U* test and Pearson product-moment correlation.

**Results:** There were 30 (88.2 %) males and 4 (11.8 %) females (male/female = 15:2) aged between 25 and 40 years. The origin of the sublingual artery was mainly from the lingual artery (73.5 %), the submental artery (17.6 %), or an anastomotic branch from the two arteries (8.9 %). The mean distance between the mandibular midline lingual foramen (MMLF) and the inferior border of the mandible was 15.58 mm (range 11.03–19.62 mm). The mean thickness of the mandible at the level of the MMLF was 10.89 mm (range 8.00–12.91 mm). No statistically significant difference was found between the two genders with regard to the morphometric measurements.

**Conclusions:** The sublingual artery that enters the MMLF was found to be the sublingual artery as either a branch of the lingual artery (73.5 %), the submental artery (17.6 %) or an anastomosis of the lingual and submental arteries (8.9 %).

**Keywords:** Sublingual artery; Dental implant; Mandibular midline foramen; Haemorrhage

## Background

The inter-foraminal region of the human mandible is a common elective area for several dental surgery procedures due to its favourable anatomic conditions [1, 2]. Some of the procedures done in this region include insertion of endosseous dental implants, bone harvesting from the chin, genioplasty in orthognathic surgery and placement of screws during plating in management of facial fractures [3].

There have been reported cases of near fatal upper airway obstruction due to haemorrhage following implant placement in this area [4, 5]. Majority of them have been attributed to transection of the sublingual artery when a misdirected drill perforates the lingual cortex and damages the blood vessel within the surrounding soft tissues [5] as it enters the mandibular midline lingual foramen (MMLF). This vessel retracts into the floor of the mouth where a haematoma forms in the sublingual and submandibular spaces leading to a compromise of the airway, by swelling and pushing of the tongue against the palate [5, 6].

This foramen is a constant finding and has an intraosseous part, midline mandibular lingual canal (MMLC), which contains a blood vessel that is prone to transection during routine dental implant placement [7–11]. It has been found that vessels travelling horizontal to the direction of an implant drill, but perpendicular to the

* Correspondence: josegaks@gmail.com
[1]Department of Conservative and Prosthetic Dentistry, University of Nairobi, P.O. Box 54954-00200, Nairobi, Kenya
Full list of author information is available at the end of the article

spin of the drill, are at the greatest risk of laceration and transection [6, 7].

A higher risk of trauma exists in some situations like where the alveolar ridge is severely resorbed, or where trimming of the ridge has to be done either to reduce excess bone or to create a flat site for drilling, because this procedure brings the MMLC closer to the superior aspect of the mandible [11]. Drilling deeper into an extraction socket to obtain primary implant stability is now an acceptable procedure which increases the risk of bleeding. Some clinical protocols require inter-foraminal implant placement, which may lead to placement of an implant in the mandibular midline position [12].

There are two main sources of arterial blood supply to the anterior lingual area of the mandible: the submental and the lingual arteries. There is however lack of consensus as to the origin of the artery that enters the MMLF. Some authors have reported that it is a branch of the lingual artery and others the submental artery, while others have found that the vessel is an anastomosis of the two arteries [2, 6, 7, 9, 13]. The possibility of existence of anastomoses and the lack of consensus as to the source of the artery that enters the MMLF pose a dilemma of whether the submental or the lingual artery should be ligated first in the event an extra-oral approach is required to control haemorrhage [7].

There is hardly any published data on the artery that enters the MMLF. This study aimed at determining the source of the artery that enters the MMLF. It was hoped that this finding would help the surgeon to precisely ligate the feeder vessel, should there be haemorrhage during placement of an inter-foraminal dental implant.

## Methods

This was a cadaveric dissection study involving 34 human adult cadavers of indigenous Kenyan descent carried out at the Department of Human Anatomy, University of Nairobi. Majority of these cadavers are unclaimed bodies in the city of Nairobi, whose demographics are hardly known. Approval to conduct the study was obtained from the Kenyatta National Hospital/University of Nairobi Ethics, Research and Standards Committee (P694/11/2014).

The procedure involved exposure of the lingual and facial arteries, beginning from the external carotid artery and following them to determine which one of them ended as the sublingual artery. This was followed by bilateral resection of the mandible at the position of the lateral incisors.

The bucco-lingual thickness of the mandible at the level of the MMLF and the distance from the inferior border of the mandible to the MMLF were measured. All photographs were taken using a HTC digital camera (Xindian, Taiwan) with dual 4 MP, 2688 × 1520 pixels and dual-LED flash. Morphometric measurements were taken with a Pittsburgh 6-in. digital calliper (Pittsburgh, China).

Data collected were analysed using SPSS version 17 (SPSS Inc., Chicago, IL) statistical software. Probabilities that were ≤0.05 were accepted as significant. Descriptive parameters were expressed as minimum, maximum and mean ± standard deviation. The statistical significance of gender differences was determined using the Mann-Whitney *U* test.

## Results

A total of 34 human cadavers were dissected in this study of which 30 (88.2 %) were males and 4 (11.8 %) were females (male/female, 15:2) aged between 25 and 40 years. The linear distance between the MMLF and the inferior border of the mandible ranged from 11.03 to 19.62 mm (mean = 15.58 mm ± 2.12 SD). The mesio-buccal thickness of the mandible at the level of the MMLF ranged between 8.00 and 12.91 mm (mean = 10.89 mm ± 1.24 SD). The

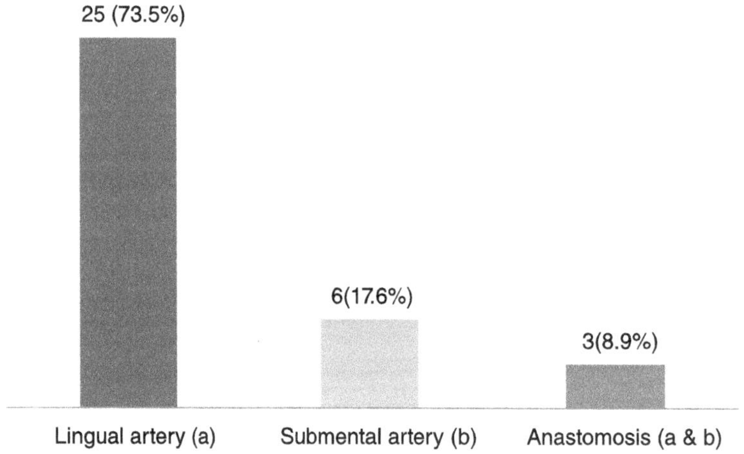


**Fig. 1** Distribution of cadavers according to source of artery entering the MMLF (*n* = 34)

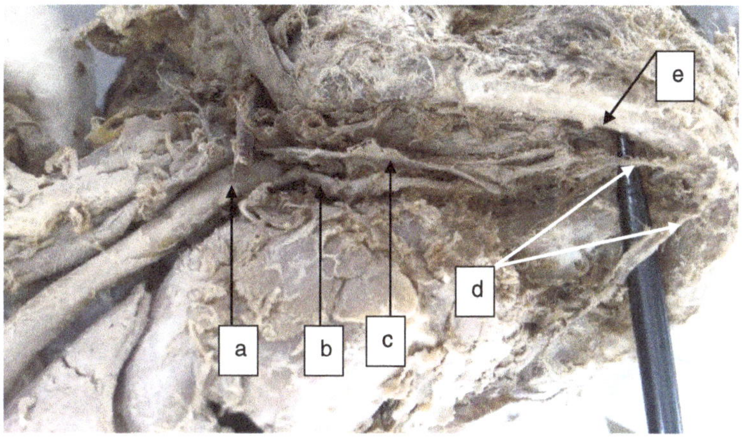


**Fig. 2** Lingual artery as the origin of the sublingual artery entering the MMLF: *a* external carotid artery, *b* lingual artery, *c* hypoglossal nerve, *d* right and left sublingual arteries originating from the ipsilateral lingual arteries and *e* inferior border of the mandible

source of the artery entering the MMLF came from either a branch of the lingual artery (73.5 %, $n = 25$) or submental artery (17.6 %, $n = 6$), or their anastomotic branch (8.9 %, $n = 3$) (Figs. 1, 2, 3 and 4).

A Mann-Whitney $U$ test did not elicit a statistically significant difference between males and females with regard to the distance from the MMLF to the inferior border of the mandible (Table 1) or the mesio-buccal width of the mandible at the level of the MMLF (Table 2). A Pearson product-moment correlation did not elicit a statistically significant association between distance from the MMLF to the inferior border of the mandible and mesio-buccal width of the mandible at the level of the MMLF ($r$ (1) = 0.062, $P = 0.803$ (two-tailed)).

## Discussion

The MMLF is a consistent structure through which the sublingual artery enters the mandible [8, 11]. Perforation of the lingual plate by an implant drill poses a high risk of trauma to this vessel especially when the sublingual fossa is very pronounced because this vessel courses closely to the gland and fossa [13]. When this artery is of a significant size, it is possible for 420 mL of blood to escape in 30 min leading to haematoma formation in the sublingual and submandibular spaces and leading to a compromise of the airway, by swelling and pushing of the tongue against the palate [5, 6, 14].

In a review of literature, Kalpidis et al. [7] concluded that when the haematoma is large and non-restrictive,

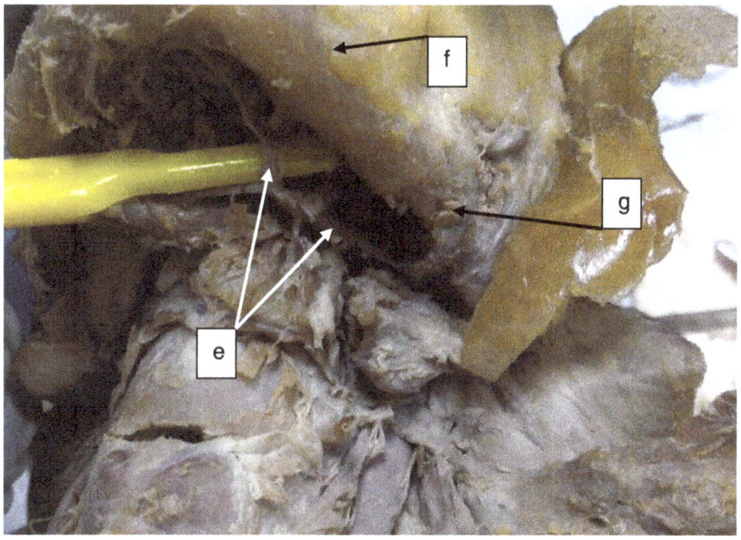


**Fig. 3** Submental artery as the source of the sublingual artery entering the MMLF: *e* submental artery, *f* inferior border of the mandible, and *g* facial artery

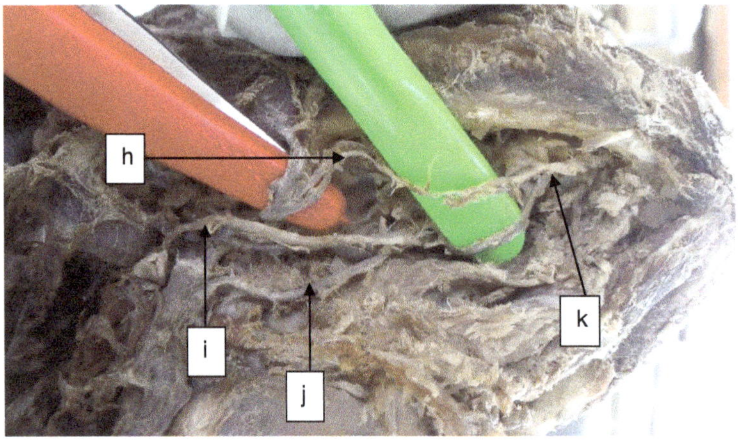


**Fig. 4** Sublingual artery originating from an anastomotic branch of the lingual and submental arteries: *h* submental artery, *i* hypoglossal artery, *j* lingual artery, and *k* anastomosis of the lingual and submental arteries

extra-oral ligation of the feeder vessel should be applied. They did not establish the exact vessel that should be ligated to arrest bleeding. This was due to the differences in study findings on the prevalence of either the submental or the lingual artery as the main source of blood supply to the floor of the mouth. They thus suggested that in every case, the decision to ligate the facial or the lingual artery should be guided by the operator's judgment.

In the present study, the sublingual artery appeared to originate mainly from the lingual artery (73.5 %) which was similar to the findings of Hofschneider et al. [13] (70 %, $n = 17$) and Loukas et al. [6] (73 %, $n = 100$). Our results however contradict those of previous studies that found the sublingual artery to originate from the lingual artery in 100 % of the cadavers dissected [2, 8, 9, 15]. The results of these previous studies should however be interpreted with caution because a majority of them examined one to two cadavers.

In a cadaveric study by Bavitz et al. [16], it was found that the submental artery was the main arterial blood supply to the floor of the mouth (53 %). Consequently, they suggested that the submental artery should be ligated first during extra-oral ligation to control haemorrhage in the floor of the mouth. Conversely, the sublingual artery appeared to originate from the submental artery in less than a quarter (17.6 %) of the cadavers in the present study. Our results are similar to those of Loukas et al. [6] (27 %).

The sublingual and submental arteries normally anastomose through their muscular mylohyoid branches [7]. Loukas et al. [6] only identified anastomotic patterns between sublingual and submental arteries in 40 % of the dissected cadavers, with no case where the two terminate as a single sublingual artery. We found three (8.9 %) cases of an anastomotic branch of the submental and lingual artery forming a single sublingual artery just before entering the MMLF.

The distance from the MMLF to the inferior border of the mandible in our study ranged from 11.03 to 19.62 mm (mean = 15.58 mm ± 2.12 SD) with no statistically significant difference between the two genders ($U = 46.000$, $P = 0.454$). Oettle et al. [11] reported a distance ranging from 10.83 to 12.874 mm in a dry mandible study of both black and white South Africans. In their study, cone beam computed tomography (CBCT) was used to scan the mandibles. Their study did not find a statistically significant difference according to sex or race. Soft tissue remnants on the surface of the mandibles in our study could explain the higher morphometric measurements.

A critical buccal bone thickness of 2 mm is recommended to prevent vertical resorption [17]. A minimum bone thickness of 6 mm would be required for successful placement of a standard-sized ±4-mm-diameter implant [11]. In the current study, the bucco-lingual thickness of the mandible at the level of the MMLF ranged from 8.00 to 12.91 mm (mean = 10.89 mm ± 1.24 SD). Thus, all the cadavers in our study had adequate bone thickness needed for implant placement without perforating the lingual cortical plate and traumatizing the sublingual artery.

**Table 1** Distribution of distance (in mm) from MMLF to the inferior border of the mandible by gender

| Gender | Number | Mean | Mann-Whitney *U* test | *P* |
|---|---|---|---|---|
| Male | 30 | 17.97 | 46.000 | 0.454 |
| Female | 4 | 14.00 | | |

**Table 2** Distribution of mesio-buccal width (in mm) of the mandible at the level of the MMLF by gender

| Gender | Number | Mean | Mann-Whitney *U* test | *P* |
|---|---|---|---|---|
| Male | 30 | 17.55 | 58.500 | .936 |
| Female | 4 | 17.13 | | |

A notable limitation in our study was a lower number of female cadavers available. Most of these cadavers are unclaimed bodies from mortuaries in Kenya. Generally, there are more male unclaimed bodies than female bodies. The Mann-Whitney *U* test was therefore used to compare the two genders.

## Conclusions

Within the limitations of this study, the sublingual artery that enters the MMLF was found to be the sublingual artery as either a branch of the lingual artery (73.5 %), the submental artery (17.6 %) or an anastomosis of the lingual and submental arteries (8.9 %). We suggest that extra-oral ligation of the lingual artery should be done first followed by ligation of the submental artery (or its parent facial artery) in case of continued bleeding. Studies with a larger sample of females should be conducted to confirm the findings of this study.

### Competing interests

Joseph Gakonyo, Fawzia Butt, Philip Mwachaka and Evelyn Wagaiyu declare that they have no competing interest.

### Authors' contributions

EW participated in the design of the study and helped to draft the manuscript. PM participated in the study design and dissection of the cadavers and helped conduct the statistical analysis. FB participated in the study design and dissection of the cadavers and helped draft the manuscript. JG conceived the idea for the study, participated in its design and coordination, and helped draft the manuscript. All authors have read and approved the final manuscript.

### Acknowledgements

The authors wish to thank the department of Human Anatomy at the University of Nairobi for enabling the conduction of this study. We thank Desmond K'Owino of the University of Nairobi for his assistance with data analysis and Dr. Antony Muthee for his assistance with typesetting. This study was financed through the University of Nairobi, Deans Committee Research Grant 2014–2015.

### Author details

[1]Department of Conservative and Prosthetic Dentistry, University of Nairobi, P.O. Box 54954-00200, Nairobi, Kenya. [2]Department of Human Anatomy, University of Nairobi, P.O. Box 25361-00603, Nairobi, Kenya. [3]Department of Periodontology/Community and Preventive Dentistry, University of Nairobi, P.O. Box 30197, Nairobi, Kenya.

### References

1. Longoni S, Sartori M, Braun M, Bravetti P, Lapi A, Baldoni M, et al. Lingual vascular canals of the mandible: the risk of bleeding complications during implant procedures. Implant Dent. 2007;16(2):131–8.
2. Tepper G, Hofschneider UB, Gahleitner A, Ulm C. Computed tomographic diagnosis and localization of bone canals in the mandibular interforaminal region for prevention of bleeding complications during implant surgery. Int J Oral Maxillofac Implants. 2001;16:68–72.
3. Liang X, Jacobs R, Lambrichts I. An assessment on spiral CT scan of the superior and inferior genial spinal foramina and canals. Surg Radiol Anat. 2006;28:98 104.
4. Niamtu 3rd J. Near-fatal airway obstruction after routine implant placement. Oral Surg Oral Med Oral Pathol Oral Radiol Endod. 2001;92:597–600.
5. Flanagan D. Important arterial supply of the mandible, control of an arterial hemorrhage, and report of a hemorrhagic incident. J Oral Implantol. 2003;29:165–73.
6. Loukas M, Kinsella Jr CR, Kapos T, Tubbs RS, Ramachandra S. Anatomical variation in arterial supply of the mandible with special regard to implant placement. Int J Oral Maxillofac Surg. 2008;37:367–71.
7. Kalpidis CD, Setayesh RM. Hemorrhaging associated with endosseous implant placement in the anterior mandible: a review of the literature. J Periodontol. 2004;75:631–45.
8. McDonnell D, Reza Nouri M, Todd ME. The mandibular lingual foramen: a consistent arterial foramen in the middle of the mandible. J Anat. 1994;184:363–9.
9. Tagaya A, Matsuda Y, Nakajima K, Seki K, Okano T. Assessment of the blood supply to the lingual surface of the mandible for reduction of bleeding during implant surgery. Clin Oral Implants Res. 2009;20:351–5.
10. Katakami K, Mishima A, Kuribayashi A, Shimoda S, Hamada Y, Kobayashi K. Anatomical characteristics of the mandibular lingual foramina observed on limited cone-beam CT images. Clin Oral Implants Res. 2009;20:386–90.
11. Oettle AC, Fourie J, Human-Baron R, van Zyl AW. The midline mandibular lingual canal: importance in implant surgery. Clin Implant Dent Relat Res. 2015;17(1):93–101.
12. Misch CE. The edentulous mandible: an organized approach to implant-supported overdentures. In: Misch CE, editor. Contemporary implant dentistry. 3rd ed. St. Louis: Mosby Elsevier; 2008. p. 293–313.
13. Hofschneider UB, Tepper G, Gahleitner A, Ulm C. Assessment of the blood supply to the mental region for reduction of bleeding complications during implant surgery in the interforaminal region. Int J Oral Maxillofac Implants. 1999;14:379–83.
14. Lustig JP, London D, Dor BL, Yanko R. Ultrasound identification and quantitative measurement of blood supply to the anterior part of the mandible. Oral Surg Oral Med Oral Pathol Oral Radiol Endod. 2003;96:625–9.
15. Kawai T, Sato I, Yosue T, Takamori H, Sunohara M. Anastomosis between the inferior alveolar artery branches and submental artery in human mandible. Surg Radiol Anat. 2006;28:308–10.
16. Bavitz JB, Harn SD, Homze EJ. Arterial supply to the floor of the mouth and lingual gingiva. Oral Surg Oral Med Oral Pathol. 1994;77(3):232–5.
17. Merheb J, Quirynen M, Teughels W. Critical buccal bone dimensions along implants. Periodontol. 2014;66:97–105.

# Dental implant treatment in a young woman after marginal mandibulectomy for treatment of mandibular gingival carcinoma: a case report

Kazuki Takaoka*, Emi Segawa, Michiyo Yamamura, Yusuke Zushi, Masahiro Urade and Hiromitsu Kishimoto

**Abstract**

Dental implants play an important role in postoperative rehabilitation after surgical treatment of oral cancer through the provision of prosthetic tooth replacement. Two major implant prosthesis designs are available: fixed implant-supported prostheses and implant-supported overdentures. We herein report a case of a 16-year-old female patient who underwent alveolar ridge resection for treatment of mandibular gingival carcinoma. Following surgery, oral rehabilitation was attempted using an implant-supported overdenture on a gold bar retainer splinting four implants. However, the patient was not satisfied with this prosthesis because of mucosal pain and discomfort, and she gradually ceased its use. Consequently, contact with the opposing teeth caused wear of the prosthetic screws. We elected to replace the implant-supported overdenture with an implant-fixed prosthesis approximately 16 years after insertion of the overdenture to prevent further wear of the prosthetic screws. The patient was highly satisfied with the improved stability of the implant-fixed prosthesis. This case report indicates that the clinician must occasionally re-evaluate and sometimes alter the direction of treatment, even after definitive therapy has been completed.

**Keywords:** Postoperative rehabilitation; Oral cancer; Implant-fixed prosthesis; Implant-supported overdenture

## Background

Surgical treatment of oral cancer may lead to significant disability, including facial deformity, loss of hard and soft tissue, and impaired function of speech, swallowing, and mastication [1]. Bone resection because of surgical treatment of a large mandibular tumor can cause long-term defects. Rehabilitation with a removable prosthesis can be difficult or impossible due to the distorted post-surgical anatomy, especially for edentulous patients, for whom provision of a removable prosthesis is almost impossible. Dental implants are useful to improve the stability and support of a prosthesis, and dental implants have recently gained an important role in the rehabilitation of patients with oral cancer by facilitating the provision of a stable prosthesis [1]. Two major implant prosthesis designs are available: fixed implant-supported prostheses and implant-supported overdentures. Several factors affect the choice between fixed and removable implant prostheses, such as the interforaminal space, interjaw relationship, oral hygiene, cost, and patient preference [2]. Zani et al. [3] reported that both fixed implant-supported prostheses and implant-supported overdentures were perceived to be equally satisfactory by mandibular edentulous patients and that the condition of the prostheses did not influence individual satisfaction in terms of rehabilitation. In this clinical case, an implant-supported overdenture that was delivered to rehabilitate the edentulous mandibular region following marginal mandibulectomy for treatment of mandibular gingival carcinoma was replaced by an implant-fixed prosthesis. Different treatment pathways should be prepared during the treatment planning stage.

The purpose of this paper is to present a case report of dental implant placement in a 17-year-old female patient after marginal mandibulectomy for treatment of

* Correspondence: ktaka@hyo-med.ac.jp
Department of Oral and Maxillofacial Surgery, Hyogo College of Medicine, 1-1 Mukogawa-cho, Nishinomiya, Hyogo 663-8501, Japan

mandibular gingival carcinoma, subsequent prosthodontic treatment, and an almost 22-year follow-up after dental implant placement.

## Case presentation

A 16-year-old female patient developed slight tenderness of the gingiva in the left mandibular premolar region, and her dentist referred her to our clinic in April 1992. Oral examination showed erythematous granular swellings that bled easily on the alveolar gingiva involving the area extending from the right second premolar to the left second molar (Fig. 1). The lesion showed extensive, superficial growth but was largely confined to the attached gingiva. Radiographic examination showed notable alveolar bone resorption in the left mandibular premolar region and slight resorption in the right mandibular canine region (Fig. 2). The lesion was biopsied, and histopathological examination showed diffuse unencapsulated proliferation of moderately to poorly differentiated squamoid tumor cells with occasional mitotic figures and keratinization as well as tumor nests comprising intermediate and clear cells. Few duct-like structures were observed, but microcysts were occasionally noted (Fig. 3). The specimen histologically resembled a mucoepidermoid carcinoma [4], but presented as a rare gingival carcinoma of the mandible. Treatment in May 1992 involved resection of the alveolar ridge between the right and left second molar regions, preserving the right inferior alveolar nerve, followed by bilateral upper neck dissection and transplantation of a lateral tongue flap to cover the alveolar ridge defect (Fig. 4). Histopathological examination of the surgical specimens showed bilateral submandibular lymph node metastases. Two courses of postoperative chemotherapy were performed to prevent local recurrence and distant metastasis.

There was no evidence of recurrence or metastasis at 1 year 3 months after surgery, and an International Team for Implantology (ITI) implant system (Institut Straumann AG, Basel, Switzerland) and prosthetic appliance were provided for cosmetic improvement and recovery of masticatory function. Four implants (three measuring 4.1 × 10 mm, one measuring 4.1 × 8 mm) were placed in the mandible in August 1993 (Fig. 5). Three months later, these implants were connected by three gold U-shaped Dolder bars soldered to gold copings and made to fit passively. The overdenture incorporated three corresponding riders/clips acting as matrices on the intaglio surface, providing attachments to the bar retainer. The implant-supported overdenture was inserted and adjusted until the patient felt no pain (Fig. 6). The patient was given oral hygiene instructions and scheduled for follow-up appointments. However, she was not satisfied with the prosthesis; she experienced denture discomfort and developed a decubital ulcer in the tongue flap area, and she gradually ceased use of the denture. The patient was followed for more than 10 years on a regular basis to examine recurrence or metastasis of the gingival carcinoma. Mild erythema and swelling of the mandibular and implant-surrounding mucosa secondary to stimulation during mastication were found (Fig. 7a), and contact with the opposing teeth resulted in wear of the prosthetic screws (Fig. 7b). In this case, the opposing occlusion involved the natural teeth, and the bone loss around the implants was negligible during the 15 years of follow-up (Fig. 8). We had previously proposed replacing the overdenture with an implant-fixed prosthesis; however, at that time, the patient elected not to proceed with this option because of the additional economic burden. Eventually, however, the patient opted for rehabilitation with a fixed implant-supported prosthesis. The patient was not willing to undergo extensive surgical intervention, including preprosthetic surgery and placement of additional implants. Therefore, we elected to replace the implant-supported overdenture with an implant-fixed prosthesis in May 2010.

After the impressions were taken, the implant-fixed prosthesis was fabricated with a cantilever design comprising two dental units. The mandibular prosthesis was then inserted in February 2011, and the final occlusion was verified and adjusted (Figs. 9a, b). The prosthesis was attached to the implants using prosthetic screws. The screw holes were filled with a dental temporary material overlaid with light-curable composite resin. The patient was highly satisfied with the improvement in oral

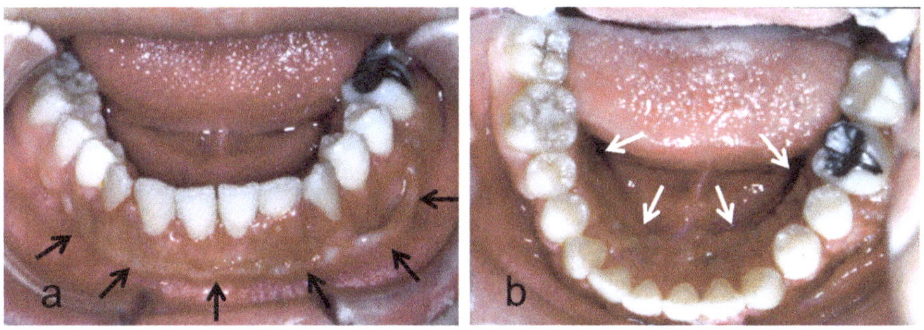


**Fig. 1** Intraoral photograph showing diffuse tumor formation on the alveolar gingiva (arrows)

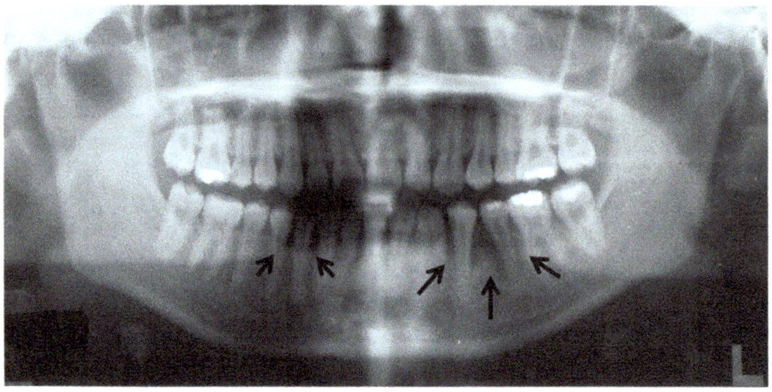

**Fig. 2** Panoramic radiograph showing notable alveolar bone resorption in the left mandibular premolar region and slight resorption in the right mandibular canine region (arrows)

rehabilitation as a result of the new prosthesis. She was instructed on brushing techniques and reviewed every 6 months. Neither dental plaque nor calculus beneath the prosthesis was detected, and there was no mucosal erythema or bone loss around the implants (Fig. 9c), which remained healthy almost 4 years after insertion of the final prosthesis.

## Conclusions

Prosthetic rehabilitation of edentulous patients after surgical management of oral cancer is difficult and therefore often avoided. However, adequate prosthetic rehabilitation is a pivotal factor for patients to regain oral function [5]. In terms of the masticatory rehabilitation of these patients, the application of a removable prosthesis unsupported by implants may be difficult or even impossible because of the postsurgical anatomical alteration [6]. The benefits of implant-supported prostheses have been recognized for several years [7]. Dental implants may improve denture retention and stability without unnecessary loading of the vulnerable mucosa. Function, comfort, esthetics, and eventually quality of life can be improved [8]. Two different options for oral rehabilitation using dental implants exist. One of these is the fixed prosthesis supported by implants, which does not involve any contact with the oral mucosa, thereby preventing frictional ulcers. The other option is an implant-supported overdenture, which allows improved oral hygiene [6]. Barão et al. [9] reported that patients with implant-supported overdentures exhibited a higher degree of stress on the supporting mucosa than those with fixed implant-supported prostheses. In those with fixed implant-supported prostheses, the prosthesis is completely supported by the implants, with no mucosal contact; therefore, fixed implant-supported prostheses limit the degree of mechanical irritation to the soft tissue.

Based on the clinical and histological findings, our case was considered to be an intermediate-grade mucoepidermoid carcinoma. Because wide local surgical excision is critical in the treatment of this tumor, we performed entire resection of the alveolar ridge, also considering her age and esthetic concerns. Loss of the alveolar ridge led to severe masticatory dysfunction. In the present case, the patient refused further surgical intervention following surgical removal of the gingival carcinoma, and we adopted an implant-supported overdenture because of its relative simplicity, ease of self-maintenance, and affordability. According to the literature, in patients with malignancies involving the lower

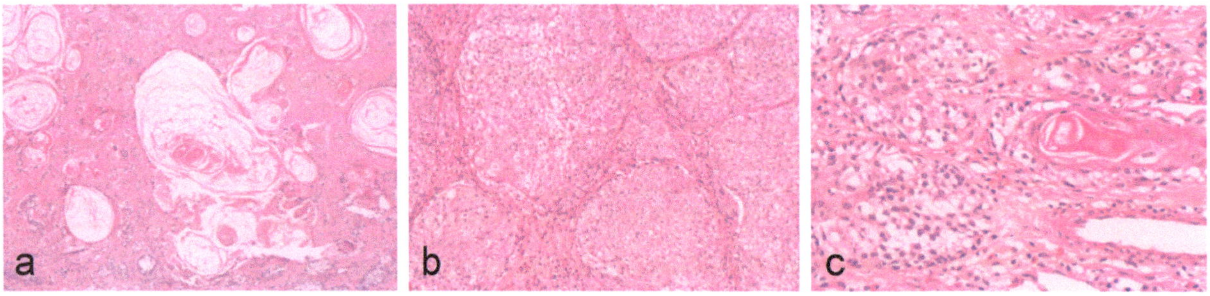


**Fig. 3** Photomicrographs of the biopsy specimen showing the intermingling of (**a**), (**b**), and (**c**). **a** Moderately differentiated epidermoid tumor cells with a duct-like structure (hematoxylin and eosin [H&E], original magnification × 100). **b** Intermediate cells (H&E, original magnification × 100). **c** Clear cells (H&E, original magnification × 100)

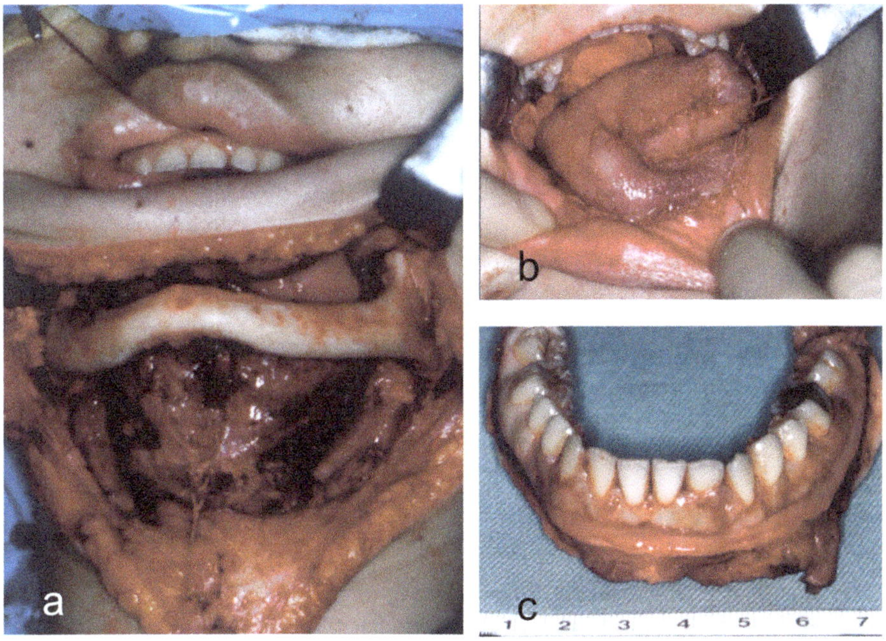


**Fig. 4 a** Intraoperative photograph of resection of the alveolar ridge and bilateral upper neck dissection. **b** Transplantation of a lateral tongue flap to cover the alveolar ridge defect. **c** Surgical specimen

region of the oral cavity, a minimum of four implants is needed to achieve maximal implant support for the prosthesis and to relieve the vulnerable underlying soft tissues [10, 11]. We inserted an implant-supported overdenture on a gold bar retainer splinting four implants. However, the patient was not satisfied with this prosthesis because of the mucosal pain and discomfort that developed over time. In such cases, prosthetic loading of atrophic mucosa is often not well tolerated. As such, we proposed replacement with an implant-fixed prosthesis. Initially, the patient elected not to proceed with this option because of the additional economic

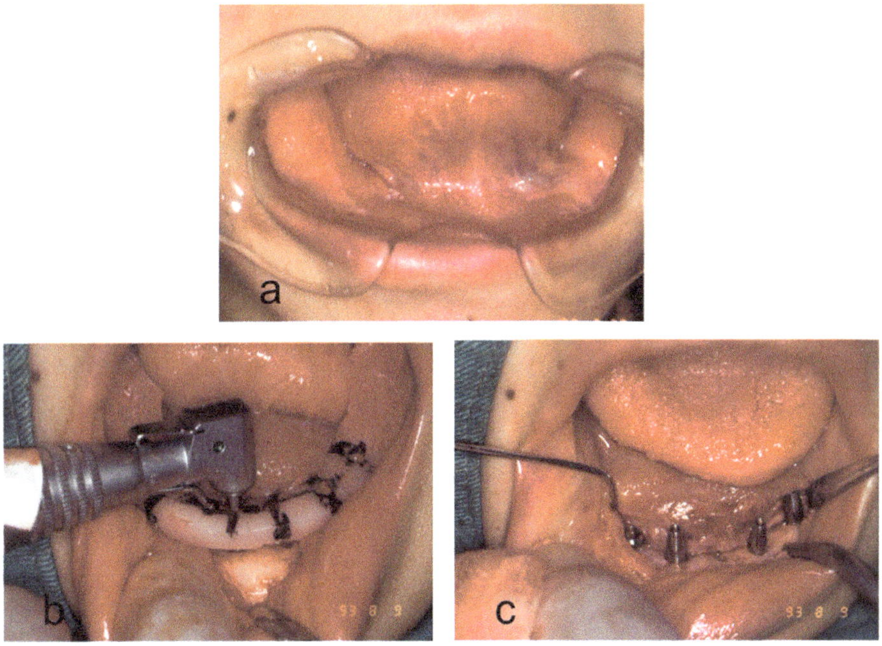


**Fig. 5** Preoperative intraoral photograph of implant placement

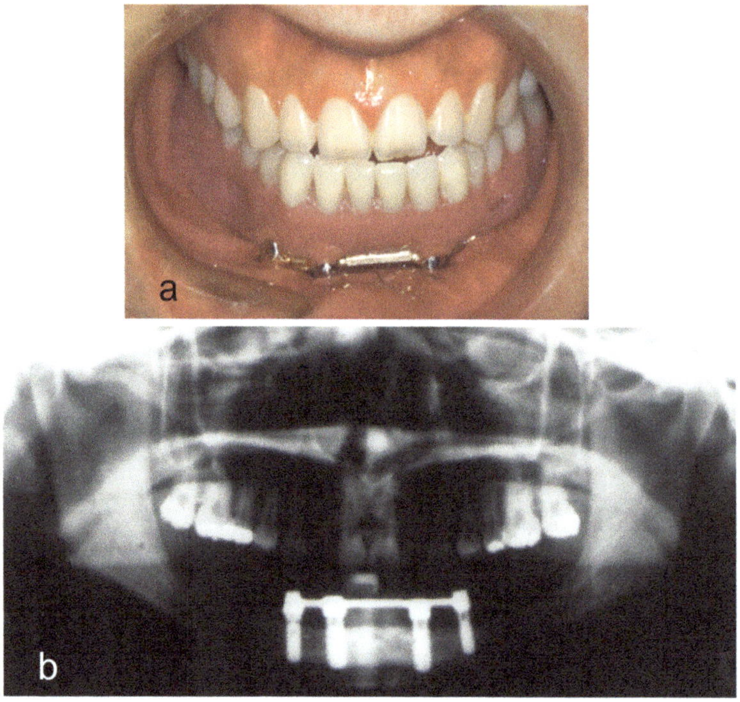


**Fig. 6 a** Mandibular implant-supported overdenture inserted into the mouth. **b** Panoramic radiograph after insertion of the prosthesis

burden. However, the patient eventually opted for rehabilitation with a fixed implant-supported prosthesis, as this provided the psychological advantage of a prosthesis that felt similar to the natural teeth. In this case, an implant-supported overdenture, which was provided to rehabilitate the edentulous mandibular region after marginal mandibulectomy for treatment of gingival carcinoma of the mandible, was replaced by an implant-fixed prosthesis.

Pjetursson et al. [12] performed a systematic review of the survival and complication rates of implant-fixed

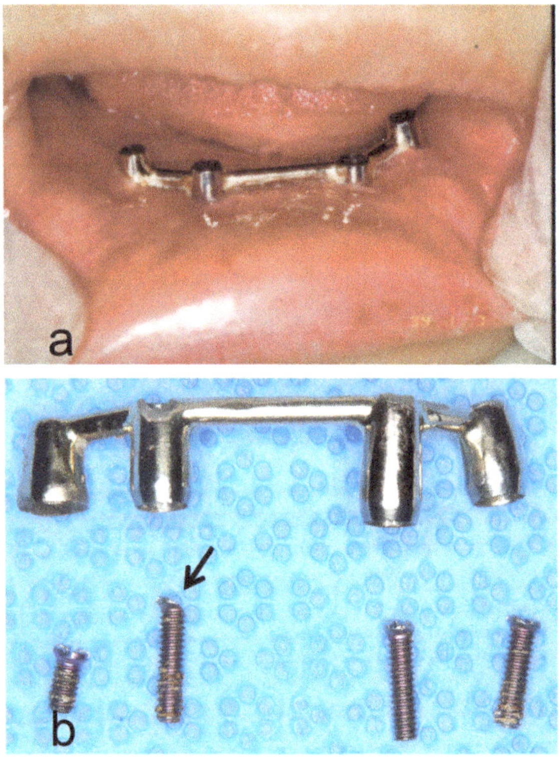


**Fig. 7 a** Intraoral photograph. **b** Gold Dolder bar and screws; marked wear of a prosthetic screw (arrow)

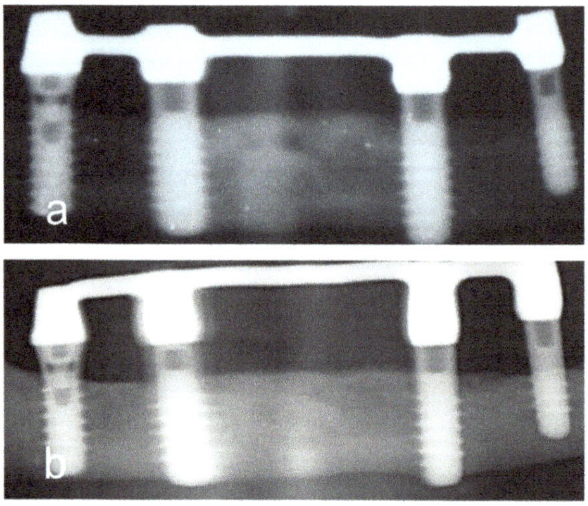


**Fig. 8** Periapical radiographs of the implants. **a** Postoperative, 1 year. **b** Postoperative, 16 years

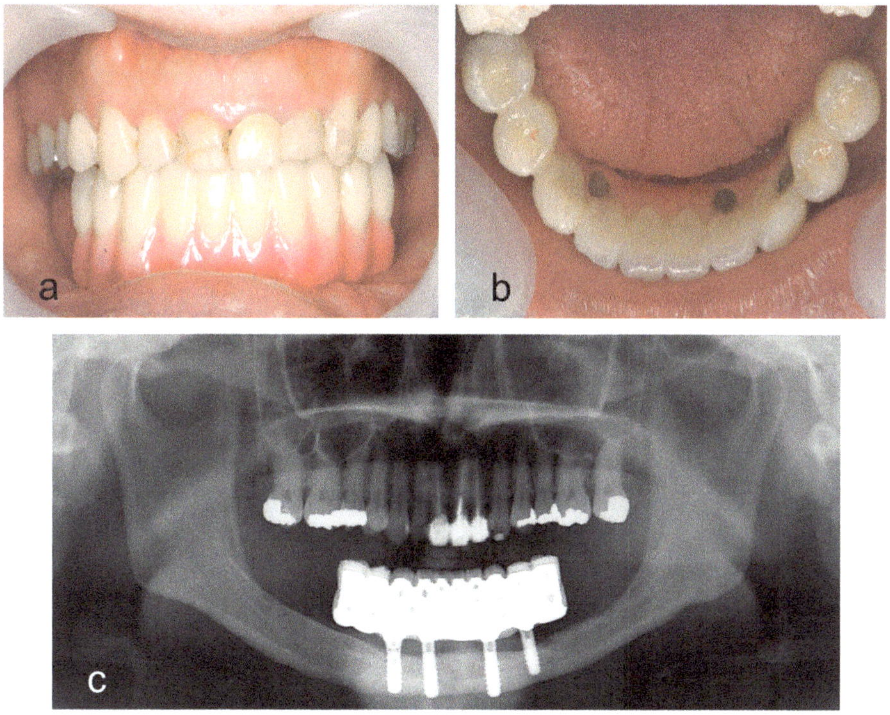


**Fig. 9** **a** Mandibular implant-fixed prosthesis inserted into the mouth. **b** Occlusal view of the implant-fixed prosthesis. **c** Panoramic radiograph 3 years 11 months after insertion of the fixed implant-supported prosthesis

prostheses after a mean observation period of at least 5 years. They concluded that implant-fixed prostheses are a safe and predictable treatment method with high survival rates. However, biological and technical complications were frequent in their review (33.6 %). To minimize the incidence of complications, dental professionals should make great effort to choose reliable components and materials for implant-fixed prostheses, and patients should undergo a well-structured maintenance protocol after treatment. In the present case, professional teeth cleaning with individual instruction every 3 months improved the patient's oral hygiene. Maintenance care may have motivated the patient to improve her oral home care regimen. This case report indicates that occasionally, even after definitive therapy has been completed, the clinician must reevaluate and sometimes alter the direction of treatment to provide the best possible outcome for the patient. In conclusion, we have herein reported a case illustrating our long-term clinical experience and the concept of switching therapy.

## Consent

Written informed consent was obtained from the patient for publication of this case report and any accompanying images. A copy of the written consent is available for review by the Editor-in-Chief of this journal.

### Competing interests

Kazuki Takaoka, Emi Segawa, Michiyo Yamamura, Yusuke Zushi, Masahiro Urade and Hiromitsu Kishimoto declare that they have no competing interests.

### Authors' contributions

KT participated in the study design and drafting of the manuscript. ES participated in the study design and data acquisition. MY and YZ participated in the data acquisition. MU participated in the surgical treatment. HK participated in the manuscript review. All authors read and approved the final manuscript.

### Authors' information

KT is an associate professor of the Department of Oral and Maxillofacial Surgery, Hyogo College of Medicine. ES is a specialist in oral and maxillofacial surgery. MY and YZ are assistant professors of the Department of Oral and Maxillofacial Surgery, Hyogo College of Medicine. MU is a professor emeritus of Hyogo College of Medicine. HK is a professor of the Department of Oral and Maxillofacial Surgery, Hyogo College of Medicine.

### Acknowledgements

Dr. Angie Smaranda (La Trobe University, Melbourne, Australia) and Dr. Angela Morben (University of Minnesota, MN, USA), language editors, provided professional English-language editing of this article.

### References

1. Barrowman RA, Wilson PR, Wiesenfeld D. Oral rehabilitation with dental implants after cancer treatment. Aust Dent J. 2011;56:160–5.
2. Stellingsma C, Vissink A, Meijer HJ, Kuiper C, Raghoebar GM. Implantology and the severely resorbed edentulous mandible. Crit Rev Oral Biol Med. 2004;15:240–8.

3. Zani SR, Rivaldo EG, Frasca SF, Caye LF. Oral health impact profile and prosthetic condition in edentulous patients rehabilitated with implant-supported overdentures and fixed prostheses. J Oral Sci. 2009;51:535–43.
4. Urade M, Sakurai K, Kawanaka M, Yoshioka W. Unusual presentation of carcinoma of the mandibular gingiva: report of a case. J Oral Maxillofac Surg. 1997;55:1007–10.
5. Kamstra JI, Jager-Wittenaar H, Dijkstra PU, Huisman PM, van Oort RP, van der Laan BF, et al. Oral symptoms and functional outcome related to oral and oropharyngeal cancer. Support Care Cancer. 2011;19:1327–33.
6. Carini F, Francesconi M, Saggese V, Monai D, Porcaro G. Implant-supported rehabilitation of a patient with mandibular ameloblastoma. Ann Stomatol. 2012;32:21–5.
7. Schoen PJ, Raghoebar GM, Bouma J, Reintsema H, Burlage FR, Roodenburg JL, et al. Prosthodontic rehabilitation of oral function in head-neck cancer patients with dental implants placed simultaneously during ablative tumour surgery: an assessment of treatment outcomes and quality of life. Int J Oral Maxillofac Surg. 2008;37:8–16.
8. Chan MF, Hayter JP, Cawood JI, Howell RA. Oral rehabilitation with implant-retained prostheses following ablative surgery and reconstruction with free flaps. Int J Oral Maxillofac Implants. 1997;12:820–7.
9. Barão VA, Delben JA, Lima J, Cabral T, Assunção WG. Comparison of different designs of implant-retained overdentures and fixed full-arch implant-supported prosthesis on stress distribution in edentulous mandible–a computed tomography-based three-dimensional finite element analysis. J Biomech. 2013;26:1312–20.
10. Roumanas ED, Markowitz BL, Lorant JA, Calcaterra TC, Jones NFJ, Beumer 3rd J. Reconstructed mandibular defects: fibula free flaps and osseointegrated implants. Plast Reconstr Surg. 1997;99:356–65.
11. Weischer T, Schettler D, Mohr C. Concept of surgical and implant-supported prostheses in the rehabilitation of patients with oral cancer. Int J Oral Maxillofac Implants. 1996;11:775–81.
12. Pjetursson BE, Thoma D, Jung R, Zwahlen M, Zembic A. A systematic review of the survival and complication rates of implant-supported fixed dental prostheses (FDPs) after a mean observation period of at least 5 years. Clin Oral Implants Res. 2012;23 Suppl 6:22–38.

# A meta-analysis on the effect of implant characteristics on the survival of the wide-diameter implant

Miriam Ting[1], Matthew Palermo[1*], David P. Donatelli[1], John P. Gaughan[2], Jon B. Suzuki[1] and Steven R. Jefferies[1]

**Abstract**

The purposes of the study are to study the implant survival of the wide-diameter implant and to analyze if the length, the implant surface, or the placement location has any effect on its survival. Electronic databases were searched from inception to Dec 2014. Studies included in the review had implants placed in areas of adequate bone width and had clear inclusion and exclusion criteria for patient selection. Immediately placed and immediately loaded implants were excluded. A meta-analysis was done using the "random effects" model on the included studies. And, a meta-regression was used to evaluate the effects of location, length, and surface on the implant survival. Of the six studies selected, three evaluated surface-treated implants and three machined implants. The overall pooled survival rate of the wide implant is 96.3 %. The meta-regression showed that when using a wide implant, neither its surface nor its length nor its position in the maxilla or mandible adversely affected its survival ($P > 0.05$). This meta-analysis concluded that the location, length, and surface of the wide-diameter implant did not affect its survival and therefore suggested that when the conditions of the implant site corresponded to the inclusion criteria of our meta-analysis, choosing a wide-diameter implant in the posterior mandible or maxilla, where implant length may be limited by the nerve or the sinus, the use of a short implant regardless of its surface would not affect its survival.

**Keywords:** Wide-diameter implants, Surface-treated or machined implants, Short implants or long implants, Implants in the mandible or maxilla

## Review

### Introduction

Endosseous implants were used reliably in the treatment of various degrees of edentulism [1–7]. In restoring the edentulous ridge, the clinician could be faced with difficult bony situations. The wide-diameter implant could be used in these situations to improve primary stability by increasing the surface area available for osteointegration [8–10]. Biomechanically, the wide-diameter implant engaged maximal bone, increased initial stability, and improved stress distribution in the supporting bone [11]. In restoring a large molar, the wide implant has the added advantage of increasing the load bearing capacity and emergence profile of the final restoration [10]. It has been shown to be three to six times stronger than the standard implant [12]. Wide-diameter implants were also used as rescue fixtures to replace fractured or non-integrated implants [8]. Thus, the wide-diameter implants could become the implant of choice when faced with these challenging situations.

The aims of this review were to research the literature published till Dec. 15, 2014, on wide-diameter implants and to perform a meta-analysis to study (1) the wide-diameter implant survival of different lengths, (2) the wide-diameter implant survival of modified surface compared to machined surface, and (3) the implant survival of wide-diameter implants placed in the maxilla compared to the mandible.

### Materials and methods

#### *Focused question*

1. Does length of the wide-diameter implant influence its survival?

* Correspondence: palermom@temple.edu
[1]Kornberg School of Dentistry, Temple University, 3223 North Broad Street, Philadelphia, PA 19140, USA
Full list of author information is available at the end of the article

2. Does the surface modification influence its survival compared to machined implant surfaces?
3. Does the implant placement in the maxilla or the mandible influence its survival?

### *Literature search and study design*

The database on PubMed, Web of Science, and Cochrane Central Register of Controlled Trials was searched from inception to December 15, 2014. The keywords for the search were "dental implants or dental implant" and "wide," and a reference librarian was consulted as to the most effective strategy. Gray literature was also searched on Google Scholar using advance search to find articles with all of the words "wide, dental, implants, endosseous, clinical, patients, survival" and without the words "animal, graft, augmentation, immediate, review". Hand searching was conducted on the reference lists of identified wide-diameter implant articles and was limited to articles not already identified in the above search strategy. Implant representatives of implant manufacturers were also contacted for any ongoing research pertaining to wide-diameter implants, and researchers were invited to clarify research information.

### *Inclusion/exclusion criteria*

1. Randomized controlled trials, controlled clinical trials, cohort, and case series reporting on the implant survival of wide-diameter endosseous titanium implants with different surface modifications were included. Only prospective data were included. Case reports, conventional reviews, and systemic reviews were excluded.
2. Implant diameter greater or equal to 4.7 mm were considered wide-diameter implants.
3. Only articles with specific documentation for wide-diameter implants were included. This documentation includes implant length, location/site, loading times, and specific failure data such as length, location, and timing of failure for wide-diameter implants.
4. Articles with information on implants placed in sites deemed to have adequate bone height and width, and did not require site development, were included. Articles with grafted sites and/or unclear description of how sites were selected were excluded.
5. Only articles with data on wide implants loaded after least 1–3 months of healing after implant placement were included; data on immediate placement in extraction sites and immediately loading implants were not covered in this review.
6. Wide-diameter implants used in immediate replacement of failed implants were excluded.
7. Studies with at least 1-year follow-up and included at least 10 implants regardless of diameter and length were included.
8. Patients with adequate health to undergo implant surgery and patients with controlled medical conditions were not excluded.
9. Smoking status of subjects was not considered a criterion for exclusion.
10. Non-English articles or articles without English translations were excluded due to language limitations.

### *Screening and selection*

Two reviewers participated in selection of studies (MT and MP). At the initial phase of selection, abstracts and titles of articles were screened by one reviewer (MT) to exclude articles that clearly were not related to wide-diameter dental implants. The previously described inclusion and exclusion criteria were applied when including articles for full-text screening. When there was a doubt as to the relevance of the article, due to insufficient information in the abstract, the full-text article was analyzed together with a second reviewer (MP).

### *Search results*

The search yielded 553 potentially relevant articles in PubMed, 303 in Web of Science, 35 in Cochrane Central Register of Controlled Trials, 64 from Google Scholar, and 19 not identified in the above search strategies from hand searching of reference lists of selected articles (Fig. 1). After screening the abstracts of the articles, 38 articles were selected for full-text screening from PubMed, 26 from Web of Science, 6 from Cochrane Central Register of Controlled Trials, 16 from Google Scholar, and 17 from hand searching of reference list. After elimination of duplicate articles, a total of 57 articles were selected for full-text screening.

Predetermined inclusion and exclusion criteria were applied to the selected full text by two reviewers (MT and MP); article selection was completed independently and then in unison. Areas of ambiguity were resolved through discussion. As for two articles that needed clarification of patient selection criteria, the authors were contacted via email and given 2 weeks to respond. One author responded with the requested information. Six articles remained for further review.

A total of 51 studies were excluded after the full-text review. These included 19 studies that did not document different lengths of wide implants studied, 15 studies that used graft materials in or around the implant sites, 4 studies that immediately placed implants in extraction sites or upon removal of failed implants, 2 studies that immediately loaded the implants, 10 studies that were

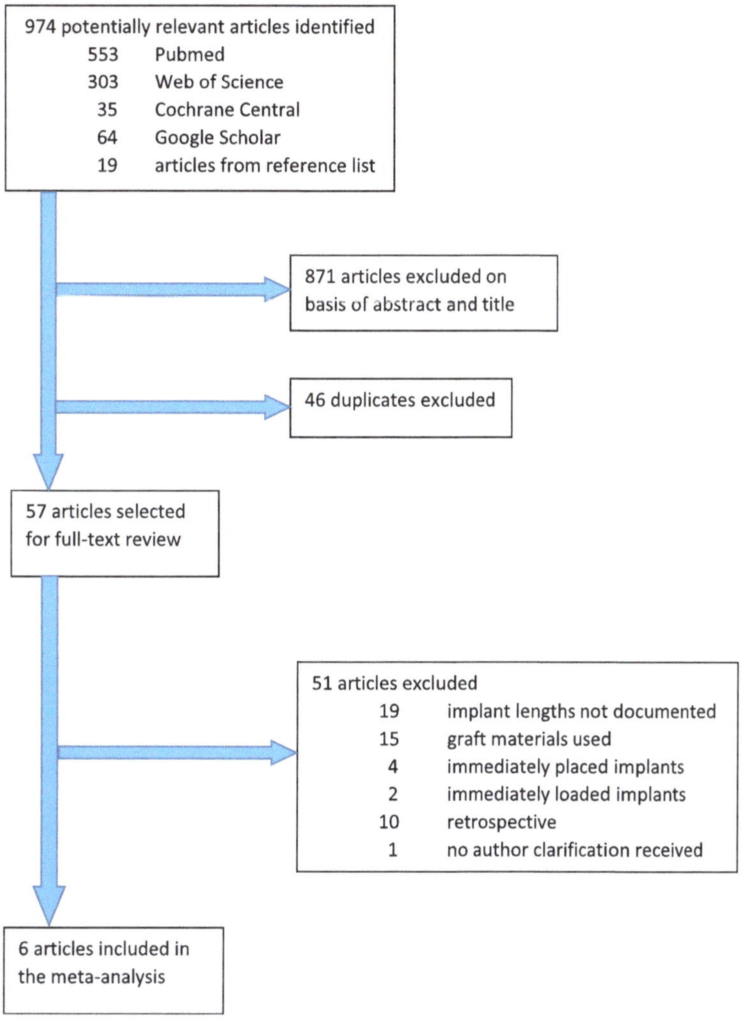


**Fig. 1** Study selection for wide-diameter implant articles

**Table 1** Wide-diameter implants

| Implant diameter (mm) | Implant lengths | No. of implants (total) | Implant type | Implant surface | Prospective clinical study | Placement follow-up/ mean (range) | Implant survival (%) | Age range (years) |
|---|---|---|---|---|---|---|---|---|
| 4.7 | 8, 10, 13, 16 | 117 | Zimmer (Screw vent, Paragon) | Acid-etched, uncoated | Khayat et al. 2001 [13] | Healing 3–6 months plus 17 months loading (11–21 months) | 95 | – |
| 5.0 | 7 | 14 | Endopore (Innova Corp) | Sintered porous | Deporter et al. 2001 [18] | 32.6 months | 100 | 25–76 (53.7) |
| 5.0 | 8.5, 10, 11.5 | 15 | Mark III WP (Nobel Biocare) | Ti-unite | Schincaglia et al. 2008 [17] | 3–4 months healing plus 12 months loading | 100 | 35–68 (49.2) |
| 5.0 | 6 | 13 | Brånemark (Nobel Biocare) | Machined | Friberg et al. 2000 [14] | 8 years (1–14 years) | 100 | 38–93 (63) |
| 5.0 | 6, 7, 8, 8.5, 10 | 109 | Brånemark (Nobel Biocare) | Machined | Tawil and Younan 2003 [15] | Healing plus 24 months loading | 94.5 | 22–80 (53.6) |
| 5.0 | 7, 8.5, 10, 11.5 | 38 | Brånemark (Nobel Biocare) | Machined | Polizzi et al. 2000 [16] | 36 months | 92 | 29–69 |

**Table 2** Wide surface-treated Implants

| Study | Implant surface | Implant type | Implant length | No. of implants | No. failed | % survived |
|---|---|---|---|---|---|---|
| Khayat et al. 2001 [13] | Acid-etched, uncoated | Zimmer (Screw vent, Paragon) | 8 | 29 | 2 | 93.1 |
| | | | 10 | 45 | 4 | 91.1 |
| | | | 13 | 28 | 0 | 100 |
| | | | 16 | 15 | 0 | 100 |
| Deporter et al. 2001 [18] | Sintered porous | Endopore (Innova Corp) | 7 | 14 | 0 | 100 |
| Schincaglia et al. 2008 [17] | Ti-unite | Mark III WP (Nobel Biocare) | 8.5 | 5 | 0 | 100 |
| | | | 10 | 5 | 0 | 100 |
| | | | 11.5 | 5 | 0 | 100 |

retrospective, and 1 study that did not receive a clarification from the author.

### *Data extraction*

One researcher (MT) extracted the data, and a second researcher (DPD) independently checked the data extraction for accuracy and completeness. The disagreements were resolved by discussion. The data extraction form was pilot tested on a representative sample before applying it to the selected articles.

### *Statistical analysis*

The forest plot was used to determine pooled wide-diameter implant survival rate of the selected studies. The funnel plot was used to determine the possibility of publication bias of the selected studies. Heterogeneity of the data was analyzed to determine if the data from the selected studies can be analyzed and if the random effects model can be used in the meta-analysis. In addition, a meta-regression (type III test of fixed effects) was used to evaluate the effects of location, length, and surface on the implant survival.

## Results

Of the six studies selected, three evaluated surface-treated implants and three machined implants (Table 1). The included studies all used similar criteria for implant survival, which was defined as the absence of mobility, pain, and radiolucent lesions. The implant survival was based on the percentage of implants evaluated, and the implant lengths in the studies range from 6 to 16 mm (Tables 2 and 3). The number of patients receiving wide implants was not specified in three studies which also evaluated other diameter implants [13–15]. Only data on the wide-diameter implants in those studies were included in the meta-analysis. Three studies evaluated only wide-diameter implants. The number of patients evaluated in these studies was as follows: Khayat et al. [13] studied 71 patients, Polizzi et al. [16] studied 34 patients, and Schincaglia et al. [17] studied 15 patients. Schincaglia et al.'s study was a randomized controlled trial evaluating immediate-loading versus delay-loading of wide-diameter implants; only data of the control group that was not immediately loaded was included in the meta-analysis. The mean patient follow-up of the six studies ranged from 1 to 8 years. The location of the implants placed in the selected studies (Table 4) was as follows: two studies evaluated implants placed in the posterior mandible [17, 18], one study in the edentulous mandible [14], and three studies in various areas of the maxilla and mandible [13, 15, 16].

The forest plot (Fig. 2) showed a pooled wide implant survival rate of 96.3 % (Table 5). The funnel plot (Fig. 3)

**Table 3** Wide machined implants

| Study | Implant surface | Implant type | Implant length | No. of implants | No. failed | % survived |
|---|---|---|---|---|---|---|
| Polizzi et al. 2000 [16] | Machined | Brånemark (Nobel Biocare) | 7 | 2 | 0 | 100 |
| | | | 8.5 | 8 | 1 | 87.5 |
| | | | 10 | 15 | 1 | 93.3 |
| | | | 11.5 | 13 | 1 | 92.3 |
| Friberg et al. 2000 [14] | Machined | Brånemark (Nobel Biocare) | 6 | 13 | 0 | 100 |
| Tawil and Younan 2003 [15] | Machined | Brånemark (Nobel Biocare) | 6 | 16 | 0 | 100 |
| | | | 7 | 3 | 0 | 100 |
| | | | 8 | 27 | 1 | 96.3 |
| | | | 8.5 | 8 | 2 | 75.0 |
| | | | 10 | 55 | 3 | 94.5 |

**Table 4** Implants used in the maxilla and mandible

| Study | Implant surface | Implant type | No. of implants in maxilla (no. failed) | No. of implants in mandible (no. failed) | % survived in maxilla | % survived in mandible |
|---|---|---|---|---|---|---|
| Khayat et al. 2001 [13] | Acid-etched, uncoated | Zimmer (Screw vent, Paragon) | 49 (2) | 62 (4) | 95.9 | 93.5 |
| Deporter et al. 2001 [18] | Sintered porous | Endopore (Innova Corp) | 0 | 14 (0) | – | 100 |
| Schincaglia et al. 2008 [17] | Ti-Unite | Mark III WP (Nobel Biocare) | 0 | 15 (0) | – | 100 |
| Polizzi et al. 2000 [16] | Machined | Brånemark (Nobel Biocare) | 4 (0) | 34 (3) | 100 | 91.2 |
| Friberg et al. 2000 [14] | Machined | Brånemark (Nobel Biocare) | 0 | 13 (0) | – | 100 |
| Tawil and Younan 2003 [15] | Machined | Brånemark (Nobel Biocare) | 22 (2) | 87 (4) | 90.9 | 95.4 |

was analyzed for publication bias. No publication bias was found in the selected studies. The meta-analysis heterogeneity statistics were shown in Table 6. The Q statistic was a measure of the total variance of the studies and along with the p-value showed that the studies do not differ significantly from the mean effect. The $I^2$ statistic along with the 95 % uncertainty interval measured the degree of inconsistency among the studies and showed no inconsistencies among the studies. $\tau^2$ was a measure of the between study variance and was defined as 0 if the Q value was less than the expected variance (Number of studies -1). The results showed no significant heterogeneity among the included studies. Within the meta-analysis using a random effects model, a meta-regression showed that the fixed effects of location, length and surface did not have a significant effect ($P > 0.05$) on survival (Table 7).

## Discussion

The present meta-analysis was limited to prospective clinical studies and utilized a rigorous inclusion and exclusion criteria. Studies included in the analysis were limited to cases in which implants placed in sites with adequate bone volume without grafting. Implants were placed in healed sites and loaded after at least 1–3 months of healing. All studies had at least 1-year follow-up. Patients were required to have adequate health to undergo implant surgery. Controlled medical conditions and smoking status were not excluded. Excluded were studies where implants were placed in sites that were initially deemed to have adequate bone; however, at the time of implant surgery, required the use of bone graft. Data from these studies could not be analyzed due to unclear documentation of which implants were grafted, thus preventing separation of the data for the analysis [19, 20]. The data from some

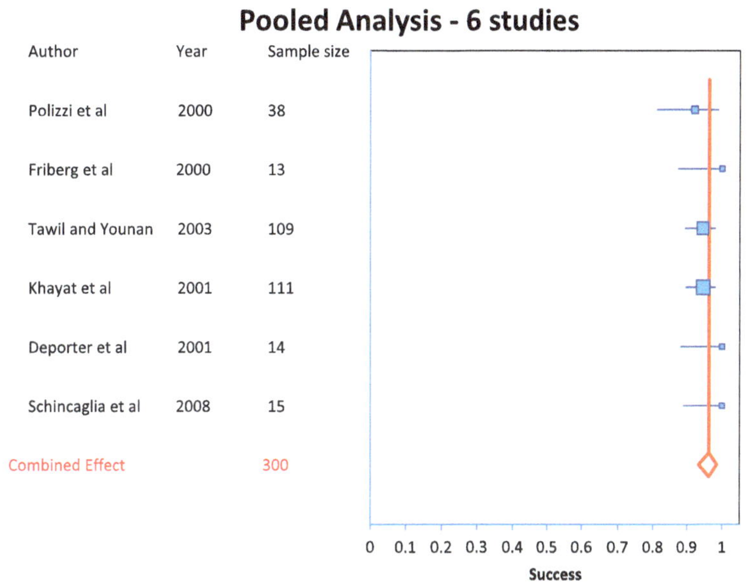


**Fig. 2** Forest plot

**Table 5** Meta-analysis implant data—pooled analysis

| Authors | Number | Success | ci− | ci+ | Weight (%) |
|---|---|---|---|---|---|
| Polizzi et al. [16] | 38 | 0.921 | 0.810 | 0.990 | 12.71 |
| Friberg et al. [14] | 13 | 1.000 | 0.872 | 1.000 | 4.46 |
| Tawil and Younan [15] | 109 | 0.945 | 0.893 | 0.981 | 36.14 |
| Khayat et al. [13] | 111 | 0.946 | 0.895 | 0.982 | 36.80 |
| Deporter et al. [18] | 14 | 1.000 | 0.881 | 1.000 | 4.79 |
| Schincaglia et al. [17] | 15 | 1.000 | 0.888 | 1.000 | 5.12 |
| | 300 | 0.963 | 0.934 | 0.985 | 100 |

**Table 6** Heterogeneity statistics

| $Q$ | $P$ | |
|---|---|---|
| 2.7008 | 0.7460 | |
| $I^2$ | ci− | ci+ |
| 0.00 % | 0.00 % | 74.62 % |
| $\tau^2$ | ci− | ci+ |
| 0.0000 | 0.0000 | 0.0069 |

of the survival studies were not able to be analyzed due to the lack of a clear description of implant length. The exclusion of these studies along with the rigorous inclusion criteria limited our meta-analysis to six studies. These six studies were well-documented with clear data on implant length, surface, and location.

The overall survival rate of wide-diameter implants based on the pooled data of the included six studies was 96.3 %, and this was within the reported range of wide-diameter [21] and regular-diameter [22] implant survival rates. Machined implants functionally integrate with the surrounding bone via a macroscopic interlock of the implant threads with the bone. Surface treatment of the machined threads increases the effectiveness of the interlock resulting in an improved bone-to-implant interface [23, 24]. However, our meta-analysis found no significant difference between the implant survivals of machined compared to surface-treated wide-diameter implants. Similarly, Al-Nawas et al. [25] also reported no significant difference between machined and double-etched surface-treated standard-diameter implant survival. Conversely, Maló and Araújo Nobre [26] reported significantly more failures for machined compared to surface-treated narrow (3.3-mm diameter) implants. This suggests that the implant surface characteristics may have an impact on implant survival rate based on the implant diameter, and as the diameter of the implant is increased, as in the wide-diameter implant, this impact may not be statistically significant. It should be noted that stringent inclusion criteria were applied including non-grafted sites, controlled medical conditions, and adequate bone volume.

In the present meta-analysis, the location of wide-diameter implants did not impact survival. This was in agreement with Degidi et al. [27] whose study did not find a statistically significant difference in the survival of wide-diameter implants in varying bone densities in the maxilla and mandible. However, this was contrary to some studies [16, 28] that reported a lower wide-diameter implant survival in the posterior mandible compared to the maxilla. This was postulated to be due to the low marginal bone vascularity of the mandible [29, 30]. And, this was also contrary to some other studies [31, 32], which reported a better outcome for immediately placed implants placed in the mandible because of better bone density and quality.

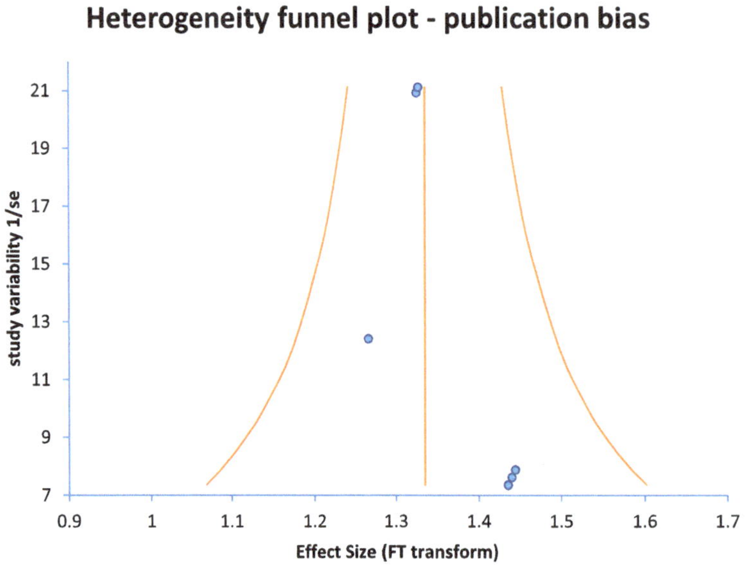


**Fig. 3** Funnel plot

**Table 7** Meta-regression—effect of surface and lengths

| Type III tests of fixed effects | | | | |
|---|---|---|---|---|
| | Num | Den | | |
| Effect | DF | DF | *F* value | *P* |
| Surface | 1 | 11 | 0.84 | 0.3787 |
| Length | 7 | 11 | 0.97 | 0.4951 |
| Location | 1 | 11 | 0.00 | 0.9868 |

Degree of free (DF) contributes to the determination of *P* value

The various lengths of wide implants used in the six selected study ranged from 6 to 16 mm, and the following implant lengths assessed in the meta-regression were 6, 7, 8, 8.5, 10, 11.5, 13, and 16 mm. Unlike our meta-analysis which focused solely on the wide-diameter implant, very few studies looked at the effects of different lengths on the survival rate specific to the wide-diameter implant. Most studies reported survival rates of the shorter implant lengths (≤10 mm) with varying diameter implants (3.75, 4, 5, and 6 mm) [33]. Studies by Deporter et al. [18, 34] included different diameter implants and were not limited to only wide-diameter implants; these studies also found no significant effect of implant length on implant performance. Conversely, Olate et al. [35], who also included different diameter implants, observed the largest failure in their short implants compared to long or medium implants. However, Olate et al. evaluated 1649 implants retrospectively, 295 were wide-diameter implants (17.9 %), 1217 were regular-diameter (73.8 %), and 137 were narrow-diameter implants (8.3 %). Thus, their conclusion would pertain more to the regular-diameter implants which makes up the majority of implant evaluated in their study. This would seem to indicate that length may have an effect on regular-diameter implant survival, but this would require further investigation. Our meta-regression, which evaluated the prospective data of a total of 306 wide-diameter implants with lengths ranging from 6 to 16 mm, concluded that wide-diameter implants ranging in length from 6 to 16 mm would not have any significant effect on the implant survival. It should be stressed that stringent inclusion criteria were applied for study selection, and hence, these results cannot be generalized to patients with medical or oral compromise.

## Conclusions

This meta-analysis concluded that the location, length, and surface treatment of the wide-diameter implant do not significantly affect its survival. It is therefore suggested with caution that when the conditions of the implant site corresponds to the inclusion criteria used in our meta-analysis, choosing a wide implant in the posterior mandible or maxilla, where implant length may be limited by the nerve or the sinus, the use of a short implant regardless of the implant surface would not adversely affect its survival.

**Competing interests**
MT, MP, DPD, JPG, and JBS declare that they have no competing interests as to the content of the manuscript. SRJ holds common stock in the company DENTSPLY International, York, PA, USA, which markets various dental implant systems. Nevertheless, the author does not believe that the abovementioned disclosure presents any apparent conflict of interest with respect to the content and subject matter of this systematic review.

**Authors' contributions**
MT, MP, DPD, JBS, and SRJ contributed to the design of the study. MT, MP, and DPD contributed to study selection and data extraction. JPG formulated and performed the statistical analysis. All authors read, revised, and approved the final manuscript.

**Authors' information**
1. Miriam Ting, BDS, MS, Cert. Advanced Periodontology (USC), is in the Advance standing program at the Temple University Kornberg School of Dentistry.
2. Matthew Palermo, DMD, is an associate professor from the Department of Restorative Dentistry at the Temple University Kornberg School of Dentistry.
3. David P. Donatelli, DDS, is an assistant professor from the Department of Restorative Dentistry at Temple University Kornberg School of Dentistry.
4. John P. Gaughan, MS, PhD, MBA, is an associate professor (emeritus) and a statistician at the Temple University School of Medicine.
5. Jon B. Suzuki, DDS, PhD, MBA is a professor, chairman, and program director from the Department of Periodontology and Oral Implantology at the Temple University Kornberg School of Dentistry.
6. Steven R. Jefferies, DDS, MS, PhD, is a professor from the Department of Restorative Dentistry at the Temple University Kornberg School of Dentistry.

**Acknowledgements**
The meta-analysis by the statistician was funded by the Temple University Research Fund.

**Author details**
[1]Kornberg School of Dentistry, Temple University, 3223 North Broad Street, Philadelphia, PA 19140, USA. [2]School of Medicine, Temple University, 3420 N Broad St, Philadelphia, PA 19140, USA.

**References**
1. Adell R, Lekholm U, Rockler B, Branemark PI. A 15-year study of osseointegrated implants in the treatment of the edentulous jaw. Int J Oral Surg. 1981;10(6):387–416.
2. Adell R, Eriksson B, Lekholm U, Branemark PI, Jemt T. Long-term follow-up study of osseointegrated implants in the treatment of totally edentulous jaws. Int J Oral Maxillofac Implants. 1990;5(4):347–59.
3. Albrektsson T. On long-term maintenance of the osseointegrated response. Australian Prosthodontic J Australian Prosthodontic Soc. 1993;7(Suppl):15–24.
4. Engquist B, Bergendal T, Kallus T, Linden U. A retrospective multicenter evaluation of osseointegrated implants supporting overdentures. Int J Oral Maxillofac Implants. 1988;3(2):129–34.
5. Jemt T, Lekholm U, Adell R. Osseointegrated implants in the treatment of partially edentulous patients: a preliminary study on 876 consecutively placed fixtures. Int J Oral Maxillofac Implants. 1989;4(3):211–7.
6. Albrektsson T. A multicenter report on osseointegrated oral implants. J Prosthet Dent. 1988;60(1):75–84.
7. Albrektsson T, Dahl E, Enbom L, Engevall S, Engquist B, Eriksson AR, et al. Osseointegrated oral implants: a Swedish multicenter study of 8139 consecutively inserted Nobelpharma implants. J Periodontol. 1988;59(5):287–96. doi:10.1902/jop.1988.59.5.287.
8. Langer B, Langer L, Herrmann I, Jorneus L. The wide fixture: a solution for special bone situations and a rescue for the compromised implant. Part 1. Int J Oral Maxillofac Implants. 1993;8(4):400–8.

9. Graves SL, Jansen CE, Siddiqui AA, Beaty KD. Wide diameter implants: indications, considerations and preliminary results over a two-year period. Australian Prosthodontic J Australian Prosthodontic Soc. 1994;8:31–7.
10. Lazzara RJ. Criteria for implant selection: surgical and prosthetic considerations. Pract Periodontics Aesthet Dent. 1994;6(9):55–62. quiz 4.
11. Lee JH, Frias V, Lee KW, Wright RF. Effect of implant size and shape on implant success rates: a literature review. J Prosthet Dent. 2005;94(4):377–81. doi:10.1016/j.prosdent.2005.04.018.
12. Sullivan DY. Wide implants for wide teeth. Dental Econ Oral Hygiene. 1994;84(3):82–3.
13. Khayat PG, Hallage PG, Toledo RA. An investigation of 131 consecutively placed wide screw-vent implants. Int J Oral Maxillofac Implants. 2001;16(6):827–32.
14. Friberg B, Grondahl K, Lekholm U, Branemark PI. Long-term follow-up of severely atrophic edentulous mandibles reconstructed with short Branemark implants. Clin Implant Dent Relat Res. 2000;2(4):184–9.
15. Tawil G, Younan R. Clinical evaluation of short, machined-surface implants followed for 12 to 92 months. Int J Oral Maxillofac Implants. 2003;18(6):894–901.
16. Polizzi G, Rangert B, Lekholm U, Gualini F, Lindstrom H. Branemark System wide platform implants for single molar replacement: clinical evaluation of prospective and retrospective materials. Clin Implant Dent Relat Res. 2000;2(2):61–9.
17. Schincaglia GP, Marzola R, Giovanni GF, Chiara CS, Scotti R. Replacement of mandibular molars with single-unit restorations supported by wide-body implants: immediate versus delayed loading. A randomized controlled study. Int J Oral Maxillofac Implants. 2008;23(3):474–80.
18. Deporter D, Pilliar RM, Todescan R, Watson P, Pharoah M. Managing the posterior mandible of partially edentulous patients with short, porous-surfaced dental implants: early data from a clinical trial. Int J Oral Maxillofac Implants. 2001;16(5):653–8.
19. Attard NJ, Zarb GA. Implant prosthodontic management of partially edentulous patients missing posterior teeth: the Toronto experience. J Prosthet Dent. 2003;89(4):352–9. doi:10.1067/mpr.2003.91.
20. Tawil G, Mawla M, Gottlow J. Clinical and radiographic evaluation of the 5-mm diameter regular-platform Branemark fixture: 2- to 5-year follow-up. Clin Implant Dent Relat Res. 2002;4(1):16–26.
21. Davarpanah M, Martinez H, Kebir M, Etienne D, Tecucianu JF. Wide-diameter implants: new concepts. Int J Periodontics Restorative Dent. 2001;21(2):149–59.
22. Javed F, Romanos GE. Role of implant diameter on long-term survival of dental implants placed in posterior maxilla: a systematic review. Clin Oral Investig. 2015;19(1):1–10. doi:10.1007/s00784-014-1333-z.
23. Khang W, Feldman S, Hawley CE, Gunsolley J. A multi-center study comparing dual acid-etched and machined-surfaced implants in various bone qualities. J Periodontol. 2001;72(10):1384–90. doi:10.1902/jop.2001.72.10.1384.
24. Cochran DL. A comparison of endosseous dental implant surfaces. J Periodontol. 1999;70(12):1523–39. doi:10.1902/jop.1999.70.12.1523.
25. Al-Nawas B, Hangen U, Duschner H, Krummenauer F, Wagner W. Turned, machined versus double-etched dental implants *in vivo*. Clin Implant Dent Relat Res. 2007;9(2):71–8. doi:10.1111/j.1708-8208.2007.00030.x.
26. Malo P, de Araujo Nobre M. Implants (3.3 mm diameter) for the rehabilitation of edentulous posterior regions: a retrospective clinical study with up to 11 years of follow-up. Clin Implant Dent Relat Res. 2011;13(2):95–103. doi:10.1111/j.1708-8208.2009.00188.x.
27. Degidi M, Piattelli A, Iezzi G, Carinci F. Wide-diameter implants: analysis of clinical outcome of 304 fixtures. J Periodontol. 2007;78(1):52–8. doi:10.1902/jop.2007.060139.
28. Ivanoff CJ, Grondahl K, Sennerby L, Bergstrom C, Lekholm U. Influence of variations in implant diameters: a 3- to 5-year retrospective clinical report. Int J Oral Maxillofac Implants. 1999;14(2):173–80.
29. von Wowern N. Variations in structure within the trabecular bone of the mandible. Scand J Dent Res. 1977;85(7):613–22.
30. von Wowern N. Variations in bone mass within the cortices of the mandible. Scand J Dent Res. 1977;85(6):444–55.
31. Balshi TJ, Wolfinger GJ. Immediate loading of Branemark implants in edentulous mandibles: a preliminary report. Implant Dent. 1997;6(2):83–8.
32. Randow K, Ericsson I, Nilner K, Petersson A, Glantz PO. Immediate functional loading of Branemark dental implants. An 18-month clinical follow-up study. Clin Oral Implants Res. 1999;10(1):8–15.
33. Hagi D, Deporter DA, Pilliar RM, Arenovich T. A targeted review of study outcomes with short (< or = 7 mm) endosseous dental implants placed in partially edentulous patients. J Periodontol. 2004;75(6):798–804. doi:10.1902/jop.2004.75.6.798.
34. Deporter DA, Todescan R, Watson PA, Pharoah M, Pilliar RM, Tomlinson G. A prospective human clinical trial of Endopore dental implants in restoring the partially edentulous maxilla using fixed prostheses. Int J Oral Maxillofac Implants. 2001;16(4):527–36.
35. Olate S, Lyrio MC, de Moraes M, Mazzonetto R, Moreira RW. Influence of diameter and length of implant on early dental implant failure. J Oral Maxillofac Surg. 2010;68(2):414–9. doi:10.1016/j.joms.2009.10.002.

# Efficacy of alternative or adjunctive measures to conventional treatment of peri-implant mucositis and peri-implantitis: a systematic review and meta-analysis

Frank Schwarz*, Andrea Schmucker and Jürgen Becker

**Abstract**

In patients with peri-implant mucositis and peri-implantitis, what is the efficacy of nonsurgical (i.e. referring to peri-implant mucositis and peri-implantitis) and surgical (i.e. referring to peri-implantitis) treatments with alternative or adjunctive measures on changing signs of inflammation compared with conventional nonsurgical (i.e. mechanical/ultrasonic debridement) and surgical (i.e. open flap debridement) treatments alone? After electronic database and hand search, a total of 40 publications (reporting on 32 studies) were finally considered for the qualitative and quantitative assessment. The weighted mean changes (WM)/ and WM differences (WMD) were estimated for bleeding on probing scores (BOP) and probing pocket depths (PD) (random effect model). Peri-implant mucositis: WMD in BOP and PD reductions amounted to −8.16 % [SE = 4.61] and −0.15 mm [SE = 0.13], not favouring adjunctive antiseptics/antibiotics (local and systemic) over control measures ($p > 0.05$). Peri-implantitis (nonsurgical): WMD in BOP scores amounted to −23.12 % [SE = 4.81] and −16.53 % [SE = 4.41], favouring alternative measures (glycine powder air polishing, Er:YAG laser) for plaque removal and adjunctive local antibiotics over control measures ($p < 0.001$), respectively. Peri-implantitis (surgical): WMD in BOP and PD reductions did not favour alternative over control measures for surface decontamination. WM reductions following open flap surgery (±resective therapy) and adjunctive augmentative therapy amounted to 34.81 and 50.73 % for BOP and 1.75 and 2.20 mm for PD, respectively. While mechanical debridement alone was found to be effective for the management of peri-implant mucositis, alternative/adjunctive measures may improve the efficacy over/of conventional nonsurgical treatments at peri-implantitis sites. Adjunctive resective and/or augmentative measures are promising; however, their beneficial effect on the clinical outcome of surgical treatments needs to be further investigated.

## Review

### Background

Peri-implant mucositis describes an inflammatory lesion that resides in the soft tissues compartment, while at peri-implantitis sites, this lesion has extended and also affects the implant supporting bone [1]. The 11th European Workshop on Periodontology has pointed to an "estimated weighted mean prevalence of peri-implant mucositis and peri-implantitis of 43 and 22 %, respectively" [2].

The main etiology of peri-implant mucositis refers to plaque accumulation [3, 4], and the conversion from mucositis to peri-implantitis was, particularly in the absence of a supportive maintenance care [5], positively correlated with the function time [2]. However, the presence of some independent systemic/patient-related (i.e. smoking) and local (i.e. residual cement, dimension of the keratinized tissue, surface roughness) risk indicators may increase the probability of the disease occurring [3].

* Correspondence: Frank.Schwarz@med.uni-duesseldorf.de
Department of Oral Surgery, Westdeutsche Kieferklinik, Universitätsklinikum Düsseldorf, D-40225 Düsseldorf, Germany

According to the cause-related concept of therapy, professionally administered plaque removal is a key strategy for the prevention and management of peri-implant diseases [6]. In previous years, several alternative or adjunctive measures (e.g. local antibiotics, air polishing, laser application) have been proposed to improve the efficacy of nonsurgical treatment approaches [7–9]. At peri-implantitis sites, surgical protocols may involve different decontamination protocols, that may also be combined with resective (e.g. pocket elimination, bone re-contouring, implantoplasty) and/or augmentative approaches (e.g. bone substitutes or autografts with or without a supporting barrier membrane) [7, 10]. Accordingly, there is a need to identify the most effective interventions for the treatment of peri-implant diseases.

The aim of this systematic review was therefore to address the following focused question: in patients with peri-implant mucositis and peri-implantitis, what is the efficacy of nonsurgical (i.e. referring to peri-implant mucositis and peri-implantitis) and surgical (i.e. referring to peri-implantitis) treatments with alternative or adjunctive measures on changing signs of inflammation compared with conventional nonsurgical and surgical treatments alone?

## Methods

This systematic review was structured and conducted according to the preferred reporting items of the PRISMA statement [11].

### *Focused question*

The focused question serving for literature search was structured according to the PICO format [12]: "In patients with peri-implant mucositis and peri-implantitis, what is the efficacy of nonsurgical (i.e. referring to peri-implant mucositis and peri-implantitis) and surgical (i.e. referring to peri-implantitis) treatments with alternative or adjunctive measures on changing signs of inflammation compared with conventional nonsurgical and surgical treatments alone?".

Population: patients with peri-implant mucositis and peri-implantitis based on case definitions used in respective publications

Intervention: alternative or adjunctive measures to nonsurgical and surgical treatments

Comparison: conventional measures for nonsurgical and surgical treatments

Outcome: changes in peri-implant mucosal inflammation

### *Search strategy*

The PubMed database of the U.S. National Library of Medicine and the Web of Knowledge of Thomson Reuters were used as electronic databases to perform a systematic search for relevant articles published in the dental literature between 1992 up to April 30, 2015. A commercially available software program (Endnote X7, Thomson, London, UK) was used for electronic title management. Screening was performed independently by two authors (F.S. and A.S.). Disagreement regarding inclusion during the first and second stage of study selection was resolved by discussion.

The combination of key words (i.e. Medical Subject Headings MeSH) and free text terms included:

"treatment" OR "nonsurgical treatment" OR "non-surgical treatment" OR "surgical treatment" OR "regenerative treatment" OR "augmentative treatment" OR "resective treatment" OR "reconstructive treatment" OR "therapy" OR "nonsurgical therapy" OR "non-surgical therapy" OR "surgical therapy" OR "regenerative therapy" OR "augmentative therapy" OR "resective therapy" OR "reconstructive therapy" OR "antiseptic treatment" OR "antibiotic treatment" OR "adjunctive treatment" OR "antiseptic therapy" OR "antibiotic therapy" OR "adjunctive therapy"

AND

"peri-implant disease" OR "periimplant disease" OR "peri-implant infection" OR "periimplant infection" OR "mucositis" (MeSH) OR "peri-implant mucositis" OR "periimplant mucositis" OR "Periimplantitis" (MeSH) OR "peri-implantitis".

Electronic search was complemented by a hand search of the following journals:

*Clinical Implant Dentistry and Related Research; Clinical Oral Implants Research; International Journal of Oral and Maxillofacial Implants; Journal of Clinical Periodontology; Journal of Periodontology*. Finally, the references of all selected full-text articles and related reviews were scanned. If required, the corresponding authors were contacted and requested to provide missing data or information.

### *Study inclusion and exclusion criteria*

During the first stage of study selection, the titles and abstracts were screened and evaluated according to the following inclusion criteria:

1) English language.
2) Prospective randomized controlled (RCT), or non-randomized controlled (CCT) studies (split-mouth or parallel group designs) in humans comparing alternative (i.e. for biofilm removal) or adjunctive measures (i.e. for biofilm removal, or adjunctive antiseptic/antibiotic therapy, or regenerative/resective approaches) to conventional nonsurgical (i.e. mechanical/ultrasonic debridement) or surgical (i.e. open flap debridement) treatments.
3) Data on the clinical changes in mucosal inflammation (i.e. bleeding scores) and probing

pocket depths (PD) following nonsurgical (referring to peri-implant mucositis and peri-implantitis) or surgical (referring to peri-implantitis) treatments in respective groups.

At the second stage of selection, all full-text articles identified during the first stage were acquired. During this procedure, the pre-selected publications were evaluated according to the following exclusion criteria:

1) Inclusion of less than five patients
2) Inadequate case definition [13]
3) Lack of clinical data on the changes in mucosal inflammation and PD

#### *Quality assessment of selected studies*

A quality assessment of all selected full-text articles was performed according to the Cochrane collaborations tool for assessing risk of bias (low, high, unclear) including the following domains: random sequence generation, allocation concealment, blinding of participants and personnel, blinding of outcome assessment, and incomplete outcome data [14]. Quality assessment was performed in two different phases. In particular, during phase I, quality assessment was based on the published full-text article performed independently by both authors. In phase II, disagreements were resolved by discussion.

#### *Data extraction and method of analysis*

A data extraction template was generated and based on the study design, population, case definition, observation period, interventions, comparisons, and primary and secondary outcomes as well as the study quality. For data analysis, the bleeding index (BI)/bleeding on probing (BOP) and PD scores after respective healing periods were defined as primary outcomes. Secondary outcomes included changes in marginal bone levels, immunological/microbiological parameters and the resolution of peri-implant diseases, based on case definitions used in respective publications. RCTs and CCTs not implementing appropriate control measures but reporting on changes in primary outcomes were used for the estimation of the overall efficacy of treatments.

Heterogeneity between RCTs, meta-analysis (i.e. weighted mean changes/differences and 95 % confidence intervals, random effect model to account for potential methodological differences between studies), forest plots and publication bias (Egger's regression to quantify the bias captured by funnel plots) were assessed using a commercially available software program (Comprehensive Meta-Analysis V2, Biostat, Englewood, NJ 07631 USA).

### Results

#### *Study selection*

A total of 368 potentially relevant titles and abstracts were found during the electronic and manual search. During the first stage of study selection, 319 publications were excluded based on title and abstract. For the second phase, the complete full-text articles of the remaining 49 publications were thoroughly evaluated. A total of 19 papers had to be excluded at this stage because they did not fulfil the inclusion criteria of the present systematic review (Table 1).

Finally, a total of 40 publications (reporting on 32 studies) were considered for the qualitative and quantitative assessment (Fig. 1).

#### *Quality and risk of bias assessment of selected studies*

The review author's judgement about each risk of bias item for each included RCT is presented in Table 2. In particular, the percentages across all included studies for high, low and unclear risk of bias items were 34.1, 54.8 and 11.1 %, respectively (Table 2).

#### *Subdivision of selected studies*

All selected publications were subdivided according to differences in the treatment protocol:

- o Nonsurgical treatment of peri-implant mucositis—-alternative or adjunctive measures for biofilm removal (2 RCTs and 1 CCT) (Table 3)
- o Nonsurgical treatment of peri-implant mucositis—-adjunctive antispectic therapy (3 RCTs) (Table 4)
- o Nonsurgical treatment of peri-implant mucositis—-adjunctive antibiotic therapy (2 RCTs) (Table 5).
- o Nonsurgical treatment of peri-implantitis—alternative measures for biofilm removal (6 RCTs) (Table 6)
- o Nonsurgical treatment of peri-implantitis—adjunctive antiseptic therapy (1 RCT) (Table 7)
- o Nonsurgical treatment of peri-implantitis—adjunctive antibiotic therapy (4 RCTs) (Table 8)
- o Surgical treatment of peri-implantitis—alternative measures for surface decontamination (3 RCTs and 1 CCT) (Table 9)
- o Surgical treatment of peri-implantitis—adjunctive resective therapy (1 RCT) (Table 10)
- o Surgical treatment of peri-implantitis—adjunctive augmentative therapy (4 RCTs, 4 CCTs) (Table 11)

#### *Nonsurgical treatment of peri-implant mucositis*

The case definitions markedly differed among the studies investigated. While three studies considered mucosal inflammation in the absence of radiographic bone loss [15–17], four studies also accepted a bone resorption of up to 3 mm for defining peri-implant mucositis [18–21]. Moreover, these studies used several clinical parameters

**Table 1** Excluded clinical studies at the second stage of selection and the reason for exclusion

| Publication | Reason for exclusion |
|---|---|
| Lavigne et al. [63] | Experimental sites without BOP at baseline |
| Ciancio et al. [64] | Homecare plaque control protocol |
| Felo et al. [65] | Homecare plaque control protocol |
| Bach et al. [66] | Lack of clinical data defined for the present systematic review |
| Dörtbudak et al. [67] | Lack of a conventional control treatment |
| Khoury and Buchmann [68] | Changes in mucosal inflammation not reported |
| Roos-Jansaker et al. [69] | Observational study |
| Duarte et al. [70] | Observational study reporting on the same study population as [71] |
| Maximo et al. [71] | Observational study |
| Ramberg et al. [72] | Homecare plaque control protocol |
| Corbella et al. [73] | Prevention of peri-implant diseases |
| Heitz-Mayfield et al. [74] | Homecare plaque control protocol |
| Costa et al. [5] | Observational study |
| De Angelis et al. [75] | Lack of subgroup analyses |
| Salvi et al. [76] | Observational study |
| Deppe et al. [59] | Observational study |
| De Siena et al. [77] | Homecare plaque control protocol |
| McKenna et al. [78] | Case definition not reported |
| Flichy-Fernandez et al. [79] | Cross-over study design |

to assess mucosal inflammation, employed various oral hygiene instructions (OHI) and defined different intervals for maintenance care. Despite significant improvements in all of the clinical parameters investigated, test (i.e. alternative or adjunctive methods for biofilm removal, adjunctive antiseptic therapy, or adjunctive antibiotic therapy) and control treatments were commonly associated with residual gingival index (GI), BI, and/or BOP scores at 3 to 12 months after therapy (Tables 3, 4 and 5).

**Alternative or adjunctive measures for biofilm removal** Three studies reported on alternative or adjunctive measures for biofilm removal (Table 3).

In particular, one RCT and one CCT compared the clinical efficacy of adjunctive air polishing (glycine powder) to OHI and mechanical debridement using either ultrasonic scalers or hand instruments [15, 18]. Both test and control groups were associated with significant improvements in mean BI and PD scores after therapy. When evaluating absolute values at 6 months, mean BI and PD scores were significantly lower following adjunctive air polishing to teflon curettes [18]. One RCT compared a repeated (3 and 6 months) monotherapy using an air abrasive device to ultrasonic scaling. After a healing period of 12 months, both groups revealed comparable BOP reductions and frequencies of diseased sites [21] (Table 3).

**Adjunctive antiseptic therapy** Three RCTs reported on the adjunctive antispectic therapy to OHI and mechanical debridement [17, 20, 22] (Table 4).

In particular, one RCT assessed the adjunctive application of phosphoric acid gel to carbon curettes and rubber cup polishing, which was provided once every month in both groups. At 5 months, test sites revealed a significantly higher reduction in mean gingival index (GI) (modified, but not specified) and colony-forming units when compared with control sites, respectively [22]. Porras et al. [20] compared OHI + mechanical debridement with and without local pocket irrigation using chlorhexidine digluconate (CHX) + topical CHX gel application + CHX mouthwash (twice for 10 days). At 3 months, mean mucosal bleeding (mBI), BOP scores and microbiological parameters did not significantly differ between test and control groups. However, the test group revealed a significantly higher change in mean PD scores [20]. In another RCT, topical CHX gel application + full mouth disinfection + CHX mouthrinse (2×/day) and tonsil spraying (1×/day) for 14 days was compared with OHI + mechanical debridement (plastic scaler + polyetheretherketone-coated ultrasonic instruments) + full mouth scaling alone. While both treatment procedures were associated with significant PD reductions at 8 months, the BOP scores did not significantly differ to baseline in both groups [17] (Table 4).

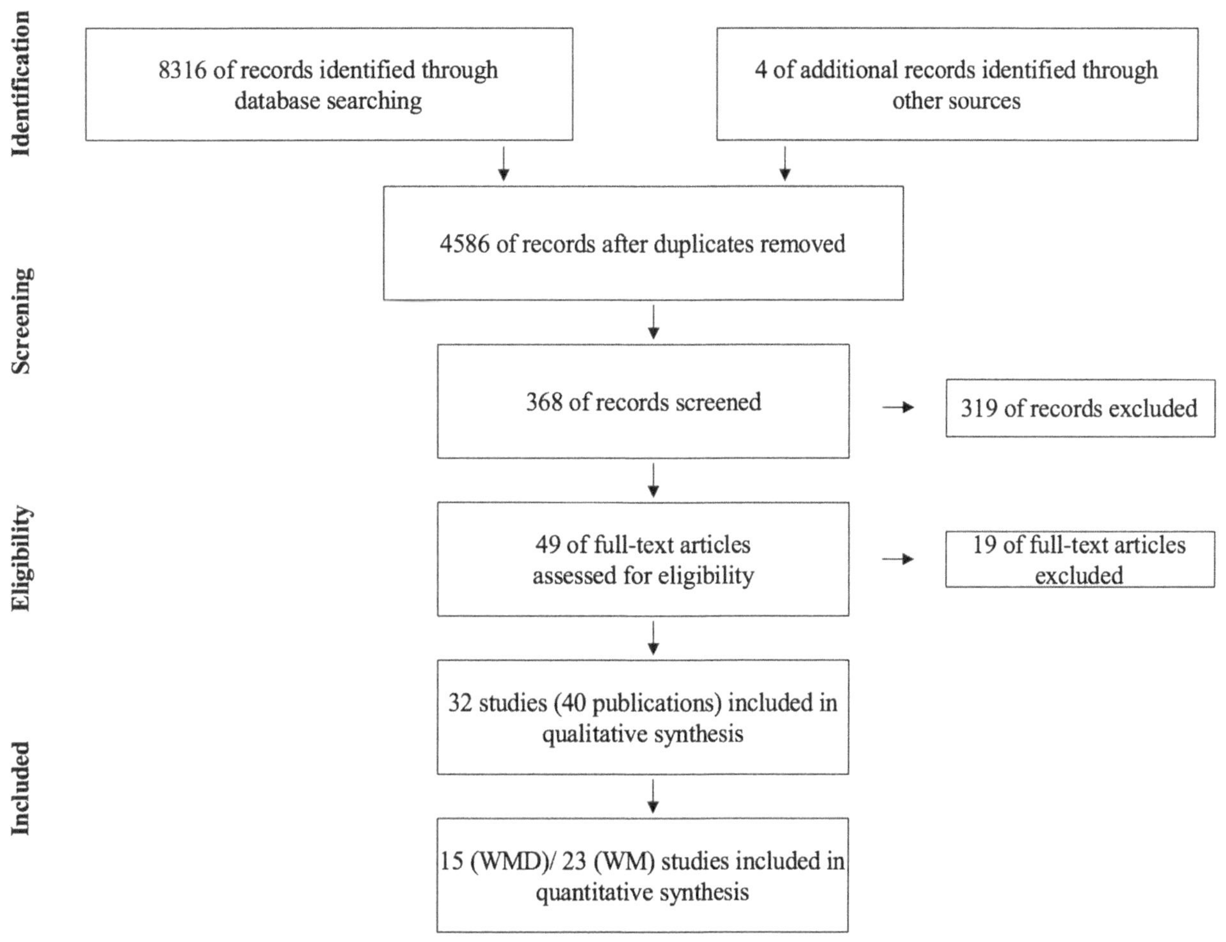


**Fig. 1** Flow diagram of literature search and inclusion

**Adjunctive antibiotic therapy** Two studies reported on the adjunctive antibiotic (i.e. local or systemic) therapy to OHI and mechanical debridement [16, 19] (Table 5).

In particular, one RCT compared the adjunctive local delivery of tetracycline HCl (25 %) fibres for 10 days (test) to mechanical debridement alone (control). A complete or partial fibre loss was noted at three implants after 7 to 10 following application. While test sites were associated with marked BOP improvements, control sites revealed a further increase of BOP scores at 3 months [16]. In another RCT, a total of 45 patients were randomly allocated to either OHI + mechanical debridement (titanium curettes + rubber polishing) + systemic antibiotic medication (Azithromycin® 500 mg day 1 and 250 mg days 2–4) (test), or OHI + mechanical debridement alone (control). The subject-based, per-protocol analysis at 6 months did not reveal any significant differences between test and control groups for all clinical and microbiological parameters investigated [19] (Table 5).

### *Nonsurgical treatment of peri-implantitis*

In all studies investigated, peri-implantitis was commonly defined by BOP and a radiographic bone loss. However, the reference points (i.e. baseline radiographs) and thresholds used to identify bone level changes were either not specified [23–25] or exhibited large variations [26–34]. Radiographic bone level changes as treatment outcome were merely assessed in three studies [28–30].

Despite significant improvements in all of the clinical and microbiological parameters investigated, test (i.e. alternative methods for biofilm removal, adjunctive antiseptic therapy, or adjunctive antibiotic therapy) and control treatments were commonly associated with residual BI and BOP scores at 3 to 12 months after therapy (Tables 6, 7 and 8).

**Alternative measures for biofilm removal** Six RCTs (corresponding to 7 publications) reported on the efficacy of alternative measures for biofilm removal (Table 6). In particular, two studies employed the same type of an ultrasonic device used with a hydroxyapatite

**Table 2** Risk of bias summary for finally selected randomized studies

| | Random sequence generation | Allocation concealment | Blinding of participants and personnel | Blinding of outcome assessment | Incomplete outcome data |
|---|---|---|---|---|---|
| Schenk et al. [16] | ? | – | – | – | + |
| Strooker et al. [22] | ? | – | – | – | + |
| Porras et al. [20] | ? | – | – | + | – |
| Büchter et al. [26] | + | – | – | ? | + |
| Romeo et al. [42, 57] | ? | – | – | – | + |
| Karring et al. [28] | ? | + | – | + | + |
| Schwarz et al. [25] | + | – | – | + | + |
| Renvert et al. [32] | + | + | – | + | + |
| Schwarz et al. [24] | + | – | – | + | + |
| Schwarz et al. [48, 51, 54] | + | – | – | + | + |
| Renvert et al. [29] | + | + | – | + | + |
| Renvert et al. [31] | + | ? | – | + | + |
| Renvert et al. [30] | + | – | – | + | + |
| Sahm et al.; John et al. [27, 33] | + | – | – | + | + |
| Thone-Mühling et al. [17] | – | ? | – | – | + |
| Hallström et al. [19] | + | ? | – | – | + |
| Schwarz et al. [49, 50, 52] | + | – | – | + | + |
| Aghanzadeh et al. [43] | ? | ? | – | + | + |
| Machtei et al. [23] | + | + | ? | + | + |
| Wohlfahrt et al. [55, 58] | + | + | – | + | + |
| deWaal et al. [38] | + | + | ? | + | + |
| McKenna et al. [78] | + | – | + | + | – |
| Schär et al.; Bassetti et al. [34, 37] | + | – | – | + | |
| deWaal et al. [39] | + | + | ? | + | + |
| Ji et al. [15] | + | ? | – | + | + |
| Papadopoulos et al. [41] | + | – | – | + | + |
| Riben Grundström et al. [21] | + | + | – | + | + |

+ low, – high, ? unclear

fluid polish [28, 31], while two studies reported on erbium-doped yttrium aluminum garnet (Er:YAG) laser monotherapy [24, 25] and two publications on glycine powder air polishing [27, 33]. One study compared Er:YAG laser monotherapy versus air polishing [30].

At 3 months after therapy, nonsurgical ultrasonic debridement was associated with a reduction in mean BOP scores, whereas these values further increased at control sites (i.e. carbon fibre curettes). However, these differences, as well as those noted for mean PD and radiographic bone level changes, did not reach statistical significance between groups [28]. Similarly, when comparing ultrasonic scaling with mechanical debridement using titanium curettes, Renvert et al. [31] also failed to identify any significant between group differences in mean BI and PD reductions at 6 months. Furthermore, both procedures did not reduce bacterial load [35] (Table 6).

In two RCTs, the efficacy of Er:YAG laser monotherapy was compared to that of mechanical debridement using carbon fibre curettes + adjunctive local antiseptic CHX irrigation/application [24, 25]. After 6 months of healing, Er:YAG laser application was associated with significantly lower mean BOP scores than the control treatment. However, these improvements failed to reach statistical significance at 12 months, particularly at advanced sites [24, 25] (Table 6). In one RCT, glycine powder air polishing resulted in a significantly higher reduction of mean BOP scores at 3, 6, and 12 months

**Table 3** Included studies—nonsurgical treatment of peri-implant mucositis: alternative or adjunctive measures for biofilm removal

| Publication | Design | Population | Case definition | Period | Test | Control | Mean (SD) outcome |
|---|---|---|---|---|---|---|---|
| Ji et al. [15] | RCT, parallel | 24 patients | PD ≥4 mm, BOP + no radiographic bone loss compared with baseline (i.e. immediately after prosthesis installation) | 3 months | OHI + mechanical debridement (ultrasonic scaler with carbon fibre tips) + air abrasive device, glycine powder (sites with PD ≥4 mm) | OHI + mechanical debridement (ultrasonic scaler with carbon fibre tips) | Test |
| | | 33 implants | | | | | BI: 1.4 (0.57) (BL) to 1.1 (0.58) (3 months, subject level) |
| | | Molar/premolar sites | | | | | BI: 1.7 (0.93) (BL) to 1.1 (0.98) (3 months, implant level) |
| | | 1 implant system | | | | | Sites without bleeding: 29.3 % |
| | | | | | | | PD: 3.6 (0.47) (BL) to 3.2 (0.48) mm (3 months, subject level) |
| | | | | | | | Control |
| | | | | | | | BI: 1.5 (0.65) (BL) to 1.0 (0.85) (3 months, subject level) |
| | | | | | | | BI: 1.7 (1.0) (BL) to 0.9 (1.1) (3 months, implant level) |
| | | | | | | | Sites without bleeding: 42 % |
| | | | | | | | PD: 3.5 (0.5) (BL) to 3.1 (0.38) mm (3 months, subject level) |
| De Siena et al. [18] | CCT, parallel | 30 patients | BOP or spontaneous bleeding with local swelling | 6 months | OHI + mechanical debridement Teflon curettes, polishing) + air abrasive device, glycine powder | OHI + mechanical debridement Teflon curettes, polishing) | Test |
| | | No information on number and types of implants | PD ≤3.5 mm | | | | PD: 3.0 (0.4) (BL) to 2.4 (0.5) mm (6 months, subject level) |
| | | | Bone loss ≤ 3.0 mm | | | | 13 patients did not present bleeding at 6 months |
| | | | | | | | Control |
| | | | | | | | PD: 2.9 (0.4) (BL) to 3.0 (0.6) mm (6 months, subject level) |
| | | | | | | | 9 patients did not present bleeding at 6 months |

**Table 3** Included studies—nonsurgical treatment of peri-implant mucositis: alternative or adjunctive measures for biofilm removal *(Continued)*

| | | | | | | | |
|---|---|---|---|---|---|---|---|
| | | | | | | | BI and PD scores sign. lower in the test group at 6 months |
| Riben Grundström et al. [21] | RCT, parallel | 37 patients | PD ≥4 mm, BOP + with or without suppuration | 12 months | OHI + air abrasive device, glycine powder | OHI + mechanical debridement (ultrasonic scaler with plastic coated tips) | Test |
| | | One implant per subject used | Bone loss ≤2 mm from implant shoulder | | Repeated treatment at 3 and 6 months | Repeated treatment at 3 and 6 months | BOP: 43.9 (7.3) (BL) to 12.1 (3.8) % (12 months, subject level) |
| | | Test $N = 19$ | | | | | Number of diseased sites (pocket depth ≥4 mm with bleeding/ suppuration) |
| | | Control $N = 18$ | | | | | 38 % (BL) to 8 % (12 months, subject level) |
| | | | | | | | Control |
| | | | | | | | BOP: 53.7 (7.9) (BL) to 18.6 (6.4) % (12 months, subject level) |
| | | | | | | | Number of diseased sites (pocket depth ≥4 mm with bleeding/ suppuration) |
| | | | | | | | 52 % (BL) to 17 % (12 months, subject level) |
| | | | | | | | No significant differences between groups for either reduction of |
| | | | | | | | BOP or of diseased sites |

*BI* bleeding index, *BL* baseline, *BOP* bleeding on probing, *CCT* non-randomized controlled clinical study, *OHI* oral hygiene instructions, *PD* probing pocket depth, *RCT* randomized controlled clinical study

**Table 4** Included studies—nonsurgical treatment of peri-implant mucositis: adjunctive antiseptic therapy

| Publication | Design | Population | Case definition | Period | Test | Control | Mean (SD) outcome |
|---|---|---|---|---|---|---|---|
| Strooker et al. [22] | RCT Split-mouth design | 16 patients each with 4 mandibular implants and bar retained over denture | Not reported | 5 months | Supra-/subgingival scaling (carbon curettes) + polishing (rubber cup) + phosphoric acid gel (35 %) in sulcus for 1 min | Supra-/subgingival scaling (carbon curettes) + polishing (rubber cup) Once every month | Test (subject level) |
| | | | | | Once every month | | BOP: 30.5 (27.5) (BL) to 9.7 (10.97) % (5 months) |
| | | | | | | | GI: 0.92 (0.75) (BL) to 0.34 (0.38) (5 months) |
| | | | | | | | PD: 2.97 (0.68) (BL) to 2.34 (0.54) mm (5 months) |
| | | | | | | | Control (subject level) |
| | | | | | | | BOP: 29.2 (29.44) (BL) to 14.3 (22.47) % (5 months) |
| | | | | | | | GI: 0.82 (0.8) (BL) to 0.57 (0.6) (5 months) |
| | | | | | | | PD: 2.83 (0.57) (BL) to 2.48 (0.49) mm (5 months) |
| | | | | | | | Sign. between group difference in mean GI values and colony-forming units at 5 months |
| Porras et al. [20] | RCT, parallel | 16 patients | Supra- and subgingival plaque | 3 months | OHI + mechanical cleansing (plastic scaler, rubber cups, polishing paste) + local irrigation CHX (0.12 %) and topical CHX gel application + 0.12 % CHX mouthrinse twice for 10 days | OHI + mechanical cleansing (plastic scaler, rubber cups, polishing paste) | mBI and BOP (%) scores: no sign. differences between groups at 1 and 3 months |
| | | 28 implants | PD ≤5 mm BOP + "incipient" radiographic lesion | | | | PD values: |
| | | 3 implant types (plasma-sprayed Ti/ cp Ti (HA-coated Ti) | | | | | Test: 3.27 (0.81) (BL) to 2.71 (0.70) mm (3 months) |
| | | | | | | | Control: 3.48 (0.61) (BL) to 2.55 (0.72) mm (3 months) |
| | | | | | | | Changes in mean PD between test and control groups at 3 months were statistically significant (0.56 vs. 0.93 mm) |
| | | | | | | | Microbiological improvements in both groups |

**Table 4** Included studies—nonsurgical treatment of peri-implant mucositis: adjunctive antiseptic therapy *(Continued)*

| | | | | | | | |
|---|---|---|---|---|---|---|---|
| Thone-Mühling et al. [17] | RCT, parallel | 11 patients | BOP + and/or GI ≥1 absence of radiographic bone loss during the last 2 years | 8 months | OHI + mechanical cleansing (plastic scaler and polyetheretherketone-coated ultrasonic instruments) + topical CHX gel application once + full mouth disinfection (deep scaling in one session + CHX disinfection of tongue and tonsils) + 0.2 % CHX mouthrinse 2×/day and tonsil spraying 1×/day for 14 days | OHI + mechanical cleansing (plastic scaler and polyetheretherketone-coated ultrasonic instruments) + full mouth scaling in one session | Test |
| | | 36 implants | | | | | BOP: 0.22 (0.11) (BL) to 0.16 (0.09) % (8 months) |
| | | 2 implant types | | | | | GI: 0.6 (0.24) (BL) to 0.44 (0.23) (8 months) |
| | | | | | | | PD: 3.4 (0.68) (BL) to 2.82 (0.59) mm (8 months) |
| | | | | | | | Control |
| | | | | | | | BOP: 0.17 (0.19) (BL) to 0.17 (0.11) % (8 months) |
| | | | | | | | GI: 0.62 (0.36) (BL) to 0.43 (0.37) (8 months) |
| | | | | | | | PD: 3.49 (0.78) (BL) to 2.84 (0.64) mm (8 months) |
| | | | | | | | Bacterial recolonization over time |

*BL* baseline, *BOP* bleeding on probing, *GI* modified gingival index, *mBI* modified bleeding index, *OHI* oral hygiene instructions, *PD* probing pocket depth, *RCT* randomized controlled clinical study

**Table 5** Included studies—nonsurgical treatment of peri-implant mucositis: adjunctive antibiotic therapy

| Publication | Design | Population | Case definition | Period | Test | Control | Mean (SD) outcome |
|---|---|---|---|---|---|---|---|
| Schenk et al. [16] | RCT Split-mouth design | 8 patients | PD >4 mm BOP on at least 1 site per implant ± mucosal hyperplasia no radiographic bone loss | 3 months | Supra-/subgingival scaling (steel curettes) + polishing (rubber cup) + locally delivered tetracycline HCl (25 %) fibre for 10 days +0.2 % CHX mouthrinse twice for 10 days | Supra-/subgingival scaling (steel curettes) + polishing (rubber cup) + +0.2 % CHX mouthrinse twice for 10 days | ΔBOP (3 months, subject level) |
| | | 24 implants | | | | | Test: −17 ± 25 % |
| | | 1 implant type (endossous part: titanium and zirconoxide/transmucosal part: titanium oxinitride) | | | | | Control: 15 ± 37 % |
| | | | | | | | PD/CAL values without significant changes in both groups |
| | | | | | | | No adverse events |
| | | | | | | | Partial/complete fibre loss at three sites |
| Hallström et al. [19] | RCT, parallel | 45 patients | PD ≥4 mm BOP + and/or pus | 6 months | OHI + mechanical cleansing (titanium curettes + rubber cups + polishing paste) + Azithromycin® 500 mg day 1 and 250 mg days 2–4 | OHI + mechanical cleansing (titanium curettes + rubber cups + polishing paste) | Test |
| | | 3 implant systems | Radiographic bone loss ≤2 mm | | | | BOP: 82.6 (24.4) (BL) to 27.3 (18.8) % (6 months, subject level) |
| | | | | | | | PD at worst site: 5.5 (0.8) (BL) to 4.1 (1.2) mm (6 months, subject level) |
| | | | | | | | Control |
| | | | | | | | BOP: 80.0 (25.0) (BL) to 47.5 (32.3) % (6 months, subject level) |
| | | | | | | | PD at worst site: 5.7 (0.8) (BL) to 4.9 (1.1) mm (6 months, subject level) |
| | | | | | | | Odds ratio of a positive treatment outcome (PD ≤ 4.0 mm and BOP ≤ 1) was 4.5:1 (test vs. control) |
| | | | | | | | Comparable reductions in bacterial counts |

*BL* baseline, *BOP* bleeding on probing, *CAL* clinical attachment level, *OHI* oral hygiene instructions, *PD* probing pocket depth, *RCT* randomized controlled clinical study

**Table 6** Included studies—nonsurgical treatment of peri-implantitis: alternative measures for biofilm removal

| Publication | Design | Population | Case definition | Period | Test | Control | Mean (SD) outcome |
|---|---|---|---|---|---|---|---|
| Karring et al. [28] | | 11 patients | PD ≥5 mm, BOP + bone loss >1.5 mm and exposed threads | 3 months | OHI + ultrasonic device with hydroxyapatite fluid polish | OHI + mechanical debridement (carbon fibre curettes) | Test |
| | | 22 implants machined and medium-rough surfaces | | | | | BOP: 63.6 (BL) to 36.4 % (3 months, subject level) |
| | | | | | | | PD: 5.8 (1.1) (BL) to 5.8 (1.2) mm (3 months, subject level) |
| | | | | | | | Radiographic bone level changes: 0.1 (0.5) mm (3 months, subject level) |
| | | | | | | | Control |
| | | | | | | | BOP: 72.7 (BL) to 81.8 % (3 months, subject level) |
| | | | | | | | PD: 6.2 (1.6) (BL) to 6.3 (2.2) mm (3 months, subject level) |
| | | | | | | | Radiographic bone level changes: −0.2 (1.2) mm (3 months, subject level) |
| | | | | | | | Absence of BOP at 7/11 (test) and 2/11 (control) sites |
| Schwarz et al. [25] | RCT, parallel | 20 patients | PD ≥4 mm, BOP + and pus | 6 months | OHI + Er:YAG laser device (cone-shaped glass fibre tip) at 12.7 J/cm$^2$ | OHI + mechanical debridement (plastic curettes), 0.2 % CHX pocket irrigation and 0.2 % CHX gel | Test |
| | | 32 implants rough and medium-rough surfaces | Radiographic bone loss | | | | BOP: 83.2 (17.2) (BL) to 31.1 (10.1) % (6 months, subject level) |
| | | | | | | | PD: 5.4 (1.2) (BL) to 4.6 (1.1) mm (6 months, subject level) |
| | | | | | | | Control |
| | | | | | | | BOP: 81.3 (19.0) (BL) to 58.3 (16.9) % (6 months, subject level) |
| | | | | | | | PD: 5.5 (1.5) (BL) to 4.8 (1.4) mm (6 months, subject level) |
| | | | | | | | BOP scores at 6 months were significantly lower in the test group |

**Table 6** Included studies—nonsurgical treatment of peri-implantitis: alternative measures for biofilm removal *(Continued)*

| | | | | | | | |
|---|---|---|---|---|---|---|---|
| Schwarz et al. [24] | RCT, parallel | 20 patients | PD ≥4 mm, BOP + and pus | 12 months | OHI + Er:YAG laser device (cone-shaped glass fibre tip) at 12.7 J/cm$^2$ | OHI + mechanical debridement (plastic curettes), 0.2 % CHX pocket irrigation and 0.2 % CHX gel | Test |
| | | 40 implants rough and medium-rough surfaces | Radiographic bone loss | | | | Moderately deep sites |
| | | | | | | | BOP: 81.7 (6.7) (BL) to 35.0 (6.3) % (12 months, subject level) |
| | | | | | | | PD: 4.5 (1.4) (BL) to 4.0 (0.1) mm (12 months, subject level) |
| | | | | | | | Deep sites |
| | | | | | | | BOP: 79.9 (4.8) (BL) to 55.0 (6.5) % (12 months, subject level) |
| | | | | | | | PD: 5.9 (0.1) (BL) to 5.4 (0.1) mm (12 months, subject level) |
| | | | | | | | Control |
| | | | | | | | Moderately deep sites |
| | | | | | | | BOP: 81.6 (5.2) (BL) to 53.3 (7.3) % (12 months, subject level) |
| | | | | | | | PD: 4.4 (0.2) (BL) to 4.3 (0.1) mm (12 months, subject level) |
| | | | | | | | Deep sites |
| | | | | | | | BOP: 88.3 (3.5) (BL) to 66.6 (5.5) % (12 months, subject level) |
| | | | | | | | PD: 5.9 (0.3) (BL) to 5.5 (0.2) mm (12 months, subject level) |
| | | | | | | | No significant differences between groups at 12 months |
| Renvert et al. [31] | RCT, parallel | 31 patients | PD ≥4 mm, BOP + and/or pus | 6 months | OHI + ultrasonic device with hydroxyapatite fluid polish | OHI + mechanical debridement (titanium curettes) | Test |
| | | 31 implants machined and medium-rough surfaces | Bone loss <2.5 mm | | | | BI: 1.7 (0.6) (BL) to 1.2 (0.7) (6 months, subject level) |
| | | | | | | | PD: 4.3 (0.6) (BL) to 3.9 (0.8) mm (6 months, subject level) |
| | | | | | | | Control |
| | | | | | | | BI: 1.7 (0.9) (BL) to 1.4 (1.0) (6 months, subject level) |

**Table 6** Included studies—nonsurgical treatment of peri-implantitis: alternative measures for biofilm removal *(Continued)*

| | | | | | | | |
|---|---|---|---|---|---|---|---|
| | | | | | | | PD: 6.2 (1.6) (BL) to 6.3 (2.2) mm (6 months, subject level) |
| | | | | | | | No significant differences between groups |
| Renvert et al. [30] | RCT, parallel | 42 patients | PD ≥5 mm, BOP + and/or pus | 6 months | OHI + air abrasive device, glycine powder | OHI + Er:YAG laser device (cone-shaped glass fibre tip, 12.7 J/cm$^2$) | Test |
| | | 90 implants machined and medium-rough surfaces | Bone loss >3 mm | | | | PD changes: 0.9 (0.8) mm (6 months, implant level) |
| | | | | | | | Radiographic bone level change: −0.3(0.9) mm (6 months, subject level) |
| | | | | | | | Positive treatment outcome: 47 % |
| | | | | | | | Control |
| | | | | | | | PD changes: 0.8 (0.5) mm (6 months, implant level) |
| | | | | | | | Radiographic bone level change: −0.1(0.8) mm (6 months, subject level) |
| | | | | | | | Positive treatment outcome: 44 % |
| | | | | | | | No significant differences between groups |
| Sahm et al.; John et al. [27, 33] | RCT, parallel | 32 patients (BL) | PD ≥4 mm, BOP + with suppuration | 12 months | OHI + air abrasive device, glycine powder | OHI + mechanical debridement (carbon curettes + 0.1 % CHX) | Test |
| | | 25 patients (12 months) | Bone loss ≤33 % | | | | BOP: 99.0 (4.1) (BL) to 57.8 (30.7) % (12 months, subject level) |
| | | 36 implants | | | | | PD: 3.7 (1.0) (BL) to 3.2 (1.1) mm (12 months, subject level) |
| | | 8 implant systems | | | | | Control |
| | | | | | | | BOP: 94.7 (13.7) (BL) to 78.1 (30.0) % (12 months, subject level) |
| | | | | | | | PD: 3.9 (1.1) (BL) to 3.5 (1.2) mm (12 months, subject level) |
| | | | | | | | BOP: significant difference between groups at 3, 6 and 12 months |

*BI* bleeding index, *BL* baseline, *BOP* bleeding on probing, *CHX* chlorhexidine digluconate, *OHI* oral hygiene instructions, *PD* probing pocket depth, *RCT* randomized controlled clinical study

**Table 7** Included studies—nonsurgical treatment of peri-implantitis: adjunctive antiseptic therapy

| Publication | Design | Population | Case definition | Period | Test | Control | Mean (SD) outcome |
|---|---|---|---|---|---|---|---|
| Machtei et al. [23] | Multicentre RCT, parallel | 60 patients | PD = 6–10 mm and BOP + radiographic bone loss | 6 months | OHI + ultrasonic debridement + matrix containing 2.5-mg CHX chips (i.e. up to 4 per implant site) | OHI + ultrasonic debridement + biodegradable crosslinked gelatin matrix chip | Test |
| | | 77 implants | | | Repeated application at sites with PD ≥6 mm at 2, 4, 6, 8, 12 and 18 weeks | Repeated application at sites with PD ≥6 mm at 2, 4, 6, 8, 12 and 18 weeks | BOP: 100 (0.0) (BL) to 42.5 (50.0) % (6 months, subject level) |
| | | | | | | | PD: 7.6 (1.1) (0.0) to 5.47 (1.86) mm (6 months, subject level) |
| | | | | | | | Control |
| | | | | | | | BOP: 100 (0.0) (BL) to 54.5 (50.5) % (6 months, subject level) |
| | | | | | | | PD: 7.21 (1.08) (BL) to 5.48 (1.25) mm (6 months, subject level) |
| | | | | | | | BOP and PD reductions at 6 months not sign. different between groups |

*BL* baseline, *BOP* bleeding on probing, *CHX* chlorhexidine digluconate, *OHI* oral hygiene instructions, *PD* probing pocket depth, *RCT* randomized controlled clinical study

when compared with mechanical debridement + local antiseptic therapy using CHX. The application of this specific air abrasive device was not associated with any emphysema formation or complications in peri-implant wound healing [27, 33]. At more advanced sites, Er:YAG laser monotherapy and glycine powder air polishing resulted in comparable BOP/PD reductions and crestal bone level changes, but failed to reduce bacterial load [36] (Table 6).

**Adjunctive antiseptic therapy** One multicenter RCT reported on the adjunctive antispective therapy to ultrasonic debridement (Table 7). In particular, a CHX containing matrix was repeatedly applied at 2, 4, 6, 8, 12 and 18 weeks until PD was reduced to ≤5 mm. At 6 months, CHX chips resulted in a significantly higher PD reduction than the placebo chips [23].

**Adjunctive antibiotic therapy** Three RCTs reported on the adjunctive local antibiotic therapy to mechanical debridement (Table 8). In particular, minocycline microspheres were either applied once [32] at baseline or repeatedly [29] at 30 and 90 days and compared with local antispectic therapy using CHX gel (1.0 %). At 12 months, minocycline was associated with significantly higher BOP (refers to a repeated application) and PD (refers to a single application) reductions when compared with the control group. The radiographic (refers to a repeated application) and microbiological analyses failed to reveal any significant differences between both groups. Similar clinical outcomes were also noted when doxycycline hyclate was used as an adjunct to mechanical debridement [26].

In one RCT, adjunctive local antibiotic therapy (minocycline microspheres) was compared to adjunctive antimicrobial photodynamic therapy. At 12 months, both test and control groups were associated with significant but comparable clinical, microbiological and immunological improvements [34, 37] (Table 8).

The weighted mean (WM) BOP and PD reductions following conventional nonsurgical treatment (referring to the control groups in respective studies) [23–27] amounted to 31.12 % [SE = 9.14; 95 % CI (12.20, 49.05)] and 0.71 mm [SE = 0.32; 95 % CI (0.07, 1.35)], respectively. The weighted mean (WM) BOP and PD reductions for alternative/adjunctive measures (i.e. air polishing, aPDT, CHX chip, doxycycline, Er:YAG laser) [23–27] amounted to 42.85 % [SE = 9.24; 95 % CI (24.70, 60.97)] and 0.87 mm [SE = 0.29; 95 % CI (0.29, 1.44)], respectively.

**Table 8** Included studies—nonsurgical treatment of peri-implantitis: adjunctive antibiotic therapy

| Publication | Design | Population | Case definition | Period | Test | Control | Mean (SD) outcome |
|---|---|---|---|---|---|---|---|
| Büchter et al. [26] | RCT, parallel | 28 patients | PD >5 mm | 18 weeks | OHI + mechanical debridement (plastic curettes) + 0.2 % CHX pocket irrigation + 8 % doxycycline hyclate | OHI + mechanical debridement (plastic curettes) + 0.2 % CHX pocket irrigation | Test |
| | | 48 implants medium-rough surfaces | Bone loss >50 % | | | | BOP: 0.54 (0.07) (BL) to 0.27 (0.06) % (18 weeks, subject level) |
| | | | | | | | PD: 5.64 (0.32) (BL) to 4.49 (0.29) mm (18 weeks, subject level) |
| | | | | | | | Control |
| | | | | | | | BOP: 0.63 (0.06) (BL) to 0.50 (0.07) % (18 weeks, subject level) |
| | | | | | | | PD: 5.68 (0.28) (BL) to 5.4 (0.34) mm (18 weeks, subject level) |
| | | | | | | | BOP and PD reductions sign. higher in the test group |
| Renvert et al. [32] | RCT, parallel | 32 patients | PD ≥4 mm, BOP + with suppuration | 12 months | OHI + mechanical debridement (scalers + rubber cup + polishing) + 1 mg minoycycline microspheres | OHI + mechanical debridement (scalers + rubber cup + polishing) + 1.0 % chlorhexidine gel | Test |
| | | 1–5 (test)/1–6 (control) implants per patient machined surfaces | Bone loss ≤3 threads | | | | BOP: 88 (12) (BL) to 71 (22) % (12 months, subject level) |
| | | | Presence of anaerobic bacteria | | | | PD: 3.9 (0.7) (BL) to 3.6 (0.6) mm (12 months, subject level) |
| | | | | | | | Control |
| | | | | | | | BOP: 86 (14) (BL) to 78 (13) % (12 months, subject level) |
| | | | | | | | PD: 3.9 (0.3) (BL) to 3.9 (0.4) mm (12 months, subject level) |
| | | | | | | | PD reductions at 12 months sign. higher in the test group |
| | | | | | | | Comparable microbiological improvements in both groups |
| Renvert et al. [29] | RCT, parallel | 32 patients | PD ≥4 mm, BOP + with suppuration | 12 months | OHI + mechanical debridement + 1 mg minoycycline microspheres | OHI + mechanical debridement + 0.5 ml of 1.0 % CHXgel | Test |
| | | 95 implants machined surfaces | Bone loss ≤3 threads | | Treatment was repeated at days 30 and 90 | Treatment was repeated at days 30 and 90 | BOP: 86.5 (20.1) (BL) to 48.1 (20.7) % (12 months, implant level) |
| | | | Presence of anaerobic bacteria | | | | PD: 3.85 (1.04) (BL) to 3.55 (0.98) mm (12 months, implant level) |

**Table 8** Included studies—nonsurgical treatment of peri-implantitis: adjunctive antibiotic therapy *(Continued)*

| | | | | | | | |
|---|---|---|---|---|---|---|---|
| | | | | | | | Radiographic bone levels: 0.77 (0.85) (BL) to 0.7 (0.85) mm (12 months, implant level) |
| | | | | | | | Control |
| | | | | | | | BOP: 39.2 (17.2) (BL) to 63.5 (19.2) % (12 months, implant level) |
| | | | | | | | PD: 3.87 (1.16) (BL) to 3.72 (1.02) mm (12 months, implant level) |
| | | | | | | | Radiographic bone levels: 0.41 (0.7) (BL) to 0.46 (0.76) mm (12 months, implant level) |
| | | | | | | | BOP reductions at 12 months sign. higher in the test group |
| | | | | | | | Comparable microbiological improvements in both groups |
| Schär et al.; Bassetti et al. [34, 37] | RCT, parallel | 40 patients | PD = 4–6 mm, BOP + bone loss = 0.5–2 mm | 12 months | OHI + mechanical debridement (titanium curettes + glycin powder air polishing, pocket irrigation using 3 % hydrogen peroxide) + aPDT (660 nm, phenothiazine chloride dye) | OHI + mechanical debridement (titanium curettes + glycin powder air polishing, pocket irrigation using 3 % hydrogen peroxide) + minocycline microspheres | Test |
| | | 40 implants medium-rough surfaces | | | | | BOP change: 57 % (12 months, subject level) |
| | | | | | | | PD changes: 0.56 mm (12 months, subject level) |
| | | | | | | | Complete resolution of mucosal inflammation: 31.6 % |
| | | | | | | | Control |
| | | | | | | | BOP change: 65 % (12 months, subject level) |
| | | | | | | | PD changes: 0.11 mm (12 months, subject level) |
| | | | | | | | Complete resolution of mucosal inflammation: 35.0 % |
| | | | | | | | No significant differences in clinical, microbiological and immunological parameters between groups |

*aPDT* antimicrobial photodynamic therapy, *BL* baseline, *BOP* bleeding on probing, *CHX* chlorhexidine digluconate, *OHI* oral hygiene instructions, *PD* probing pocket depth, *RCT* randomized controlled clinical study

**Table 9** Included studies—surgical treatment of peri-implantitis: alternative measures for surface decontamination

| Publication | Design | Population | Case definition | Period | Test | Control | Mean (SD) outcome |
|---|---|---|---|---|---|---|---|
| Deppe et al. [40] | CCT, parallel | 32 patients | PD ≥5 mm, BOP + progressive vertical bone loss | 5 years | OHI + open flap[a] surgery + air polishing + carbon dioxide laser (cw mode, 2.5 W, 12 × 5 s) decontamination + soft tissue resection | OHI + open flap[b] surgery + air polishing + soft tissue resection | Test |
| | | 73 implants machined, rough- and medium-rough surfaces | | | | | SBI: 0.6 (0.3) (BL) to 1.8 (1.1) (48 months, implant level) |
| | | | | | | | PD: 6.1 (1.6) (BL) to 3.4 (1.5) mm (48 months, implant level) |
| | | | | | | | Control |
| | | | | | | | SBI: 0.7 (0.8) (BL) to 1.1 (1.2) (48 months, implant level) |
| | | | | | | | PD: 5.1 (1.3) (BL) to 4.3 (1.2) mm (48 months, implant level) |
| | | | | | | | Comparable outcomes in both groups |
| De Waal et al. [38] | RCT, parallel | 30 patients | PD ≥5 mm, BOP + and/or suppuration | 12 months | OHI/mechanical debridement + resective therapy (apical re-positioned flap + bone re-contouring) + surface debridement using surgical gauzes soaked in saline + decontamination using 0.12 % CHX + 0.05 % cetylpyridinium chloride CPC | OHI/mechanical debridement + resective therapy (apical re-positioned flap + bone re-contouring) + surface debridement using surgical gauzes soaked in saline + decontamination using placebo solution | Test |
| | | 79 implants machined, rough- and medium-rough surfaces | Bone loss ≥2 mm | | | | BOP: 80.4 (26.5) (BL) to 60.5 (30.1) % (12 months, implant level) |
| | | | | | | | PD: 6.6 (1.6) (BL) to 4.3 (2.1) mm (12 months, implant level) |
| | | | | | | | MBL: 4.3 (2.1) (BL) to 5.0 (2.5) mm (12 months, implant level) |
| | | | | | | | Control |
| | | | | | | | BOP: 79.7 (28.1) (BL) to 57.2 (29.0) % (12 months, implant level) |
| | | | | | | | PD: 5.5 (1.4) (BL) to 3.7 (0.8) mm (12 months, implant level) |

**Table 9** Included studies—surgical treatment of peri-implantitis: alternative measures for surface decontamination *(Continued)*

| | | | | | | | |
|---|---|---|---|---|---|---|---|
| | | | | | | | MBL: 3.6 (1.9) (BL) to 3.9 (2.0) mm (12 months, implant level)<br>No sign. differences in BOP and PD reductions between groups |
| De Waal et al. [39] | RCT, parallel | 44 patients | PD ≥5 mm, BOP + and/or suppuration | 12 months | OHI/mechanical debridement + resective therapy (apical re-positioned flap + bone re-contouring) + surface debridement using surgical gauzes soaked in saline + decontamination using 0.12 % CHX + 0.05 % cetylpyridinium chloride | OHI/mechanical debridement – resective therapy (apical re-positioned flap + bone re-contouring) + surface debridement using surgical gauzes soaked in saline + decontamination using 2.0 % CHX | Test |
| | | 108 implants machined, rough- and medium-rough surfaces | Bone loss ≥2 mm | | | | BOP: 82.1 (23.9) (BL) to 42.7 (34.2) % (12 months, implant level)<br>PD: 4.7 (1.0) (BL) to 3.0 (0.7) mm (12 months, implant level)<br>MBL: 4.0 (1.5) (BL) to 4.3 (1.7) mm (12 months, implant level)<br>Control<br>BOP: 74.2 (27.8) (BL) to 37.0 (35.5) % (12 months, implant level)<br>PD: 5.0 (1.2) (BL) to 2.9 (0.7) mm (12 months, implant level)<br>MBL: 4.1 (1.6) (BL) to 4.1 (1.7) mm (12 months, implant level)<br>No sign. differences in BOP and PD reductions between groups |

**Table 9** Included studies—surgical treatment of peri-implantitis: alternative measures for surface decontamination *(Continued)*

| | | | | | | | |
|---|---|---|---|---|---|---|---|
| Papadopoulos et al. [41] | RCT, parallel | 16 patients | PD ≥6 mm, BOP + and/or suppuration | 6 months | Mechanical debridement + open flap surgery + mechanical debridement (plastic curettes) and cotton swabs soaked in saline | Mechanical debridement + open flap surgery + mechanical debridement (plastic curettes) and cotton swabs soaked in saline + 980 nm diode laser application | Test |
| | | 16 implants | Radiographic bone loss ≥2 mm | | | | BOP: 81.2 (BL) to 23.8 % (6 months, implant level)<br>PD: 5.92 (BL) to 4.44 mm (6 months, implant level)<br>Control<br>BOP: 81.2 (BL) to 23.8 % (6 months, implant level)<br>PD: 5.52 (BL) to 4.31 mm (6 months, implant level)<br>Sign. BOP and PD reductions in both groups at 6 months |

*BL* baseline, *BOP* bleeding on probing, *CCT* non-randomized controlled clinical study, *CHX* chlorhexidine digluconate, *MBL* marginal bone level, *OHI* oral hygiene instructions, *PD* probing pocket depth, *RCT* randomized controlled clinical study, *SBI* sulcus bleeding index

[a]Subgroup analysis of $n = 17$ implants

[b]Subgroup analysis of $n = 16$ implants

**Table 10** Included studies—surgical treatment of peri-implantitis: adjunctive resective therapy

| Publication | Design | Population | Case definition | Period | Test | Control | Mean (SD) outcome |
|---|---|---|---|---|---|---|---|
| Romeo et al. [42, 57] | RCT, parallel | 17 patients | Suppuration or sulcus bleeding, PD >4 mm horizontal peri-implant translucency | 36 months systemic antibiotic medication (Amoxicillin for 8 days) | Full mouth disinfection/ mechanical debridement + resective therapy (apical re-positioned flap + bone re-contouring) + decontamination using metronida zole + tetracycline hydro chloride (3 min) + implanto plasty using diamond and arkansas burs/silicone polishers | Full mouth disinfection/ mechanical debridement + resective therapy (apical re-positioned flap + bone re-contouring) + decontam ination using metronidazole + tetracycline hydrochloride (3 min) | Test |
| | | 22 implants rough surfaces | | | | | BOP: 2.83 (0.47) (BL) to 0.5 (0.69) (24 months[a], implant level)PD: 5.79 (1.69) (BL) to 3.58 (1.06) mm (24 months[a], implant level) |
| | | | | | | | MBL: 0.0–0.01 mm (36 months, implant level) |
| | | | | | | | Control |
| | | | | | | | BOP: 2.86 (0.35) (BL) to 2.33 (0.74) (24 months[a], implant level) |
| | | | | | | | PD: 6.52 (1.62) (BL) to 5.5 (1.47) mm (24 months[a], implant level) |
| | | | | | | | MBL: 1.44–1.54 mm (36 months, implant level) |

*BL* baseline, *BOP* bleeding on probing, *MBL* marginal bone loss, *PD* probing pocket depth, *RCT* randomized controlled clinical study
[a]All patients of the control group were discontinued from the study due to persistent clinical signs of inflammation

***Surgical treatment of peri-implantitis***

Twelve studies (18 publications) reported on the surgical treatment of peri-implantitis, employing either alternative measures for surface decontamination (3 RCTs and 1 CCT) [38–41], adjunctive resective (1 RCT) [42] or augmentative (4 RCTs and 4 CCTs) [40, 43–55] therapy. In these studies, peri-implantitis was commonly defined by BOP and a radiographic bone level changes. However, the thresholds used to assess bone loss revealed large variations and defect configurations (i.e. supra-/intrabony defects) [56] were rarely reported (Tables 9, 10 and 11).

**Alternative measures for surface decontamination** In one CCT, Deppe et al. [40] assessed the clinical efficacy of carbon dioxide laser decontamination used as an adjunct to resective flap surgery + air polishing (control). While the test treatment improved the clinical outcomes over the control measure at 4 months, mean SBI and PD values were comparable in both groups at about 5 years (Table 9).

In further two studies, De Waal et al. [38, 39] employed an open flap debridement using gauzes soaked in sterile saline + bone re-contouring + apical flap re-positioning and compared one test (0.12 % CHX + 0.05 % cetylpyridinium chloride) and two control (placebo solution or 2.0 % CHX) measures for surface decontamination. At 12 months, the test and both control procedures were associated with marked but comparable reductions in mean BOP and PD scores, respectively. Furthermore, between group comparisons

**Table 11** Included studies—surgical treatment of peri-implantitis: adjunctive augmentative therapy

| Publication | Design | Population | Case definition | Period | Test | Control | Mean (SD) outcome |
|---|---|---|---|---|---|---|---|
| Schwarz et al. [48, 51, 54] | RCT, parallel | 20 patients | PD >6 mm, BOP + and/ or pus | 4 years nonsubmerged healing | OHI + initial nonsurgical therapy | OHI + initial nonsurgical therapy | Test |
| | | 21 implants machined and medium-rough surfaces | Intrabony defect >3 mm | | Open flap surgery + mechanical debridement (plastic curettes) + nanocrystalline hydroxyapatite paste | Open flap surgery + mechanical debridement (plastic curettes) + bovine-derived xenograft + native collagen barrier membrane | BOP reduction: 32 % (4 years, subject level) |
| | | | | | | | PD reduction: 2.5 (0.9) mm (4 years, subject level) |
| | | | | | | | Control |
| | | | | | | | BOP reduction: 51 % (4 years, subject level) |
| | | | | | | | PD reduction: 1.1 (0.3) mm (4 years, subject level) |
| | | | | | | | BOP and PD reductions sign. higher at control sites |
| Deppe et al. [40] | CCT, parallel | 32 patients | PD ≥5 mm, BOP + progressive vertical bone loss | 5 years | Group 2 OHI + open flap[a] surgery + air polishing + carbon dioxide laser (cw mode, 2.5 W, 12 × 5 s) decontamination + beta tricalcium phosphate + cortical bone chips harvested from the retromoar area (50:50) + nonresorbable synthetic barrier membrane | Group 4 OHI + open flap[b] surgery + air polishing + beta tricalcium phosphate + cortical bone chips harvested from the retromoar area (50:50) + nonresorbable synthetic barrier membrane | Test |
| | | 73 implants machined, rough- and medium-rough surfaces | | | | | SBI: 0.5 (0.8) (BL) to 2.1 (1.4) (48 months, implant level) |
| | | | | | | | PD: 4.8 (1.4) (BL) to 2.5 (1.1) mm (48 months, implant level) |
| | | | | | | | Control |
| | | | | | | | SBI: 1.2 (0.6) (BL) to 1.9 (1.0) (48 months, implant level) |
| | | | | | | | PD: 5.7 (1.4) (BL) to 2.5 (1.4) mm (48 months, implant level) |

**Table 11** Included studies—surgical treatment of peri-implantitis: adjunctive augmentative therapy *(Continued)*

| | | | | | | | |
|---|---|---|---|---|---|---|---|
| | | | | | | | Comparable outcomes in both groups |
| Roos-Jansaker et al. [45–47] | CCT, parallel | 25 patients | BOP + and/or pus | 5 years transmucosal healing systemic antibiotic medication (amoxicillin + metronidazole for 10 days) | Removal of the suprastructure | Removal of the suprastructure | Test |
| | | 45 implants machined and medium-rough surfaces | Bone loss ≥3 threads one- to four-wall defects | | Open flap surgery + debridement + decontamination using hydrogen peroxide 3 % algae derived xenograft + resorbable synthetic barrier membrane | Open flap surgery + debridement + decontamination using hydrogen peroxide 3 % algae derived xenograft + | PD reduction: 3.0 (2.4) mm (5 years, implant level) |
| | | | | | | | Radiographic defect fill: 0.1 (0.5) mm (5 years, implant level) |
| | | | | | | | Control |
| | | | | | | | PD reduction: 3.3 (2.0) mm (5 years, implant level) |
| | | | | | | | Radiographic defect fill: 0.1 (0.5) mm (5 years, implant level) |
| | | | | | | | Comparable defect fill and BOP reductions in both groups |
| Schwarz et al. [53] | CCT, parallel | 27 patients | PD >6 mm, BOP + and/or pus | 12 months nonsubmerged healing | Circumferential-type (Ie) defects OHI + initial nonsurgical therapy | Buccal dehiscence-type defects with a semicircular (Ib) or circular component (Ic) | Test Ib |
| | | 27 implants machined and medium-rough surfaces | Intrabony defect >3 mm | | Open flap surgery + mechanical debridement (carbon curettes) + decontamination (cotton pellets soaked in saline) | OHI + initial nonsurgical therapy Open flap surgery + Mechanical debridement (carbon curettes) + decontamination (cotton pellets soaked in saline) | BOP reduction: 38.9 (16.6) % (12 months, subject level) |
| | | | Supracrestal component ≤1 mm | | Bovine-derived xenograft + native collagen barrier membrane | Bovine-derived xenograft + native collagen barrier membrane | PD reduction: 1.6 (0.9) mm (12 months, subject level) |
| | | | | | | | Test Ic |
| | | | | | | | BOP reduction: 25.9 (14.7) % (12 months, subject level) |
| | | | | | | | PD reduction: 1.6 (0.7) mm (12 months, subject level) |
| | | | | | | | Control Ie |
| | | | | | | | BOP reduction: 61.1 (16.7) % (12 months, subject level) |

**Table 11** Included studies—surgical treatment of peri-implantitis: adjunctive augmentative therapy *(Continued)*

| | | | | | | | |
|---|---|---|---|---|---|---|---|
| | | | | | | | PD reduction: 2.7 (0.7) mm (12 months, subject level) |
| | | | | | | | Sign. difference in BOP reductions between Ic and Ie |
| Rocuzzo et al. [44] | CCT, parallel | 26 patients | PD ≥6 mm | 12 months nonsubmerged healing simultaneous connective tissue graft at sites lacking keratinized mucosa systemic antibiotic medication (amoxicillin + clavulanic acid for 6 days) | SLA surfaced implants | TPS surfaced implants | Test |
| | | 26 implants rough and medium-rough surfaces | Crater-like (intrabony) defects | | OHI | OHI | BOP reduction: 60.4 % (12 months, subject level) |
| | | | | | Open flap surgery + mechanical debridement (plastic curettes) + decontamination (24 % EDTA and 1 % CHX gel) + bovine-derived xenograft | Open flap surgery + mechanical debridement (plastic curettes) + decontamination (24 % EDTA and 1 % CHX gel) + bovine-derived xenograft | PD reduction: 3.4 (1.7) mm (12 months, subject level) |
| | | | | | | | Radiographic defect fill: 1.9 (1.3) mm (12 months, subject level) |
| | | | | | | | Control |
| | | | | | | | BOP reduction: 33.9 % (12 months, subject level) |
| | | | | | | | PD reduction: 2.1 (1.2) mm (12 months, subject level) |
| | | | | | | | Radiographic defect fill: 1.6 (0.7) mm (12 months, subject level) |
| | | | | | | | BOP and PD reductions sign. higher in the test group |

**Table 11** Included studies—surgical treatment of peri-implantitis: adjunctive augmentative therapy *(Continued)*

| | | | | | | | |
|---|---|---|---|---|---|---|---|
| Schwarz et al. [49, 50, 52] | RCT, parallel | 17 patients | PD >6 mm, BOP + and/ or pus | 4 years nonsubmerged healing | OHI + initial nonsurgical therapy | OHI + initial nonsurgical therapy | Test |
| | | 17 implants machined and medium-rough surfaces | Intrabony defect >3 mm | | Open flap surgery + debridement + decontamination using an Er:YAG laser device (cone-shaped glass fibre tip) at 11.4 J/cm$^2$ implantoplasty at bucally and supracrestally exposed implant parts | Open flap surgery + Mechanical debridement (plastic curettes) + decontamination (cotton pellets soaked in saline) implantoplasty at bucally and supracrestally exposed implant parts | BOP reduction: 71.6 (24.9) % (4 years, subject level) |
| | | | Supracrestal component >1 mm | | Bovine-derived xenograft + native collagen barrier membrane at intrabony components | Bovine-derived xenograft + native collagen barrier membrane at intrabony components | PD reduction: 1.3 (1.8) mm (4 years, subject level) |
| | | | | | | | Control |
| | | | | | | | BOP reduction: 85.2 (16.4) % (4 years, subject level) |
| | | | | | | | PD reduction: 1.2 (1.9) mm (4 years, subject level) |
| | | | | | | | BOP and PD reductions comparable in both groups |
| Aghanzadeh et al. [43] | RCT, parallel | 45 patients | PD ≥2 mm, BOP + and pus | 12 months nonsubmerged healing systemic antibiotic medication (Azithromycin for 4 days) | Open flap surgery + mechanical debridement (titanium instruments) + decontamination using hydrogen peroxide 3 % cortical bone chips harvested from the mandibular ramus + resorbable synthetic barrier membrane | Open flap surgery + mechanical debridement (titanium instruments) + decontamination using hydrogen peroxide 3 % bovine-derived xenograft + resorbable synthetic barrier membrane | Test |
| | | 75 implants medium-rough surfaces | Bone loss ≥2 mm | | | | BOP reduction: 44.8 (6.3) % (12 months, implant level) |
| | | | Angular defects ≥3 mm in depth | | | | PD reduction: 2.0 (0.3) mm (12 months, implant level) |
| | | | | | | | Radiographic bone level gain: 0.2 (0.3) mm (12 months, implant level) |
| | | | | | | | Control |
| | | | | | | | BOP reduction: 50.4 (5.3 %) (12 months, implant level) |
| | | | | | | | PD reduction: 3.1 (0.2)mm (12 months, implant level) |

**Table 11** Included studies—surgical treatment of peri-implantitis: adjunctive augmentative therapy *(Continued)*

| | | | | | | | | |
|---|---|---|---|---|---|---|---|---|
| | | | | | | | | Radiographic bone level gain: 0.8 (0.4) mm (12 months, implant level) |
| | | | | | | | | PD reductions and bone level gains were significantly higher at control sites |
| Wohlfahrt et al. [55, 58] | RCT, parallel | 33 patients | PD ≥5 mm, BOP + intrabony defects ≥4 mm | 12 months submerged healing for 6 months | | Open flap surgery + mechanical debridement (titanium curettes) + conditioning using 24 % ethylenediaminetetraacetic acid gel (2 min) + augmentation of intrabony defect components using porous titanium granules | Open flap surgery + mechanical debridement (titanium currettes) + conditioning using 24 % ethylenediaminetetraacetic acid gel (2 min) | Test |
| | | 33 implants medium-rough surfaces | | | | | | BOP reduction: 0.38 (2.1) % (12 months, implant level) |
| | | | | | | | | PD reduction: 1.7 (1.7) mm (12 months, implant level) |
| | | | | | | | | Radiographic defect fill: 57.0 (45.1) % (12 months, implant level) |
| | | | | | | | | Control |
| | | | | | | | | BOP reduction: 0.56 (2.9) % (12 months, implant level) |
| | | | | | | | | PD reduction: 2.0 (2.3) mm (12 months, implant level) |
| | | | | | | | | Radiographic defect fill: −14.8 (83.4) % (12 months, implant level) no sign. reductions in BOP scores in both groups comparable reductions in MMP-8 and bone level markers |

*BL* baseline, *BOP* bleeding on probing, *CCT* non-randomized controlled clinical study, *CHX* chlorhexidine dugluconate, *MMP-8* matrixmetalloproteinase-8, *PD* probing pocket depth, *RCT* randomized controlled clinical study, *SBI* sulcus bleeding index, *SLA* sand blasted and acid etched, *TPS* titanium plasma flamed

[a]Subgroup analysis of $n = 11$ implants

[b]Subgroup analysis of $n = 13$ implants

failed to reveal any significant differences in mean marginal bone loss after therapy [38, 39]. Similarly, Papadopoulos et al. [41] also failed to reveal any significant clinical improvements in mean BOP and PD scores at 6 months, when a 980-nm diode laser was used as an adjunct to mechanical open flap debridement (Table 9).

**Adjunctive resective therapy** One study assessed the clinical efficacy of an implantoplasty (diamond/arkansas burs + silicone polishers) when used as an adjunct to open flap debridement + bone re-contouring + apical flap re-positioning [42]. At 24 months, all patients from the control group had to be discontinued from the study due to persistent active signs of peri-implant inflammation. This was associated with elevated mBI and PD scores when compared with the test group. On the contrary, resective therapy resulted in significantly higher mean mucosal recessions (1.64 ± 1.29 vs. 2.3 ± 1.45 mm) but no pseudopocket formation [42], while test sites were associated with stable radiographic bone levels at 3 years, the interproximal bone loss at control sites amounted to 1.45–1.54 mm [57] (Table 10).

The calculated WM BOP [38, 39, 55] and PD [38–40, 55] reductions following surgical treatment (i.e. open flap with and without soft tissue resection) amounted to 34.81 % [SE = 8.95; 95 % CI (17.25, 52.37)] and 1.75 mm [SE = 0.34; 95 % CI (1.08, 2.42)].

**Adjunctive augmentative therapy** The clinical efficacy of adjunctive augmentative therapy to open flap debridement (titanium curettes + conditioning using 24 % ethylenediaminetetraacetic acid gel + submerged healing for 6 months) was merely assessed in one study [55]. Notably, 12/16 control and 13/16 test sites revealed a premature exposure during the submerged healing phase of 6 months. At 12 months after therapy, the application of porous titanium granules to the intrabony defect components resulted in a significantly higher percentage of radiographic defect fill when compared with open flap surgery alone. Moreover, the test group was associated with an increase in implant stability quotient, whereas these values further decreased at control sites. However, both groups revealed comparable PD reductions and only minor improvements in mean BOP scores [55]. The immunological analysis did not reveal any significant between differences in the reduction of MMP-8 levels or bone level markers [58] (Table 11). Four RCTs and four CCTs compared different augmentation protocols employing various methods for surface decontamination, bone fillers (i.e. alloplastic, xenogenic, autogenous) and barrier membranes (synthetic, native collagen) over a period of up to 5 years [40, 43–55]. The majority of these studies considered PD and BOP reductions as primary outcomes but also reported on radiographic defect fill (Table 11).

WM BOP [43, 49, 51, 53, 55] and PD [40, 43–55] reductions following adjunctive augmentative therapy amounted to 50.73 % [SE = 3.5; 95 % CI (43.87, 57.59)] and 2.20 mm [SE = 0.22; 95 % CI (1.76, 2.64)], respectively. The outcomes of therapy was mainly influenced by the type of bone filler (i.e. a slowly resorbing bovine-derived mineral was superior to autogenous bone and an alloplastic material), defect characteristics (i.e. circumferential-type defects were superior to dehiscence-type defects) and implant surface characteristics (i.e. moderately rough surfaces were superior to rough surfaces) (Table 11).

#### *Meta-analysis*

Meta-analysis to estimate the weighted mean difference (WMD) between test and control treatments was conducted on RCTs reporting on similar assessments of either absolute BOP or PD scores.

**Nonsurgical treatment of peri-implant mucositis—adjunctive antiseptics/antibiotics** Based on four and four studies, WMD in BOP [16, 17, 19, 22] and PD [17, 19, 20, 22] scores amounted to −8.16 % [SE = 4.61; $p > 0.05$; 95 % CI (−17.20, 0.88)] and −0.15 mm [SE = 0.13; $p > 0.05$; 95 % CI (−0.42, 0.11)], not favouring local antiseptic or antibiotic (i.e. local and systemic) therapy as an adjunct to mechanical debridement ($p$ value for heterogeneity: 0.42, $I^2 = 0.0$ % = low heterogeneity; $p$ value for heterogeneity: 0.45, $I^2 = 0.0$ % = low heterogeneity, respectively) (Fig. 2a, b).

Egger's linear regression method revealed symmetrical plots for changes in BOP ($p = 0.51$) and PD ($p = 0.69$) thus suggesting the absence of publication bias.

**Nonsurgical treatment of peri-implantitis—alterna tive methods for biofilm removal** Based on three studies [24, 25, 27], WMD in BOP scores between test and control groups amounted to −23.12 % [SE = 4.81; $p < 0.001$; 95 % CI (−32.56, −13.69)] favouring alternative methods (i.e. Er:YAG laser, glycine air polishing,) for biofilm removal over mechanical debridement ($p$ value for heterogeneity: 0.55, $I^2 = 0.0$ % = low heterogeneity; 0.39) (Fig. 3a). Based on five studies [24, 25, 27, 28, 31], WMD in PD scores between test and control groups amounted to −0.49 mm [SE = 0.21; $p < 0.05$; 95 % CI (−0.91, −0.08)] not favouring alternative methods (i.e. Er:YAG laser, glycine air polishing, ultrasonic system) for biofilm removal over mechanical debridement ($p$ value for heterogeneity: 0.029, $I^2 = 62.8$ % = substantial heterogeneity; 0.39) (Fig. 3b).

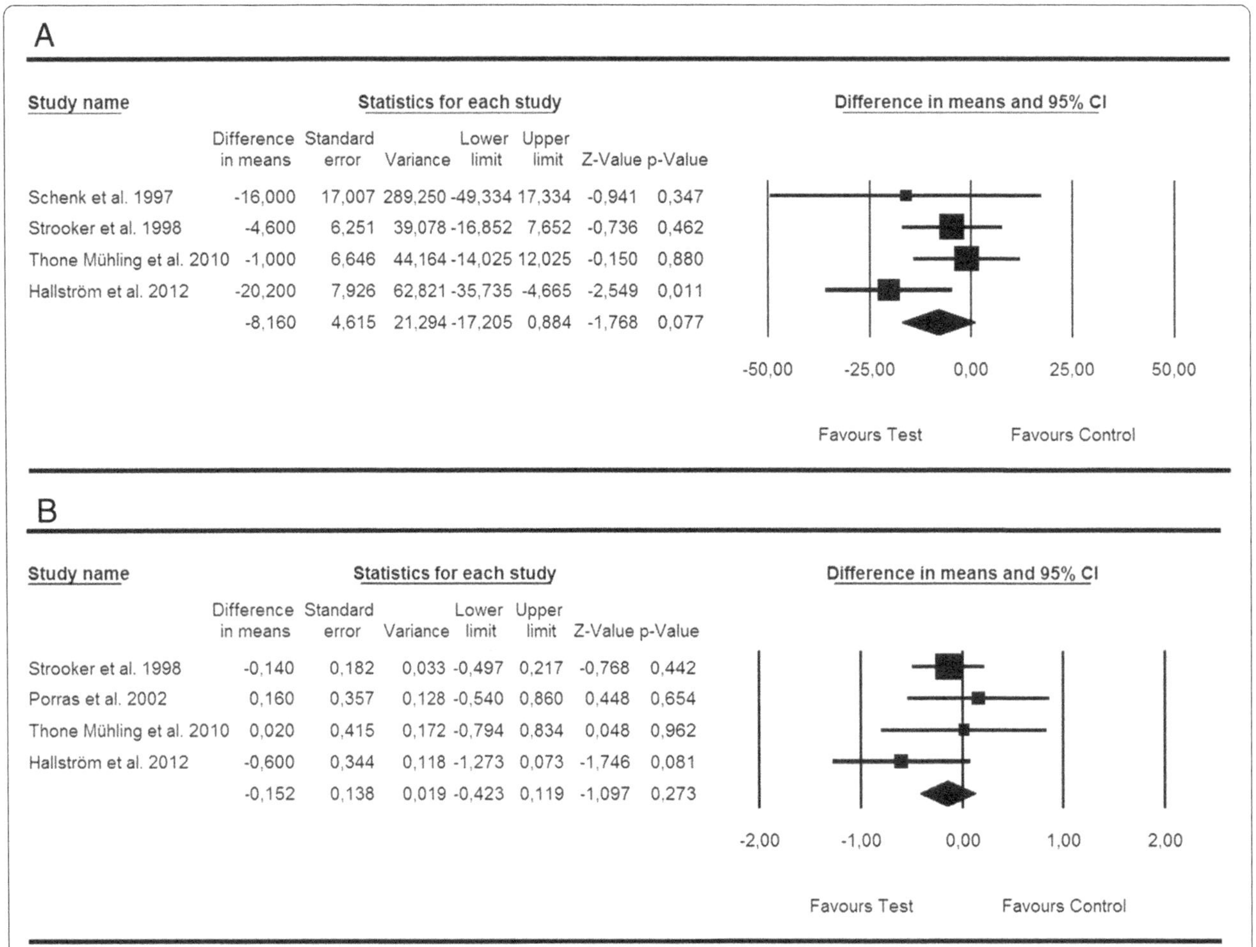


A

| Study name | Difference in means | Standard error | Variance | Lower limit | Upper limit | Z-Value | p-Value |
|---|---|---|---|---|---|---|---|
| Schenk et al. 1997 | -16,000 | 17,007 | 289,250 | -49,334 | 17,334 | -0,941 | 0,347 |
| Strooker et al. 1998 | -4,600 | 6,251 | 39,078 | -16,852 | 7,652 | -0,736 | 0,462 |
| Thone Mühling et al. 2010 | -1,000 | 6,646 | 44,164 | -14,025 | 12,025 | -0,150 | 0,880 |
| Hallström et al. 2012 | -20,200 | 7,926 | 62,821 | -35,735 | -4,665 | -2,549 | 0,011 |
| | -8,160 | 4,615 | 21,294 | -17,205 | 0,884 | -1,768 | 0,077 |

B

| Study name | Difference in means | Standard error | Variance | Lower limit | Upper limit | Z-Value | p-Value |
|---|---|---|---|---|---|---|---|
| Strooker et al. 1998 | -0,140 | 0,182 | 0,033 | -0,497 | 0,217 | -0,768 | 0,442 |
| Porras et al. 2002 | 0,160 | 0,357 | 0,128 | -0,540 | 0,860 | 0,448 | 0,654 |
| Thone Mühling et al. 2010 | 0,020 | 0,415 | 0,172 | -0,794 | 0,834 | 0,048 | 0,962 |
| Hallström et al. 2012 | -0,600 | 0,344 | 0,118 | -1,273 | 0,073 | -1,746 | 0,081 |
| | -0,152 | 0,138 | 0,019 | -0,423 | 0,119 | -1,097 | 0,273 |

**Fig. 2** Forest plot indicating weighted mean difference (95 % CI) in the reduction of primary outcomes following nonsurgical treatment of peri-implant mucositis. **a** Adjunctive antiseptic/antibiotic therapy—BOP. **b** Adjunctive antiseptic/antibiotic therapy—PD

Egger's linear regression method revealed symmetrical plots for changes in BOP ($p = 0.41$) and PD ($p = 0.39$) thus suggesting the absence of any publication bias.

**Nonsurgical treatment of peri-implantitis—adjunctive antiseptic/antibiotic therapy** Based on four studies [23, 26, 29, 32], WMD in BOP scores between test and control groups amounted to −16.53 % [SE = 4.41; $p < 0.001$; 95 % CI (−25.18, −7.89)] favouring local antibiotic therapy as an adjunct to mechanical debridement ($p$ value for heterogeneity: 0.113, $I^2 = 49.77$ % = moderate heterogeneity) (Fig. 3c). WMD in PD scores between test and control groups amounted to −0.829 mm [SE = 0.51; $p > 0.05$; 95 % CI (−1.84, 0.18)] not favouring antiseptic/antibiotic therapy as an adjunct to mechanical debridement ($p$ value for heterogeneity: 0.000, $I^2 = 87.37$ % = considerable heterogeneity) (Fig. 3d).

Egger's linear regression method revealed symmetrical plots for changes in BOP ($p = 0.17$) and PD ($p = 0.07$) thus suggesting the absence of any publication bias.

**Surgical treatment of peri-implantitis - alternative measures for surface decontamination** Based on two studies [38, 39], WMD in BOP and PD scores between test and control groups amounted to 5.61 % [SE = 7.68; $p > 0.05$; 95 % CI (−9.44, 20.68)] and 0.22 mm [SE = 0.22; $p > 0.05$; 95 % CI (−0.20, 0.65)] not favouring alternative (i.e. CHX + CPC) over conventional (i.e. CHX) measures for surface decontamination ($p$ value for heterogeneity: 0.76, $I^2 = 0.0$ % = low heterogeneity; 0.60, $I^2 = 0.0$ % = low heterogeneity, respectively) (Fig. 4a, b).

## Discussion

The present systematic review and meta-analysis was conducted to address the following focused question: "In patients with peri-implant mucositis and peri-implantitis, what is the efficacy of nonsurgical (i.e. referring to peri-implant mucositis and peri-implantitis) and surgical (i.e. referring to peri-implantitis) treatments with alternative or adjunctive measures on changing signs of inflammation compared with conventional nonsurgical and surgical treatments alone?".

a

| Study name | Difference in means | Standard error | Variance | Lower limit | Upper limit | Z-Value | p-Value |
|---|---|---|---|---|---|---|---|
| Schwarz et al. 2005 | -27,200 | 6,226 | 38,762 | -39,403 | -14,997 | -4,369 | 0,000 |
| Schwarz et al. 2006 | -15,000 | 9,730 | 94,673 | -34,070 | 4,070 | -1,542 | 0,123 |
| John et al. 2015 | -20,300 | 12,144 | 147,487 | -44,103 | 3,503 | -1,672 | 0,095 |
| | -23,129 | 4,815 | 23,180 | -32,565 | -13,692 | -4,804 | 0,000 |

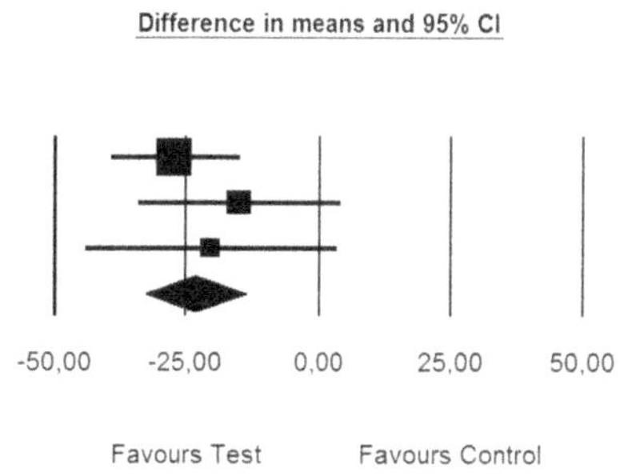


b

| Study name | Difference in means | Standard error | Variance | Lower limit | Upper limit | Z-Value | p-Value |
|---|---|---|---|---|---|---|---|
| Karring et al. 2005 | -0,500 | 0,792 | 0,628 | -2,053 | 1,053 | -0,631 | 0,528 |
| Schwarz et al. 2005 | -0,200 | 0,563 | 0,317 | -1,304 | 0,904 | -0,355 | 0,722 |
| Schwarz et al. 2006 | -0,200 | 0,313 | 0,098 | -0,814 | 0,414 | -0,639 | 0,523 |
| Renvert et al. 2009 | -2,400 | 0,621 | 0,385 | -3,616 | -1,184 | -3,867 | 0,000 |
| John et al. 2015 | -0,300 | 0,462 | 0,213 | -1,205 | 0,605 | -0,650 | 0,516 |
| | -0,499 | 0,212 | 0,045 | -0,915 | -0,084 | -2,355 | 0,019 |

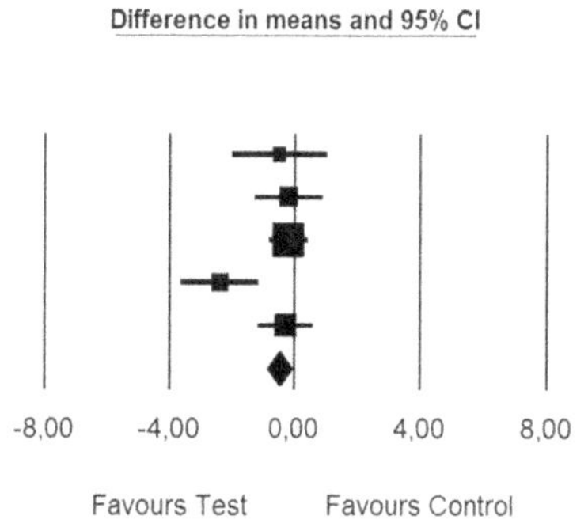


c

| Study name | Difference in means | Standard error | Variance | Lower limit | Upper limit | Z-Value | p-Value |
|---|---|---|---|---|---|---|---|
| Büchter et al. 2004 | -23,000 | 2,464 | 6,071 | -27,829 | -18,171 | -9,334 | 0,000 |
| Renvert et al. 2006 | -7,000 | 6,726 | 45,234 | -20,182 | 6,182 | -1,041 | 0,298 |
| Renvert et al. 2008 | -15,400 | 7,090 | 50,266 | -29,296 | -1,504 | -2,172 | 0,030 |
| Machtei et al. 2012 | -12,000 | 13,397 | 179,487 | -38,258 | 14,258 | -0,896 | 0,370 |
| | -16,536 | 4,411 | 19,458 | -25,182 | -7,890 | -3,749 | 0,000 |

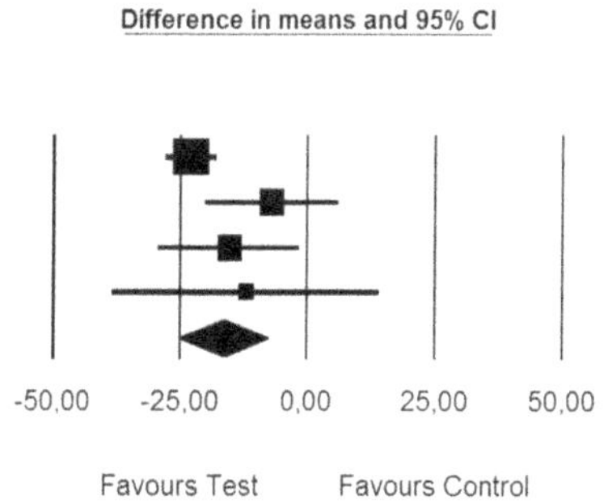


d

| Study name | Difference in means | Standard error | Variance | Lower limit | Upper limit | Z-Value | p-Value |
|---|---|---|---|---|---|---|---|
| Büchter et al. 2004 | -0,910 | 0,119 | 0,014 | -1,144 | -0,676 | -7,619 | 0,000 |
| Renvert et al. 2006 | -0,300 | 0,189 | 0,036 | -0,671 | 0,071 | -1,586 | 0,113 |
| Renvert et al. 2008 | -0,170 | 0,354 | 0,125 | -0,864 | 0,524 | -0,480 | 0,631 |
| Machtei et al. 2012 | -0,010 | 0,430 | 0,185 | -0,854 | 0,834 | -0,023 | 0,981 |
| | -0,430 | 0,238 | 0,057 | -0,896 | 0,036 | -1,807 | 0,071 |

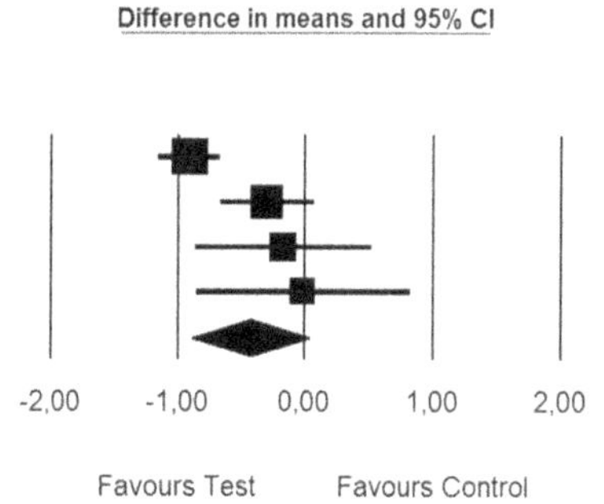


**Fig. 3** Forest plot indicating weighted mean difference (95 % CI) in the reduction of primary outcomes following nonsurgical treatment of peri-implantitis. **a** Alternative measures for biofilm removal—BOP. **b** Alternative measures for biofilm removal—PD. **c** Adjunctive antibiotic therapy—BOP. **d** Adjunctive antiseptic/antibiotic therapy—PD

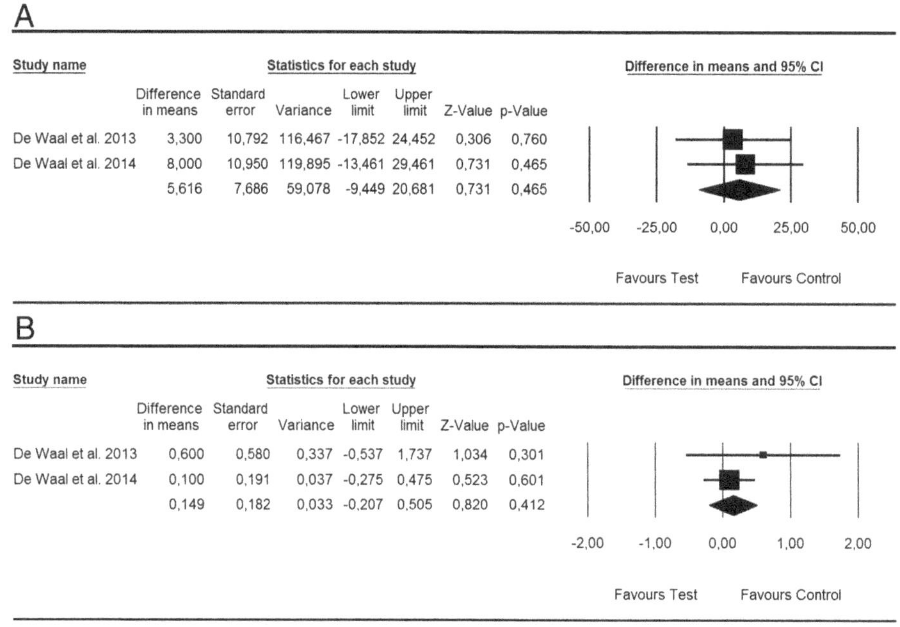


**Fig. 4** Forest plot indicating weighted mean difference (95 % CI) in the reduction of primary outcomes following surgical treatment of peri-implantitis. **a** Alternative measures for surface decontamination—BOP. **b** Alternative measures for surface decontamination—PD

Basically, the literature search revealed that only a few studies considered appropriate test and control treatments needed to address the aforementioned focused question. In particular, this was true for 8 (7 RCTs and 1 CCT) [15–22] and 9 (9 RCTs) [23–26, 28, 29, 31–33] studies reporting on the nonsurgical treatment of peri-implant mucositis and peri-implantitis, as well as 5 RCTs [38, 39, 41, 42, 55] reporting on the surgical treatment of peri-implantitis. In addition, 5 RCTs and 4 CCTs not implementing appropriate control measures (i.e. mechanical/ultrasonic debridement or open flap debridement alone) but reporting on changes in primary outcomes were included for the estimation of the overall efficacy (referring to WM changes in BOP and PD scores) of nonsurgical [30, 34] and surgical [40, 43, 44, 46, 48, 52, 53] treatments of peri-implantitis. Moreover, it must be emphasized that the percentage across all included studies for high risk of bias items was 34.1 %, thus pointing to a need to improve the quality of reporting in future studies.

Within these limitations, the current data synthesis revealed that for the nonsurgical treatment of peri-implant mucositis, WMD in BOP [16, 17, 19, 22] and PD [15, 17, 19, 20, 22] scores amounted to −8.16 % and −0.15 mm, not favouring local antiseptic or antibiotic (i.e. local and systemic) therapy as an adjunct to mechanical debridement alone. Basically, these data corroborate the findings of a recent systematic review and meta-analysis, also indicating that adjunctive therapy may not improve the efficacy of professionally administered plaque removal in reducing BOP (i.e. local antiseptic or local/systemic antibiotics), GI and PD (i.e. local antiseptics, systemic antibiotics, air abrasive device) scores at mucositis sites [9]. When considering the present narrative data synthesis on the adjunctive [15] or alternative use of glycine powder air polishing [21], it was also noted that this device did not reveal any major improvements in BI/BOP scores or disease resolution over the respective control measures. In this context, it must be emphasized that BOP is the key parameter for the diagnosis of peri-implant mucositis [1], and the "resolution of peri-implant mucosal inflammation as evidenced by the absence of BOP" was the suggested endpoint following nonsurgical treatment of mucositis lesions [13]. All these data, taken together with the present findings support the view that OHI and mechanical debridement with or without polishing tools may be defined as a current standard of care for the management of peri-implant mucositis [6].

In contrast, for the nonsurgical treatment of peri-implantitis, WMD in BOP scores amounted to −16.53 % [23, 26, 29, 32] and 23.12 % [24, 25, 27], thus favouring either adjunctive local antibiotic therapy or alternative measures for plaque removal (i.e. Er:YAG laser or glycine powder air polishing) over respective control treatments. However, these improvements were not observed when analysing WMD in PD scores between test and control groups. Basically, these observations were also supported by the differences in the estimated WM BOP (31.12 vs.

42.85 %) and PD (0.71 vs. 0.87 mm) reductions noted following nonsurgical treatment of peri-implantitis using either conventional [23–27] or alternative/adjunctive measures (i.e. air polishing, aPDT, CHX chip, doxycycline, Er:YAG laser) [23–27], respectively.

Since the suggested endpoint following nonsurgical treatment of peri-implantitis is a "composite outcome of disease resolution including the absence of deep PD with bleeding and suppuration" [13], one has to critically emphasize the limited efficacy at "deep sites". In particular, several studies reported on increasing BOP scores between 3 and 12 months following nonsurgical treatment of "severe" peri-implantitis sites using either mechanical debridement, adjunctive aPDT, Er:YAG laser monotherapy or glycine powder air polishing. The efficacy of all treatment procedures investigated was higher at "moderately" deep sites [24, 27, 33, 59]. In this context, however, one also has to realize that PD scores at implant sites may be influenced by a variety of different local factors, including the soft tissue thickness, vertical implant positioning, or a specific design of the implant-abutment connection (e.g. platform-switching). Accordingly, the classification of a "deep" pocket needs to be accomplished on an individual basis and disease severity should also consider "proportions of affected implants per patient in the presence of multiple implants" [6].

When further analysing the present results, it was also noted that nonsurgical treatment of peri-implantitis commonly failed to result in major microbiological improvements [32, 34–37], thus potentially explaining the frequency of residual BOP scores at respective sites.

At the time being, there is a lack of clinical studies aimed at comparing the efficacy of nonsurgical and surgical treatments of peri-implantitis. However, a preclinical study employing the ligature model has indicated that open flap debridement was associated with significant histological improvements in osseous defect fill and establishment of a new bone-to-implant when compared with nonsurgical treatments. The latter outcome was mainly influenced by the method of surface decontamination [60]. Accordingly, a "proven method of decontaminating the implant surface" has been defined as a critical component in surgical therapy [13]. However, the present qualitative and quantitative analysis has indicated that the clinical, radiographical and microbiological outcomes following either open flap debridement or surgical augmentative therapy were not influenced by the decontamination protocol, including chemical or photothermal (i.e. carbon dioxide, diode- or Er:YAG laser radiation) approaches [38–41, 49, 50, 52]. Moreover, two RCTs [38, 39] reported on an additional bone loss at 6 and 12 months after open flap debridement, thus indicating that disease resolution (i.e. "absence of deep probing pocket depths with bleeding and suppuration and no additional bone loss") [13] was commonly not achieved.

The present data synthesis also revealed a lack of RCTs/CCTs implementing appropriate test and control groups to assess the efficacy of adjunctive resective or augmentative measures over open flap debridement alone. The available studies have indicated that resective surgery (i.e. apical re-positioned flap + bone contouring) + implantoplasty was more effective in obtaining and maintaining disease resolution over resective surgery alone [42, 57]. In contrast, surgical augmentative therapy of the intrabony defect component using porous titanium granules was associated with a significantly higher radiographic defect fill, but failed to improve a reduction in mean BOP and PD scores over the control treatment [55]. When considering the estimated WM BOP (50.73 vs. 34.81 %) [38, 39, 43, 49, 51, 53, 55] and PD (2.20 vs. 1.75 mm) [38–40, 43–55] reductions, the clinical outcomes obtained following adjunctive augmentative therapy tended to be improved when compared with surgical measures alone. However, it has to be realized that for the data synthesis in the latter group, surgical procedures with and without soft tissue resection were combined, and therefore, the interpretation of the overall performance of surgical measures without augmentative measures on PD reductions is difficult. Moreover, obvious variations in the surgical procedures, including different decontamination protocols, administration of prophylactic systemic antibiotics, and modes of healing (i.e. open vs. submerged) may not allow for a direct comparison of these estimated outcomes. Basically, the estimated WM BOP and PD reductions corroborate those calculations reported in a recent systematic review on reconstructive procedures for the management of peri-implantitis. When also case series were included in the meta-analysis, these values amounted to 45.8 and 2.97 mm [61]. Furthermore, the present qualitative analysis of the available data on surgical augmentative therapy have indicated, that the outcomes of therapy may be influenced by several local factors, mainly including the physicochemical properties of the bone filler [43, 48, 51, 54], the defect configuration [53], as well as implant surface characteristics [44]. Any beneficial effect of a resorbable synthetic barrier membrane could not be identified [45–47]. Nevertheless, the available evidence did not allow for any conclusive statements on the potential superiority of any particular augmentation protocol.

Finally, it must be emphasized that laser therapy, the application of bone grafts and barrier membranes were reported to be associated with the highest cost-effectiveness ratio (i.e. costs and proportions of lost implants) among 11 treatment procedures investigated [62].

## Conclusions

While OHI + mechanical debridement alone was found to be effective for the management of peri-implant mucositis, alternative/adjunctive measures may improve the efficacy over/of conventional treatments at peri-implantitis sites. Adjunctive resective and/or augmentative measures are promising; however, their beneficial effect on the clinical outcome of surgical treatments needs to be further investigated.

#### Abbreviations
aPDT: antimicrobial photodynamic therapy; BOP: bleeding on probing; CAL: clinical attachment level; CCD: controlled clinical study; CHX: chlorhexidine digluconate; Er:YAG laser: erbium-doped yttrium aluminum garnet laser; GI: gingival index; mBI: (modified) bleeding index; MMP: matrixmetalloproteinase; MR: mucosal recession; OHI: oral hygiene instructions; PD: probing pocket depth; RCT: randomized controlled clinical study; WM: weighted mean changes; WMD: weighted mean differences.

#### Competing interests
Frank Schwarz and Jürgen Becker received lecture fees and/or unrestricted research grants from Geistlich Biomaterials, Rooth, Switzerland; Osteology Foundation, Lucerne, Switzerland; EMS, Nyon, Switzerland. Frank Schwarz, Andrea Schmucker and Jürgen Becker declare that they have no competing interests related to this systematic review.

#### Authors' contributions
FS and JB have made substantial contributions to study conception and interpretation of data as well as manuscript preparation. AS and FS were involved in the literature search and data management as well as the statistical analysis. All authors read and approved the final manuscript.

#### Acknowledgements
The authors appreciate the additional information provided during the process of "contact" with the following authors:
Herbert Deppe, Department of Oral and Maxillofacial Surgery at the Klinikum Rechts Der Isar, Technische Universität München, Munich, Germany; Eli Machtei, Department of Periodontology, School of Graduate Dentistry, Rambam HCC, Technion - Israeli Institute of Technology, Haifa, Israel; Giovanni Salvi, Department of Periodontology, School of Dental Medicine, University of Bern, Bern, Switzerland; Yvonne de Waal, Center for Dentistry and Oral Hygiene, University of Groningen, University Medical Center Groningen, Groningen, The Netherlands.

#### References
1. Lang NP, Berglundh T. Periimplant diseases: where are we now? Consensus of the Seventh European Workshop on Periodontology. J Clin Periodontol. 2011;38 Suppl 11:178–81.
2. Derks J, Tomasi C. Peri-implant health and disease. A systematic review of current epidemiology. J Clin Periodontol. 2015;42 Suppl 16:158–71.
3. Renvert S, Polyzois I. Risk indicators for peri-implant mucositis: a systematic literature review. J Clin Periodontol. 2015;42 Suppl 16:172–86.
4. Schwarz F, Mihatovic I, Golubovich V, Eick S, Iglhaut T, Becker J. Experimental peri-implant mucositis at different implant surfaces. J Clin Periodontol. 2014;41:513–20.
5. Costa FO, Takenaka-Martinez S, Cota LO, Ferreira SD, Silva GL, Costa JE. Peri-implant disease in subjects with and without preventive maintenance: a 5-year follow-up. J Clin Periodontol. 2012;39:173–81.
6. Jepsen S, Berglundh T, Genco R, Aass AM, Demirel K, Derks J, et al. Primary prevention of peri-implantitis: managing peri-implant mucositis. J Clin Periodontol. 2015;42 Suppl 16:152–7.
7. Heitz-Mayfield LJ, Mombelli A. The therapy of peri-implantitis: a systematic review. Int J Oral Maxillofac Implants. 2014;29(Suppl):325–45.
8. Klinge B, Meyle J. Working G. Peri-implant tissue destruction. The Third EAO Consensus Conference 2012. Clin Oral Implants Res. 2012;23 Suppl 6:108–10.
9. Schwarz F, Becker K, Sager M. Efficacy of professionally administered plaque removal with or without adjunctive measures for the treatment of peri-implant mucositis. A systematic review and meta-analysis. J Clin Periodontol. 2015;42 Suppl 16:202–13.
10. Claffey N, Clarke E, Polyzois I, Renvert S. Surgical treatment of peri-implantitis. J Clin Periodontol. 2008;35:316–32.
11. Moher D, Liberati A, Tetzlaff J, Altman DG, Group P. Preferred reporting items for systematic reviews and meta-analyses: the PRISMA statement. PLoS Med. 2009;6:e1000097.
12. Miller SA, Forrest JL. Enhancing your practice through evidence-based decision making: PICO, learning how to ask good questions. J Evid Base Dent Pract. 2001;1:136–41.
13. Sanz M, Chapple IL, Working Group 4 of the VEWoP. Clinical research on peri-implant diseases: consensus report of Working Group 4. J Clin Periodontol. 2012;39 Suppl 12:202–6.
14. Higgins JPT, Green S. Cochrane Handbook for Systematic Reviews of Interventions Version 5.1.0 [updated March 2011]. The Cochrane Collaboration, 2011. Available from http://www.cochrane-handbook.org. 2011.
15. Ji YJ, Tang ZH, Wang R, Cao J, Cao CF, Jin LJ. Effect of glycine powder air-polishing as an adjunct in the treatment of peri-implant mucositis: a pilot clinical trial. Clin Oral Implants Res. 2014;25:683–9.
16. Schenk G, Flemmig TF, Betz T, Reuther J, Klaiber B. Controlled local delivery of tetracycline HCl in the treatment of periimplant mucosal hyperplasia and mucositis. A controlled case series. Clin Oral Implants Res. 1997;8:427–33.
17. Thone-Mühling M, Swierkot K, Nonnenmacher C, Mutters R, Flores-de-Jacoby L, Mengel R. Comparison of two full-mouth approaches in the treatment of peri-implant mucositis: a pilot study. Clin Oral Implants Res. 2010;21:504–12.
18. De Siena F, Corbella S, Taschieri S, Del Fabbro M, Francetti L. Adjunctive glycine powder air-polishing for the treatment of peri-implant mucositis: an observational clinical trial. Int J Dent Hyg. 2014;14. doi:10.1111/idh.12114.
19. Hallström H, Persson GR, Lindgren S, Olofsson M, Renvert S. Systemic antibiotics and debridement of peri-implant mucositis. A randomized clinical trial. J Clin Periodontol. 2012;39:574–81.
20. Porras R, Anderson GB, Caffesse R, Narendran S, Trejo PM. Clinical response to 2 different therapeutic regimens to treat peri-implant mucositis. J Periodontol. 2002;73:1118–25.
21. Riben Grundström C, Norderyd O, Andre U, Renvert S. Treatment of peri-implant mucositis using a glycine powder air-polishing or ultrasonic device. A randomized clinical trial. J Clin Periodontol. 2015;42:462–9.
22. Strooker H, Rohn S, Van Winkelhoff AJ. Clinical and microbiologic effects of chemical versus mechanical cleansing in professional supportive implant therapy. Int J Oral Maxillofac Implants. 1998;13:845–50.
23. Machtei EE, Frankenthal S, Levi G, Elimelech R, Shoshani E, Rosenfeld O, et al. Treatment of peri-implantitis using multiple applications of chlorhexidine chips: a double-blind, randomized multi-centre clinical trial. J Clin Periodontol. 2012;39:1198–205.
24. Schwarz F, Bieling K, Bonsmann M, Latz T, Becker J. Nonsurgical treatment of moderate and advanced periimplantitis lesions: a controlled clinical study. Clin Oral Investig. 2006;10:279–88.
25. Schwarz F, Sculean A, Rothamel D, Schwenzer K, Georg T, Becker J. Clinical evaluation of an Er : YAG laser for nonsurgical treatment of peri-implantitis: a pilot study. Clin Oral Implants Res. 2005;16:44–52.
26. Büchter A, Meyer U, Kruse-Losler B, Joos U, Kleinheinz J. Sustained release of doxycycline for the treatment of peri-implantitis: randomised controlled trial. Br J Oral Maxillofac Surg. 2004;42:439–44.
27. John G, Sahm N, Becker J, Schwarz F. Nonsurgical treatment of peri-implantitis using an air-abrasive device or mechanical debridement and local application of chlorhexidine. Twelve-month follow-up of a prospective, randomized, controlled clinical study. Clin Oral Investig. 2015. doi:10.1007/s00784-015-1406-7.
28. Karring ES, Stavropoulos A, Ellegaard B, Karring T. Treatment of peri-implantitis by the VectorR system. A pilot study. Clin Oral Implants Res. 2005;16:288–93.
29. Renvert S, Lessem J, Dahlen G, Renvert H, Lindahl C. Mechanical and repeated antimicrobial therapy using a local drug delivery system in the treatment of peri-implantitis: a randomized clinical trial. J Periodontol. 2008;79:836–44.
30. Renvert S, Lindahl C, Roos Jansker A-M, Persson GR. Treatment of peri-implantitis using an Er:YAG laser or an air-abrasive device: a randomized clinical trial. J Clin Periodontol. 2011;38:65–73.
31. Renvert S, Samuelsson E, Lindahl CPersson GR. Mechanical non-surgical treatment of peri-implantitis: a double-blind randomized longitudinal clinical study. I: clinical results. J Clin Periodontol. 2009;36:604–9.
32. Renvert S, Lessem J, Dahlen G, Lindahl C, Svensson M. Topical minocycline microspheres versus topical chlorhexidine gel as an adjunct to mechanical

debridement of incipient peri-implant infections: a randomized clinical trial. J Clin Periodontol. 2006;33:362–9.
33. Sahm N, Becker J, Santel T, Schwarz F. Non-surgical treatment of peri-implantitis using an air-abrasive device or mechanical debridement and local application of chlorhexidine: a prospective, randomized, controlled clinical study. J Clin Periodontol. 2011;38:872–8.
34. Schär D, Ramseier CA, Eick S, Arweiler NB, Sculean A, Salvi GE. Anti-infective therapy of peri-implantitis with adjunctive local drug delivery or photodynamic therapy: six-month outcomes of a prospective randomized clinical trial. Clin Oral Implants Res. 2013;24:104–10.
35. Persson GR, Samuelsson E, Lindahl C, Renvert S. Mechanical non-surgical treatment of peri-implantitis: a single-blinded randomized longitudinal clinical study. II Microbiological results. J Clin Periodontol. 2010;37:563–73.
36. Persson GR, Roos-Jansker AM, Lindahl C, Renvert S. Microbiologic results after non-surgical erbium-doped:yttrium, aluminum, and garnet laser or air-abrasive treatment of peri-implantitis: a randomized clinical trial. J Periodontol. 2011;82:1267–78.
37. Bassetti M, Schär D, Wicki B, Eick S, Ramseier CA, Arweiler NB, et al. Anti-infective therapy of peri-implantitis with adjunctive local drug delivery or photodynamic therapy: 12-month outcomes of a randomized controlled clinical trial. Clin Oral Implants Res. 2013;25:279–87.
38. de Waal YC, Raghoebar GM, Huddleston Slater JJ, Meijer HJ, Winkel EG, van Winkelhoff AJ. Implant decontamination during surgical peri-implantitis treatment: a randomized, double-blind, placebo-controlled trial. J Clin Periodontol. 2013;40:186–95.
39. de Waal YC, Raghoebar GM, Meijer HJ, Winkel EG, van Winkelhoff AJ. Implant decontamination with 2% chlorhexidine during surgical peri-implantitis treatment: a randomized, double-blind, controlled trial. Clin Oral Implants Res. 2014. doi:10.1111/clr.12419.
40. Deppe H, Horch HH, Neff A. Conventional versus CO2 laser-assisted treatment of peri-implant defects with the concomitant use of pure-phase beta-tricalcium phosphate: a 5-year clinical report. Int J Oral Maxillofac Implants. 2007;22:79–86.
41. Papadopoulos CA, Vouros I, Menexes G, Konstantinidis A. The utilization of a diode laser in the surgical treatment of peri-implantitis. A randomized clinical trial. Clin Oral Investig. 2015. doi:10.1007/s00784-014-1397-9.
42. Romeo E, Ghisolfi M, Murgolo N, Chiapasco M, Lops D, Vogel G. Therapy of peri-implantitis with resective surgery. A 3-year clinical trial on rough screw-shaped oral implants. Part I: clinical outcome. Clin Oral Implants Res. 2005;16:9–18.
43. Aghazadeh A, Persson GR, Renvert S. A single-centre randomized controlled clinical trial on the adjunct treatment of intra-bony defects with autogenous bone or a xenograft: results after 12 months. J Clin Periodontol. 2012;39(7):666–73.
44. Roccuzzo M, Bonino F, Bonino L, Dalmasso P. Surgical therapy of peri-implantitis lesions by means of a bovine-derived xenograft: comparative results of a prospective study on two different implant surfaces. Surgical treatment of peri-implantitis. J Clin Periodontol. 2011;38(8):738–45.
45. Roos-Jansaker AM, Persson GR, Lindahl C, Renvert S. Surgical treatment of peri-implantitis using a bone substitute with or without a resorbable membrane: a 5-year follow-up. J Clin Periodontol. 2014;41:1108–14.
46. Roos-Jansaker AM, Renvert H, Lindahl C, Renvert S. Surgical treatment of peri-implantitis using a bone substitute with or without a resorbable membrane: a prospective cohort study. J Clin Periodontol. 2007;34:625–32.
47. Roos-Jansker A-M, Lindahl C, Pesson GR, Renvert S. Long-term stability of surgical bone regenerative procedures of peri-implantitis lesions in a prospective case–control study over 3 years. J Clin Periodontol. 2011;38:590–7.
48. Schwarz F, Bieling K, Latz T, Nuesry E, Becker J. Healing of intrabony peri-implantitis defects following application of a nanocrystalline hydroxyapatite (Ostim) or a bovine-derived xenograft (Bio-Oss) in combination with a collagen membrane (Bio-Gide). A case series. J Clin Periodontol. 2006;33:491–9.
49. Schwarz F, Hegewald A, John G, Sahm N, Becker J. Four-year follow-up of combined surgical therapy of advanced peri-implantitis evaluating two methods of surface decontamination. J Clin Periodontol. 2013;40:962–7.
50. Schwarz F, John G, Mainusch S, Sahm N, Becker J. Combined surgical therapy of peri-implantitis evaluating two methods of surface debridement and decontamination. A two-year clinical follow up report. J Clin Periodontol. 2012;39:789–97.
51. Schwarz F, Sahm N, Bieling K, Becker J. Surgical regenerative treatment of peri-implantitis lesions using a nanocrystalline hydroxyapatite or a natural bone mineral in combination with a collagen membrane: a four-year clinical follow-up report. J Clin Periodontol. 2009;36:807–14.
52. Schwarz F, Sahm N, Iglhaut G, Becker J. Impact of the method of surface debridement and decontamination on the clinical outcome following combined surgical therapy of peri-implantitis: a randomized controlled clinical study. J Clin Periodontol. 2011;38:276–84.
53. Schwarz F, Sahm N, Schwarz K, Becker J. Impact of defect configuration on the clinical outcome following surgical regenerative therapy of peri-implantitis. J Clin Periodontol. 2010;37:449–55.
54. Schwarz F, Sculean A, Bieling K, Ferrari D, Rothamel D, Becker J. Two-year clinical results following treatment of peri-implantitis lesions using a nanocrystalline hydroxyapatite or a natural bone mineral in combination with a collagen membrane. J Clin Periodontol. 2008;35:80–7.
55. Wohlfahrt JC, Lyngstadaas SP, Ronold HJ, Saxegaard E, Ellingsen JE, Karlsson S, et al. Porous titanium granules in the surgical treatment of peri-implant osseous defects: a randomized clinical trial. Int J Oral Maxillofac Implants. 2012;27:401–10.
56. Schwarz F, Herten M, Sager M, Bieling K, Sculean A, Becker J. Comparison of naturally occurring and ligature-induced peri-implantitis bone defects in humans and dogs. Clin Oral Implants Res. 2007;18:161–70.
57. Romeo E, Lops D, Chiapasco M, Ghisolfi M, Vogel G. Therapy of peri-implantitis with resective surgery. A 3-year clinical trial on rough screw-shaped oral implants. Part II: radiographic outcome. Clin Oral Implants Res. 2007;18:179–87.
58. Wohlfahrt JC, Aass AM, Granfeldt F, Lyngstadaas SP, Reseland JE. Sulcus fluid bone marker levels and the outcome of surgical treatment of peri-implantitis. J Clin Periodontol. 2014;41:424–31.
59. Deppe H, Mucke T, Wagenpfeil S, Kesting M, Sculean A. Nonsurgical antimicrobial photodynamic therapy in moderate vs severe peri-implant defects: a clinical pilot study. Quintessence Int. 2013;44:609–18.
60. Schwarz F, Jepsen S, Herten M, Sager M, Rothamel D, Becker J. Influence of different treatment approaches on non-submerged and submerged healing of ligature induced peri-implantitis lesions: an experimental study in dogs. J Clin Periodontol. 2006;33:584–95.
61. Khoshkam V, Chan HL, Lin GH, Mac Eachern MP, Monje A, Suarez F, et al. Reconstructive procedures for treating peri-implantitis: a systematic review. J Dent Res. 2013;92:131S–8.
62. Schwendicke F, Tu YK, Stolpe M. Preventing and treating peri-implantitis: a cost-effectiveness analysis. J Periodontol. 2015;9:1–15.
63. Lavigne SE, Krust-Bray KS, Williams KB, Killoy WJ, Theisen F. Effects of subgingival irrigation with chlorhexidine on the periodontal status of patients with HA-coated integral dental implants. Int J Oral Maxillofac Implants. 1994;9:156–62.
64. Ciancio SG, Lauciello F, Shibly O, Vitello M, Mather M. The effect of an antiseptic mouthrinse on implant maintenance: plaque and peri-implant gingival tissues. J Periodontol. 1995;66:962–5.
65. Felo A, Shibly O, Ciancio SG, Lauciello FR, Ho A. Effects of subgingival chlorhexidine irrigation on peri-implant maintenance. Am J Dent. 1997;10:107–10.
66. Bach G, Neckel C, Mall C, Krekeler G. Conventional versus laser-assisted therapy of periimplantitis: a five-year comparative study. Implant Dent. 2000;9:247–51.
67. Dörtbudak O, Haas R, Bernhart T, Mailath-Pokorny G. Lethal photosensitization for decontamination of implant surfaces in the treatment of peri-implantitis. Clin Oral Implants Res. 2001;12:104–8.
68. Khoury F, Buchmann R. Surgical therapy of peri-implant disease: a 3-year follow-up study of cases treated with 3 different techniques of bone regeneration. J Periodontol. 2001;72:1498–508.
69. Roos-Jansaker AM, Renvert H, Lindahl C, Renvert S. Submerged healing following surgical treatment of peri- implantitis: a case series. J Periodontol. 2001;72:1498–508.
70. Duarte PM, de Mendonca AC, Maximo MB, Santos VR, Bastos MF, Nociti FH. Effect of anti-infective mechanical therapy on clinical parameters and cytokine levels in human peri-implant diseases. J Periodontol. 2009;80:234–43.
71. Maximo MB, de Mendonca AC, Renata Santos V, Figueiredo LC, Feres M, Duarte PM. Short-term clinical and microbiological evaluations of peri-implant diseases before and after mechanical anti-infective therapies. Clin Oral Implants Res. 2009;20:99–108.
72. Ramberg P, Lindhe J, Botticelli D, Botticelli A. The effect of a triclosan dentifrice on mucositis in subjects with dental implants: a six-month clinical study. J Clin Dent. 2009;20:103–7.

73. Corbella S, Del Fabbro M, Taschieri S, De Siena F, Francetti L. Clinical evaluation of an implant maintenance protocol for the prevention of peri-implant diseases in patients treated with immediately loaded full-arch rehabilitations. Int J Dent Hyg. 2011;9:216–22.
74. Heitz-Mayfield LJ, Salvi GE, Botticelli D, Mombelli A, Faddy M, Lang NP, et al. Anti-infective treatment of peri-implant mucositis: a randomised controlled clinical trial. Clin Oral Implants Res. 2011;22:237–41.
75. De Angelis N, Felice P, Grusovin MG, Camurati A, Esposito M. The effectiveness of adjunctive light-activated disinfection (LAD) in the treatment of peri-implantitis: 4-month results from a multicentre pragmatic randomised controlled trial. Eur J Oral Implantol. 2012;5:321–31.
76. Salvi GE, Aglietta M, Eick S, Sculean A, Lang NP, Ramseier CA. Reversibility of experimental peri-implant mucositis compared with experimental gingivitis in humans. Clin Oral Implants Res. 2012;23:182–90.
77. De Siena F, Francetti L, Corbella S, Taschieri S, Del Fabbro M. Topical application of 1% chlorhexidine gel versus 0.2% mouthwash in the treatment of peri-implant mucositis. An observational study. Int J Dent Hyg. 2013;11:41–7.
78. McKenna DF, Borzabadi-Farahani A, Lynch E. The effect of subgingival ozone and/or hydrogen peroxide on the development of peri-implant mucositis: a double-blind randomized controlled trial. Int J Oral Maxillofac Implants. 2013;28:1483–9.
79. Flichy-Fernandez AJ, Ata-Ali J, Alegre-Domingo T, Candel-Marti E, Ata-Ali F, Palacio JR, et al. The effect of orally administered probiotic lactobacillus reuteri-containing tablets in peri-implant mucositis: a double-blind randomized controlled trial. J Periodontal Res. 2015. doi:10.1111/jre.12264.

# Permissions

All chapters in this book were first published in IJID, by Springer; hereby published with permission under the Creative Commons Attribution License or equivalent. Every chapter published in this book has been scrutinized by our experts. Their significance has been extensively debated. The topics covered herein carry significant findings which will fuel the growth of the discipline. They may even be implemented as practical applications or may be referred to as a beginning point for another development.

The contributors of this book come from diverse backgrounds, making this book a truly international effort. This book will bring forth new frontiers with its revolutionizing research information and detailed analysis of the nascent developments around the world.

We would like to thank all the contributing authors for lending their expertise to make the book truly unique. They have played a crucial role in the development of this book. Without their invaluable contributions this book wouldn't have been possible. They have made vital efforts to compile up to date information on the varied aspects of this subject to make this book a valuable addition to the collection of many professionals and students.

This book was conceptualized with the vision of imparting up-to-date information and advanced data in this field. To ensure the same, a matchless editorial board was set up. Every individual on the board went through rigorous rounds of assessment to prove their worth. After which they invested a large part of their time researching and compiling the most relevant data for our readers.

The editorial board has been involved in producing this book since its inception. They have spent rigorous hours researching and exploring the diverse topics which have resulted in the successful publishing of this book. They have passed on their knowledge of decades through this book. To expedite this challenging task, the publisher supported the team at every step. A small team of assistant editors was also appointed to further simplify the editing procedure and attain best results for the readers.

Apart from the editorial board, the designing team has also invested a significant amount of their time in understanding the subject and creating the most relevant covers. They scrutinized every image to scout for the most suitable representation of the subject and create an appropriate cover for the book.

The publishing team has been an ardent support to the editorial, designing and production team. Their endless efforts to recruit the best for this project, has resulted in the accomplishment of this book. They are a veteran in the field of academics and their pool of knowledge is as vast as their experience in printing. Their expertise and guidance has proved useful at every step. Their uncompromising quality standards have made this book an exceptional effort. Their encouragement from time to time has been an inspiration for everyone.

The publisher and the editorial board hope that this book will prove to be a valuable piece of knowledge for researchers, students, practitioners and scholars across the globe.

# List of Contributors

**Martin Gosau**
Department of Cranio- and Maxillofacial Surgery, Hospital of the University of Regensburg, Franz-Josef-Strauss-Allee 11, 93053 Regensburg, Germany
Department of Oral and Maxillofacial Surgery, Paracelsus Medical University Nuernberg, Breslauer Str., 201, 90471 Nürnberg, Germany

**Sandra Viale-Bouroncle, Hannah Eickhoff, Esthera Prateeptongkum, Anja Reck, Christoph Klingelhöffer, Steffen Müller and Christian Morsczeck**
Department of Cranio- and Maxillofacial Surgery, Hospital of the University of Regensburg, Franz-Josef-Strauss-Allee 11, 93053 Regensburg, Germany

**W Götz**
Department of Orthodontics, Oral Biology Laboratory, Dental Clinic, University of Bonn, Regina-Pacis-Weg 3, 53113 Bonn, Germany

**Yoshiyuki Hagiwara, Tatsuya Narita, Yohei Shioda, Keisuke Iwasaki, Takayuki Ikeda and Shunsuke Namaki**
Implant Dentistry, Nihon University School of Dentistry, Dental Hospital, 1-8-13 Kandasurugadai, Chiyoda-ku, Tokyo 101-8310, Japan

**Thomas J Salinas**
Department of Dental Specialties, Mayo Clinic, Mayo Clinic, 200 First Street SW, Rochester, MINN 55905, USA

**Kirsten W Slagter, Gerry M Raghoebar and Arjan Vissink**
Department of Oral and Maxillofacial Surgery, University of Groningen, University Medical Center Groningen, PO Box 30.001, 9700RB Groningen, The Netherlands

**Henny J A Meijer**
Department of Oral and Maxillofacial Surgery, University of Groningen, University Medical Center Groningen, PO Box 30.001, 9700RB Groningen, The Netherlands
Department of Fixed and Removable Prosthodontics, University of Groningen, University Medical Center Groningen, PO Box 30.001, 9700RB Groningen, The Netherlands

**Motoshi Kimura and Shigeyoshi Hanano**
Hanano Dental Clinic, 4-2-3 Yamanoue, Hirakata, Osaka 573-0047, Japan

**Yoshihiro Takasugi**
Department of Anesthesiology, Kinki University Faculty of Medicine, 377-2 Ohno-Higashi, Osaka-Sayama, Osaka 589-8511, Japan

**Katsuyuki Terabe**
Terabe Dental Clinic, 4-249 Sakae-cho, Tsu, Mie 514-0004, Japan

**Yuko Kimura**
First Department of Internal Medicine, Osaka Medical College, 2-7 Daigaku-machi, Takatsuki, Osaka 569-8686, Japan

**Masayuki Fukuda, Satoru Matsunaga, Kento Odaka, Yuuya Oomine, Masaaki Kasahara, Masahito Yamamoto and Shinichi Abe**
Department of Anatomy, Tokyo Dental College, 2-9-18, Misaki-cho, Chiyoda-ku, Tokyo 101-0061, Japan

**Frank Schwarz and Andrea Hegewald**
Department of Oral Surgery, Westdeutsche Kieferklinik, Heinrich Heine University, Moorenstraße 5, D-40225 Düsseldorf, Germany

**Kathrin Becker**
Department of Orthodontics, Westdeutsche Kieferklinik, Heinrich Heine University, Moorenstraße 5, D-40225 Düsseldorf, Germany

**Sebastian Rahn, Klaus Pfeffer and Birgit Henrich**
Institute of Medical Microbiology and Hospital Hygiene, Heinrich Heine University, Universitätsstraße 1, D-40225 Düsseldorf, Germany

**Catharina Ladwein, Rainer Schmelzeisen, Katja Nelson, Tabea Viktoria Fluegge and Tobias Fretwurst**
Department of Oral and Craniomaxillofacial Surgery, Center for Dental Medicine, University Medical Center Freiburg, Hugstetter Straße 55, D-79106 Freiburg, Germany

**Eric W Meisberger and Sjoerd J G Bakker**
University Medical Center Groningen, Center for Dentistry and Oral Hygiene, Department of Fixed and Removable Prosthodontics and Biomaterials, The University of Groningen, Gebouw 3216, kamer 206, A. Deusinglaan 1, 9713 AV Groningen, The Netherlands

**Marco S Cune**
University Medical Center Groningen, Center for Dentistry and Oral Hygiene, Department of Fixed and Removable Prosthodontics and Biomaterials, The University of Groningen, Gebouw 3216, kamer 206, A. Deusinglaan 1, 9713 AV Groningen, The Netherlands
Department of Oral-Maxillofacial Surgery, Prosthodontics and Special Dental Care, St. Antonius Hospital Nieuwegein, Koekoekslaan 1, 3435 CM Nieuwegein, The Netherlands

**Elise G Zuiderveld, Arjan Vissink and Gerry M Raghoebar**
Department of Oral and Maxillofacial Surgery, University of Groningen, University Medical Center Groningen, P.O. Box 30.001, NL-9700 RB Groningen, the Netherlands

Department of Fixed and Removable Prosthodontics, University of Groningen, University Medical Center Groningen, P.O. Box 30.001, 9700RB, Groningen, the Netherlands

**Henny J A Meijer**
Department of Oral and Maxillofacial Surgery, University of Groningen, University Medical Center Groningen, P.O. Box 30.001, NL-9700 RB Groningen, the Netherlands
Department of Fixed and Removable Prosthodontics, University of Groningen, University Medical Center Groningen, P.O. Box 30.001, 9700RB, Groningen, the Netherlands

**Miyuki Omori, Yuji Sato, Noboru Kitagawa, Yuta Shimura and Manabu Ito**
Department of Geriatric Dentistry, Showa University, School of Dentistry, 2-1-1 Kitasenzoku, Ota-ku, Tokyo 145-8515, Japan

**Siddharth Shanbhag**
Department of Periodontology, Faculty of Odontology, Malmö University, Carl Gustafs väg 34, 214 21 Malmö, Sweden
Centre for Oral Rehabilitation & Implant Dentistry, 1 Laxmi Niwas, 87 Bajaj Road, Vile Parle West, Mumbai 400056, India

**Vivek Shanbhag**
Centre for Oral Rehabilitation & Implant Dentistry, 1 Laxmi Niwas, 87 Bajaj Road, Vile Parle West, Mumbai 400056, India

**Andreas Stavropoulos**
Department of Periodontology, Faculty of Odontology, Malmö University, Carl Gustafs väg 34, 214 21 Malmö, Sweden

**Federico Gelpi**
Via delle Mimose, 8 Colognola ai Colli, 37030 Verona, Italy

**Daniele De Santis**
Dental and Maxillofacial Department, University of Verona, Verona, Italy

**Simone Marconcini**
Department of surgery, University of Pisa Ist. Stomatologico, Tirreno, Italy

**Francesco Briguglio**
Messina, Italy

**Marco Finotti**
Padova, Italy

**Johann Malina-Altzinger**
Clinic of Cranio-Maxillofacial Surgery, University Hospital of Bern, Freiburgstrasse 4, 3010 Bern, Switzerland

**Georg Damerau and PD Bernd Stadlinger**
Clinic of Oral Surgery, Center of Dental Medicine, University of Zurich, Plattenstrasse 11, 8032 Zurich, Switzerland

**Klaus W Grätz**
Former Head of the Department of Cranio-Maxillofacial and Oral Surgery, University of Zurich, Plattenstrasse 11, 8032 Zurich, Switzerland

**Sho Kayumi**
Removable Prosthodontics, Hokkaido University Hospital, Hokkaido University, Kita-14, Nishi-5, Kita-Ku, Sapporo 060-8648, Japan
Department of Oral Functional Prosthodontics, Division of Oral Functional Science, Graduate School of Dental Medicine, Hokkaido University, Kita-13, Nishi-7, Kita-Ku, Sapporo 060-8648, Japan

**Yoshiyuki Takayama and Nana Ueda**
Removable Prosthodontics, Hokkaido University Hospital, Hokkaido University, Kita-14, Nishi-5, Kita-Ku, Sapporo 060-8648, Japan

**Atsuro Yokoyama**
Department of Oral Functional Prosthodontics, Division of Oral Functional Science, Graduate School of Dental Medicine, Hokkaido University, Kita-13, Nishi-7, Kita-Ku, Sapporo 060-8648, Japan

**Yukihiko Okada, Yuji Sato, Noboru Kitagawa, Keiichiro Uchida, Tokiko Osawa, Yoshiki Imamura and Mayumi Terazawa**
Department of Geriatric Dentistry, School of Dentistry Showa University, 2-1-1 Kitasenzoku, Ota Ward, Tokyo 145-8515, Japan

**Masahiro Wada, Yasutane Tsuiki, Tohru Suganami, Kazunori Ikebe, Motofumi Sogo, Ikuhisa Okuno and Yoshinobu Maeda**
Department of Prosthodontics, Gerodontology and Oral Rehabilitation, Osaka University Graduate School of Dentistry, 1-8 Yamadaoka, Suita, Osaka 565-0871, Japan

**Yasunori Hotta, Koji Ito, Shinichi Komatsu and Takashi Saito**
Aichi Implant Center, Hotta Dental Clinic, 13, Morimaki-cho, Moriyama-ku, Nagoya 463-0073, Japan

**Yoko Yamaguchi and Masahiko Ozeki**
Department of Implant Dentistry, Showa University School of Dentistry, 2-1-1 Kitasenzoku Ota-ku, Tokyo 145-8515, Japan

**Makoto Shiota and Shohei Kasugai**
Oral Implantology and Regenerative Dental Medicine, Department of Masticatory Function Rehabilitation, Division of Oral Health Sciences, Graduate School, Tokyo Medical and Dental University, 1-5-45 Yushima, Bunkyo-ku, Tokyo 113-8510, Japan

**Motohiro Munakata**
Oral Implantology Department of Prosthodontic Dentistry for Function of TMJ and Occlusion, Kanagawa Dental University, 82, Inaokachou, Yokosuka-shi, Kanagawa 238-8580, Japan

**Fumihiko Watanabe**
Department of Crown and Bridge Prosthodontics, School of Life Dentistry at Niigata, The Nippon Dental University, 951-8580 1-8 Hamaura-cho, Chuo-ku, Niigata, Japan

**Kazuhiko Hiroyasu and Kazuhiko Ueda**
Oral Implant Care Unit Niigata Hospital, The Nippon Dental University, 1-8 Hamaura-cho, Chuo-ku, Niigata, Japan

**Michael Stiller**
School of Dental Medicine, Section of Experimental Orofacial Medicine, Philipps University, Georg-Voigt-Str. 3, 35039 Marburg, Germany
Private Practice for Oral Surgery and Implantology, ECDI Center, Brahmsst. 11, 14193 Berlin, Germany

**Rainer Mengel and Barbara Peleska**
School of Dental Medicine, Department of Prosthodontics, Philipps University, Georg-Voigt-Str. 3, 35039 Marburg, Germany

**Sebastian Becher**
Practice of Oral and Maxillofacial Surgery, ECDI Center, Königsallee 68, 40212 Düsseldorf, Germany

**Bernhard Brinkmann**
Clinic ABC Bogen, ECDI Center, ABC Strasse 19, 20354 Hamburg, Germany

**Esther Kluk**
Department of Postgraduate Education - Master of Oral Implantology, Center for Oral and Maxillofacial Surgery, Johann Wolfgang Goethe University Frankfurt, Theodor-Stern-Kai 17, Frankfurt 60577, Germany
Private Practice for Oral Surgery and Implantology, ECDI Center, Brahmsst. 11, 14193 Berlin, Germany

**Natália Galvão Garcia, Francisco Barbara Abreu Barros and Denise Tostes Oliveira**
Department of Stomatology, Area of Pathology, Bauru School of Dentistry, University of São Paulo, Bauru, São Paulo, Brazil

**Márcia Maria Dalmolin Carvalho**
Dentist, Private Practice, Campinas, São Paulo, Brazil

**Mito Kobayashi**
Division of Oral Bioengineering, Institute of Medicine and Dentistry, Niigata University, Niigata, Japan
Division of Periodontology, Institute of Medicine and Dentistry, Niigata University, Niigata, Japan
Advanced Research Center, The Nippon Dental University School of Life Dentistry at Niigata, Niigata, Japan

**Tomoyuki Kawase**
Division of Oral Bioengineering, Institute of Medicine and Dentistry, Niigata University, Niigata, Japan
Advanced Research Center, The Nippon Dental University School of Life Dentistry at Niigata, Niigata, Japan

**Kazuhiro Okuda and Hiromasa Yoshie**
Division of Periodontology, Institute of Medicine and Dentistry, Niigata University, Niigata, Japan

**Larry F. Wolff**
Division of Periodontology, Department of Developmental and Surgical Sciences, University of Minnesota School of Dentistry, Minneapolis, MN, USA

**Sachiko Maeda**
Private practice limited to orthodontics, 8F Hankyu-Terminal-Bldg. 1-1-4 Shibata, Kitaku, Osaka 530-0012, Japan

**Takeshi Sasaki**
Private practice in general practice, 9F Nissei-Shinosaka-Bldg. 3-4-30 Miyahara, Yodogawa-ku, Osaka 532-0003, Japan

**Yukimori Isoda**
Unit of Oral and Maxillofacial Implantology, Tsurumi University Dental Hospital, Yokohama, Japan

**Tsubasa Akaike and Eisaku Imamura**
Department of Oral and Maxillofacial Surgery, Yokohama General Hospital, 2201-5 Kurogane-cho, Aoba-ku, Yokohama-shi, Kanagawa 225-0025, Japan

**Daisuke Ueno**
Department of Implantology and Periodontology, Graduate School of Dentistry, Kanagawa Dental University, Yokohama, Japan

**Yoshiki Hamada**
Department of Oral and Maxillofacial Surgery, Tsurumi University School of Dental Medicine, Yokohama, Japan

**Hendrik Terheyden**
Department of Oral and Maxillofacial Surgery, Red Cross Hospital, Hansteinstr. 29, D-34121 Kassel, Germany

**Falk Wüsthoff**
Department of Oral and Maxillofacial Surgery, Schleswig-Holstein University Hospital, Arnold-Heller-Straße 3, Haus 26, 2D-4105 Kiel, Germany

**Daisuke Ueno**
Department of Implantology and Periodontology, Kanagawa Dental University, Graduate School of Dentistry, 3-31-6 Tsuruya-cho, Kanagawa-ku, Yokohama, Japan

**Takashi Kurokawa and Tsuneaki Watanabe**
Unit of Oral and Maxillofacial Implantology, Tsurumi University Dental Hospital, Yokohama, Japan

**Katsuichiro Maruo**
Department of Removal Prosthodontics, Kanagawa Dental University, Graduate School of Dentistry, Yokosuka, Japan

**Jayanetti Asiri Jayawardena**
Department of General Education, Tsurumi University, School of Dental Medicine, Yokohama, Japan

**Ahmed M. Abdelhamid**
Prosthodontics Department, Faculty of Dentistry, Alexandria University, Alexandria, Egypt

**Kenda I. Hanno**
Prosthodontics, Faculty of Dentistry, Alexandria University, Alexandria, Egypt

**Mohamed H. Imam**
Physical Medicine, Rheumatology and Rehabilitation, Faculty of Medicine, Alexandria University, Alexandria, Egypt

**Joseph Gakonyo**
Department of Conservative and Prosthetic Dentistry, University of Nairobi, P.O. Box 54954-00200, Nairobi, Kenya

**Fawzia Butt and Philip Mwachaka**
Department of Human Anatomy, University of Nairobi, P.O. Box 25361-00603, Nairobi, Kenya

**Evelyn Wagaiyu**
Department of Periodontology/Community and Preventive Dentistry, University of Nairobi, P.O. Box 30197, Nairobi, Kenya

**Kazuki Takaoka, Emi Segawa, Michiyo Yamamura, Yusuke Zushi, Masahiro Urade and Hiromitsu Kishimoto**
Department of Oral and Maxillofacial Surgery, Hyogo College of Medicine, 1-1 Mukogawa-cho, Nishinomiya, Hyogo 663-8501, Japan

**Miriam Ting, Matthew Palermo, David P. Donatelli, Jon B. Suzuki and Steven R. Jefferies**
Kornberg School of Dentistry, Temple University, 3223 North Broad Street, Philadelphia, PA 19140, USA

**John P. Gaughan**
School of Medicine, Temple University, 3420 N Broad St, Philadelphia, PA 19140, USA

**Frank Schwarz, Andrea Schmucker and Jürgen Becker**
Department of Oral Surgery, Westdeutsche Kieferklinik, Universitätsklinikum Düsseldorf, D-40225 Düsseldorf, Germany